REFERENCE

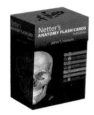

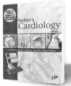

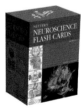
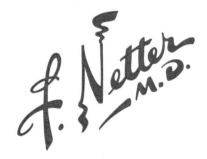

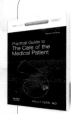

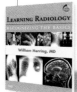

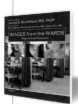

Atlas of
Human Anatomy

Fifth Edition

Frank H. Netter, MD

SAUNDERS
ELSEVIER

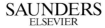

1600 John F. Kennedy Blvd.
Ste 1800
Philadelphia, PA 19103-2899

ATLAS OF HUMAN ANATOMY
Fifth Edition

Standard Edition:	978-1-4160-5951-6
International Edition:	978-0-8089-2423-4
Enhanced International Edition:	978-0-8089-2422-7
Professional Edition:	978-1-4377-0970-4

Notice

Neither the Publisher nor the Editors assume any responsibility for any loss or injury and/or damage to persons or property arising out of or related to any use of the material contained in this book. It is the responsibility of the treating practitioner, relying on independent expertise and knowledge of the patient, to determine the best treatment and method of application for the patient.

The Publisher

Previous editions copyrighted 2006, 2003, 1997, 1989.

Library of Congress Cataloging-in-Publication Data
Netter, Frank H. (Frank Henry), 1906-1991.
  Atlas of human anatomy / Frank H. Netter.—5th ed.
    p. ; cm.
  Includes index.
  ISBN 978–1–4160–5951–6
  1. Human anatomy—Atlases. I. Title.
  [DNLM: 1. Anatomy—Atlases. QS 17 N474a 2010]
  QM25.N46 2010
  611.0022'2—dc22   2009034216

Director of Netter Products: Anne Lenehan
Online Editor: Elyse O'Grady
Developmental Editor: Marybeth Thiel
Publishing Services Manager: Linda Van Pelt
Design Direction: Lou Forgione
Illustrations Manager: Karen Giacomucci
Marketing Manager: Jason Oberacker

Printed in United States of America.

Last digit is the print number: 9 8 7 6 5 4 3 2 1

Consulting Editors

John T. Hansen, PhD
Lead Editor
Professor of Neurobiology and Anatomy
Associate Dean for Admissions
University of Rochester School of Medicine and Dentistry
Rochester, New York

Brion Benninger, MD, MS
Department of Surgery
Department of Oral & Maxillofacial Surgery
Department of Integrated Biosciences
Course Director
Oregon Health Sciences University
Portland, Oregon

Jennifer K. Brueckner, PhD
Assistant Dean for Student Affairs
University of Kentucky College of Medicine
Office of the Dean, Student Affairs
Lexington, Kentucky

Stephen W. Carmichael, PhD, DSc
International Consultant
Professor Emeritus of Anatomy
Professor Emeritus of Orthopedic Surgery
Mayo Clinic
Rochester, Minnesota

Noelle A. Granger, PhD
Professor Emeritus
Department of Cell and Developmental Biology
University of North Carolina at Chapel Hill
Chapel Hill, North Carolina

R. Shane Tubbs, MS, PA-C, PhD
Pediatric Neurosurgery
Children's Hospital
Birmingham, Alabama

Acknowledgments

Brion Benninger, MD, MS

I would like to thank my wife Alison for her support and for our son Jack, who keeps it all worthwhile. I want to thank Elsevier, especially Anne Lenehan, Marybeth Thiel, and Linda Van Pelt, for their insight and direction, enabling my fellow coeditors and Carlos Machado to work in such a rich environment. I particularly want to thank my first clinical anatomy mentors, Gerald Tressidor and Harold Ellis (Guy's Hospital); my clinical mentors, Peter Bell, Chris Colton, and David deBono; all my past and future patients and students; and OHSU clinical colleagues who bring anatomy to life (DT, LL). Thanks to my colleagues in the Department of Radiology at OHSU. Lastly, I thank my mother for her love of education and my father for his inquisitive mind.

Jennifer K. Brueckner, PhD

I am eternally grateful to my fiancé Kurt and to my parents, John and Rheba, for their patience, support, encouragement, and inspiration. Many thanks to John Hansen for the kind invitation and opportunity to contribute to this premier atlas! I would also like to thank the University of Kentucky College of Medicine Class of 2012 for their excellent input and suggestions for this edition; I am so lucky to have the privilege of working with such wonderful medical students! I am indebted to Carlos Machado for making the anatomical visions in my imagination come alive on paper with his magical artwork. Last but not least, I am so thankful for the Elsevier staff for their patience and support, including Marybeth Thiel, Anne Lenehan, and Linda Van Pelt.

Stephen W. Carmichael, PhD, DSc

I would like to thank Anne Lenehan and Elyse O'Grady for their administrative support during the preparation of this edition.

Noelle A. Granger, PhD

I am deeply grateful to my husband, Gene, for his support of my efforts during the work on this new edition. I also want to acknowledge two of my colleagues from the University of North Carolina School of Medicine: James Scatliff, MD, former Chair of the Department of Radiology, and O.W. Henson, PhD, Professor Emeritus of Anatomy, who showed me the beauty and complexity of anatomy. Special recognition goes to the supremely talented Carlos Machado and the artists at Elsevier, who did such exceptional work on this edition. Lastly, thanks go to the wonderful staff at Elsevier, in particular Marybeth Thiel and Anne Lenehan, for their leadership and patience with us academics.

John T. Hansen, PhD

I would like to thank Marybeth Thiel, Developmental Editor; Anne Lenehan, Acquisitions Editor; and Linda Van Pelt, Publishing Services Manager, for their meticulous shepherding of this fifth edition of the *Atlas of Human Anatomy* through each step of the publishing process. They, along with the entire Editorial, Production, Design, Illustration, and Marketing team at Elsevier, have been the epitome of professionalism. Also, I wish to express my thanks to my teaching colleagues at Rochester, and all my past and present students who have enriched my career and taught me much more than I have taught them. Finally, I am indebted to my entire family for their continued support, and especially to my wife Paula, whose love and encouragement has been the constant in my life and is the source of all the joy I know.

R. Shane Tubbs, MS, PA-C, PhD

I am indebted to the fantastic staff at Elsevier, including Anne Lenehan, Marybeth Thiel, and Elyse O'Grady. Dr. Carlos Machado's artwork has been a most welcomed contribution. I thank my wonderful wife Susan and son Isaiah for their patience during this endeavor. Colleagues and friends that supported me during the production of this edition include Drs. W. Jerry Oakes, E. George Salter, Marios Loukas, Arthur McAdams, Mohammadali Shoja, and Aaron Cohen-Gadol, and I thank each of them. Finally, without God and His wonderful design of the human body, we, as anatomists, would be left with nothing to describe or name!

Foreword

The fifth edition of *Atlas of Human Anatomy* by Frank H. Netter, MD, has been updated by the Consulting Editor team, led by John T. Hansen, of Brion Benninger, Jennifer K. Brueckner, Stephen W. Carmichael, Noelle A. Granger, and R. Shane Tubbs. We have each reviewed, modified, and updated a section of the *Atlas*. In this new edition, the editorial team has updated the radiologic images in the print book and in the online ancillaries, bringing clinical imaging into context with anatomy. As anatomy does require new material, Carlos A.G. Machado, MD, has added outstanding new images and anatomic views to this edition. The Consulting Editor team has relied heavily on *Terminologica Anatomica* as the basis for updates to nomenclature and terminology. The genius of Dr. Netter's paintings is that the anatomy is portrayed clearly, realistically, and in a clinically relatable fashion while maintaining the balance between complexity and oversimplification. This fifth edition owes much to the consulting editors of the earlier editions, Drs. Sharon Colacino (Oberg) (first edition), Arthur F. Dalley II (second edition), and John T. Hansen (third edition), who shepherded their editions with great skill and uncompromising professionalism, making our task significantly easier. The fourth edition was the first published under Elsevier and included the contributions of Anil Walji and Thomas Gest, as well as many members of the current consulting editor team.

Overall global changes to all sections of the *Atlas* include re-organization of plate order to more accurately reflect the current practice of teaching anatomy; reduction of labeling of some images; and removal of dated clinical plates. The flow of images in each section is now oriented from superficial to deep layers. In the upper and lower limb sections, the images have been changed to reflect the orientation common for imaging anatomy. In addition, many plates throughout the book have been updated to improve the artwork for a more contemporary view of anatomic aspects. We hope you enjoy this new edition of the *Atlas of Human Anatomy* and that you find it useful for learning and for your career.

About the Online versions:

For the standard edition and enhanced international edition of the *Atlas,* we have included access to the website *www.studentconsult.com.* From student and faculty feedback, we learned that the inclusion of Netter: *Atlas of Human Anatomy* in Student Consult would further enrich this excellent site. Many of the tools that were available on *www.Netteranatomy.com* are now available on Student Consult, and there are extra features as well. In addition to the 80+ images from the print *Atlas,* there are over 250 clinical images that the Consulting Editors have added to the site, including many Netter clinical images. These images are clinical and radiologic images showing both normal anatomy and pathologic conditions. The Integration Links from Netter on Student Consult are expanded and enable the user to link to the major brands and products on this site that students and faculty love. Also on Student Consult are videos created from Interact Elsevier, *Netter's 3D Interactive Anatomy* product, and the Interactive Dissection Modules from the University of North Carolina, Chapel Hill. Additional online resources such as radiologic images, videos from UNC Dissection Modules, and many other resources are indicated by the symbol 📺. The symbol 👤 indicates videos from *Netter's 3D Interactive Anatomy.*

For the Professional edition of the Atlas, the online resource is through *www.netterreference.com,* the site for clinical Netter products. The *Atlas* online will have 80+ Netter images and the clinical images, as well as videos from *Netter's 3D Interactive Anatomy.* This site will be the jumping-off point for the new version of the Netter Presenter, which allows users to create custom Netter images.

Brion Benninger, MD, MS
Jennifer K. Brueckner, PhD
Stephen W. Carmichael, PhD, DSc
Noelle A. Granger, PhD
John T. Hansen, PhD
R. Shane Tubbs, MS, PA-C, PhD

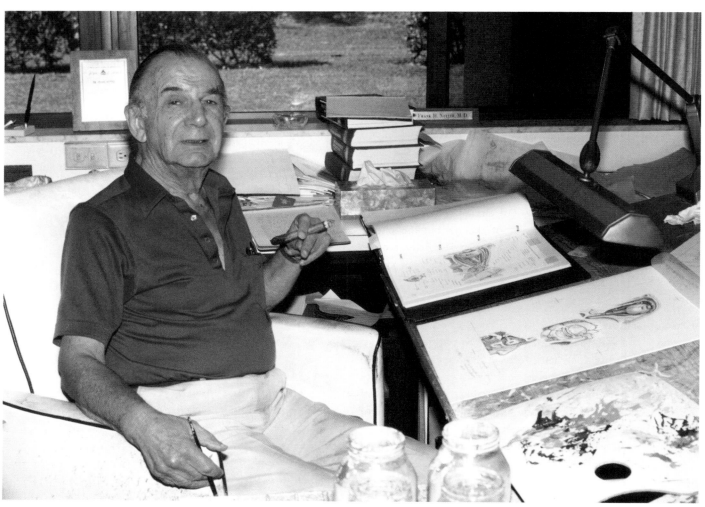

Frank H. Netter, MD

Photograph by James L. Clayton

To my dear wife, Vera

Preface to the First Edition

I have often said that my career as a medical artist for almost 50 years has been a sort of "command performance" in the sense that it has grown in response to the desires and requests of the medical profession. Over these many years, I have produced almost 4,000 illustrations, mostly for *The CIBA* (now *Netter*) *Collection of Medical Illustrations* but also for *Clinical Symposia*. These pictures have been concerned with the varied subdivisions of medical knowledge such as gross anatomy, histology, embryology, physiology, pathology, diagnostic modalities, surgical and therapeutic techniques, and clinical manifestations of a multitude of diseases. As the years went by, however, there were more and more requests from physicians and students for me to produce an atlas purely of gross anatomy. Thus, this atlas has come about, not through any inspiration on my part but rather, like most of my previous works, as a fulfillment of the desires of the medical profession.

It involved going back over all the illustrations I had made over so many years, selecting those pertinent to gross anatomy, classifying them and organizing them by system and region, adapting them to page size and space, and arranging them in logical sequence. Anatomy of course does not change, but our understanding of anatomy and its clinical significance does change, as do anatomical terminology and nomenclature. This therefore required much updating of many of the older pictures and even revision of a number of them in order to make them more pertinent to today's ever-expanding scope of medical and surgical practice. In addition, I found that there were gaps in the portrayal of medical knowledge as pictorialized in the illustrations I had previously done, and this necessitated my making a number of new pictures that are included in this volume.

In creating an atlas such as this, it is important to achieve a happy medium between complexity and simplification. If the pictures are too complex, they may be difficult and confusing to read; if oversimplified, they may not be adequately definitive or may even be misleading. I have therefore striven for a middle course of realism without the clutter of confusing minutiae. I hope that the students and members of the medical and allied professions will find the illustrations readily understandable, yet instructive and useful.

At one point, the publisher and I thought it might be nice to include a foreword by a truly outstanding and renowned anatomist, but there are so many in that category that we could not make a choice. We did think of men like Vesalius, Leonardo da Vinci, William Hunter, and Henry Gray, who of course are unfortunately unavailable, but I do wonder what their comments might have been about this atlas.

Frank H. Netter, MD
(1906–1991)

Frank H. Netter, MD

Frank H. Netter was born in New York City in 1906. He studied art at the Art Students League and the National Academy of Design before entering medical school at New York University, where he received his Doctor of Medicine degree in 1931. During his student years, Dr. Netter's notebook sketches attracted the attention of the medical faculty and other physicians, allowing him to augment his income by illustrating articles and textbooks. He continued illustrating as a sideline after establishing a surgical practice in 1933, but he ultimately opted to give up his practice in favor of a full-time commitment to art. After service in the United States Army during World War II, Dr. Netter began his long collaboration with the CIBA Pharmaceutical Company (now Novartis Pharmaceuticals). This 45-year partnership resulted in the production of the extraordinary collection of medical art so familiar to physicians and other medical professionals worldwide.

Icon Learning Systems acquired the Netter Collection in July 2000 and continued to update Dr. Netter's original paintings and to add newly commissioned paintings by artists trained in the style of Dr. Netter. In 2005, Elsevier Inc. purchased the Netter Collection and all publications from Icon Learning Systems. There are now over 50 publications featuring the art of Dr. Netter available through Elsevier Inc.

Dr. Netter's works are among the finest examples of the use of illustration in the teaching of medical concepts. The 13-book *Netter Collection of Medical Illustrations,* which includes the greater part of the more than 20,000 paintings created by Dr. Netter, became and remains one of the most famous medical works ever published. *The Netter Atlas of Human Anatomy,* first published in 1989, presents the anatomic paintings from the Netter Collection. Now translated into 16 languages, it is the anatomy atlas of choice among medical and health professions students the world over.

The Netter illustrations are appreciated not only for their aesthetic qualities, but also, more important, for their intellectual content. As Dr. Netter wrote in 1949, "Clarification of a subject is the aim and goal of illustration. No matter how beautifully painted, how delicately and subtly rendered a subject may be, it is of little value as a *medical illustration* if it does not serve to make clear some medical point." Dr. Netter's planning, conception, point of view, and approach are what inform his paintings and what make them so intellectually valuable.

Frank H. Netter, MD, physician and artist, died in 1991.

Contents

Section 1   HEAD AND NECK

Topographic Anatomy	1
Superficial Head and Neck	2-3
Bones and Ligaments	4-23
Superficial Face	24-25
Neck	26-34
Nasal Region	35-50
Oral Region	51-62
Pharynx	63-73
Thyroid Gland and Larynx	74-80
Orbit and Contents	81-91
Ear	92-98
Meninges and Brain	99-114
Cranial and Cervical Nerves	115-134
Cerebral Vasculature	135-146
Regional Scans	147-148

Section 2   BACK AND SPINAL CORD

Topographic Anatomy	149
Bones and Ligaments	150-156
Spinal Cord	157-167
Muscles and Nerves	168-172
Cross-sectional Anatomy	173-174

Section 3   THORAX

Topographic Anatomy	175
Mammary Gland	176-178
Body Wall	179-189
Lungs	190-204
Heart	205-223
Mediastinum	224-234
Regional Scans	235
Cross-sectional Anatomy	236-239

Section 4   ABDOMEN

Topographic Anatomy	240
Body Wall	241-260
Peritoneal Cavity	261-266
Viscera (Gut)	267-276
Viscera (Accessory Organs)	277-282
Visceral Vasculature	283-296
Innervation	297-307
Kidneys and Suprarenal Glands	308-322
Cross-sectional Anatomy	323-330

Section 5   PELVIS AND PERINEUM

Topographic Anatomy	331
Bones and Ligaments	332-336
Pelvic Floor and Contents	337-347
Urinary Bladder	348-351
Uterus, Vagina, and Supporting Structures	352-355
Perineum and External Genitalia: Female	356-359
Perineum and External Genitalia: Male	360-367
Homologues of Genitalia	368-369
Testis, Epididymis, and Ductus Deferens	370
Rectum	371-376
Regional Scans	377
Vasculature	378-388
Innervation	389-397
Cross-sectional Anatomy	398-399

Section 6   UPPER LIMB

Topographic Anatomy	400
Cutaneous Anatomy	401-405
Shoulder and Axilla	406-418
Arm	419-423
Elbow and Forearm	424-439
Wrist and Hand	440-459
Neurovasculature	460-467
Regional Scans	468

Section 7   LOWER LIMB

Topographic Anatomy	469
Cutaneous Anatomy	470-473
Hip and Thigh	474-493
Knee	494-500
Leg	501-510
Ankle and Foot	511-525
Neurovasculature	526-530
Regional Scans	531

Section 8   CROSS-SECTIONAL ANATOMY

Key Figures for Cross Sections	532

References
Index

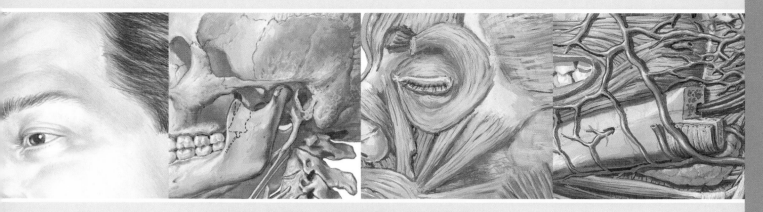

Section 1 **HEAD AND NECK**

Topographic Anatomy
Plate 1

1   Head and Neck

Superficial Head and Neck
Plates 2-3

2   Cutaneous Nerves of Head and Neck

3   Superficial Arteries and Veins of Face and Scalp

Bones and Ligaments
Plates 4-23

4   Skull: Anterior View

5   Skull: Anteroposterior Radiograph

6   Skull: Lateral View

7   Skull: Lateral Radiograph

8   Skull: Midsagittal Section

9   Calvaria

10   Cranial Base: Inferior View

11   Cranial Base: Superior View

12   Foramina and Canals of Cranial Base: Inferior View

13   Foramina and Canals of Cranial Base: Superior View

14   Skull of Newborn

15   Bony Framework of Head and Neck

16   Pterygoid Fossae: Posterior View

17   Mandible

18   Temporomandibular Joint

19   Cervical Vertebrae: Atlas and Axis

20   Cervical Vertebrae (continued)

1 HEAD AND NECK

21   Cervical Vertebrae: Uncovertebral Joints

22   External Craniocervical Ligaments

23   Internal Craniocervical Ligaments

Superficial Face
Plates 24-25

24   Facial Nerve Branches and Parotid Gland

25   Muscles of Facial Expression: Lateral View

Neck
Plates 26-34

26   Muscles of Neck: Lateral View

27   Muscles of Neck: Anterior View

28   Infrahyoid and Suprahyoid Muscles

29   Scalene and Prevertebral Muscles

30   Superficial Veins and Cutaneous Nerves of Neck

31   Nerves and Vessels of Neck

32   Nerves and Vessels of Neck (continued)

33   Carotid Arteries

34   Fascial Layers of Neck

Nasal Region
Plates 35-50

35   Nose

36   Lateral Wall of Nasal Cavity

37   Lateral Wall of Nasal Cavity (continued)

38   Medial Wall of Nasal Cavity (Nasal Septum)

39   Maxillary Artery

40   Arteries of Nasal Cavity: Nasal Septum Turned Up

41   Nerves of Nasal Cavity: Nasal Septum Turned Up

42   Nerves of Nasal Cavity (continued)

43   Autonomic Innervation of Nasal Cavity

44   Ophthalmic (V_1) and Maxillary (V_2) Nerves

45   Mandibular Nerve (V_3)

46   Orientation of Nerves and Vessels of the Cranial Base

47   Nose and Maxillary Sinus: Transverse Section

48   Paranasal Sinuses

49   Paranasal Sinuses (continued)

50   Paranasal Sinuses: Changes with Age

Oral Region
Plates 51-62

51   Inspection of Oral Cavity

52   Roof of Oral Cavity

53   Floor of Oral Cavity

54   Muscles Involved in Mastication

55   Muscles Involved in Mastication (continued)

56   Teeth

57   Teeth (continued)

58   Tongue

59   Tongue (continued)

60   Tongue and Salivary Glands: Sections

61   Salivary Glands

62   Afferent Innervation of Oral Cavity and Pharynx

Pharynx
Plates 63-73

63   Pharynx: Median Section

64   Fauces

65   Muscles of Pharynx: Sagittal Section

66   Pharynx: Opened Posterior View

67   Muscles of Pharynx: Partially Opened Posterior View

68   Muscles of Pharynx: Lateral View

69   Arteries of Oral and Pharyngeal Regions

70   Veins of Oral and Pharyngeal Regions

71   Nerves of Oral and Pharyngeal Regions

72   Lymph Vessels and Nodes of Head and Neck

73   Lymph Vessels and Nodes of Pharynx and Tongue

Thyroid Gland and Larynx
Plates 74-80

74   Thyroid Gland: Anterior View

75   Thyroid Gland and Pharynx: Posterior View

76   Parathyroid Glands

77   Cartilages of Larynx

78   Intrinsic Muscles of Larynx

79   Action of Intrinsic Muscles of Larynx

80   Nerves of Larynx

Orbit and Contents
Plates 81-91

81 Eyelids

82 Lacrimal Apparatus

83 Fasciae of Orbit and Eyeball

84 Extrinsic Eye Muscles

85 Arteries and Veins of Orbit and Eyelids

86 Nerves of Orbit

87 Eyeball

88 Anterior and Posterior Chambers of Eye

89 Lens and Supporting Structures

90 Intrinsic Arteries and Veins of Eye

91 Vascular Supply of Eye

Ear
Plates 92-98

92 Pathway of Sound Reception

93 External Ear and Tympanic Cavity

94 Tympanic Cavity

95 Bony and Membranous Labyrinths

96 Bony and Membranous Labyrinths (continued)

97 Orientation of Labyrinths in Skull

98 Auditory (Pharnygotympanic, Eustachian) Tube

Meninges and Brain
Plates 99-114

99 Meninges and Diploic Veins

100 Meningeal Arteries

101 Meninges and Superficial Cerebral Veins

102 Dural Venous Sinuses

103 Dural Venous Sinuses (continued)

104 Cerebrum: Lateral Views

105 Cerebrum: Medial Views

106 Cerebrum: Inferior View

107 Ventricles of Brain

108 Circulation of Cerebrospinal Fluid

109 Basal Nuclei (Ganglia)

110 Thalamus

111 Hippocampus and Fornix

112 Cerebellum

113 Brainstem

114 Fourth Ventricle and Cerebellum

Cranial and Cervical Nerves
Plates 115-134

115 Cranial Nerve Nuclei in Brainstem: Schema

116 Cranial Nerve Nuclei in Brainstem: Schema (continued)

117 Cranial Nerves (Motor and Sensory Distribution): Schema

118 Olfactory Nerve (I): Schema

119 Optic Nerve (II) (Visual Pathway): Schema

120 Oculomotor (III), Trochlear (IV), and Abducent (VI) Nerves: Schema

121 Trigeminal Nerve (V): Schema

122 Facial Nerve (VII): Schema

123 Vestibulocochlear Nerve (VIII): Schema

124 Glosssopharyngeal Nerve (IX): Schema

125 Vagus Nerve (X): Schema

126 Accessory Nerve (XI): Schema

127 Hypoglossal Nerve (XII): Schema

128 Cervical Plexus: Schema

129 Autonomic Nerves in Neck

130 Autonomic Nerves in Head

131 Ciliary Ganglion: Schema

132 Pterygopalatine and Submandibular Ganglia: Schema

133 Otic Ganglion: Schema

134 Taste Pathways: Schema

Cerebral Vasculature
Plates 135-146

135 Arteries to Brain and Meninges

136 Arteries to Brain: Schema

137 Arteries of Brain: Inferior Views

138 Cerebral Arterial Circle (of Willis)

139 Arteries of Brain: Frontal View and Section

140 Arteries of Brain: Lateral and Medial Views

141 Arteries of Posterior Cranial Fossa

142 Veins of Posterior Cranial Fossa

143 Deep Veins of Brain

144 Subependymal Veins of Brain

145 Hypothalamus and Hypophysis

146 Arteries and Veins of Hypothalmus and Hypophysis

Regional Scans

Plates 147-148

147 Cranial Imaging (MRV and MRA)

148 Cranial Imaging (MRI)

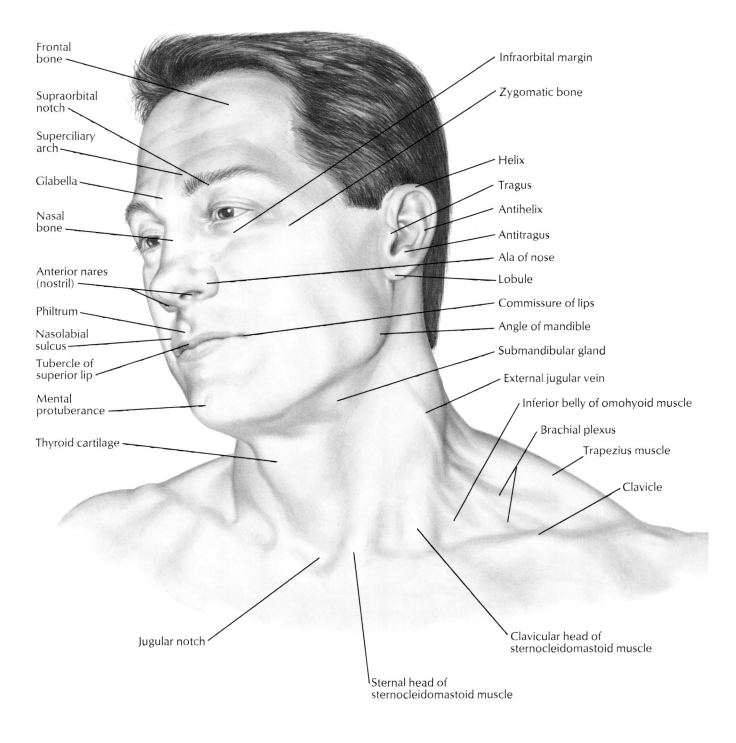

Frontal bone

Supraorbital notch

Superciliary arch

Glabella

Nasal bone

Anterior nares (nostril)

Philtrum

Nasolabial sulcus

Tubercle of superior lip

Mental protuberance

Thyroid cartilage

Infraorbital margin

Zygomatic bone

Helix

Tragus

Antihelix

Antitragus

Ala of nose

Lobule

Commissure of lips

Angle of mandible

Submandibular gland

External jugular vein

Inferior belly of omohyoid muscle

Brachial plexus

Trapezius muscle

Clavicle

Clavicular head of sternocleidomastoid muscle

Jugular notch

Sternal head of sternocleidomastoid muscle

Cutaneous Nerves of Head and Neck

See also **Plates 31, 35, 44, 45, 121, 159**

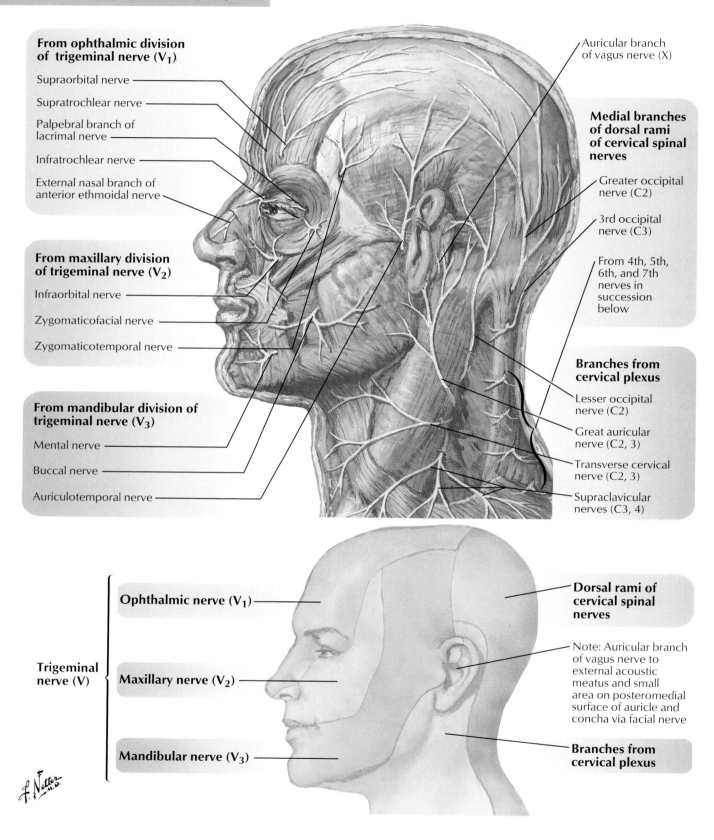

From ophthalmic division of trigeminal nerve (V₁)

Supraorbital nerve

Supratrochlear nerve

Palpebral branch of lacrimal nerve

Infratrochlear nerve

External nasal branch of anterior ethmoidal nerve

From maxillary division of trigeminal nerve (V₂)

Infraorbital nerve

Zygomaticofacial nerve

Zygomaticotemporal nerve

From mandibular division of trigeminal nerve (V₃)

Mental nerve

Buccal nerve

Auriculotemporal nerve

Auricular branch of vagus nerve (X)

Medial branches of dorsal rami of cervical spinal nerves

Greater occipital nerve (C2)

3rd occipital nerve (C3)

From 4th, 5th, 6th, and 7th nerves in succession below

Branches from cervical plexus

Lesser occipital nerve (C2)

Great auricular nerve (C2, 3)

Transverse cervical nerve (C2, 3)

Supraclavicular nerves (C3, 4)

Trigeminal nerve (V)

Ophthalmic nerve (V₁)

Maxillary nerve (V₂)

Mandibular nerve (V₃)

Dorsal rami of cervical spinal nerves

Note: Auricular branch of vagus nerve to external acoustic meatus and small area on posteromedial surface of auricle and concha via facial nerve

Branches from cervical plexus

Plate 2

Superficial Head and Neck

See also **Plates 33, 39, 69, 70, 85, 99**

Scalp {
Skin and subcutaneous tissue
Epicranial aponeurosis (galea aponeurotica) *(cut to reveal skull)*

Parietal emissary vein

Frontal
Parietal } Branches of superficial temporal artery and vein

Middle temporal artery and vein

Zygomaticoorbital artery

Anterior auricular arteries

Transverse facial artery and vein

Supraorbital artery and vein

Supratrochlear artery and vein

Nasofrontal vein

Dorsal nasal artery and vein

Zygomaticotemporal artery and vein

Angular artery and vein

Zygomatico-facial artery and vein

Infraorbital artery and vein

Deep facial vein (from pterygoid plexus)

Facial artery and vein

Mastoid emissary vein and meningeal branch of occipital artery (posterior meningeal artery)

Occipital artery and vein *(cut)*

Posterior auricular artery and vein

External jugular vein *(cut)*

Retromandibular vein

Common facial vein

Internal jugular vein

Internal carotid artery

External carotid artery

Common carotid artery

Lingual artery and vein

Sources of arterial supply of face

Black: from internal carotid artery (via ophthalmic artery)
Red: from external carotid artery

f. Netter M.D.

Skull: Anterior View

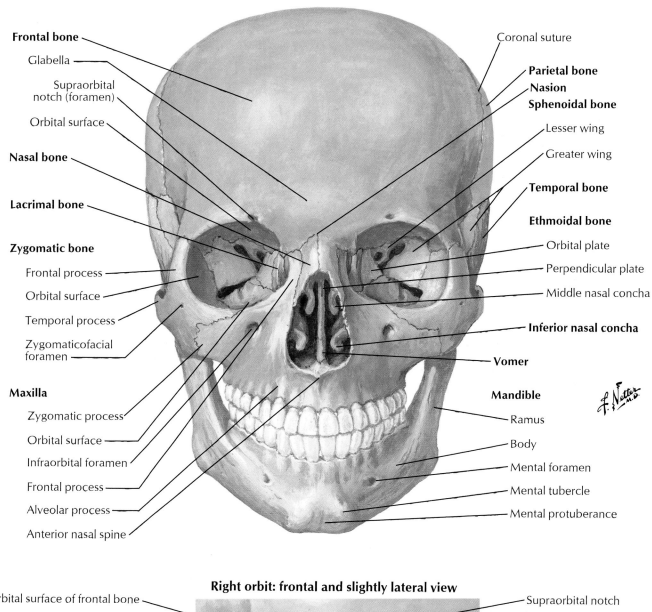

Frontal bone
Glabella
Supraorbital notch (foramen)
Orbital surface

Nasal bone

Lacrimal bone

Zygomatic bone
Frontal process
Orbital surface
Temporal process
Zygomaticofacial foramen

Maxilla
Zygomatic process
Orbital surface
Infraorbital foramen
Frontal process
Alveolar process
Anterior nasal spine

Coronal suture

Parietal bone
Nasion
Sphenoidal bone
Lesser wing
Greater wing

Temporal bone

Ethmoidal bone
Orbital plate
Perpendicular plate
Middle nasal concha

Inferior nasal concha

Vomer

Mandible
Ramus
Body
Mental foramen
Mental tubercle
Mental protuberance

F. Netter M.D.

Right orbit: frontal and slightly lateral view

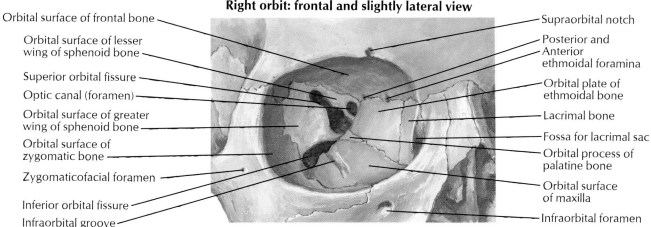

Orbital surface of frontal bone
Orbital surface of lesser wing of sphenoid bone
Superior orbital fissure
Optic canal (foramen)
Orbital surface of greater wing of sphenoid bone
Orbital surface of zygomatic bone
Zygomaticofacial foramen
Inferior orbital fissure
Infraorbital groove

Supraorbital notch
Posterior and Anterior ethmoidal foramina
Orbital plate of ethmoidal bone
Lacrimal bone
Fossa for lacrimal sac
Orbital process of palatine bone
Orbital surface of maxilla
Infraorbital foramen

Plate 4   **Bones and Ligaments**

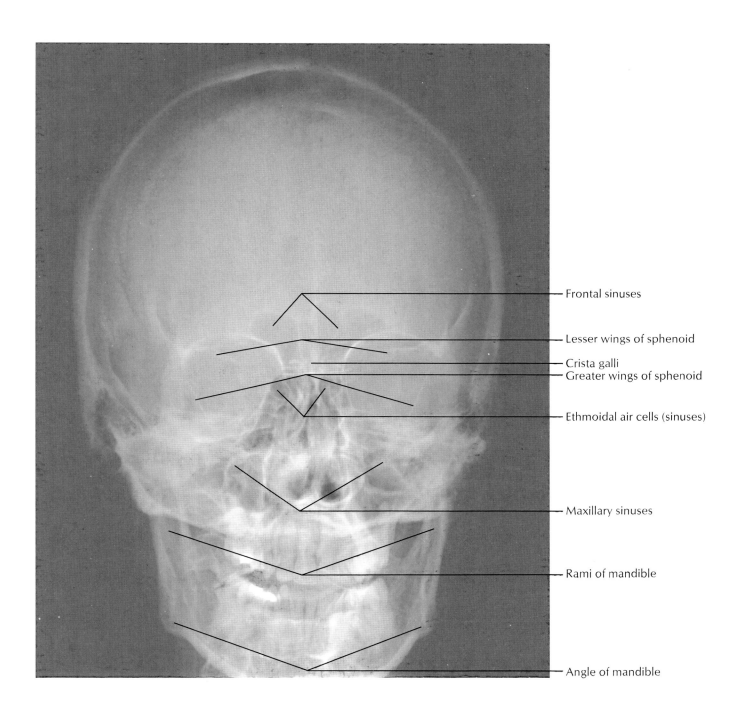

Frontal sinuses

Lesser wings of sphenoid

Crista galli
Greater wings of sphenoid

Ethmoidal air cells (sinuses)

Maxillary sinuses

Rami of mandible

Angle of mandible

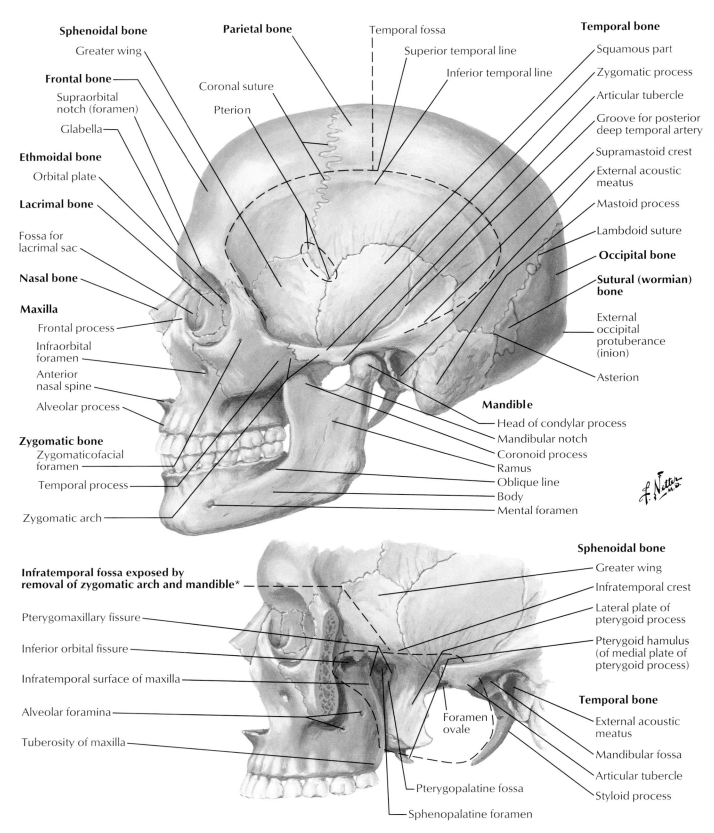

Sphenoidal bone
Greater wing

Frontal bone
Supraorbital notch (foramen)
Glabella

Ethmoidal bone
Orbital plate

Lacrimal bone
Fossa for lacrimal sac

Nasal bone

Maxilla
Frontal process
Infraorbital foramen
Anterior nasal spine
Alveolar process

Zygomatic bone
Zygomaticofacial foramen
Temporal process
Zygomatic arch

Parietal bone
Coronal suture
Pterion

Temporal fossa
Superior temporal line
Inferior temporal line

Temporal bone
Squamous part
Zygomatic process
Articular tubercle
Groove for posterior deep temporal artery
Supramastoid crest
External acoustic meatus
Mastoid process
Lambdoid suture

Occipital bone

Sutural (wormian) bone

External occipital protuberance (inion)

Asterion

Mandible
Head of condylar process
Mandibular notch
Coronoid process
Ramus
Oblique line
Body
Mental foramen

Infratemporal fossa exposed by removal of zygomatic arch and mandible*

Pterygomaxillary fissure

Inferior orbital fissure

Infratemporal surface of maxilla

Alveolar foramina

Tuberosity of maxilla

Sphenoidal bone
Greater wing
Infratemporal crest
Lateral plate of pterygoid process
Pterygoid hamulus (of medial plate of pterygoid process)

Temporal bone
External acoustic meatus
Mandibular fossa
Articular tubercle
Styloid process

Foramen ovale

Pterygopalatine fossa

Sphenopalatine foramen

*Superficially, mastoid process forms posterior boundary.

Plate 6   **Bones and Ligaments**

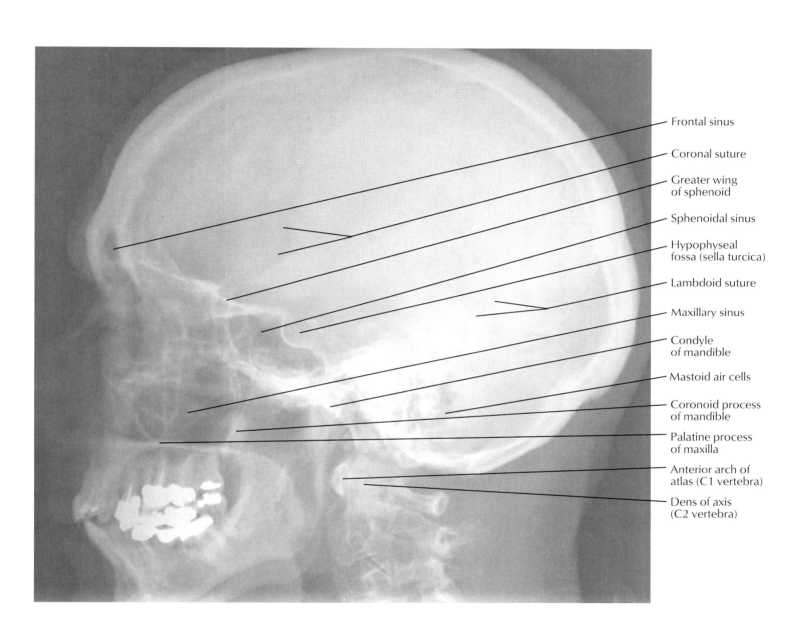

Frontal sinus

Coronal suture

Greater wing
of sphenoid

Sphenoidal sinus

Hypophyseal
fossa (sella turcica)

Lambdoid suture

Maxillary sinus

Condyle
of mandible

Mastoid air cells

Coronoid process
of mandible

Palatine process
of maxilla

Anterior arch of
atlas (C1 vertebra)

Dens of axis
(C2 vertebra)

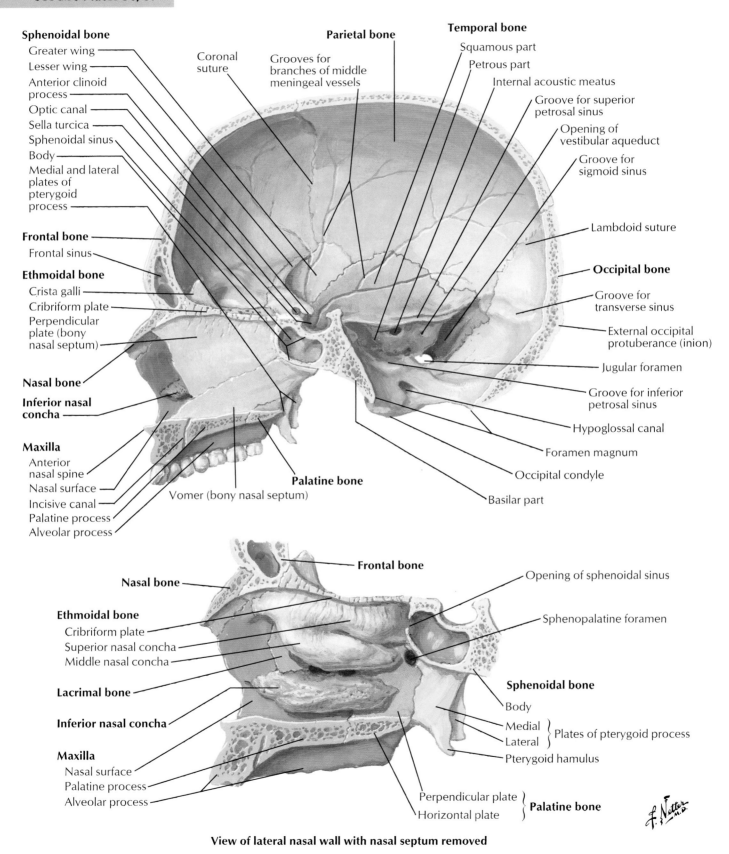

Sphenoidal bone
Greater wing
Lesser wing
Anterior clinoid process
Optic canal
Sella turcica
Sphenoidal sinus
Body
Medial and lateral plates of pterygoid process

Frontal bone
Frontal sinus

Ethmoidal bone
Crista galli
Cribriform plate
Perpendicular plate (bony nasal septum)

Nasal bone

Inferior nasal concha

Maxilla
Anterior nasal spine
Nasal surface
Incisive canal
Palatine process
Alveolar process

Coronal suture

Grooves for branches of middle meningeal vessels

Parietal bone

Temporal bone
Squamous part
Petrous part
Internal acoustic meatus
Groove for superior petrosal sinus
Opening of vestibular aqueduct
Groove for sigmoid sinus

Lambdoid suture

Occipital bone
Groove for transverse sinus
External occipital protuberance (inion)
Jugular foramen
Groove for inferior petrosal sinus
Hypoglossal canal
Foramen magnum
Occipital condyle
Basilar part

Vomer (bony nasal septum)

Palatine bone

Nasal bone

Ethmoidal bone
Cribriform plate
Superior nasal concha
Middle nasal concha

Lacrimal bone

Inferior nasal concha

Maxilla
Nasal surface
Palatine process
Alveolar process

Frontal bone

Opening of sphenoidal sinus

Sphenopalatine foramen

Sphenoidal bone
Body
Medial
Lateral } Plates of pterygoid process
Pterygoid hamulus

Perpendicular plate
Horizontal plate } **Palatine bone**

View of lateral nasal wall with nasal septum removed

Plate 8

Bones and Ligaments

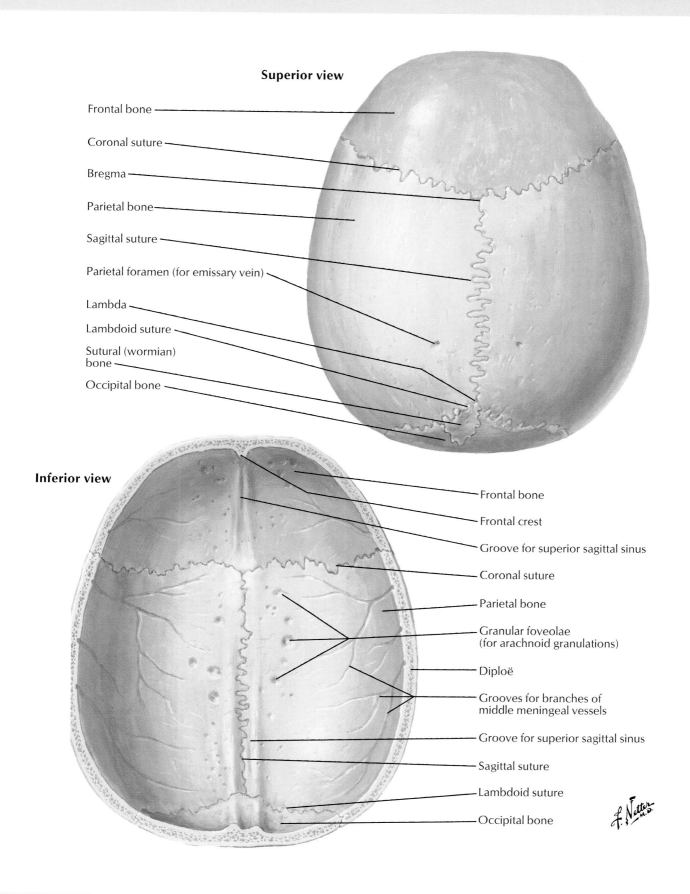

Superior view

Frontal bone

Coronal suture

Bregma

Parietal bone

Sagittal suture

Parietal foramen (for emissary vein)

Lambda

Lambdoid suture

Sutural (wormian) bone

Occipital bone

Inferior view

Frontal bone

Frontal crest

Groove for superior sagittal sinus

Coronal suture

Parietal bone

Granular foveolae (for arachnoid granulations)

Diploë

Grooves for branches of middle meningeal vessels

Groove for superior sagittal sinus

Sagittal suture

Lambdoid suture

Occipital bone

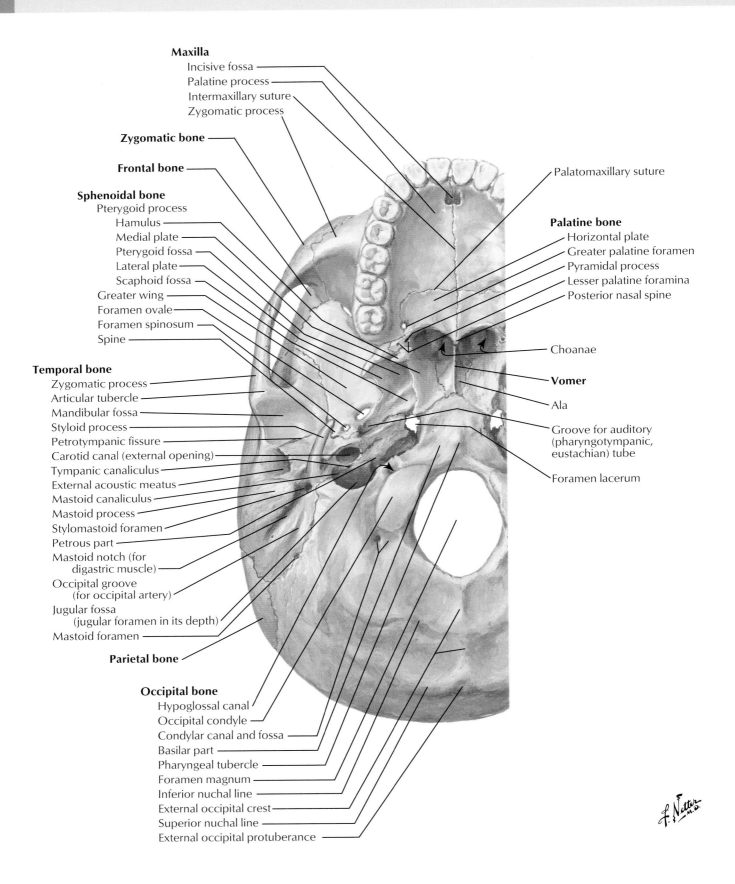

Maxilla
Incisive fossa
Palatine process
Intermaxillary suture
Zygomatic process

Zygomatic bone

Frontal bone

Sphenoidal bone
Pterygoid process
Hamulus
Medial plate
Pterygoid fossa
Lateral plate
Scaphoid fossa
Greater wing
Foramen ovale
Foramen spinosum
Spine

Temporal bone
Zygomatic process
Articular tubercle
Mandibular fossa
Styloid process
Petrotympanic fissure
Carotid canal (external opening)
Tympanic canaliculus
External acoustic meatus
Mastoid canaliculus
Mastoid process
Stylomastoid foramen
Petrous part
Mastoid notch (for
    digastric muscle)
Occipital groove
    (for occipital artery)
Jugular fossa
    (jugular foramen in its depth)
Mastoid foramen

Parietal bone

Occipital bone
Hypoglossal canal
Occipital condyle
Condylar canal and fossa
Basilar part
Pharyngeal tubercle
Foramen magnum
Inferior nuchal line
External occipital crest
Superior nuchal line
External occipital protuberance

Palatomaxillary suture

Palatine bone
Horizontal plate
Greater palatine foramen
Pyramidal process
Lesser palatine foramina
Posterior nasal spine

Choanae

Vomer

Ala

Groove for auditory
(pharyngotympanic,
eustachian) tube

Foramen lacerum

f. Netter m.d.

Plate 10 **Bones and Ligaments**

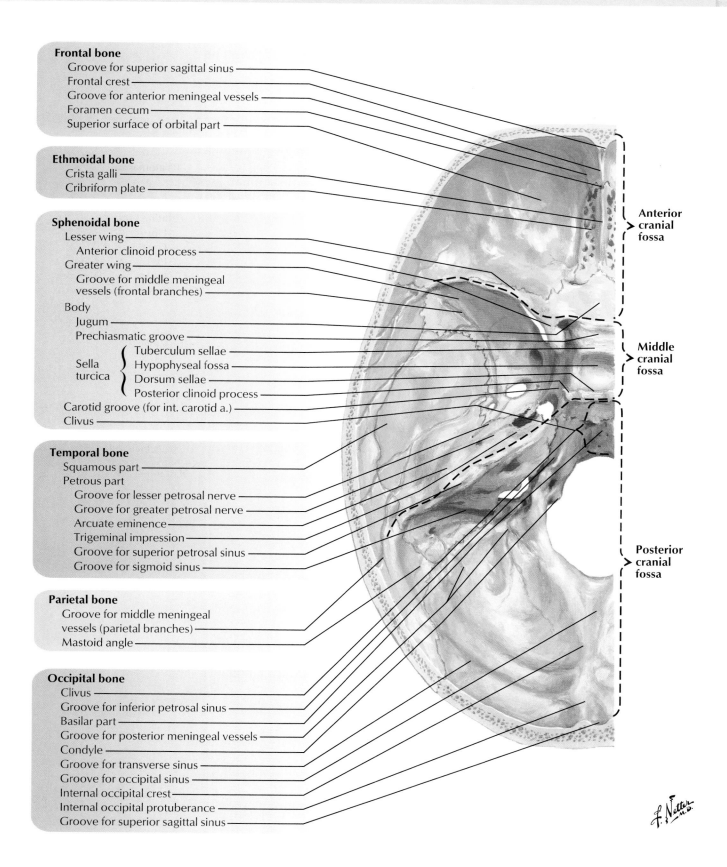

Frontal bone
Groove for superior sagittal sinus
Frontal crest
Groove for anterior meningeal vessels
Foramen cecum
Superior surface of orbital part

Ethmoidal bone
Crista galli
Cribriform plate

Sphenoidal bone
Lesser wing
Anterior clinoid process
Greater wing
Groove for middle meningeal
vessels (frontal branches)
Body
Jugum
Prechiasmatic groove
Sella turcica {
Tuberculum sellae
Hypophyseal fossa
Dorsum sellae
Posterior clinoid process
Carotid groove (for int. carotid a.)
Clivus

Temporal bone
Squamous part
Petrous part
Groove for lesser petrosal nerve
Groove for greater petrosal nerve
Arcuate eminence
Trigeminal impression
Groove for superior petrosal sinus
Groove for sigmoid sinus

Parietal bone
Groove for middle meningeal
vessels (parietal branches)
Mastoid angle

Occipital bone
Clivus
Groove for inferior petrosal sinus
Basilar part
Groove for posterior meningeal vessels
Condyle
Groove for transverse sinus
Groove for occipital sinus
Internal occipital crest
Internal occipital protuberance
Groove for superior sagittal sinus

Anterior
cranial
fossa

Middle
cranial
fossa

Posterior
cranial
fossa

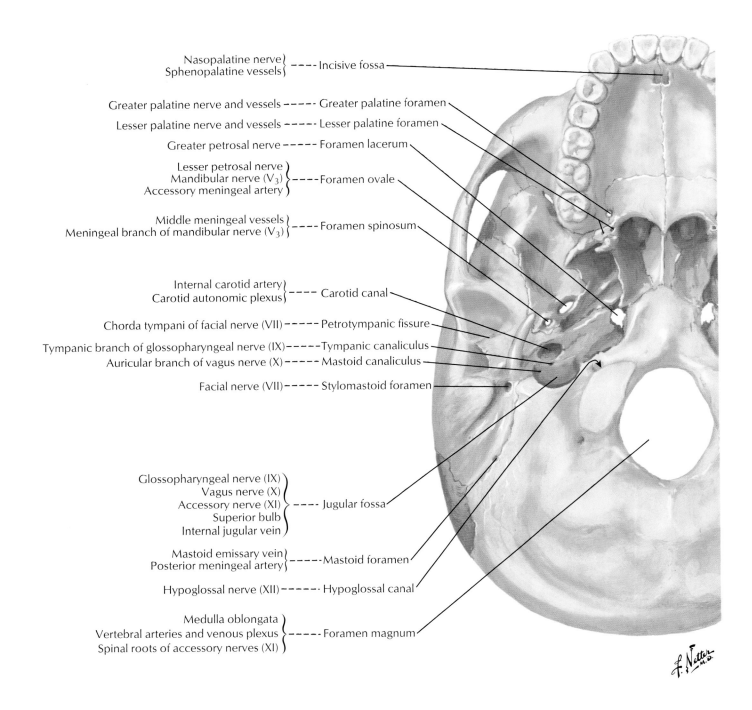

Nasopalatine nerve ⎱ ---- Incisive fossa
Sphenopalatine vessels ⎰

Greater palatine nerve and vessels ---- Greater palatine foramen

Lesser palatine nerve and vessels ---- Lesser palatine foramen

Greater petrosal nerve ---- Foramen lacerum

Lesser petrosal nerve ⎱
Mandibular nerve (V₃) ⎬ ---- Foramen ovale
Accessory meningeal artery ⎰

Middle meningeal vessels ⎱ ---- Foramen spinosum
Meningeal branch of mandibular nerve (V₃) ⎰

Internal carotid artery ⎱ ---- Carotid canal
Carotid autonomic plexus ⎰

Chorda tympani of facial nerve (VII) ---- Petrotympanic fissure

Tympanic branch of glossopharyngeal nerve (IX) ---- Tympanic canaliculus

Auricular branch of vagus nerve (X) ---- Mastoid canaliculus

Facial nerve (VII) ---- Stylomastoid foramen

Glossopharyngeal nerve (IX) ⎱
Vagus nerve (X) ⎬
Accessory nerve (XI) ⎬ ---- Jugular fossa
Superior bulb ⎬
Internal jugular vein ⎰

Mastoid emissary vein ⎱ ---- Mastoid foramen
Posterior meningeal artery ⎰

Hypoglossal nerve (XII) ---- Hypoglossal canal

Medulla oblongata ⎱
Vertebral arteries and venous plexus ⎬ ---- Foramen magnum
Spinal roots of accessory nerves (XI) ⎰

Plate 12

Bones and Ligaments

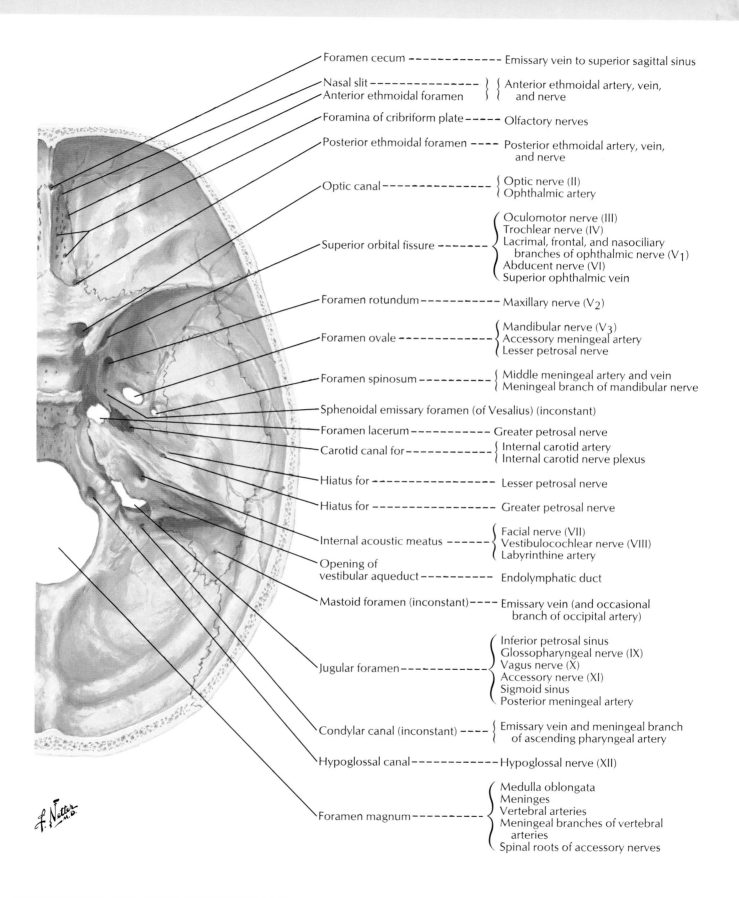

Foramen cecum – – – – – – – – – – Emissary vein to superior sagittal sinus

Nasal slit – – – – – – – – – – – – – } { Anterior ethmoidal artery, vein,
Anterior ethmoidal foramen } { and nerve

Foramina of cribriform plate – – – – – Olfactory nerves

Posterior ethmoidal foramen – – – – Posterior ethmoidal artery, vein,
and nerve

Optic canal – – – – – – – – – – – – – { Optic nerve (II)
{ Ophthalmic artery

Superior orbital fissure – – – – – – – { Oculomotor nerve (III)
Trochlear nerve (IV)
Lacrimal, frontal, and nasociliary
branches of ophthalmic nerve (V$_1$)
Abducent nerve (VI)
Superior ophthalmic vein

Foramen rotundum – – – – – – – – – – Maxillary nerve (V$_2$)

Foramen ovale – – – – – – – – – – – { Mandibular nerve (V$_3$)
Accessory meningeal artery
Lesser petrosal nerve

Foramen spinosum – – – – – – – – – – { Middle meningeal artery and vein
{ Meningeal branch of mandibular nerve

Sphenoidal emissary foramen (of Vesalius) (inconstant)

Foramen lacerum – – – – – – – – – – Greater petrosal nerve

Carotid canal for – – – – – – – – – – { Internal carotid artery
{ Internal carotid nerve plexus

Hiatus for – – – – – – – – – – – – – Lesser petrosal nerve

Hiatus for – – – – – – – – – – – – – Greater petrosal nerve

Internal acoustic meatus – – – – – – { Facial nerve (VII)
Vestibulocochlear nerve (VIII)
Labyrinthine artery

Opening of
vestibular aqueduct – – – – – – – – – Endolymphatic duct

Mastoid foramen (inconstant) – – – – Emissary vein (and occasional
branch of occipital artery)

Jugular foramen – – – – – – – – – – { Inferior petrosal sinus
Glossopharyngeal nerve (IX)
Vagus nerve (X)
Accessory nerve (XI)
Sigmoid sinus
Posterior meningeal artery

Condylar canal (inconstant) – – – – { Emissary vein and meningeal branch
of ascending pharyngeal artery

Hypoglossal canal – – – – – – – – – – Hypoglossal nerve (XII)

Foramen magnum – – – – – – – – – { Medulla oblongata
Meninges
Vertebral arteries
Meningeal branches of vertebral
arteries
Spinal roots of accessory nerves

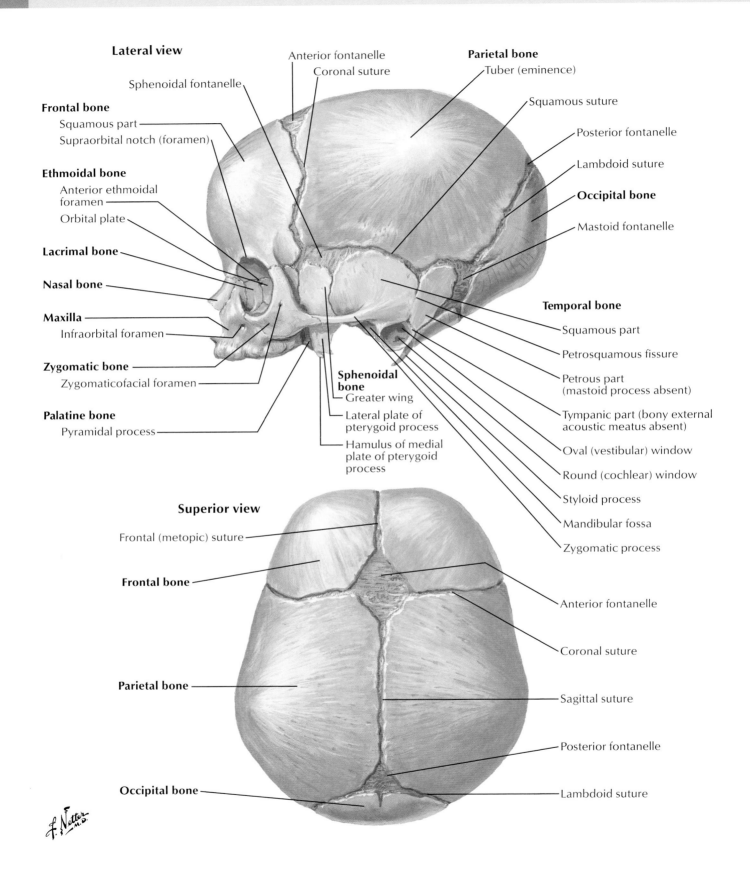

Lateral view

Anterior fontanelle

Coronal suture

Parietal bone

Tuber (eminence)

Sphenoidal fontanelle

Squamous suture

Frontal bone

Squamous part

Supraorbital notch (foramen)

Posterior fontanelle

Lambdoid suture

Ethmoidal bone

Anterior ethmoidal foramen

Occipital bone

Orbital plate

Mastoid fontanelle

Lacrimal bone

Nasal bone

Temporal bone

Maxilla

Squamous part

Infraorbital foramen

Petrosquamous fissure

Zygomatic bone

Petrous part (mastoid process absent)

Zygomaticofacial foramen

Sphenoidal bone

Greater wing

Tympanic part (bony external acoustic meatus absent)

Palatine bone

Lateral plate of pterygoid process

Oval (vestibular) window

Pyramidal process

Hamulus of medial plate of pterygoid process

Round (cochlear) window

Styloid process

Mandibular fossa

Zygomatic process

Superior view

Frontal (metopic) suture

Frontal bone

Anterior fontanelle

Coronal suture

Parietal bone

Sagittal suture

Posterior fontanelle

Occipital bone

Lambdoid suture

Plate 14 **Bones and Ligaments**

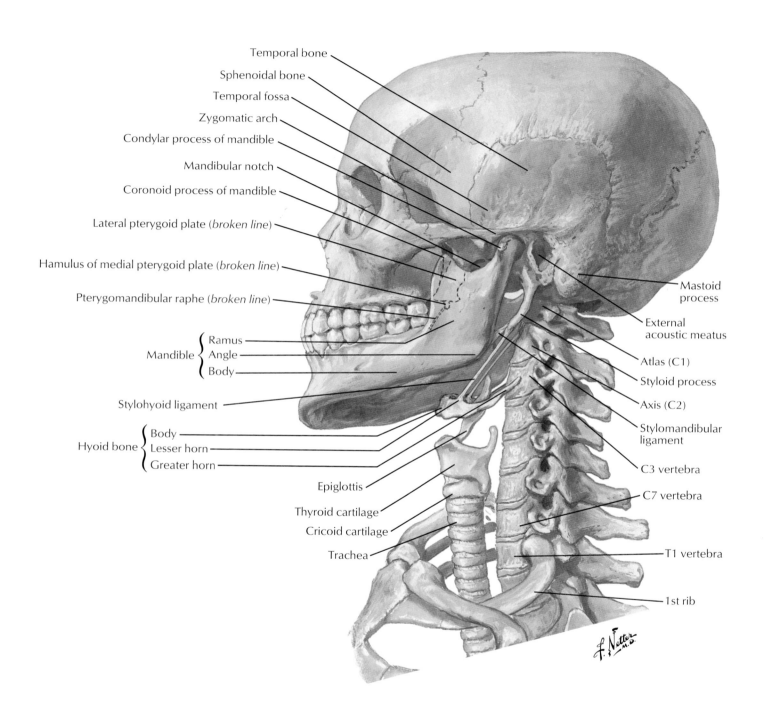

Temporal bone

Sphenoidal bone

Temporal fossa

Zygomatic arch

Condylar process of mandible

Mandibular notch

Coronoid process of mandible

Lateral pterygoid plate (*broken line*)

Hamulus of medial pterygoid plate (*broken line*)

Pterygomandibular raphe (*broken line*)

Mandible { Ramus / Angle / Body

Stylohyoid ligament

Hyoid bone { Body / Lesser horn / Greater horn

Epiglottis

Thyroid cartilage

Cricoid cartilage

Trachea

Mastoid process

External acoustic meatus

Atlas (C1)

Styloid process

Axis (C2)

Stylomandibular ligament

C3 vertebra

C7 vertebra

T1 vertebra

1st rib

F. Netter M.D.

Posterior view

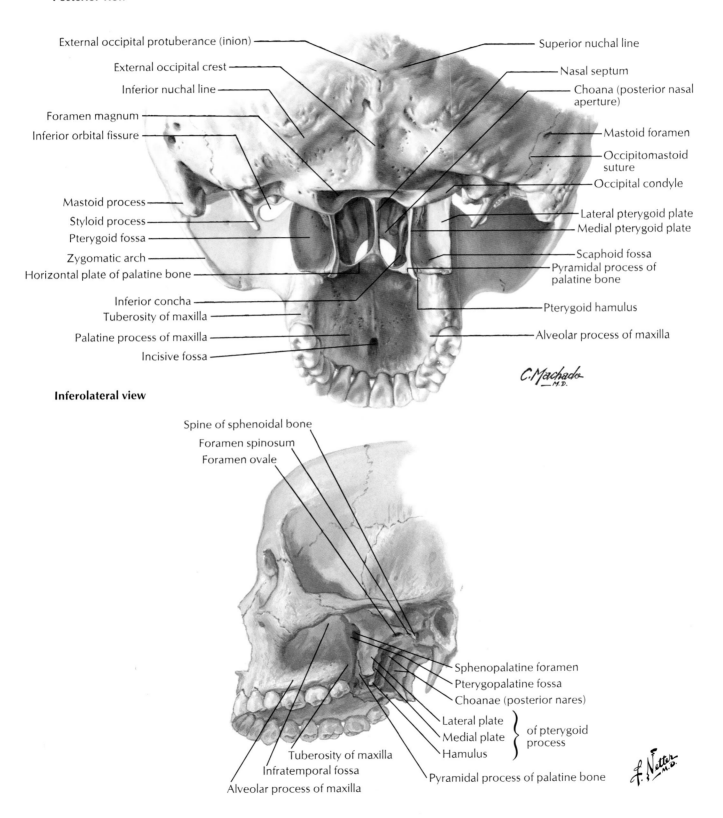

External occipital protuberance (inion)

External occipital crest

Inferior nuchal line

Foramen magnum

Inferior orbital fissure

Mastoid process

Styloid process

Pterygoid fossa

Zygomatic arch

Horizontal plate of palatine bone

Inferior concha

Tuberosity of maxilla

Palatine process of maxilla

Incisive fossa

Superior nuchal line

Nasal septum

Choana (posterior nasal aperture)

Mastoid foramen

Occipitomastoid suture

Occipital condyle

Lateral pterygoid plate

Medial pterygoid plate

Scaphoid fossa

Pyramidal process of palatine bone

Pterygoid hamulus

Alveolar process of maxilla

C. Machado M.D.

Inferolateral view

Spine of sphenoidal bone

Foramen spinosum

Foramen ovale

Sphenopalatine foramen

Pterygopalatine fossa

Choanae (posterior nares)

Lateral plate ⎫
Medial plate ⎬ of pterygoid process
Hamulus ⎭

Tuberosity of maxilla

Infratemporal fossa

Alveolar process of maxilla

Pyramidal process of palatine bone

F. Netter M.D.

Plate 16 **Bones and Ligaments**

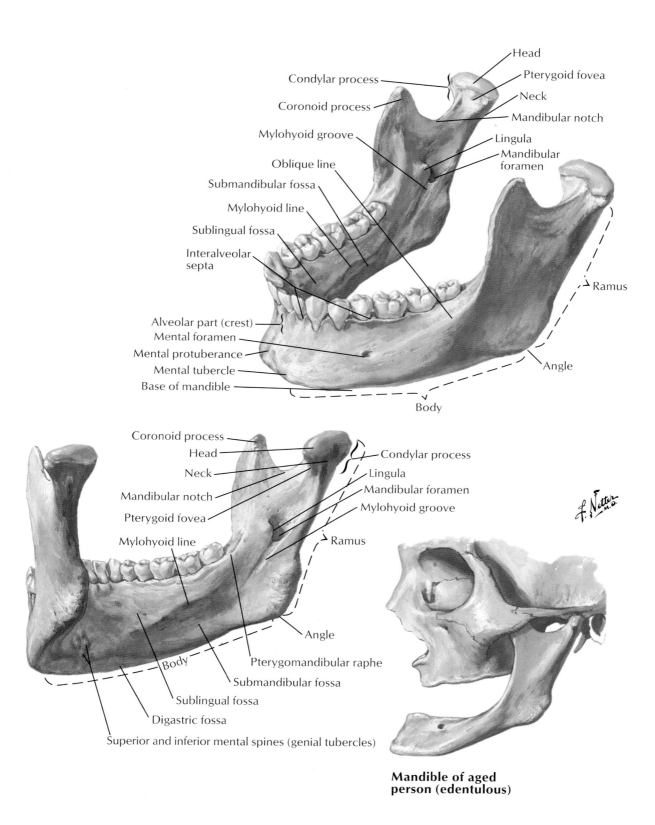

Condylar process — Head
— Pterygoid fovea
Coronoid process — Neck
— Mandibular notch
Mylohyoid groove — Lingula
— Mandibular foramen
Oblique line
Submandibular fossa
Mylohyoid line
Sublingual fossa
Interalveolar septa
— Ramus
Alveolar part (crest)
Mental foramen
Mental protuberance
Mental tubercle
Base of mandible — Angle
— Body

Coronoid process
Head — Condylar process
Neck — Lingula
Mandibular notch — Mandibular foramen
Pterygoid fovea — Mylohyoid groove
Mylohyoid line
— Ramus
— Angle
— Body
Pterygomandibular raphe
Submandibular fossa
Sublingual fossa
Digastric fossa
Superior and inferior mental spines (genial tubercles)

Mandible of aged person (edentulous)

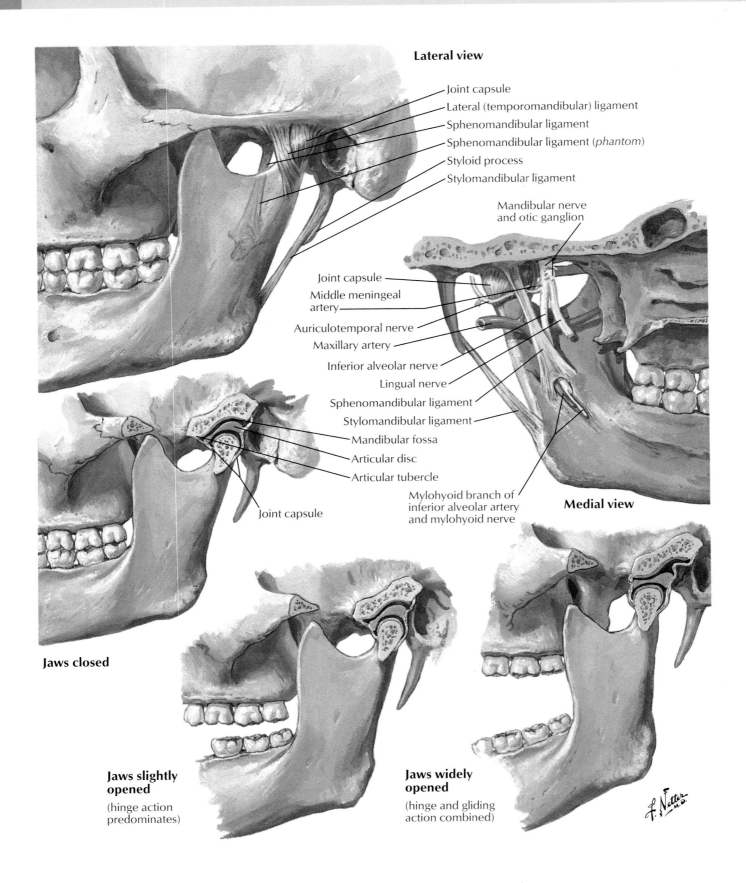

Lateral view

Joint capsule

Lateral (temporomandibular) ligament

Sphenomandibular ligament

Sphenomandibular ligament (*phantom*)

Styloid process

Stylomandibular ligament

Mandibular nerve and otic ganglion

Joint capsule

Middle meningeal artery

Auriculotemporal nerve

Maxillary artery

Inferior alveolar nerve

Lingual nerve

Sphenomandibular ligament

Stylomandibular ligament

Mandibular fossa

Articular disc

Articular tubercle

Joint capsule

Mylohyoid branch of inferior alveolar artery and mylohyoid nerve

Medial view

Jaws closed

Jaws slightly opened

(hinge action predominates)

Jaws widely opened

(hinge and gliding action combined)

Plate 18

Bones and Ligaments

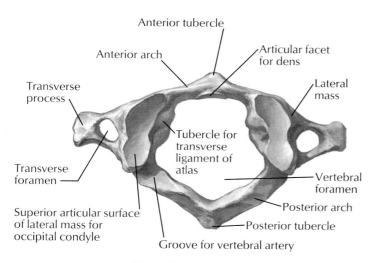

Anterior tubercle

Anterior arch

Articular facet for dens

Transverse process

Lateral mass

Transverse foramen

Tubercle for transverse ligament of atlas

Superior articular surface of lateral mass for occipital condyle

Vertebral foramen

Posterior arch

Posterior tubercle

Groove for vertebral artery

Atlas (C1): superior view

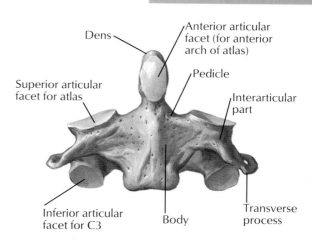

Dens

Anterior articular facet (for anterior arch of atlas)

Superior articular facet for atlas

Pedicle

Interarticular part

Inferior articular facet for C3

Body

Transverse process

Axis (C2): anterior view

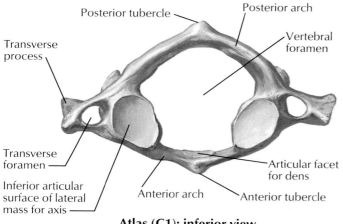

Posterior tubercle

Posterior arch

Transverse process

Vertebral foramen

Transverse foramen

Articular facet for dens

Inferior articular surface of lateral mass for axis

Anterior arch

Anterior tubercle

Atlas (C1): inferior view

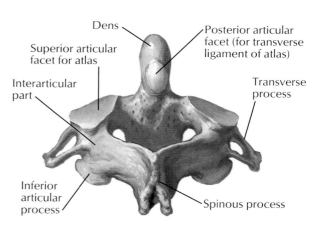

Dens

Superior articular facet for atlas

Posterior articular facet (for transverse ligament of atlas)

Interarticular part

Transverse process

Inferior articular process

Spinous process

Axis (C2): posterosuperior view

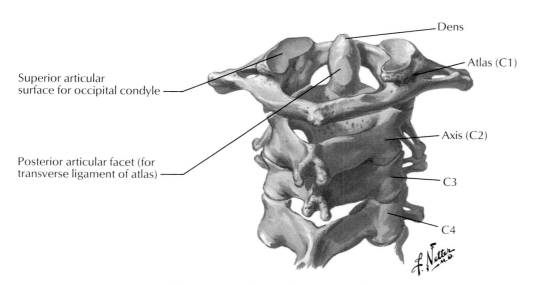

Dens

Atlas (C1)

Superior articular surface for occipital condyle

Axis (C2)

C3

Posterior articular facet (for transverse ligament of atlas)

C4

Upper cervical vertebrae, assembled: posterosuperior view

Inferior aspect of C3 and superior aspect of C4 showing the sites of the facet and uncovertebral articulations

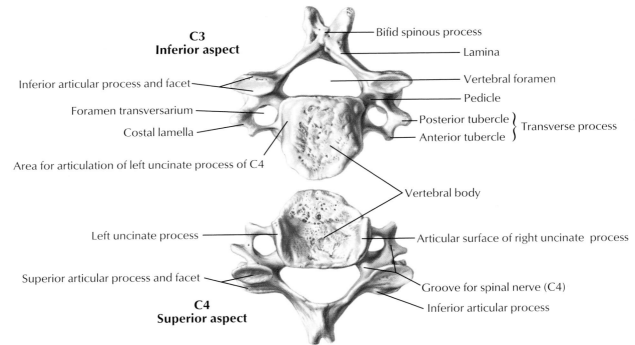

C3
Inferior aspect

Bifid spinous process

Lamina

Inferior articular process and facet

Vertebral foramen

Foramen transversarium

Pedicle

Costal lamella

Posterior tubercle ⎫
Anterior tubercle ⎬ Transverse process

Area for articulation of left uncinate process of C4

Vertebral body

Left uncinate process

Articular surface of right uncinate process

Superior articular process and facet

Groove for spinal nerve (C4)

Inferior articular process

C4
Superior aspect

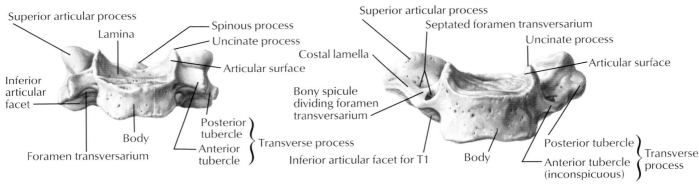

4th cervical vertebra: anterior view

Superior articular process

Lamina

Spinous process

Uncinate process

Articular surface

Inferior articular facet

Body

Foramen transversarium

Posterior tubercle ⎫
Anterior tubercle ⎬ Transverse process

7th cervical vertebra: anterior view

Superior articular process

Septated foramen transversarium

Uncinate process

Costal lamella

Articular surface

Bony spicule dividing foramen transversarium

Posterior tubercle ⎫
Anterior tubercle (inconspicuous) ⎬ Transverse process

Inferior articular facet for T1

Body

7th cervical vertebra (vertebra prominens): superior view

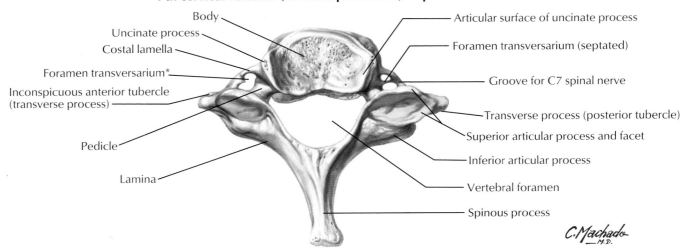

Body

Uncinate process

Costal lamella

Foramen transversarium*

Inconspicuous anterior tubercle (transverse process)

Pedicle

Lamina

Articular surface of uncinate process

Foramen transversarium (septated)

Groove for C7 spinal nerve

Transverse process (posterior tubercle)

Superior articular process and facet

Inferior articular process

Vertebral foramen

Spinous process

C. Machado
_M.D._

The foramina transversaria of C7 transmit vertebral veins, but usually not the vertebral artery, and are asymmetrical in this specimen.

Plate 20

Bones and Ligaments

Cervical vertebrae: anterior view

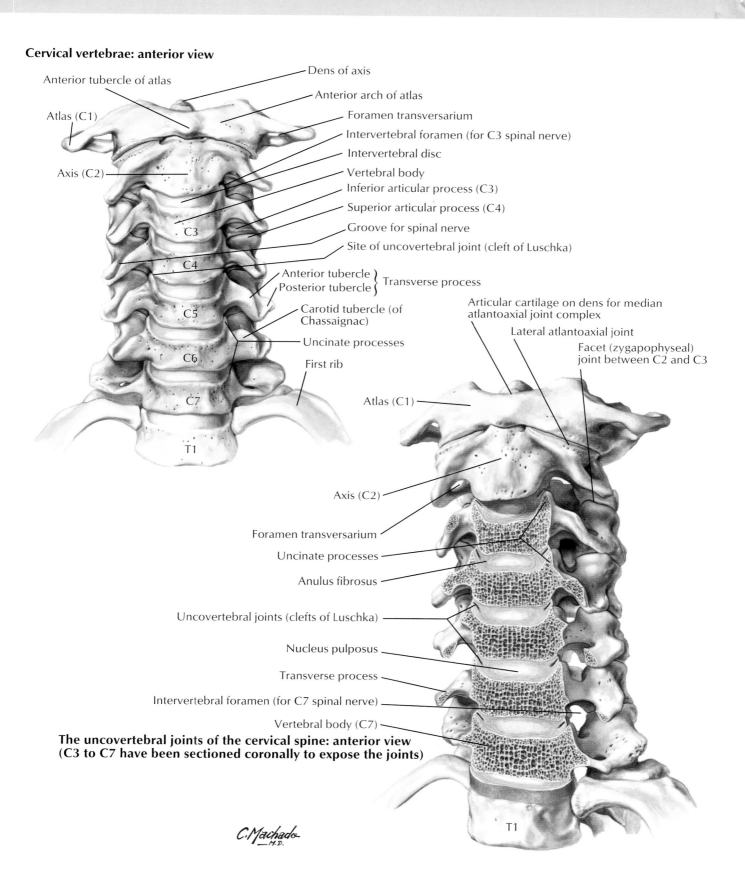

Anterior tubercle of atlas

Dens of axis

Anterior arch of atlas

Atlas (C1)

Foramen transversarium

Intervertebral foramen (for C3 spinal nerve)

Intervertebral disc

Axis (C2)

Vertebral body

Inferior articular process (C3)

Superior articular process (C4)

C3

Groove for spinal nerve

Site of uncovertebral joint (cleft of Luschka)

C4

Anterior tubercle } Transverse process
Posterior tubercle }

Articular cartilage on dens for median atlantoaxial joint complex

C5

Carotid tubercle (of Chassaignac)

Lateral atlantoaxial joint

Facet (zygapophyseal) joint between C2 and C3

C6

Uncinate processes

First rib

C7

Atlas (C1)

T1

Axis (C2)

Foramen transversarium

Uncinate processes

Anulus fibrosus

Uncovertebral joints (clefts of Luschka)

Nucleus pulposus

Transverse process

Intervertebral foramen (for C7 spinal nerve)

Vertebral body (C7)

The uncovertebral joints of the cervical spine: anterior view (C3 to C7 have been sectioned coronally to expose the joints)

C. Machado
M.D.

T1

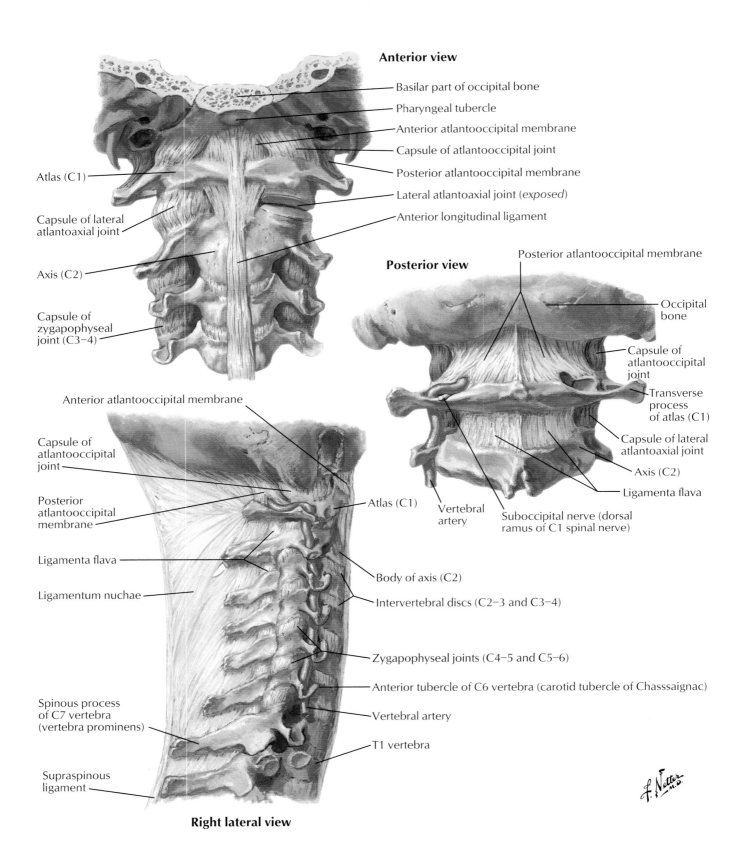

Anterior view

Basilar part of occipital bone

Pharyngeal tubercle

Anterior atlantooccipital membrane

Capsule of atlantooccipital joint

Posterior atlantooccipital membrane

Lateral atlantoaxial joint (*exposed*)

Anterior longitudinal ligament

Atlas (C1)

Capsule of lateral atlantoaxial joint

Axis (C2)

Capsule of zygapophyseal joint (C3–4)

Posterior view

Posterior atlantooccipital membrane

Occipital bone

Capsule of atlantooccipital joint

Transverse process of atlas (C1)

Capsule of lateral atlantoaxial joint

Axis (C2)

Ligamenta flava

Vertebral artery

Suboccipital nerve (dorsal ramus of C1 spinal nerve)

Anterior atlantooccipital membrane

Capsule of atlantooccipital joint

Posterior atlantooccipital membrane

Ligamenta flava

Ligamentum nuchae

Atlas (C1)

Body of axis (C2)

Intervertebral discs (C2–3 and C3–4)

Zygapophyseal joints (C4–5 and C5–6)

Anterior tubercle of C6 vertebra (carotid tubercle of Chasssaignac)

Vertebral artery

T1 vertebra

Spinous process of C7 vertebra (vertebra prominens)

Supraspinous ligament

Right lateral view

Plate 22   **Bones and Ligaments**

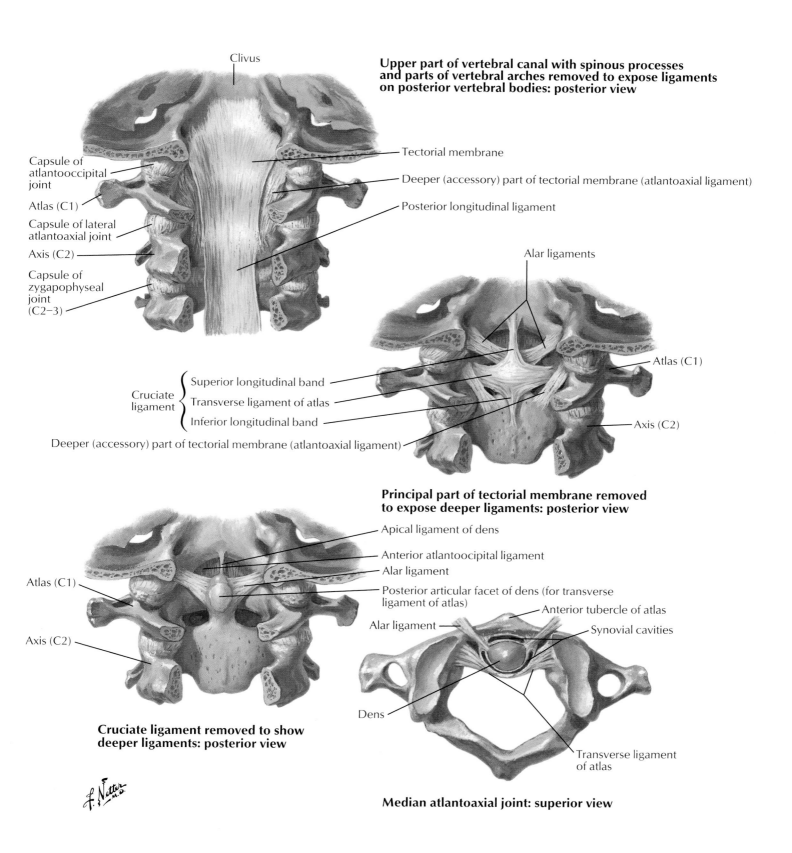

Clivus

Upper part of vertebral canal with spinous processes and parts of vertebral arches removed to expose ligaments on posterior vertebral bodies: posterior view

Tectorial membrane

Deeper (accessory) part of tectorial membrane (atlantoaxial ligament)

Posterior longitudinal ligament

Capsule of atlantooccipital joint

Atlas (C1)

Capsule of lateral atlantoaxial joint

Axis (C2)

Capsule of zygapophyseal joint (C2–3)

Alar ligaments

Atlas (C1)

Axis (C2)

Cruciate ligament:
Superior longitudinal band
Transverse ligament of atlas
Inferior longitudinal band

Deeper (accessory) part of tectorial membrane (atlantoaxial ligament)

Principal part of tectorial membrane removed to expose deeper ligaments: posterior view

Apical ligament of dens

Anterior atlantooccipital ligament

Alar ligament

Posterior articular facet of dens (for transverse ligament of atlas)

Atlas (C1)

Axis (C2)

Anterior tubercle of atlas

Alar ligament

Synovial cavities

Dens

Transverse ligament of atlas

Cruciate ligament removed to show deeper ligaments: posterior view

Median atlantoaxial joint: superior view

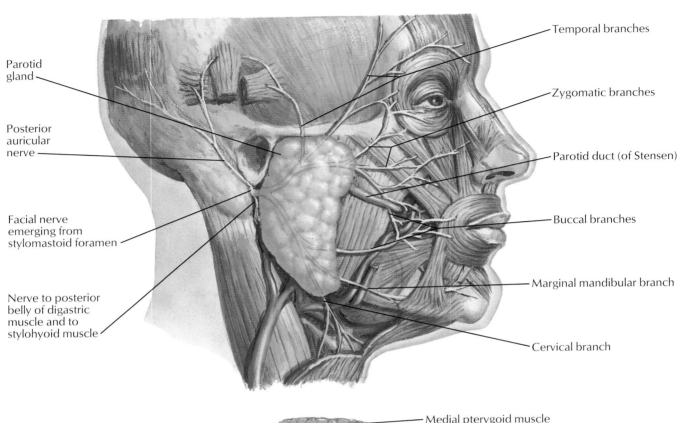

Temporal branches

Parotid gland

Zygomatic branches

Posterior auricular nerve

Parotid duct (of Stensen)

Facial nerve emerging from stylomastoid foramen

Buccal branches

Marginal mandibular branch

Nerve to posterior belly of digastric muscle and to stylohyoid muscle

Cervical branch

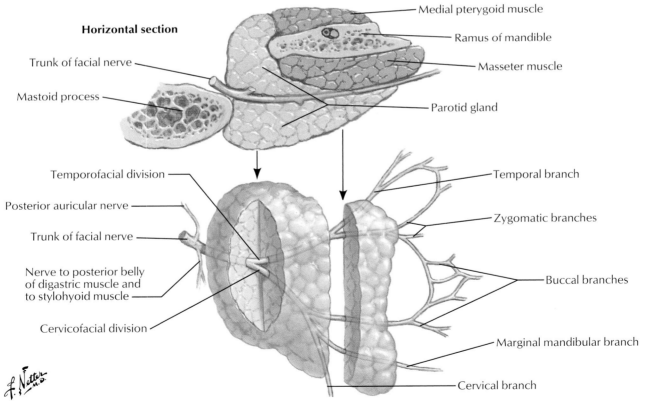

Horizontal section

Medial pterygoid muscle

Trunk of facial nerve

Ramus of mandible

Mastoid process

Masseter muscle

Parotid gland

Temporofacial division

Temporal branch

Posterior auricular nerve

Trunk of facial nerve

Zygomatic branches

Nerve to posterior belly of digastric muscle and to stylohyoid muscle

Buccal branches

Cervicofacial division

Marginal mandibular branch

Cervical branch

Plate 24

Superficial Face

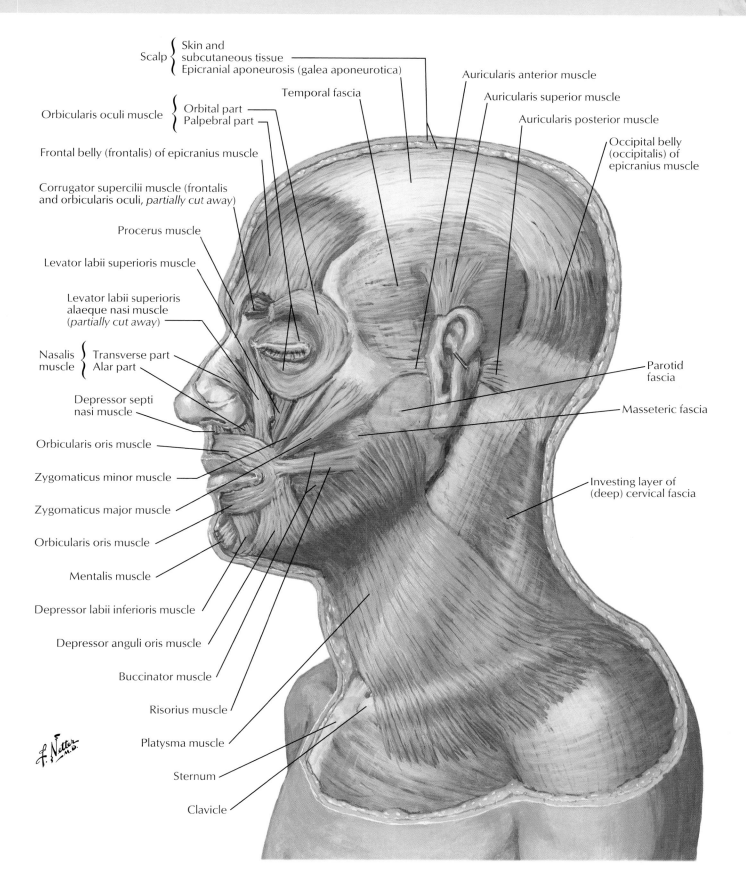

Scalp {
Skin and
subcutaneous tissue
Epicranial aponeurosis (galea aponeurotica)

Temporal fascia

Orbicularis oculi muscle { Orbital part
Palpebral part

Frontal belly (frontalis) of epicranius muscle

Corrugator supercilii muscle (frontalis and orbicularis oculi, *partially cut away*)

Procerus muscle

Levator labii superioris muscle

Levator labii superioris alaeque nasi muscle (*partially cut away*)

Nasalis muscle { Transverse part
Alar part

Depressor septi nasi muscle

Orbicularis oris muscle

Zygomaticus minor muscle

Zygomaticus major muscle

Orbicularis oris muscle

Mentalis muscle

Depressor labii inferioris muscle

Depressor anguli oris muscle

Buccinator muscle

Risorius muscle

Platysma muscle

Sternum

Clavicle

Auricularis anterior muscle

Auricularis superior muscle

Auricularis posterior muscle

Occipital belly (occipitalis) of epicranius muscle

Parotid fascia

Masseteric fascia

Investing layer of (deep) cervical fascia

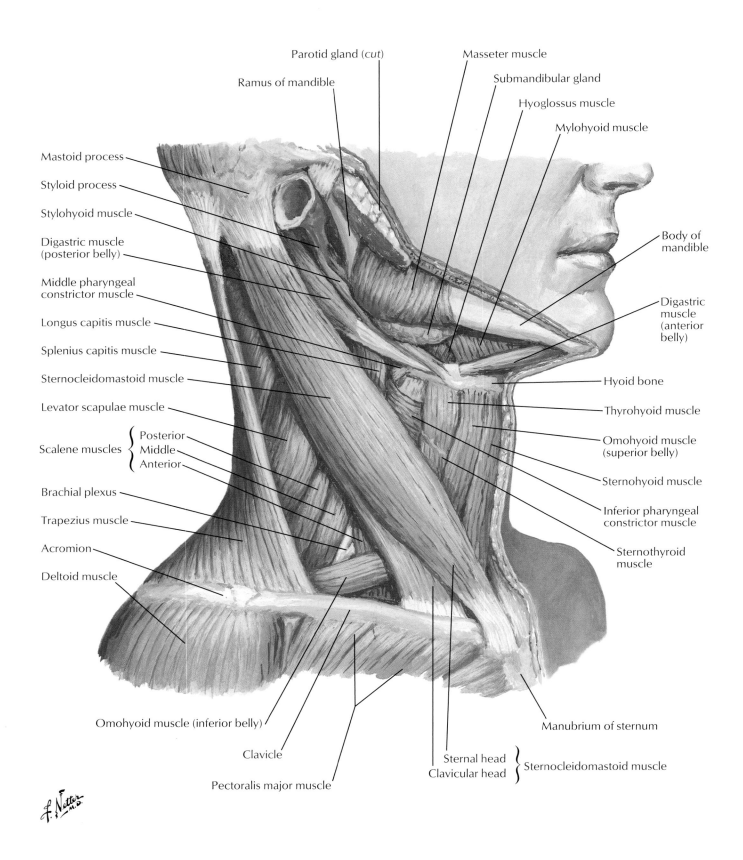

Parotid gland (*cut*)

Ramus of mandible

Masseter muscle

Submandibular gland

Hyoglossus muscle

Mylohyoid muscle

Mastoid process

Styloid process

Stylohyoid muscle

Digastric muscle (posterior belly)

Middle pharyngeal constrictor muscle

Longus capitis muscle

Splenius capitis muscle

Sternocleidomastoid muscle

Levator scapulae muscle

Scalene muscles { Posterior / Middle / Anterior

Brachial plexus

Trapezius muscle

Acromion

Deltoid muscle

Body of mandible

Digastric muscle (anterior belly)

Hyoid bone

Thyrohyoid muscle

Omohyoid muscle (superior belly)

Sternohyoid muscle

Inferior pharyngeal constrictor muscle

Sternothyroid muscle

Omohyoid muscle (inferior belly)

Clavicle

Pectoralis major muscle

Sternal head / Clavicular head } Sternocleidomastoid muscle

Manubrium of sternum

Plate 26

Neck

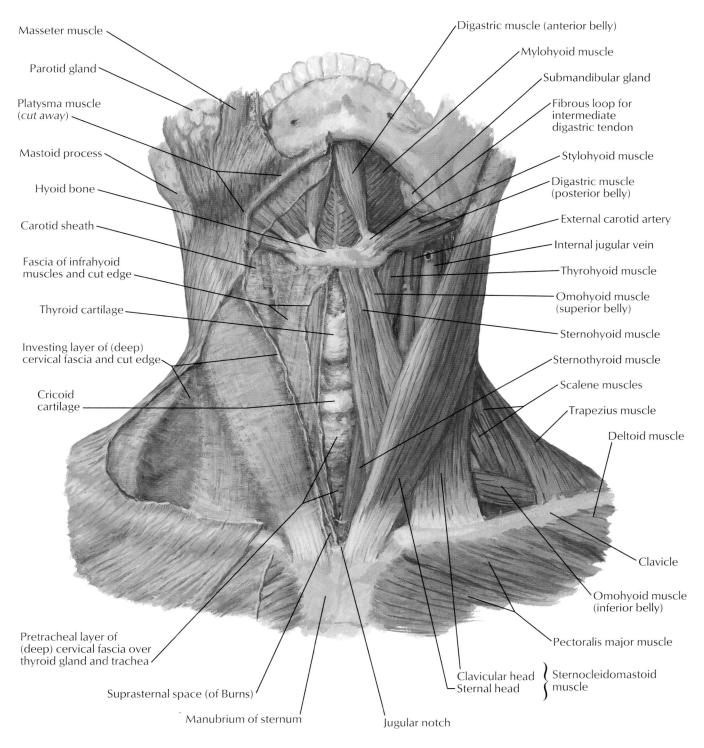

Masseter muscle

Parotid gland

Platysma muscle
(*cut away*)

Mastoid process

Hyoid bone

Carotid sheath

Fascia of infrahyoid
muscles and cut edge

Thyroid cartilage

Investing layer of (deep)
cervical fascia and cut edge

Cricoid
cartilage

Pretracheal layer of
(deep) cervical fascia over
thyroid gland and trachea

Suprasternal space (of Burns)

Manubrium of sternum

Digastric muscle (anterior belly)

Mylohyoid muscle

Submandibular gland

Fibrous loop for
intermediate
digastric tendon

Stylohyoid muscle

Digastric muscle
(posterior belly)

External carotid artery

Internal jugular vein

Thyrohyoid muscle

Omohyoid muscle
(superior belly)

Sternohyoid muscle

Sternothyroid muscle

Scalene muscles

Trapezius muscle

Deltoid muscle

Clavicle

Omohyoid muscle
(inferior belly)

Pectoralis major muscle

Clavicular head
Sternal head } Sternocleidomastoid
muscle

Jugular notch

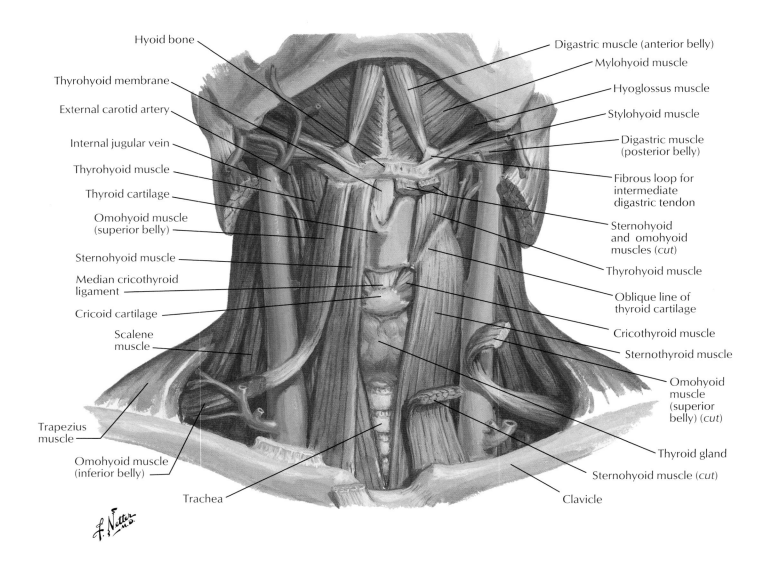

Hyoid bone

Thyrohyoid membrane

External carotid artery

Internal jugular vein

Thyrohyoid muscle

Thyroid cartilage

Omohyoid muscle (superior belly)

Sternohyoid muscle

Median cricothyroid ligament

Cricoid cartilage

Scalene muscle

Trapezius muscle

Omohyoid muscle (inferior belly)

Trachea

Digastric muscle (anterior belly)

Mylohyoid muscle

Hyoglossus muscle

Stylohyoid muscle

Digastric muscle (posterior belly)

Fibrous loop for intermediate digastric tendon

Sternohyoid and omohyoid muscles (cut)

Thyrohyoid muscle

Oblique line of thyroid cartilage

Cricothyroid muscle

Sternothyroid muscle

Omohyoid muscle (superior belly) (cut)

Thyroid gland

Sternohyoid muscle (cut)

Clavicle

Plate 28

Neck

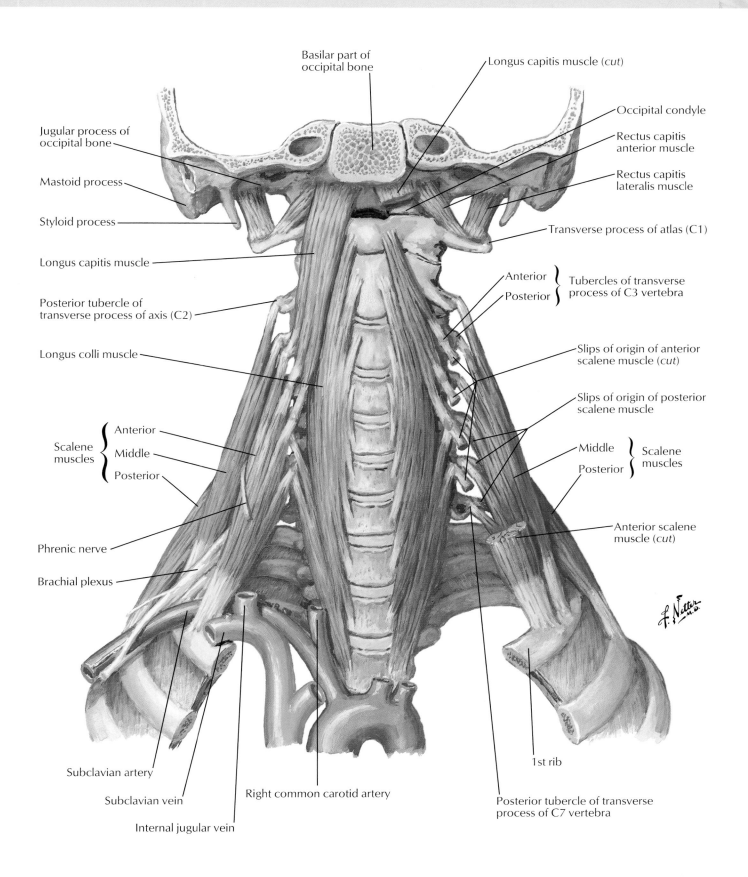

Basilar part of occipital bone

Longus capitis muscle (*cut*)

Occipital condyle

Rectus capitis anterior muscle

Rectus capitis lateralis muscle

Jugular process of occipital bone

Mastoid process

Styloid process

Transverse process of atlas (C1)

Longus capitis muscle

Anterior
Posterior } Tubercles of transverse process of C3 vertebra

Posterior tubercle of transverse process of axis (C2)

Slips of origin of anterior scalene muscle (*cut*)

Longus colli muscle

Slips of origin of posterior scalene muscle

Scalene muscles {
Anterior
Middle
Posterior

Middle
Posterior } Scalene muscles

Anterior scalene muscle (*cut*)

Phrenic nerve

Brachial plexus

Subclavian artery

Subclavian vein

Internal jugular vein

Right common carotid artery

1st rib

Posterior tubercle of transverse process of C7 vertebra

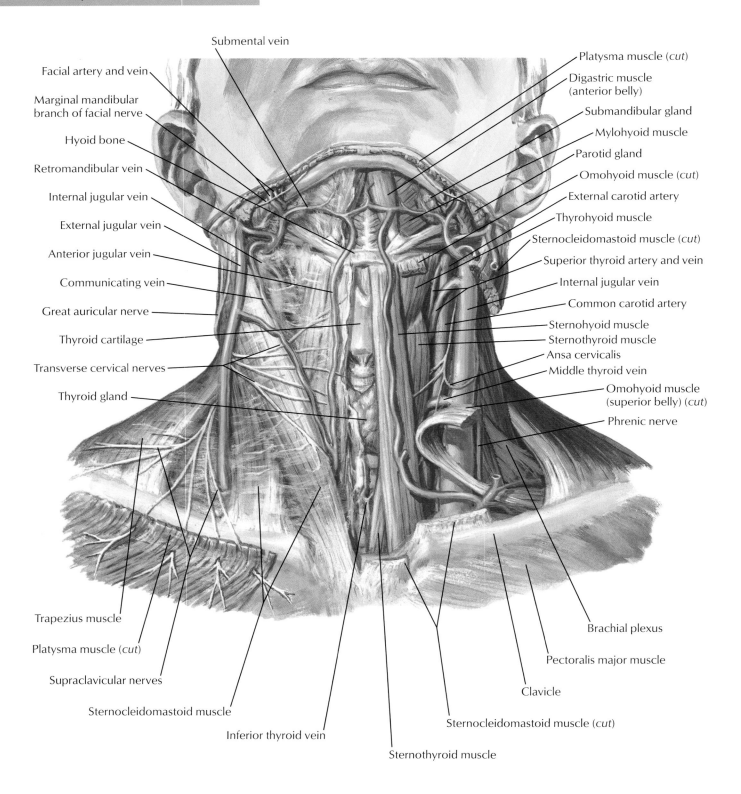

Submental vein

Facial artery and vein

Marginal mandibular branch of facial nerve

Hyoid bone

Retromandibular vein

Internal jugular vein

External jugular vein

Anterior jugular vein

Communicating vein

Great auricular nerve

Thyroid cartilage

Transverse cervical nerves

Thyroid gland

Platysma muscle (*cut*)

Digastric muscle (anterior belly)

Submandibular gland

Mylohyoid muscle

Parotid gland

Omohyoid muscle (*cut*)

External carotid artery

Thyrohyoid muscle

Sternocleidomastoid muscle (*cut*)

Superior thyroid artery and vein

Internal jugular vein

Common carotid artery

Sternohyoid muscle

Sternothyroid muscle

Ansa cervicalis

Middle thyroid vein

Omohyoid muscle (superior belly) (*cut*)

Phrenic nerve

Trapezius muscle

Platysma muscle (*cut*)

Supraclavicular nerves

Sternocleidomastoid muscle

Inferior thyroid vein

Sternothyroid muscle

Sternocleidomastoid muscle (*cut*)

Clavicle

Pectoralis major muscle

Brachial plexus

Plate 30   **Neck**

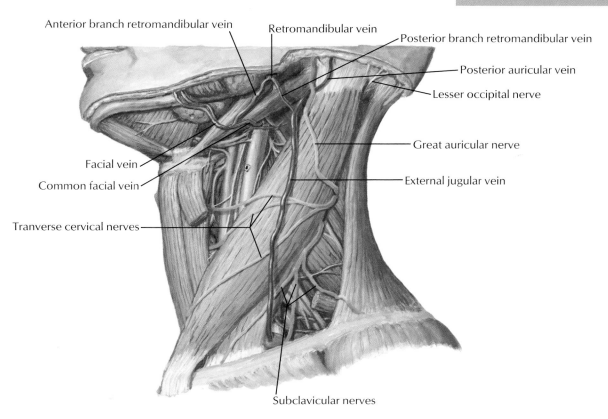

Anterior branch retromandibular vein

Retromandibular vein

Posterior branch retromandibular vein

Posterior auricular vein

Lesser occipital nerve

Facial vein

Great auricular nerve

Common facial vein

External jugular vein

Tranverse cervical nerves

Subclavicular nerves

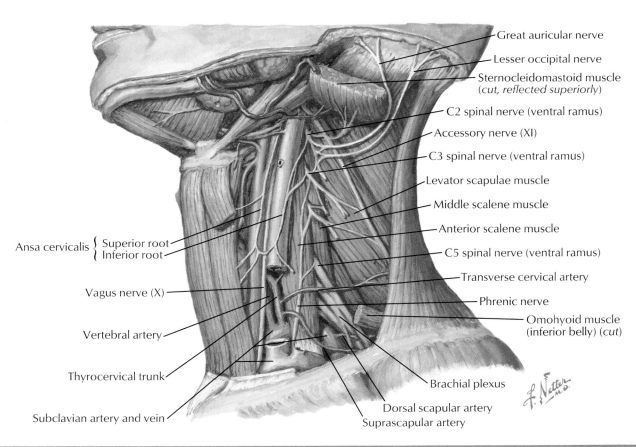

Great auricular nerve

Lesser occipital nerve

Sternocleidomastoid muscle
(cut, reflected superiorly)

C2 spinal nerve (ventral ramus)

Accessory nerve (XI)

C3 spinal nerve (ventral ramus)

Levator scapulae muscle

Middle scalene muscle

Anterior scalene muscle

C5 spinal nerve (ventral ramus)

Transverse cervical artery

Phrenic nerve

Omohyoid muscle
(inferior belly) (cut)

Ansa cervicalis { Superior root
                 { Inferior root

Vagus nerve (X)

Vertebral artery

Thyrocervical trunk

Brachial plexus

Subclavian artery and vein

Dorsal scapular artery

Suprascapular artery

Cervical plexus: schema
(S = gray ramus from superior
cervical sympathetic ganglion)

Hypoglossal nerve (XII)

S

C1

Accessory nerve (XI)

Great auricular nerve

Lesser occipital nerve

To geniohyoid muscle

To thyrohyoid muscle

Communication to vagus nerve

S

C2

To rectus capitis lateralis,
longus capitis, and rectus
capitis anterior muscles

Transverse cervical nerves

To omohyoid muscle (superior belly)

Ansa cervicalis { Superior root
Inferior root

S

C3

S

C4

To longus capitis and
longus colli muscles

To sternothyroid muscle

To sternohyoid muscle

To omohyoid muscle (inferior belly)

Supraclavicular nerves

Phrenic nerve

To scalene and levator
scapulae muscles

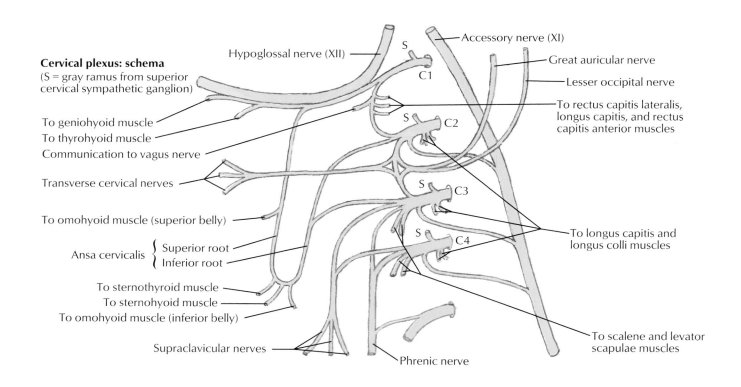

Right anterior dissection

Internal jugular vein

Common carotid artery

Ascending cervical artery

Phrenic nerve

Anterior scalene muscle

Inferior thyroid artery

Transverse cervical artery

Suprascapular artery

Dorsal scapular artery

Costocervical trunk

Thyrocervical trunk

Subclavian artery and vein

Thyroid gland (*retracted*)

Middle cervical sympathetic ganglion

Vagus nerve (X)

Vertebral artery

Common carotid artery

Recurrent laryngeal nerve

Brachiocephalic trunk

Internal jugular vein (*cut*)

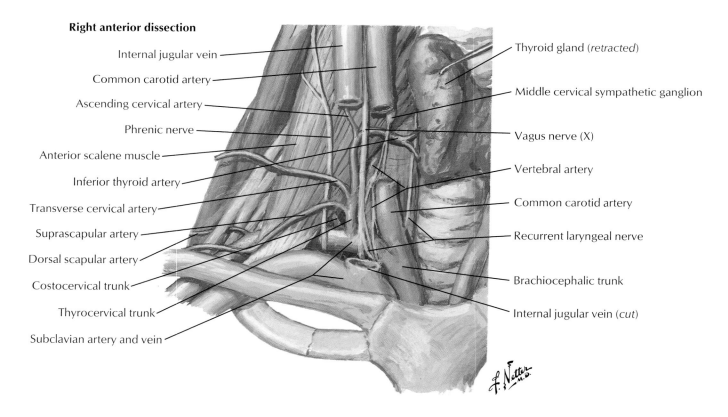

Plate 32

Neck

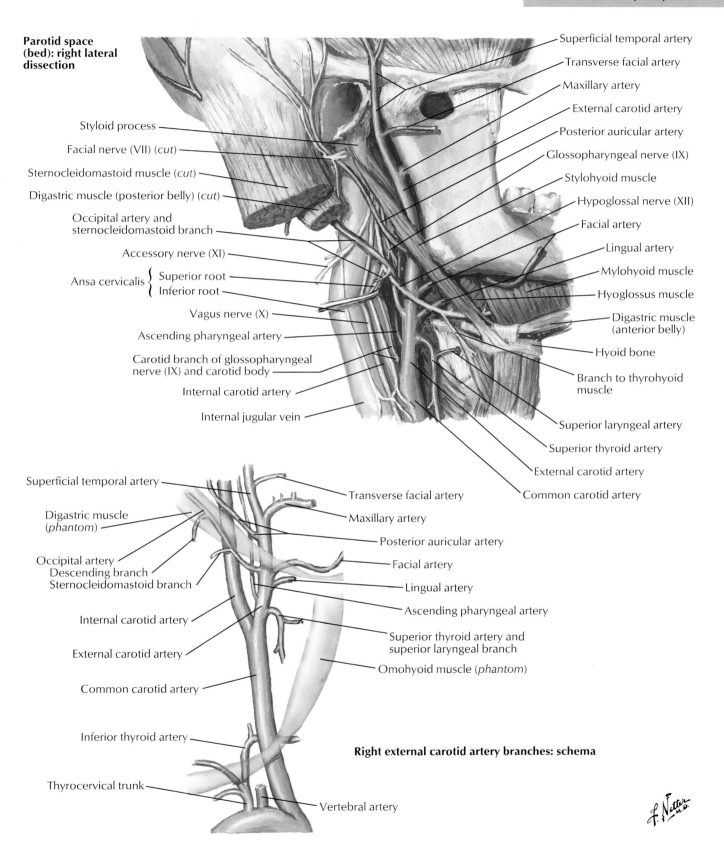

Parotid space (bed): right lateral dissection

Superficial temporal artery

Transverse facial artery

Maxillary artery

External carotid artery

Posterior auricular artery

Glossopharyngeal nerve (IX)

Stylohyoid muscle

Hypoglossal nerve (XII)

Facial artery

Lingual artery

Mylohyoid muscle

Hyoglossus muscle

Digastric muscle (anterior belly)

Hyoid bone

Branch to thyrohyoid muscle

Superior laryngeal artery

Superior thyroid artery

External carotid artery

Common carotid artery

Styloid process

Facial nerve (VII) (cut)

Sternocleidomastoid muscle (cut)

Digastric muscle (posterior belly) (cut)

Occipital artery and sternocleidomastoid branch

Accessory nerve (XI)

Ansa cervicalis { Superior root / Inferior root

Vagus nerve (X)

Ascending pharyngeal artery

Carotid branch of glossopharyngeal nerve (IX) and carotid body

Internal carotid artery

Internal jugular vein

Superficial temporal artery

Transverse facial artery

Maxillary artery

Posterior auricular artery

Facial artery

Lingual artery

Ascending pharyngeal artery

Superior thyroid artery and superior laryngeal branch

Omohyoid muscle (phantom)

Digastric muscle (phantom)

Occipital artery
Descending branch
Sternocleidomastoid branch

Internal carotid artery

External carotid artery

Common carotid artery

Inferior thyroid artery

Thyrocervical trunk

Vertebral artery

Right external carotid artery branches: schema

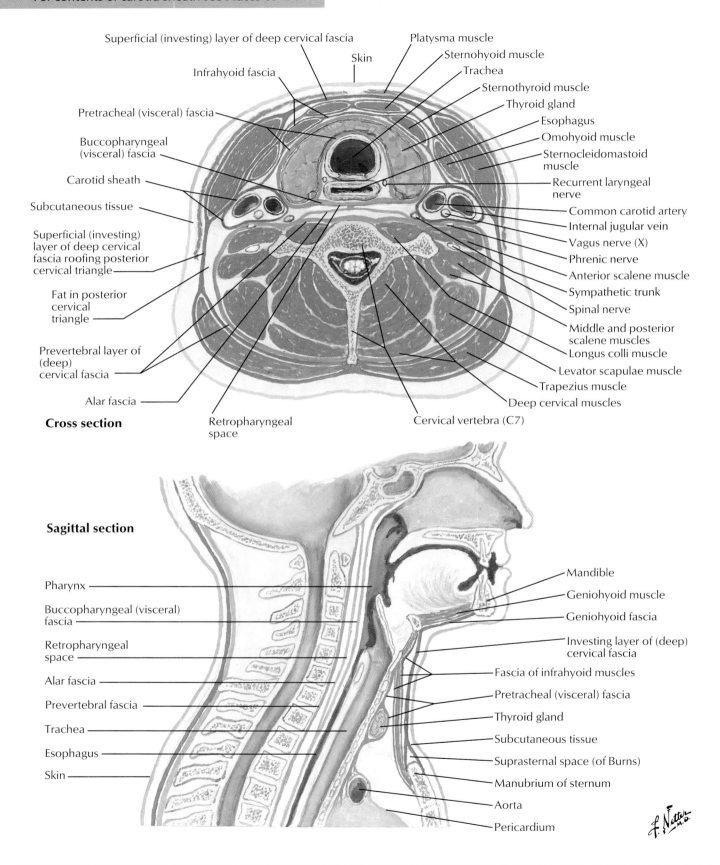

Cross section

Superficial (investing) layer of deep cervical fascia

Infrahyoid fascia

Skin

Pretracheal (visceral) fascia

Buccopharyngeal (visceral) fascia

Carotid sheath

Subcutaneous tissue

Superficial (investing) layer of deep cervical fascia roofing posterior cervical triangle

Fat in posterior cervical triangle

Prevertebral layer of (deep) cervical fascia

Alar fascia

Retropharyngeal space

Platysma muscle

Sternohyoid muscle

Trachea

Sternothyroid muscle

Thyroid gland

Esophagus

Omohyoid muscle

Sternocleidomastoid muscle

Recurrent laryngeal nerve

Common carotid artery

Internal jugular vein

Vagus nerve (X)

Phrenic nerve

Anterior scalene muscle

Sympathetic trunk

Spinal nerve

Middle and posterior scalene muscles

Longus colli muscle

Levator scapulae muscle

Trapezius muscle

Deep cervical muscles

Cervical vertebra (C7)

Sagittal section

Pharynx

Buccopharyngeal (visceral) fascia

Retropharyngeal space

Alar fascia

Prevertebral fascia

Trachea

Esophagus

Skin

Mandible

Geniohyoid muscle

Geniohyoid fascia

Investing layer of (deep) cervical fascia

Fascia of infrahyoid muscles

Pretracheal (visceral) fascia

Thyroid gland

Subcutaneous tissue

Suprasternal space (of Burns)

Manubrium of sternum

Aorta

Pericardium

Plate 34

Neck

Anterolateral view

Frontal bone

Nasal bones

Frontal process of maxilla

Lateral process of
septal nasal cartilages

Septal cartilage

Minor alar cartilage

Accessory nasal cartilage

Major alar cartilage { Lateral crus

Medial crus

Nasal septal cartilage

Anterior nasal spine of maxilla

Alar fibrofatty tissue

Infraorbital foramen

Inferior view

Major alar cartilage

Lateral
crus

Medial
crus

Alar
fibrofatty
tissue

Nasal septal
cartilage

Anterior
nasal spine
of maxilla

Intermaxillary
suture

Superficial temporal artery

Frontalis muscle

Supraorbital artery and nerve

Supratrochlear artery and nerve

Procerus muscle

Corrugator supercilii muscle

Dorsal nasal artery

Infratrochlear nerve

Angular artery

External nasal artery and nerve

Nasalis muscle (transverse part)

Infraorbital artery and nerve

Lateral nasal artery

Transverse facial artery

Nasalis muscle (alar part)

Depressor septi nasi muscle

Orbicularis oris muscle

Facial artery

Superior and inferior labial arteries

Nasal Region

Plate 35

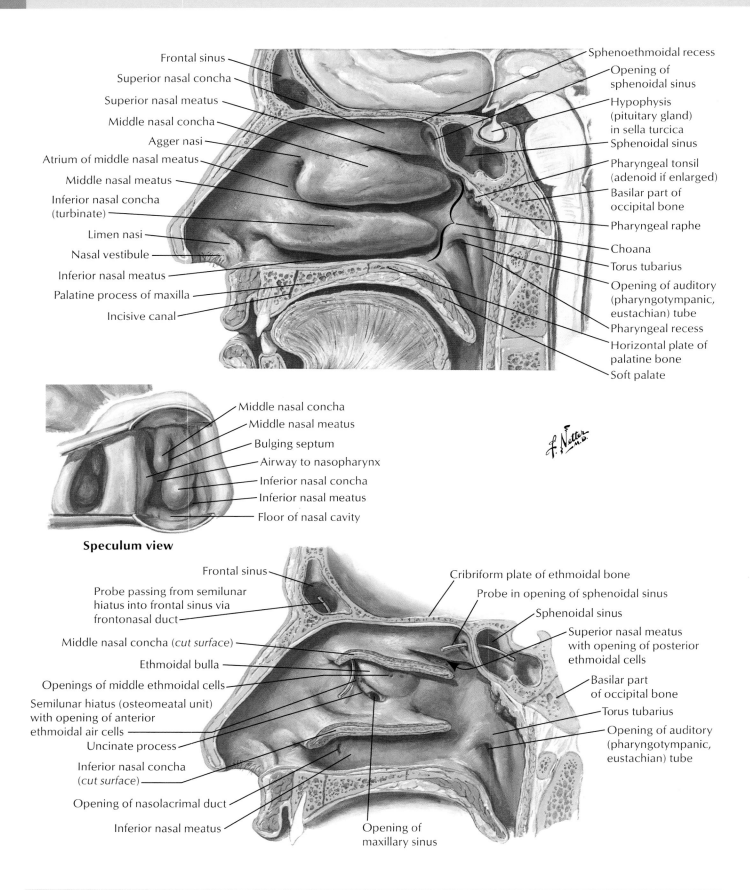

Frontal sinus

Superior nasal concha

Superior nasal meatus

Middle nasal concha

Agger nasi

Atrium of middle nasal meatus

Middle nasal meatus

Inferior nasal concha (turbinate)

Limen nasi

Nasal vestibule

Inferior nasal meatus

Palatine process of maxilla

Incisive canal

Sphenoethmoidal recess

Opening of sphenoidal sinus

Hypophysis (pituitary gland) in sella turcica

Sphenoidal sinus

Pharyngeal tonsil (adenoid if enlarged)

Basilar part of occipital bone

Pharyngeal raphe

Choana

Torus tubarius

Opening of auditory (pharyngotympanic, eustachian) tube

Pharyngeal recess

Horizontal plate of palatine bone

Soft palate

Middle nasal concha

Middle nasal meatus

Bulging septum

Airway to nasopharynx

Inferior nasal concha

Inferior nasal meatus

Floor of nasal cavity

Speculum view

Frontal sinus

Probe passing from semilunar hiatus into frontal sinus via frontonasal duct

Middle nasal concha (*cut surface*)

Ethmoidal bulla

Openings of middle ethmoidal cells

Semilunar hiatus (osteomeatal unit) with opening of anterior ethmoidal air cells

Uncinate process

Inferior nasal concha (*cut surface*)

Opening of nasolacrimal duct

Inferior nasal meatus

Cribriform plate of ethmoidal bone

Probe in opening of sphenoidal sinus

Sphenoidal sinus

Superior nasal meatus with opening of posterior ethmoidal cells

Basilar part of occipital bone

Torus tubarius

Opening of auditory (pharyngotympanic, eustachian) tube

Opening of maxillary sinus

Plate 36

Nasal Region

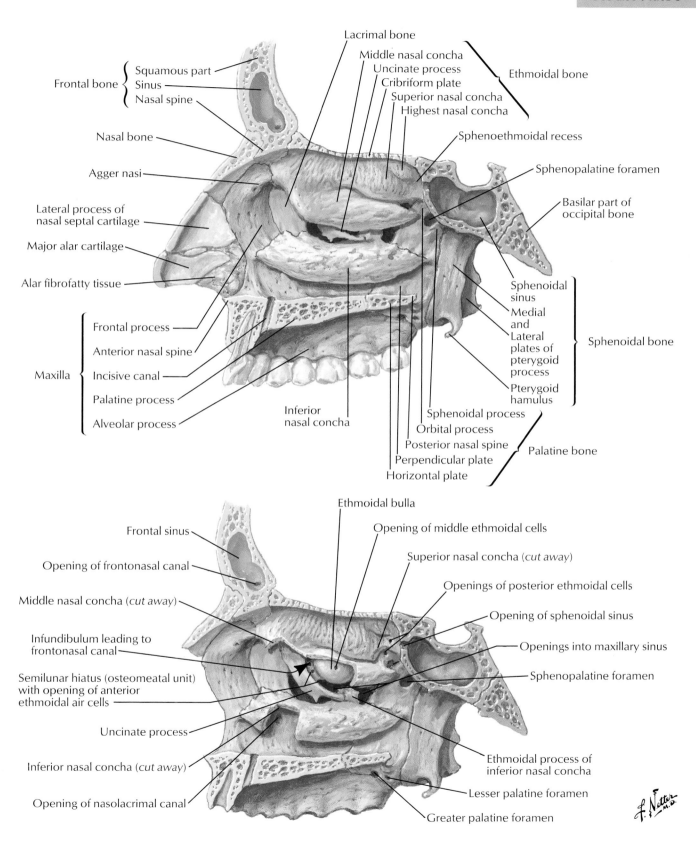

Lacrimal bone

Middle nasal concha

Uncinate process

Cribriform plate

Superior nasal concha

Highest nasal concha

Ethmoidal bone

Frontal bone { Squamous part

Sinus

Nasal spine

Nasal bone

Agger nasi

Lateral process of nasal septal cartilage

Major alar cartilage

Alar fibrofatty tissue

Sphenoethmoidal recess

Sphenopalatine foramen

Basilar part of occipital bone

Sphenoidal sinus

Medial and Lateral plates of pterygoid process

Pterygoid hamulus

Sphenoidal bone

Maxilla {

Frontal process

Anterior nasal spine

Incisive canal

Palatine process

Alveolar process

Inferior nasal concha

Sphenoidal process

Orbital process

Posterior nasal spine

Perpendicular plate

Horizontal plate

Palatine bone

Ethmoidal bulla

Opening of middle ethmoidal cells

Superior nasal concha (*cut away*)

Openings of posterior ethmoidal cells

Opening of sphenoidal sinus

Openings into maxillary sinus

Sphenopalatine foramen

Frontal sinus

Opening of frontonasal canal

Middle nasal concha (*cut away*)

Infundibulum leading to frontonasal canal

Semilunar hiatus (osteomeatal unit) with opening of anterior ethmoidal air cells

Uncinate process

Inferior nasal concha (*cut away*)

Opening of nasolacrimal canal

Ethmoidal process of inferior nasal concha

Lesser palatine foramen

Greater palatine foramen

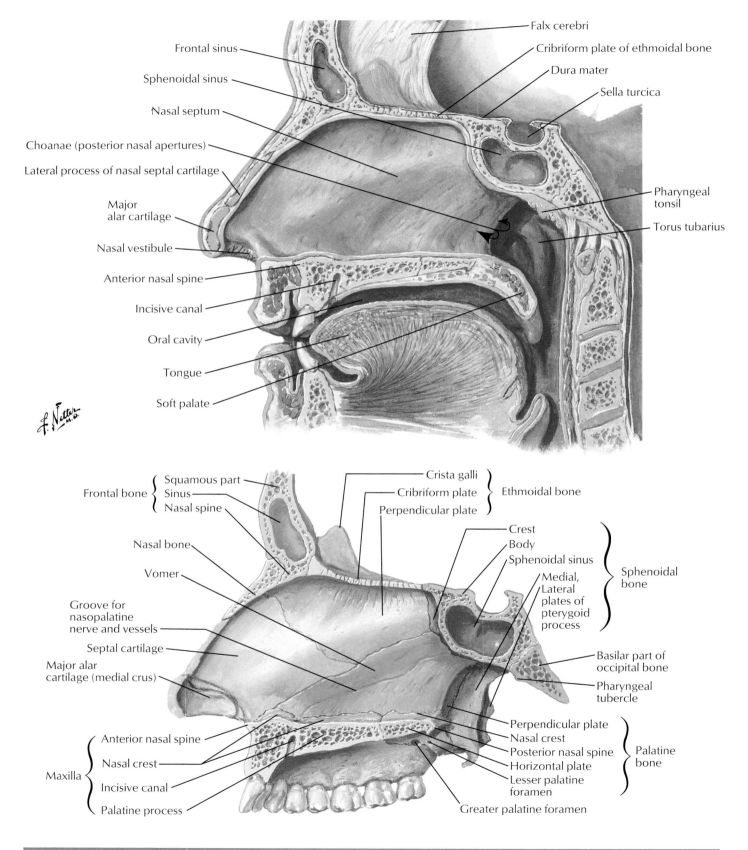

Falx cerebri

Frontal sinus

Cribriform plate of ethmoidal bone

Sphenoidal sinus

Dura mater

Nasal septum

Sella turcica

Choanae (posterior nasal apertures)

Lateral process of nasal septal cartilage

Pharyngeal tonsil

Major alar cartilage

Torus tubarius

Nasal vestibule

Anterior nasal spine

Incisive canal

Oral cavity

Tongue

Soft palate

Squamous part

Crista galli

Frontal bone — Sinus

Cribriform plate — Ethmoidal bone

Nasal spine

Perpendicular plate

Nasal bone

Crest

Body

Vomer

Sphenoidal sinus

Groove for nasopalatine nerve and vessels

Medial, Lateral plates of pterygoid process

Sphenoidal bone

Septal cartilage

Major alar cartilage (medial crus)

Basilar part of occipital bone

Pharyngeal tubercle

Anterior nasal spine

Perpendicular plate

Nasal crest

Nasal crest

Posterior nasal spine

Horizontal plate

Palatine bone

Incisive canal

Lesser palatine foramen

Maxilla

Palatine process

Greater palatine foramen

Plate 38   **Nasal Region**

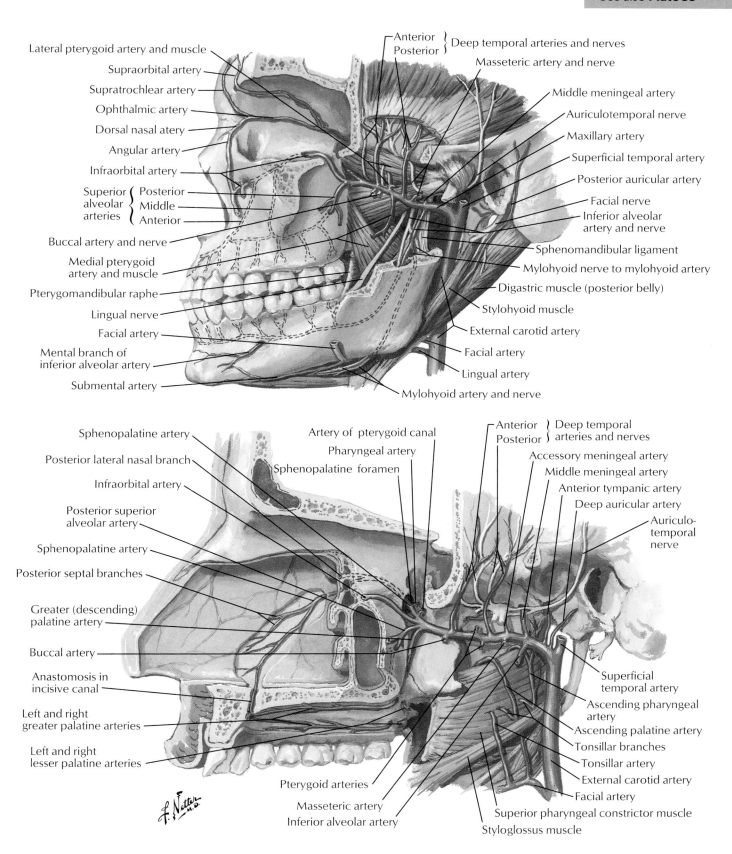

Lateral pterygoid artery and muscle

Supraorbital artery

Supratrochlear artery

Ophthalmic artery

Dorsal nasal atery

Angular artery

Infraorbital artery

Superior { Posterior
alveolar { Middle
arteries { Anterior

Buccal artery and nerve

Medial pterygoid artery and muscle

Pterygomandibular raphe

Lingual nerve

Facial artery

Mental branch of inferior alveolar artery

Submental artery

Anterior } Deep temporal arteries and nerves
Posterior }

Masseteric artery and nerve

Middle meningeal artery

Auriculotemporal nerve

Maxillary artery

Superficial temporal artery

Posterior auricular artery

Facial nerve

Inferior alveolar artery and nerve

Sphenomandibular ligament

Mylohyoid nerve to mylohyoid artery

Digastric muscle (posterior belly)

Stylohyoid muscle

External carotid artery

Facial artery

Lingual artery

Mylohyoid artery and nerve

Sphenopalatine artery

Posterior lateral nasal branch

Infraorbital artery

Posterior superior alveolar artery

Sphenopalatine artery

Posterior septal branches

Greater (descending) palatine artery

Buccal artery

Anastomosis in incisive canal

Left and right greater palatine arteries

Left and right lesser palatine arteries

Artery of pterygoid canal

Pharyngeal artery

Sphenopalatine foramen

Anterior } Deep temporal
Posterior } arteries and nerves

Accessory meningeal artery

Middle meningeal artery

Anterior tympanic artery

Deep auricular artery

Auriculo-temporal nerve

Superficial temporal artery

Ascending pharyngeal artery

Ascending palatine artery

Tonsillar branches

Tonsillar artery

External carotid artery

Facial artery

Pterygoid arteries

Masseteric artery

Inferior alveolar artery

Superior pharyngeal constrictor muscle

Styloglossus muscle

F. Netter M.D.

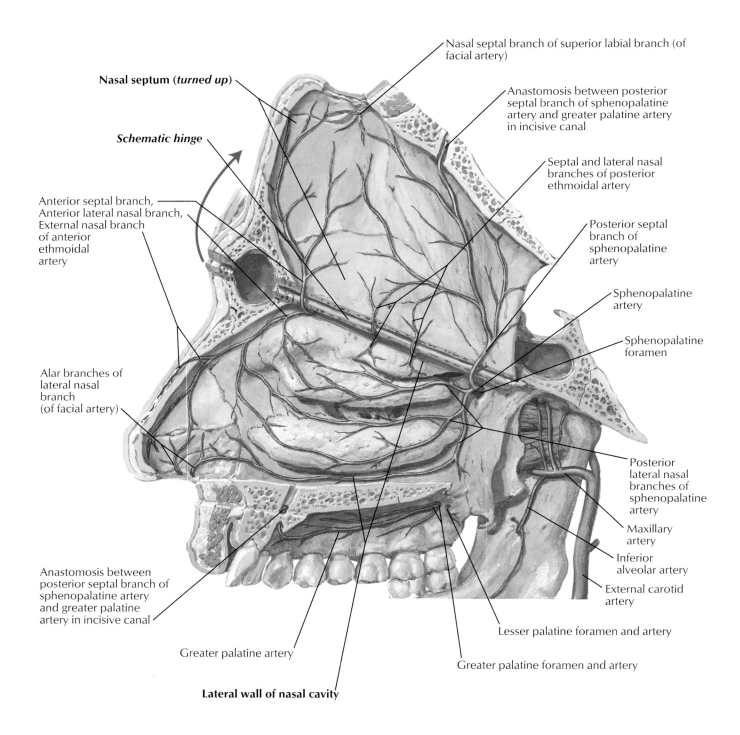

Nasal septal branch of superior labial branch (of facial artery)

Nasal septum (*turned up*)

Anastomosis between posterior septal branch of sphenopalatine artery and greater palatine artery in incisive canal

Schematic hinge

Septal and lateral nasal branches of posterior ethmoidal artery

Anterior septal branch, Anterior lateral nasal branch, External nasal branch of anterior ethmoidal artery

Posterior septal branch of sphenopalatine artery

Sphenopalatine artery

Sphenopalatine foramen

Alar branches of lateral nasal branch (of facial artery)

Posterior lateral nasal branches of sphenopalatine artery

Maxillary artery

Inferior alveolar artery

External carotid artery

Anastomosis between posterior septal branch of sphenopalatine artery and greater palatine artery in incisive canal

Lesser palatine foramen and artery

Greater palatine artery

Greater palatine foramen and artery

Lateral wall of nasal cavity

Plate 40

Nasal Region

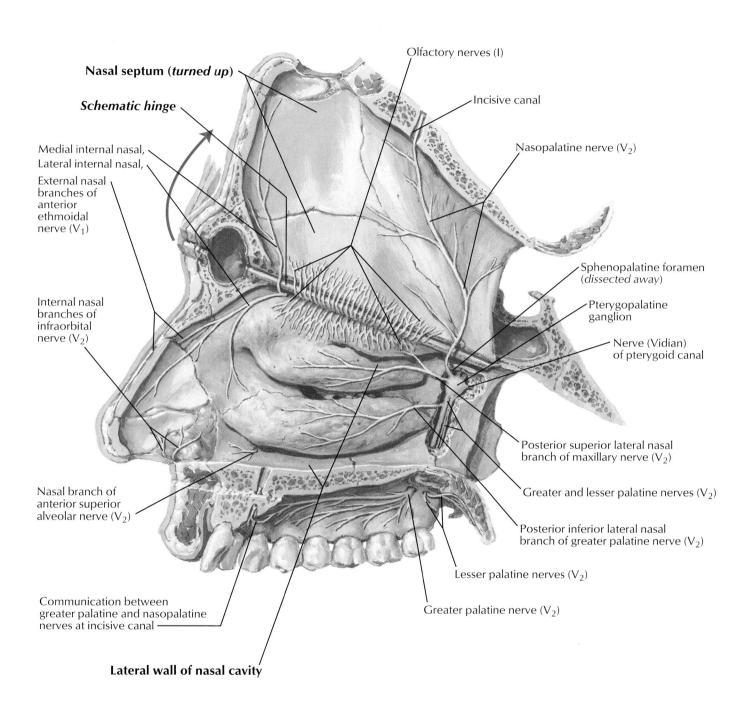

Nasal septum (*turned up*)

Schematic hinge

Medial internal nasal,
Lateral internal nasal,
External nasal
branches of
anterior
ethmoidal
nerve (V₁)

Internal nasal
branches of
infraorbital
nerve (V₂)

Nasal branch of
anterior superior
alveolar nerve (V₂)

Communication between
greater palatine and nasopalatine
nerves at incisive canal

Lateral wall of nasal cavity

Olfactory nerves (I)

Incisive canal

Nasopalatine nerve (V₂)

Sphenopalatine foramen
(*dissected away*)

Pterygopalatine
ganglion

Nerve (Vidian)
of pterygoid canal

Posterior superior lateral nasal
branch of maxillary nerve (V₂)

Greater and lesser palatine nerves (V₂)

Posterior inferior lateral nasal
branch of greater palatine nerve (V₂)

Lesser palatine nerves (V₂)

Greater palatine nerve (V₂)

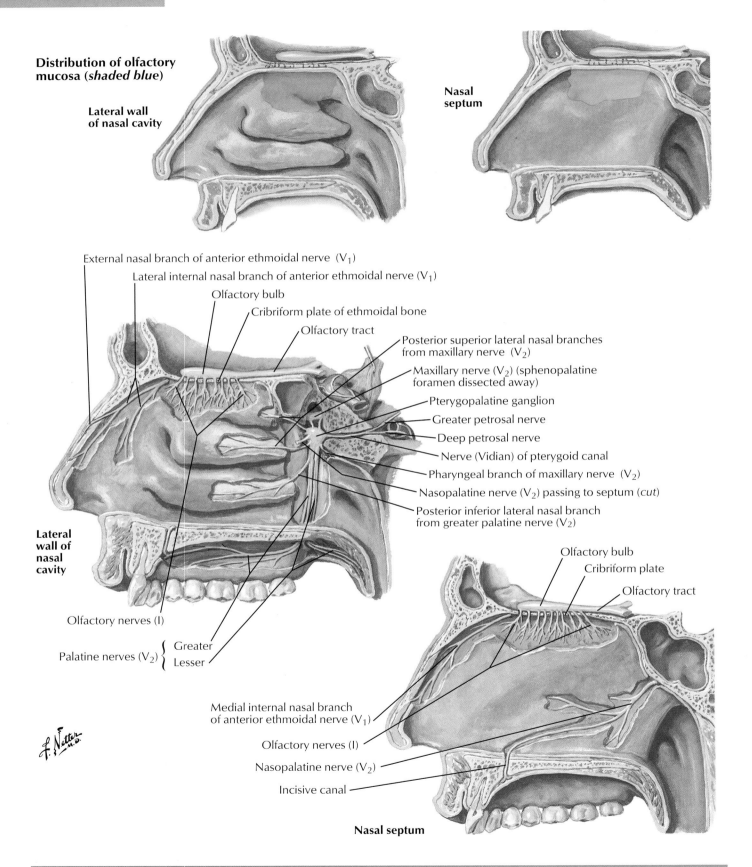

Distribution of olfactory mucosa (*shaded blue*)

Lateral wall of nasal cavity

Nasal septum

External nasal branch of anterior ethmoidal nerve (V$_1$)

Lateral internal nasal branch of anterior ethmoidal nerve (V$_1$)

Olfactory bulb

Cribriform plate of ethmoidal bone

Olfactory tract

Posterior superior lateral nasal branches from maxillary nerve (V$_2$)

Maxillary nerve (V$_2$) (sphenopalatine foramen dissected away)

Pterygopalatine ganglion

Greater petrosal nerve

Deep petrosal nerve

Nerve (Vidian) of pterygoid canal

Pharyngeal branch of maxillary nerve (V$_2$)

Nasopalatine nerve (V$_2$) passing to septum (*cut*)

Posterior inferior lateral nasal branch from greater palatine nerve (V$_2$)

Lateral wall of nasal cavity

Olfactory nerves (I)

Palatine nerves (V$_2$) { Greater Lesser

Olfactory bulb

Cribriform plate

Olfactory tract

Medial internal nasal branch of anterior ethmoidal nerve (V$_1$)

Olfactory nerves (I)

Nasopalatine nerve (V$_2$)

Incisive canal

Nasal septum

Plate 42

Nasal Region

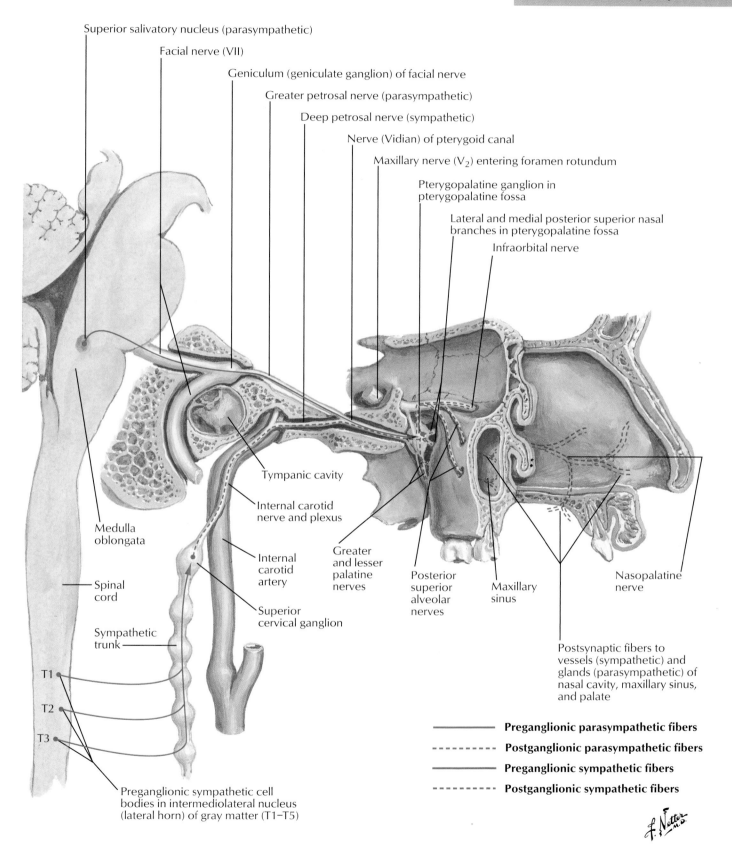

Superior salivatory nucleus (parasympathetic)

Facial nerve (VII)

Geniculum (geniculate ganglion) of facial nerve

Greater petrosal nerve (parasympathetic)

Deep petrosal nerve (sympathetic)

Nerve (Vidian) of pterygoid canal

Maxillary nerve (V$_2$) entering foramen rotundum

Pterygopalatine ganglion in pterygopalatine fossa

Lateral and medial posterior superior nasal branches in pterygopalatine fossa

Infraorbital nerve

Tympanic cavity

Internal carotid nerve and plexus

Medulla oblongata

Internal carotid artery

Greater and lesser palatine nerves

Posterior superior alveolar nerves

Maxillary sinus

Nasopalatine nerve

Spinal cord

Superior cervical ganglion

Sympathetic trunk

T1

T2

T3

Postsynaptic fibers to vessels (sympathetic) and glands (parasympathetic) of nasal cavity, maxillary sinus, and palate

Preganglionic sympathetic cell bodies in intermediolateral nucleus (lateral horn) of gray matter (T1–T5)

———————— **Preganglionic parasympathetic fibers**

- - - - - - - - **Postganglionic parasympathetic fibers**

———————— **Preganglionic sympathetic fibers**

- - - - - - - - **Postganglionic sympathetic fibers**

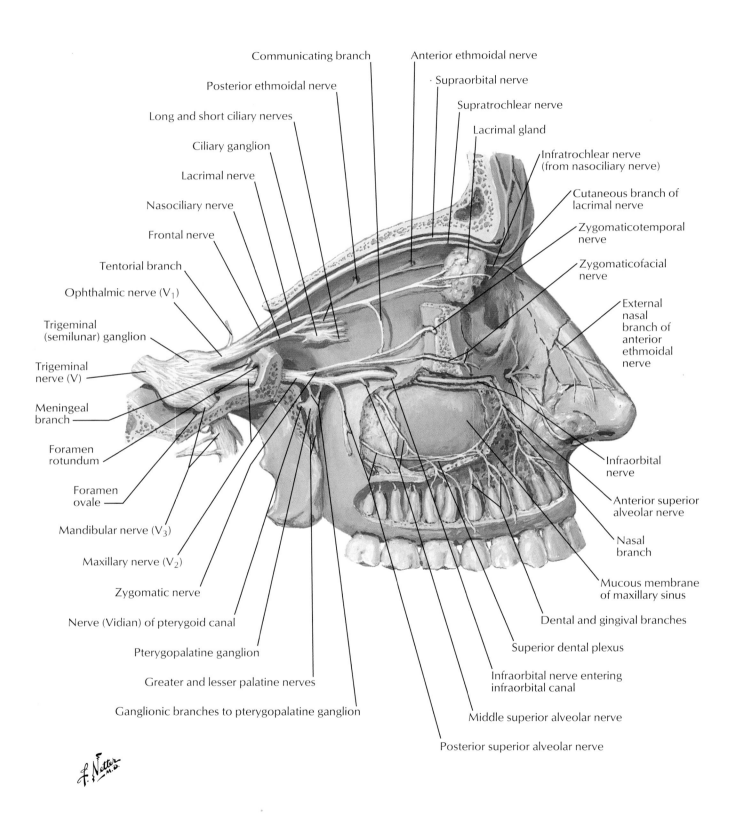

Communicating branch

Anterior ethmoidal nerve

Posterior ethmoidal nerve

Supraorbital nerve

Supratrochlear nerve

Long and short ciliary nerves

Lacrimal gland

Ciliary ganglion

Infratrochlear nerve (from nasociliary nerve)

Lacrimal nerve

Cutaneous branch of lacrimal nerve

Nasociliary nerve

Zygomaticotemporal nerve

Frontal nerve

Zygomaticofacial nerve

Tentorial branch

Ophthalmic nerve (V₁)

External nasal branch of anterior ethmoidal nerve

Trigeminal (semilunar) ganglion

Trigeminal nerve (V)

Meningeal branch

Infraorbital nerve

Foramen rotundum

Anterior superior alveolar nerve

Foramen ovale

Nasal branch

Mandibular nerve (V₃)

Mucous membrane of maxillary sinus

Maxillary nerve (V₂)

Zygomatic nerve

Dental and gingival branches

Nerve (Vidian) of pterygoid canal

Superior dental plexus

Pterygopalatine ganglion

Infraorbital nerve entering infraorbital canal

Greater and lesser palatine nerves

Middle superior alveolar nerve

Ganglionic branches to pterygopalatine ganglion

Posterior superior alveolar nerve

Plate 44

Nasal Region

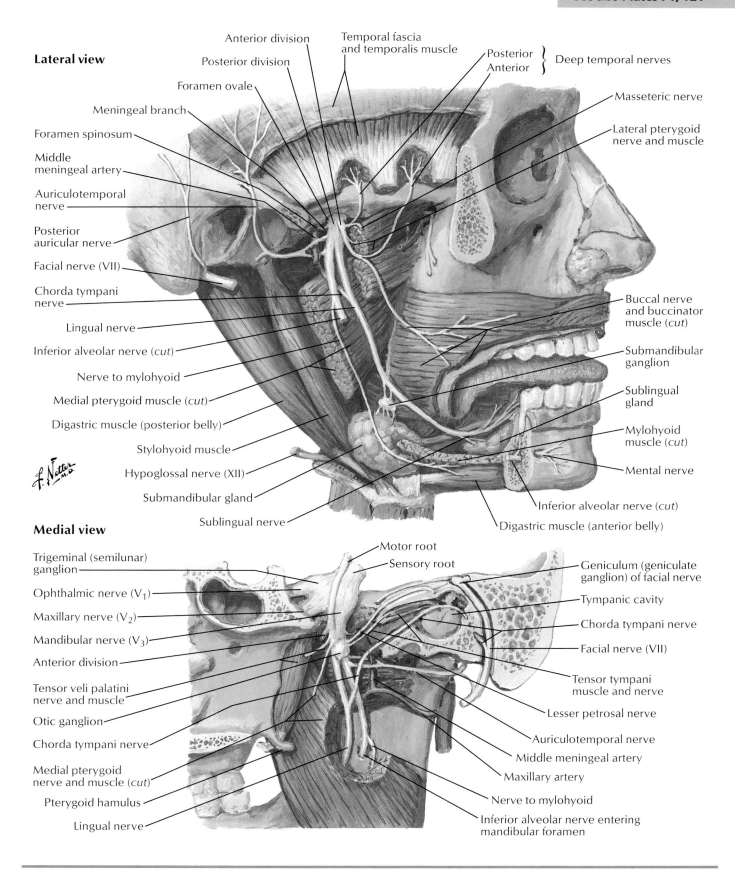

Lateral view

Anterior division
Posterior division
Temporal fascia and temporalis muscle
Foramen ovale
Posterior } Deep temporal nerves
Anterior }
Meningeal branch
Masseteric nerve
Foramen spinosum
Lateral pterygoid nerve and muscle
Middle meningeal artery
Auriculotemporal nerve
Posterior auricular nerve
Facial nerve (VII)
Buccal nerve and buccinator muscle (*cut*)
Chorda tympani nerve
Lingual nerve
Submandibular ganglion
Inferior alveolar nerve (*cut*)
Sublingual gland
Nerve to mylohyoid
Medial pterygoid muscle (*cut*)
Mylohyoid muscle (*cut*)
Digastric muscle (posterior belly)
Stylohyoid muscle
Mental nerve
Hypoglossal nerve (XII)
Inferior alveolar nerve (*cut*)
Submandibular gland
Digastric muscle (anterior belly)
Sublingual nerve

Medial view

Trigeminal (semilunar) ganglion
Motor root
Sensory root
Geniculum (geniculate ganglion) of facial nerve
Ophthalmic nerve (V₁)
Tympanic cavity
Maxillary nerve (V₂)
Chorda tympani nerve
Mandibular nerve (V₃)
Facial nerve (VII)
Anterior division
Tensor veli palatini nerve and muscle
Tensor tympani muscle and nerve
Otic ganglion
Lesser petrosal nerve
Chorda tympani nerve
Auriculotemporal nerve
Middle meningeal artery
Medial pterygoid nerve and muscle (*cut*)
Maxillary artery
Pterygoid hamulus
Nerve to mylohyoid
Lingual nerve
Inferior alveolar nerve entering mandibular foramen

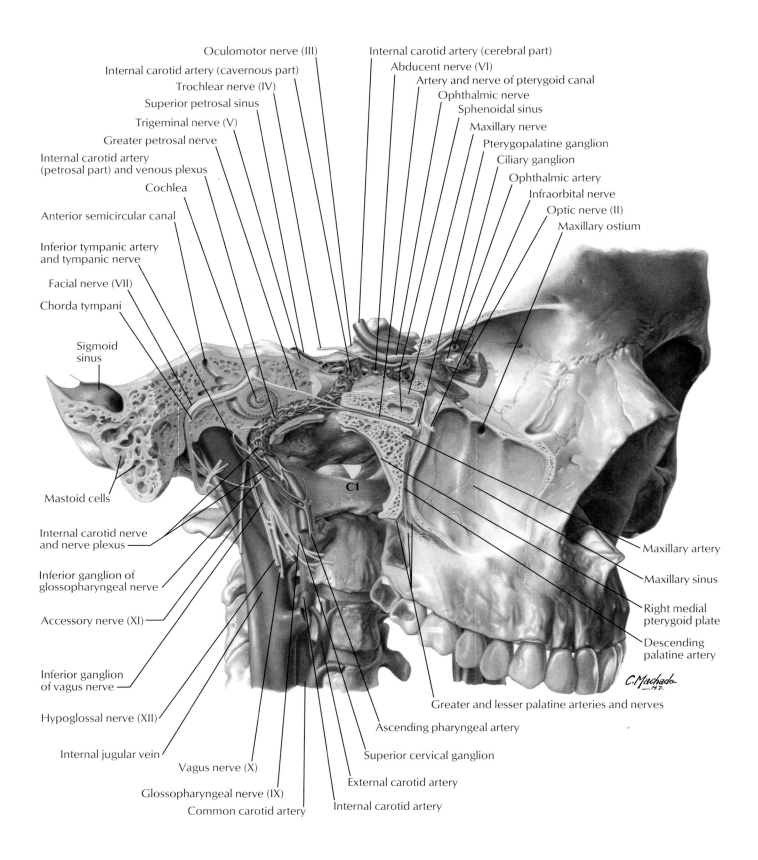

Oculomotor nerve (III)

Internal carotid artery (cavernous part)

Trochlear nerve (IV)

Superior petrosal sinus

Trigeminal nerve (V)

Greater petrosal nerve

Internal carotid artery
(petrosal part) and venous plexus

Cochlea

Anterior semicircular canal

Inferior tympanic artery
and tympanic nerve

Facial nerve (VII)

Chorda tympani

Sigmoid
sinus

Mastoid cells

Internal carotid nerve
and nerve plexus

Inferior ganglion of
glossopharyngeal nerve

Accessory nerve (XI)

Inferior ganglion
of vagus nerve

Hypoglossal nerve (XII)

Internal jugular vein

Vagus nerve (X)

Glossopharyngeal nerve (IX)

Common carotid artery

Internal carotid artery (cerebral part)

Abducent nerve (VI)

Artery and nerve of pterygoid canal

Ophthalmic nerve

Sphenoidal sinus

Maxillary nerve

Pterygopalatine ganglion

Ciliary ganglion

Ophthalmic artery

Infraorbital nerve

Optic nerve (II)

Maxillary ostium

C1

Maxillary artery

Maxillary sinus

Right medial
pterygoid plate

Descending
palatine artery

Greater and lesser palatine arteries and nerves

Ascending pharyngeal artery

Superior cervical ganglion

External carotid artery

Internal carotid artery

C.Machado
_M.D._

Plate 46 **Nasal Region**

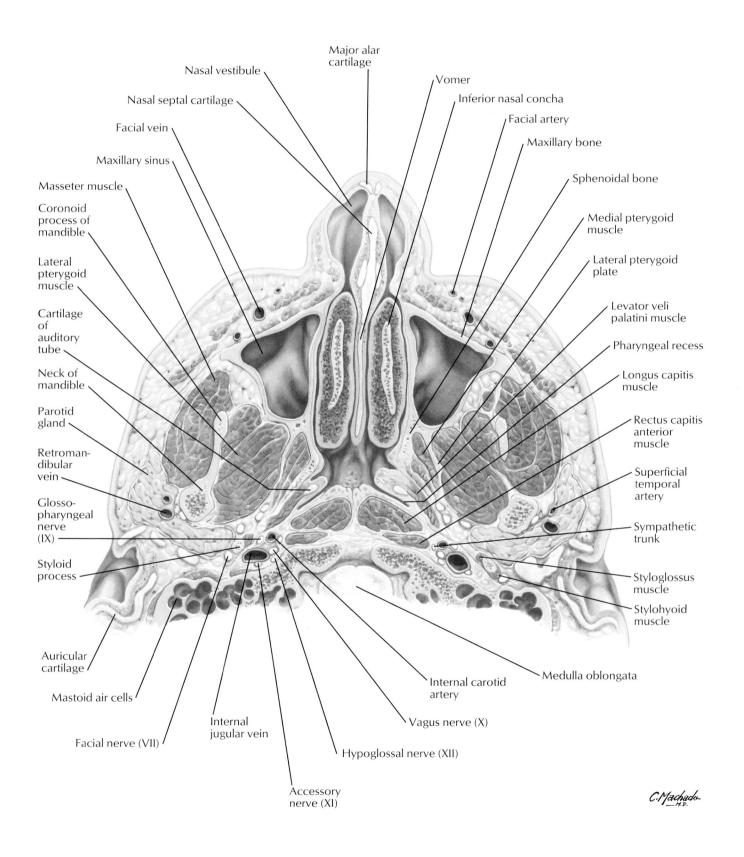

Major alar cartilage

Nasal vestibule

Vomer

Nasal septal cartilage

Inferior nasal concha

Facial vein

Facial artery

Maxillary sinus

Maxillary bone

Masseter muscle

Sphenoidal bone

Coronoid process of mandible

Medial pterygoid muscle

Lateral pterygoid muscle

Lateral pterygoid plate

Cartilage of auditory tube

Levator veli palatini muscle

Pharyngeal recess

Neck of mandible

Longus capitis muscle

Parotid gland

Rectus capitis anterior muscle

Retromandibular vein

Superficial temporal artery

Glossopharyngeal nerve (IX)

Sympathetic trunk

Styloid process

Styloglossus muscle

Stylohyoid muscle

Auricular cartilage

Medulla oblongata

Mastoid air cells

Internal carotid artery

Internal jugular vein

Vagus nerve (X)

Facial nerve (VII)

Hypoglossal nerve (XII)

Accessory nerve (XI)

C. Machado M.D.

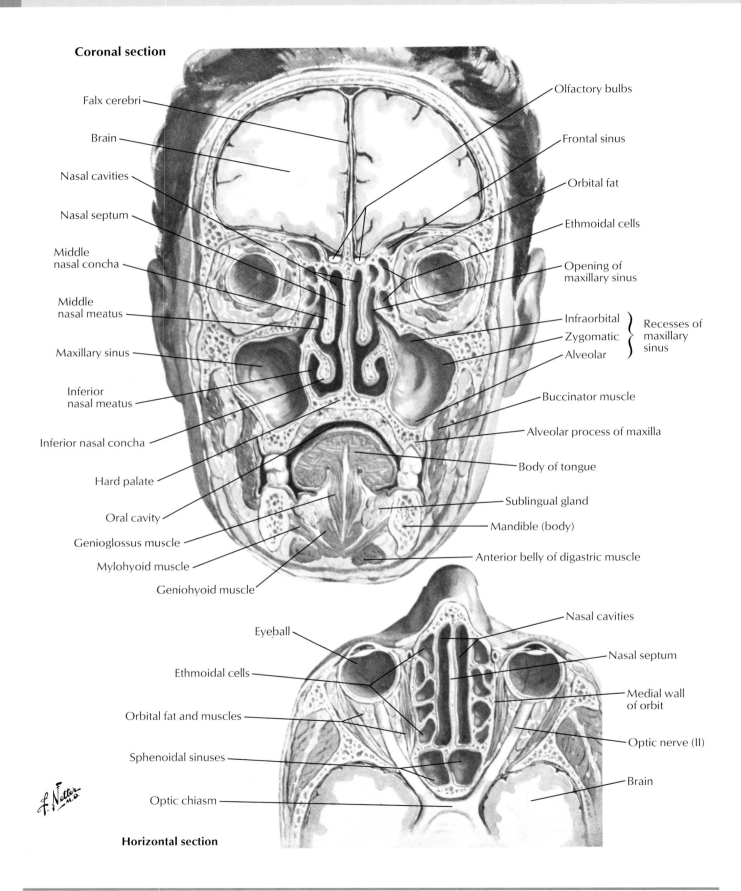

Coronal section

Falx cerebri

Brain

Nasal cavities

Nasal septum

Middle nasal concha

Middle nasal meatus

Maxillary sinus

Inferior nasal meatus

Inferior nasal concha

Hard palate

Oral cavity

Genioglossus muscle

Mylohyoid muscle

Geniohyoid muscle

Olfactory bulbs

Frontal sinus

Orbital fat

Ethmoidal cells

Opening of maxillary sinus

Infraorbital ⎫
Zygomatic ⎬ Recesses of maxillary sinus
Alveolar ⎭

Buccinator muscle

Alveolar process of maxilla

Body of tongue

Sublingual gland

Mandible (body)

Anterior belly of digastric muscle

Eyeball

Ethmoidal cells

Orbital fat and muscles

Sphenoidal sinuses

Optic chiasm

Nasal cavities

Nasal septum

Medial wall of orbit

Optic nerve (II)

Brain

Horizontal section

Plate 48

Nasal Region

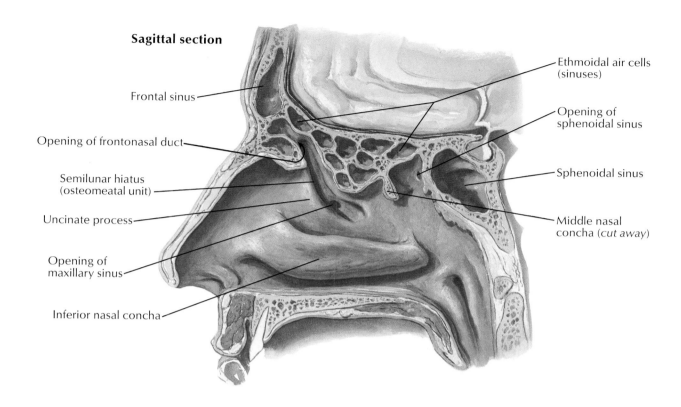

Sagittal section

Frontal sinus

Opening of frontonasal duct

Semilunar hiatus (osteomeatal unit)

Uncinate process

Opening of maxillary sinus

Inferior nasal concha

Ethmoidal air cells (sinuses)

Opening of sphenoidal sinus

Sphenoidal sinus

Middle nasal concha (*cut away*)

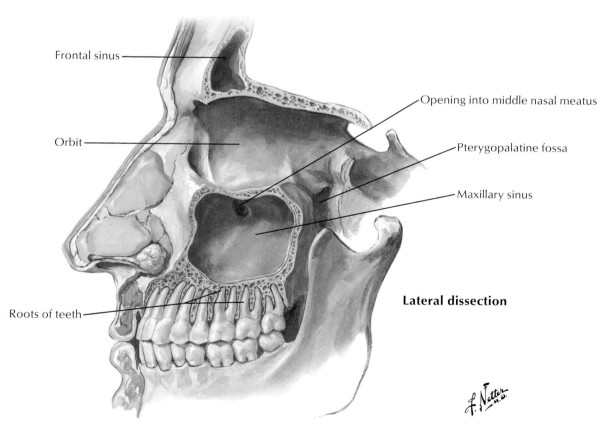

Frontal sinus

Orbit

Roots of teeth

Opening into middle nasal meatus

Pterygopalatine fossa

Maxillary sinus

Lateral dissection

F. Netter M.D.

Nasal Region

Bones of nasal cavity and paranasal sinuses at birth

Part of nasolacrimal duct that formed in depths of nasooptic furrow

Nasal bone

Lacrimal bone

Nasolacrimal foramen (becomes bony canal)

Part of nasolacrimal duct within nasal cavity with slit-like opening in inferior nasal meatus

Maxilla

Uncinate process of ethmoidal bone

Semilunar hiatus

Sinus represents one or more anterior ethmoidal cells opening into semilunar hiatus of middle nasal meatus

Sinus represents one or more middle ethmoidal cells opening into middle nasal meatus

Sinuses represent two or more posterior ethmoidal cells opening into superior nasal meatus

Sphenoidal sinus within bony shell (sphenoidal concha) located anterior and lateral to body of sphenoidal bone (broken line indicates sinus lateral to sphenoid body)

Body of sphenoidal bone

Hypophyseal fossa

Vestigial remnant of Rathke's pouch

Medial plate of pterygoid process

Lower border of highest nasal concha

Lower border of superior nasal concha

Superior nasal meatus

Middle nasal concha (*cut edge*) (inferior nasal concha completely removed)

Palatine bone

Pterygoid hamulus

Maxillary sinus with opening into semilunar hiatus (striped area represents membrane forming most of medial wall of sinus)

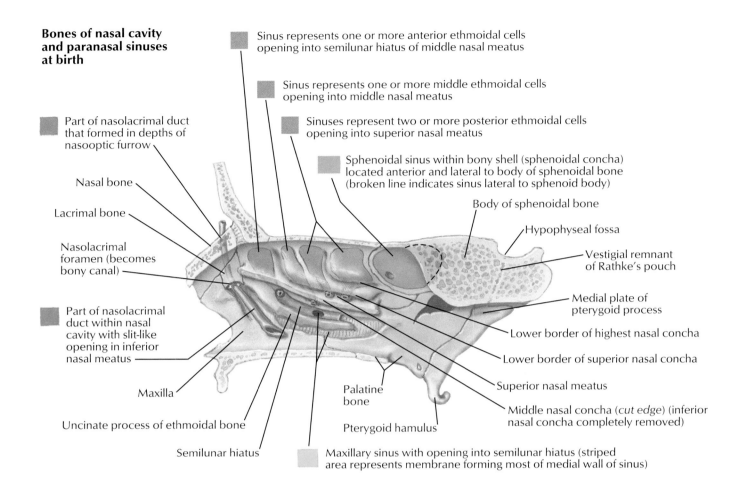

Growth of frontal and maxillary sinuses throughout life

Birth

1 year

4 years

7 years

12 years

Adult

Old age

Frontal sinus within frontal bone

Middle nasal concha

Nasal septum

Nasal cavity

Inferior nasal concha

Palate

Left orbit

Maxillary sinus within maxilla

Molar tooth

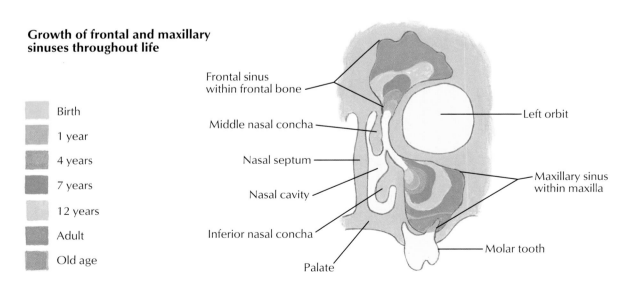

Plate 50   **Nasal Region**

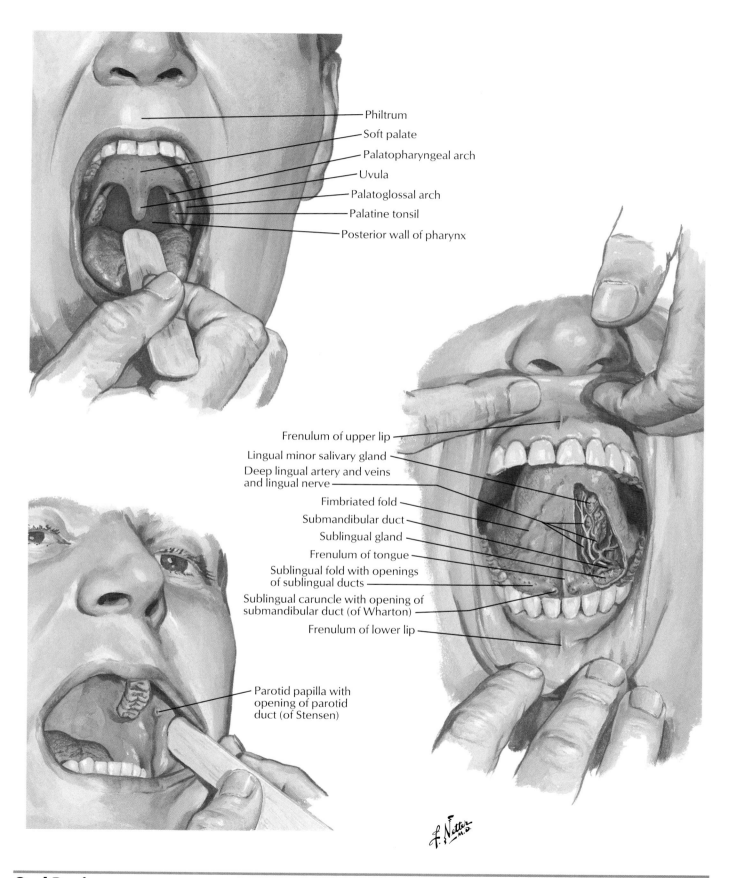

Philtrum

Soft palate

Palatopharyngeal arch

Uvula

Palatoglossal arch

Palatine tonsil

Posterior wall of pharynx

Frenulum of upper lip

Lingual minor salivary gland

Deep lingual artery and veins and lingual nerve

Fimbriated fold

Submandibular duct

Sublingual gland

Frenulum of tongue

Sublingual fold with openings of sublingual ducts

Sublingual caruncle with opening of submandibular duct (of Wharton)

Frenulum of lower lip

Parotid papilla with opening of parotid duct (of Stensen)

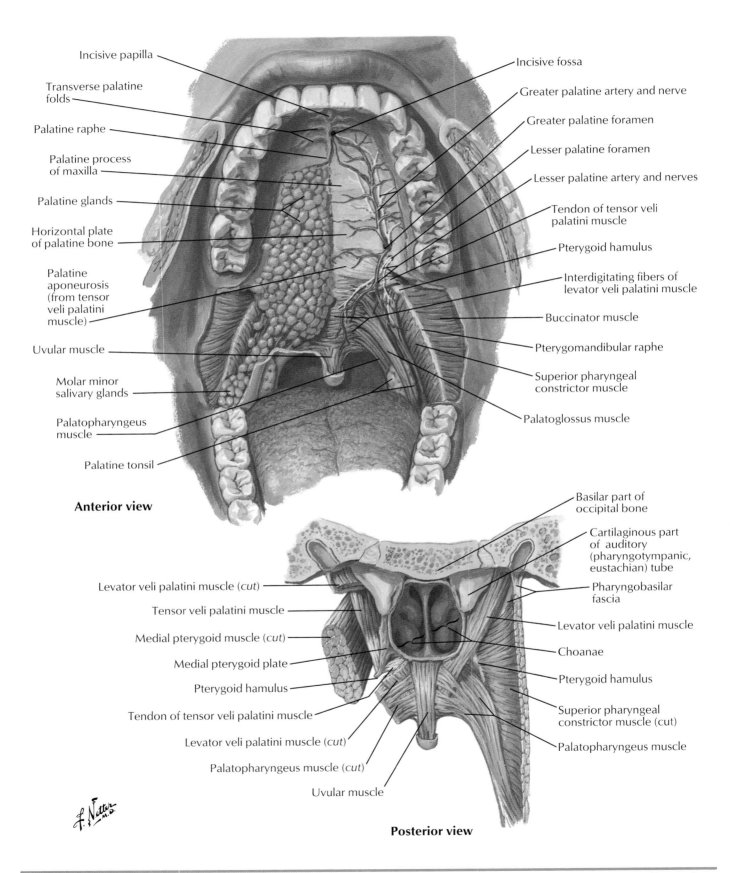

Incisive papilla

Transverse palatine folds

Palatine raphe

Palatine process of maxilla

Palatine glands

Horizontal plate of palatine bone

Palatine aponeurosis (from tensor veli palatini muscle)

Uvular muscle

Molar minor salivary glands

Palatopharyngeus muscle

Palatine tonsil

Incisive fossa

Greater palatine artery and nerve

Greater palatine foramen

Lesser palatine foramen

Lesser palatine artery and nerves

Tendon of tensor veli palatini muscle

Pterygoid hamulus

Interdigitating fibers of levator veli palatini muscle

Buccinator muscle

Pterygomandibular raphe

Superior pharyngeal constrictor muscle

Palatoglossus muscle

Anterior view

Levator veli palatini muscle (*cut*)

Tensor veli palatini muscle

Medial pterygoid muscle (*cut*)

Medial pterygoid plate

Pterygoid hamulus

Tendon of tensor veli palatini muscle

Levator veli palatini muscle (*cut*)

Palatopharyngeus muscle (*cut*)

Uvular muscle

Basilar part of occipital bone

Cartilaginous part of auditory (pharyngotympanic, eustachian) tube

Pharyngobasilar fascia

Levator veli palatini muscle

Choanae

Pterygoid hamulus

Superior pharyngeal constrictor muscle (cut)

Palatopharyngeus muscle

Posterior view

Plate 52   **Oral Region**

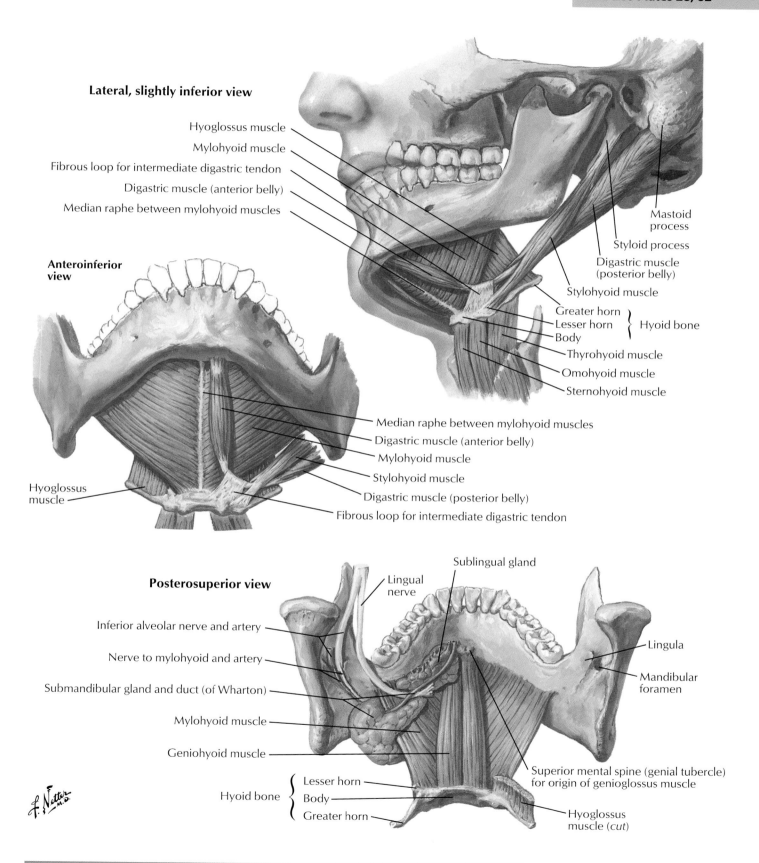

Lateral, slightly inferior view

Hyoglossus muscle
Mylohyoid muscle
Fibrous loop for intermediate digastric tendon
Digastric muscle (anterior belly)
Median raphe between mylohyoid muscles

Mastoid process
Styloid process
Digastric muscle (posterior belly)
Stylohyoid muscle
Greater horn
Lesser horn } Hyoid bone
Body
Thyrohyoid muscle
Omohyoid muscle
Sternohyoid muscle

Anteroinferior view

Median raphe between mylohyoid muscles
Digastric muscle (anterior belly)
Mylohyoid muscle
Stylohyoid muscle
Digastric muscle (posterior belly)
Fibrous loop for intermediate digastric tendon

Hyoglossus muscle

Posterosuperior view

Lingual nerve
Sublingual gland

Inferior alveolar nerve and artery
Nerve to mylohyoid and artery
Submandibular gland and duct (of Wharton)
Mylohyoid muscle
Geniohyoid muscle

Lingula
Mandibular foramen

Lesser horn
Hyoid bone { Body
Greater horn

Superior mental spine (genial tubercle) for origin of genioglossus muscle
Hyoglossus muscle (cut)

For facial muscles see **Plate 25**

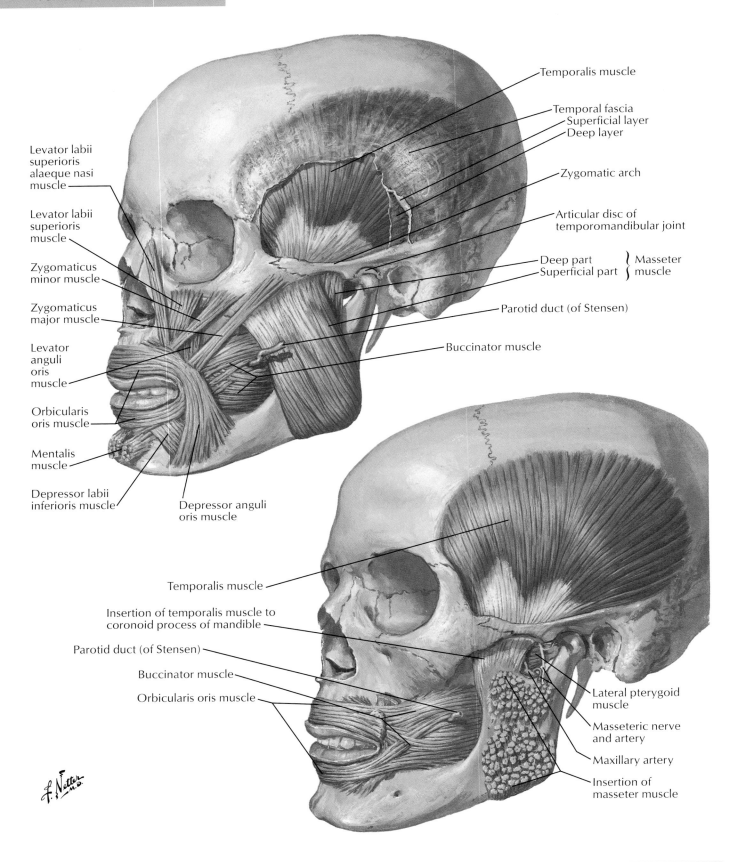

Temporalis muscle

Temporal fascia
Superficial layer
Deep layer

Zygomatic arch

Articular disc of
temporomandibular joint

Deep part } Masseter
Superficial part } muscle

Parotid duct (of Stensen)

Buccinator muscle

Levator labii
superioris
alaeque nasi
muscle

Levator labii
superioris
muscle

Zygomaticus
minor muscle

Zygomaticus
major muscle

Levator
anguli
oris
muscle

Orbicularis
oris muscle

Mentalis
muscle

Depressor labii
inferioris muscle

Depressor anguli
oris muscle

Temporalis muscle

Insertion of temporalis muscle to
coronoid process of mandible

Parotid duct (of Stensen)

Buccinator muscle

Orbicularis oris muscle

Lateral pterygoid
muscle

Masseteric nerve
and artery

Maxillary artery

Insertion of
masseter muscle

F. Netter
M.D.

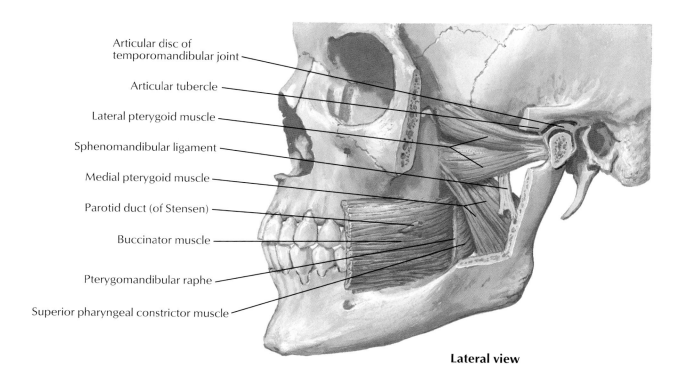

Articular disc of temporomandibular joint

Articular tubercle

Lateral pterygoid muscle

Sphenomandibular ligament

Medial pterygoid muscle

Parotid duct (of Stensen)

Buccinator muscle

Pterygomandibular raphe

Superior pharyngeal constrictor muscle

Lateral view

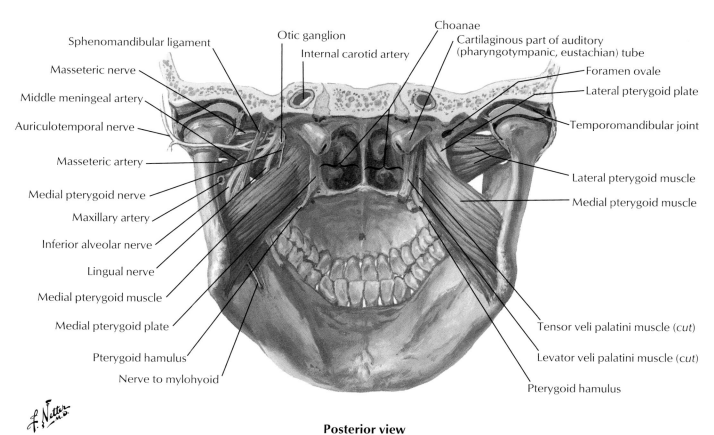

Sphenomandibular ligament

Masseteric nerve

Middle meningeal artery

Auriculotemporal nerve

Masseteric artery

Medial pterygoid nerve

Maxillary artery

Inferior alveolar nerve

Lingual nerve

Medial pterygoid muscle

Medial pterygoid plate

Pterygoid hamulus

Nerve to mylohyoid

Otic ganglion

Internal carotid artery

Choanae

Cartilaginous part of auditory (pharyngotympanic, eustachian) tube

Foramen ovale

Lateral pterygoid plate

Temporomandibular joint

Lateral pterygoid muscle

Medial pterygoid muscle

Tensor veli palatini muscle (cut)

Levator veli palatini muscle (cut)

Pterygoid hamulus

Posterior view

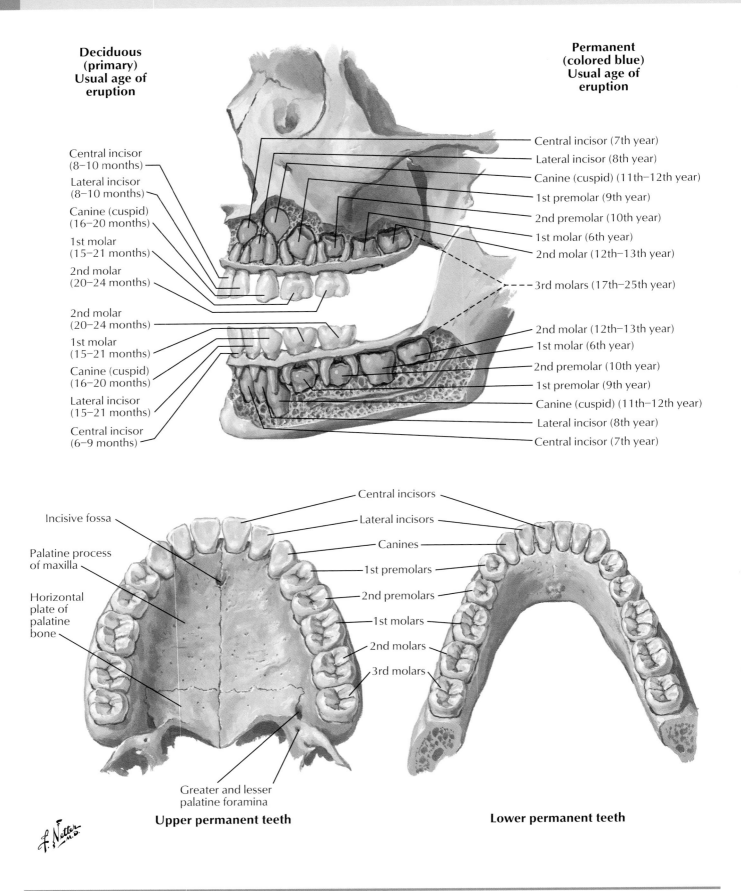

Deciduous (primary) Usual age of eruption

Central incisor (8–10 months)
Lateral incisor (8–10 months)
Canine (cuspid) (16–20 months)
1st molar (15–21 months)
2nd molar (20–24 months)

2nd molar (20–24 months)
1st molar (15–21 months)
Canine (cuspid) (16–20 months)
Lateral incisor (15–21 months)
Central incisor (6–9 months)

Permanent (colored blue) Usual age of eruption

Central incisor (7th year)
Lateral incisor (8th year)
Canine (cuspid) (11th–12th year)
1st premolar (9th year)
2nd premolar (10th year)
1st molar (6th year)
2nd molar (12th–13th year)

3rd molars (17th–25th year)

2nd molar (12th–13th year)
1st molar (6th year)
2nd premolar (10th year)
1st premolar (9th year)
Canine (cuspid) (11th–12th year)
Lateral incisor (8th year)
Central incisor (7th year)

Incisive fossa
Palatine process of maxilla
Horizontal plate of palatine bone

Central incisors
Lateral incisors
Canines
1st premolars
2nd premolars
1st molars
2nd molars
3rd molars

Greater and lesser palatine foramina

Upper permanent teeth

Lower permanent teeth

Plate 56

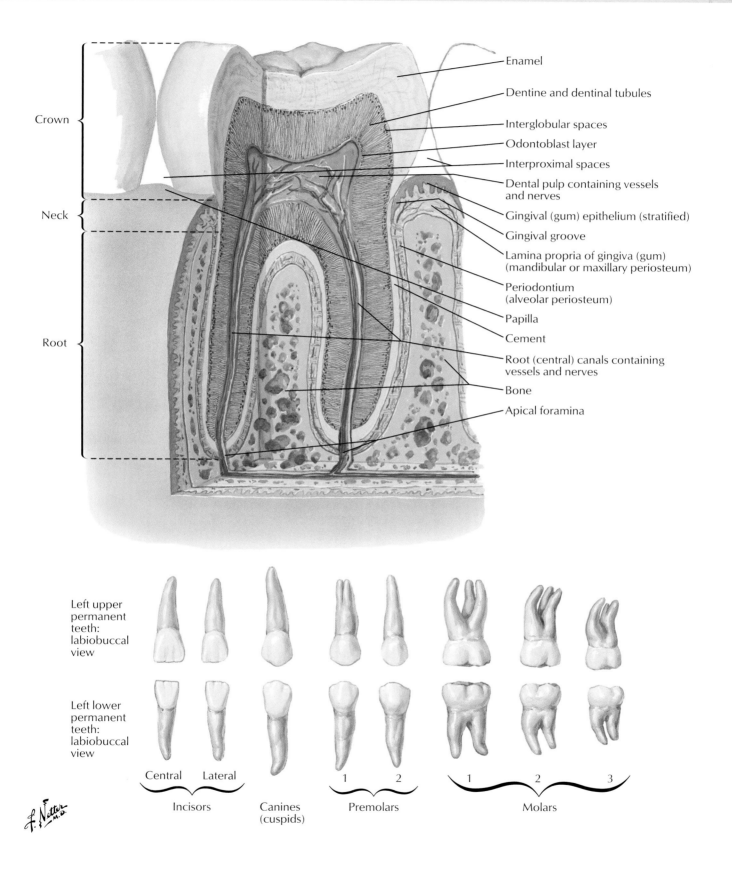

Crown

Neck

Root

Enamel

Dentine and dentinal tubules

Interglobular spaces

Odontoblast layer

Interproximal spaces

Dental pulp containing vessels and nerves

Gingival (gum) epithelium (stratified)

Gingival groove

Lamina propria of gingiva (gum) (mandibular or maxillary periosteum)

Periodontium (alveolar periosteum)

Papilla

Cement

Root (central) canals containing vessels and nerves

Bone

Apical foramina

Left upper permanent teeth: labiobuccal view

Left lower permanent teeth: labiobuccal view

Central   Lateral

Incisors

Canines (cuspids)

1   2

Premolars

1   2   3

Molars

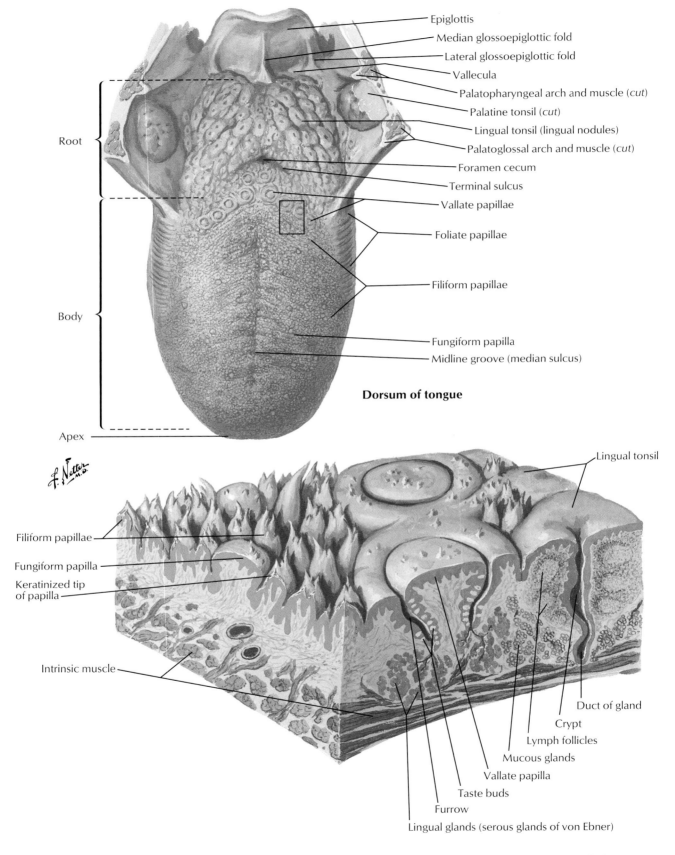

Epiglottis

Median glossoepiglottic fold

Lateral glossoepiglottic fold

Vallecula

Palatopharyngeal arch and muscle (*cut*)

Palatine tonsil (*cut*)

Lingual tonsil (lingual nodules)

Palatoglossal arch and muscle (*cut*)

Foramen cecum

Terminal sulcus

Vallate papillae

Foliate papillae

Filiform papillae

Fungiform papilla

Midline groove (median sulcus)

Root

Body

Apex

Dorsum of tongue

Lingual tonsil

Filiform papillae

Fungiform papilla

Keratinized tip
of papilla

Intrinsic muscle

Duct of gland

Crypt

Lymph follicles

Mucous glands

Vallate papilla

Taste buds

Furrow

Lingual glands (serous glands of von Ebner)

Schematic stereogram: area indicated above

Plate 58 **Oral Region**

See also **Plates 33, 53, 62, 127**

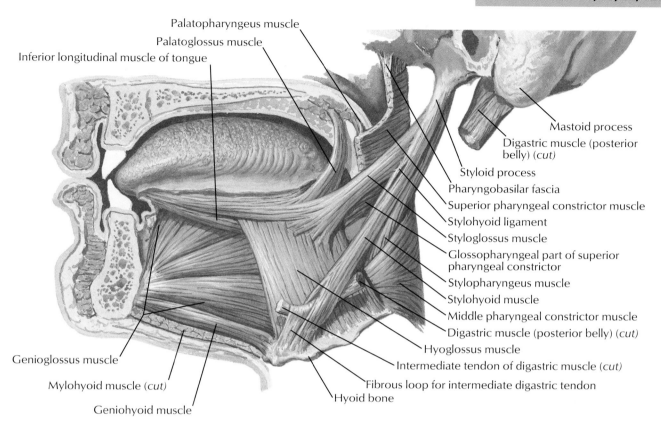

Palatopharyngeus muscle

Palatoglossus muscle

Inferior longitudinal muscle of tongue

Mastoid process

Digastric muscle (posterior belly) (*cut*)

Styloid process

Pharyngobasilar fascia

Superior pharyngeal constrictor muscle

Stylohyoid ligament

Styloglossus muscle

Glossopharyngeal part of superior pharyngeal constrictor

Stylopharyngeus muscle

Stylohyoid muscle

Middle pharyngeal constrictor muscle

Digastric muscle (posterior belly) (*cut*)

Hyoglossus muscle

Intermediate tendon of digastric muscle (*cut*)

Fibrous loop for intermediate digastric tendon

Hyoid bone

Genioglossus muscle

Mylohyoid muscle (*cut*)

Geniohyoid muscle

Lateral view

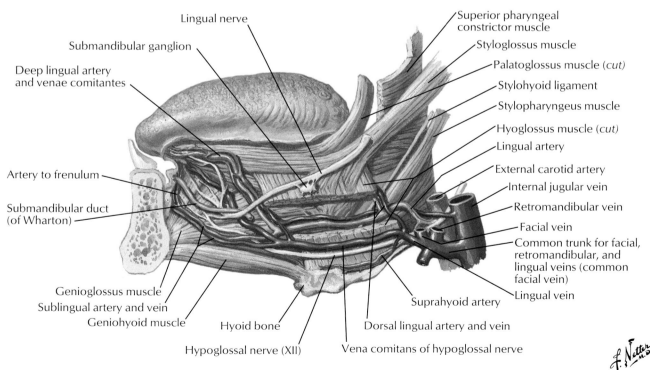

Lingual nerve

Submandibular ganglion

Deep lingual artery and venae comitantes

Artery to frenulum

Submandibular duct (of Wharton)

Superior pharyngeal constrictor muscle

Styloglossus muscle

Palatoglossus muscle (*cut*)

Stylohyoid ligament

Stylopharyngeus muscle

Hyoglossus muscle (*cut*)

Lingual artery

External carotid artery

Internal jugular vein

Retromandibular vein

Facial vein

Common trunk for facial, retromandibular, and lingual veins (common facial vein)

Lingual vein

Genioglossus muscle

Sublingual artery and vein

Geniohyoid muscle

Hyoid bone

Hypoglossal nerve (XII)

Suprahyoid artery

Dorsal lingual artery and vein

Vena comitans of hypoglossal nerve

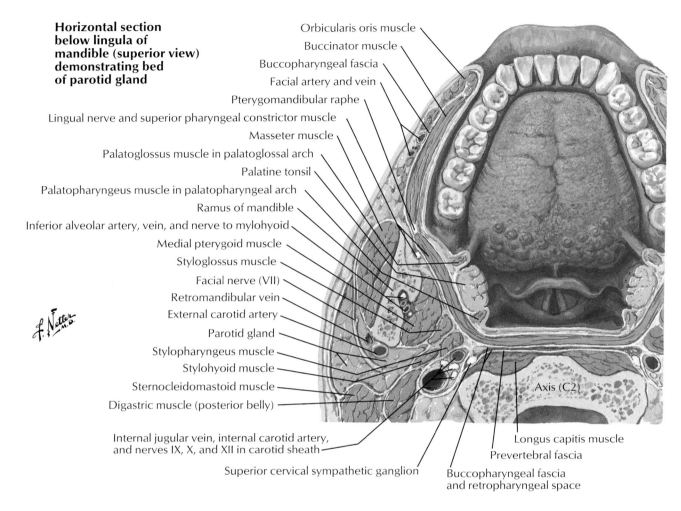

Horizontal section below lingula of mandible (superior view) demonstrating bed of parotid gland

Orbicularis oris muscle

Buccinator muscle

Buccopharyngeal fascia

Facial artery and vein

Pterygomandibular raphe

Lingual nerve and superior pharyngeal constrictor muscle

Masseter muscle

Palatoglossus muscle in palatoglossal arch

Palatine tonsil

Palatopharyngeus muscle in palatopharyngeal arch

Ramus of mandible

Inferior alveolar artery, vein, and nerve to mylohyoid

Medial pterygoid muscle

Styloglossus muscle

Facial nerve (VII)

Retromandibular vein

External carotid artery

Parotid gland

Stylopharyngeus muscle

Stylohyoid muscle

Sternocleidomastoid muscle

Digastric muscle (posterior belly)

Internal jugular vein, internal carotid artery, and nerves IX, X, and XII in carotid sheath

Superior cervical sympathetic ganglion

Axis (C2)

Longus capitis muscle

Prevertebral fascia

Buccopharyngeal fascia and retropharyngeal space

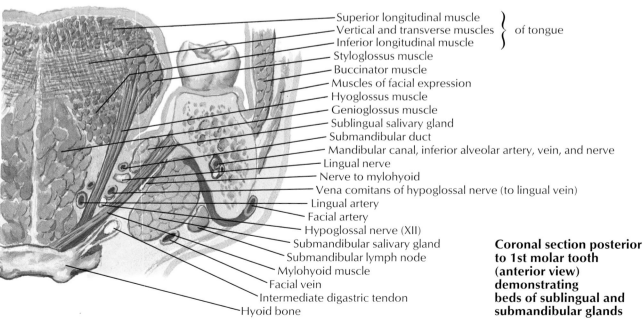

Superior longitudinal muscle ⎫
Vertical and transverse muscles ⎬ of tongue
Inferior longitudinal muscle ⎭

Styloglossus muscle

Buccinator muscle

Muscles of facial expression

Hyoglossus muscle

Genioglossus muscle

Sublingual salivary gland

Submandibular duct

Mandibular canal, inferior alveolar artery, vein, and nerve

Lingual nerve

Nerve to mylohyoid

Vena comitans of hypoglossal nerve (to lingual vein)

Lingual artery

Facial artery

Hypoglossal nerve (XII)

Submandibular salivary gland

Submandibular lymph node

Mylohyoid muscle

Facial vein

Intermediate digastric tendon

Hyoid bone

Coronal section posterior to 1st molar tooth (anterior view) demonstrating beds of sublingual and submandibular glands

Plate 60   **Oral Region**

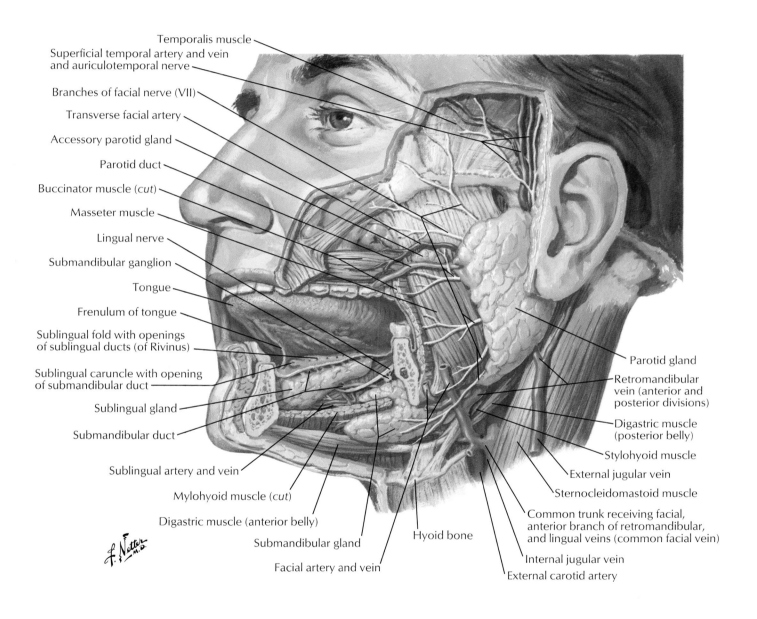

Temporalis muscle

Superficial temporal artery and vein and auriculotemporal nerve

Branches of facial nerve (VII)

Transverse facial artery

Accessory parotid gland

Parotid duct

Buccinator muscle (*cut*)

Masseter muscle

Lingual nerve

Submandibular ganglion

Tongue

Frenulum of tongue

Sublingual fold with openings of sublingual ducts (of Rivinus)

Sublingual caruncle with opening of submandibular duct

Sublingual gland

Submandibular duct

Sublingual artery and vein

Mylohyoid muscle (*cut*)

Digastric muscle (anterior belly)

Submandibular gland

Facial artery and vein

Hyoid bone

Parotid gland

Retromandibular vein (anterior and posterior divisions)

Digastric muscle (posterior belly)

Stylohyoid muscle

External jugular vein

Sternocleidomastoid muscle

Common trunk receiving facial, anterior branch of retromandibular, and lingual veins (common facial vein)

Internal jugular vein

External carotid artery

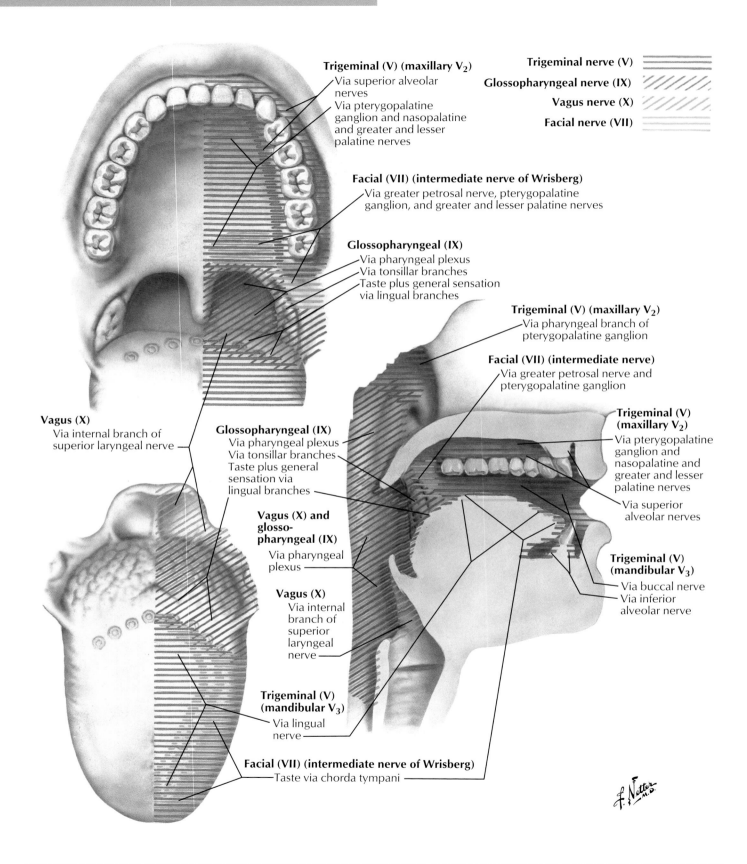

Trigeminal (V) (maxillary V₂)
Via superior alveolar nerves
Via pterygopalatine ganglion and nasopalatine and greater and lesser palatine nerves

Trigeminal nerve (V)
Glossopharyngeal nerve (IX)
Vagus nerve (X)
Facial nerve (VII)

Facial (VII) (intermediate nerve of Wrisberg)
Via greater petrosal nerve, pterygopalatine ganglion, and greater and lesser palatine nerves

Glossopharyngeal (IX)
Via pharyngeal plexus
Via tonsillar branches
Taste plus general sensation via lingual branches

Trigeminal (V) (maxillary V₂)
Via pharyngeal branch of pterygopalatine ganglion

Facial (VII) (intermediate nerve)
Via greater petrosal nerve and pterygopalatine ganglion

Vagus (X)
Via internal branch of superior laryngeal nerve

Glossopharyngeal (IX)
Via pharyngeal plexus
Via tonsillar branches
Taste plus general sensation via lingual branches

Trigeminal (V) (maxillary V₂)
Via pterygopalatine ganglion and nasopalatine and greater and lesser palatine nerves
Via superior alveolar nerves

Vagus (X) and glosso-pharyngeal (IX)
Via pharyngeal plexus

Vagus (X)
Via internal branch of superior laryngeal nerve

Trigeminal (V) (mandibular V₃)
Via buccal nerve
Via inferior alveolar nerve

Trigeminal (V) (mandibular V₃)
Via lingual nerve

Facial (VII) (intermediate nerve of Wrisberg)
Taste via chorda tympani

Plate 62

Oral Region

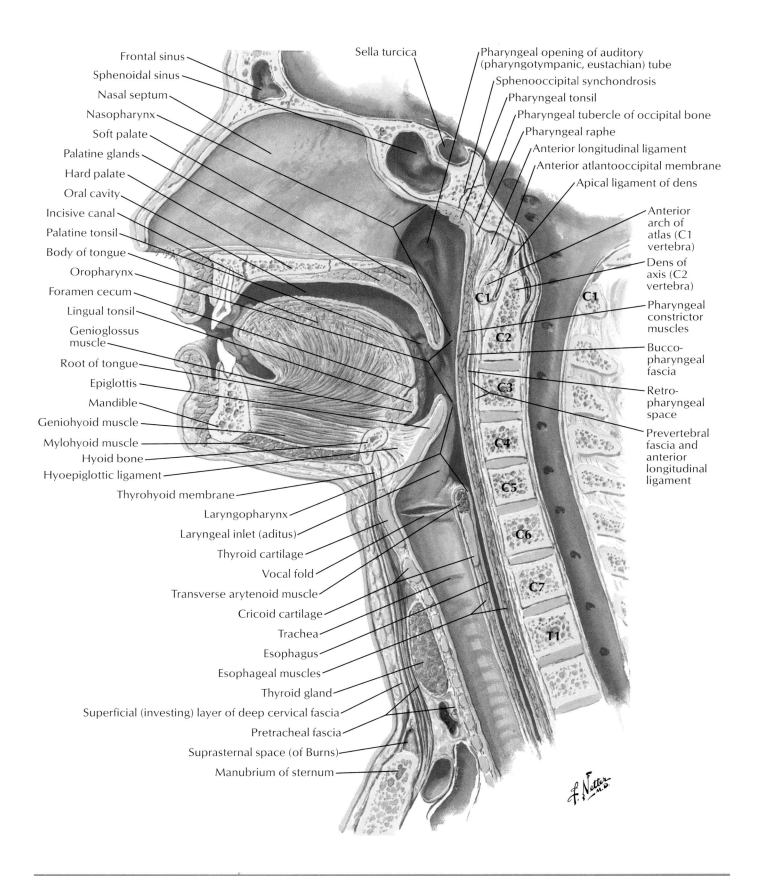

Frontal sinus

Sphenoidal sinus

Nasal septum

Nasopharynx

Soft palate

Palatine glands

Hard palate

Oral cavity

Incisive canal

Palatine tonsil

Body of tongue

Oropharynx

Foramen cecum

Lingual tonsil

Genioglossus muscle

Root of tongue

Epiglottis

Mandible

Geniohyoid muscle

Mylohyoid muscle

Hyoid bone

Hyoepiglottic ligament

Thyrohyoid membrane

Laryngopharynx

Laryngeal inlet (aditus)

Thyroid cartilage

Vocal fold

Transverse arytenoid muscle

Cricoid cartilage

Trachea

Esophagus

Esophageal muscles

Thyroid gland

Superficial (investing) layer of deep cervical fascia

Pretracheal fascia

Suprasternal space (of Burns)

Manubrium of sternum

Sella turcica

Pharyngeal opening of auditory (pharyngotympanic, eustachian) tube

Sphenooccipital synchondrosis

Pharyngeal tonsil

Pharyngeal tubercle of occipital bone

Pharyngeal raphe

Anterior longitudinal ligament

Anterior atlantooccipital membrane

Apical ligament of dens

Anterior arch of atlas (C1 vertebra)

Dens of axis (C2 vertebra)

Pharyngeal constrictor muscles

Buccopharyngeal fascia

Retropharyngeal space

Prevertebral fascia and anterior longitudinal ligament

C1

C2

C3

C4

C5

C6

C7

T1

C1

**Medial view
sagittal section**

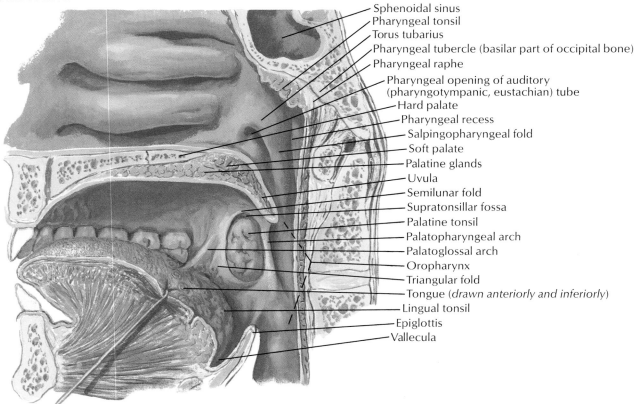

Sphenoidal sinus
Pharyngeal tonsil
Torus tubarius
Pharyngeal tubercle (basilar part of occipital bone)
Pharyngeal raphe
Pharyngeal opening of auditory (pharyngotympanic, eustachian) tube
Hard palate
Pharyngeal recess
Salpingopharyngeal fold
Soft palate
Palatine glands
Uvula
Semilunar fold
Supratonsillar fossa
Palatine tonsil
Palatopharyngeal arch
Palatoglossal arch
Oropharynx
Triangular fold
Tongue (*drawn anteriorly and inferiorly*)
Lingual tonsil
Epiglottis
Vallecula

Pharyngeal mucosa removed

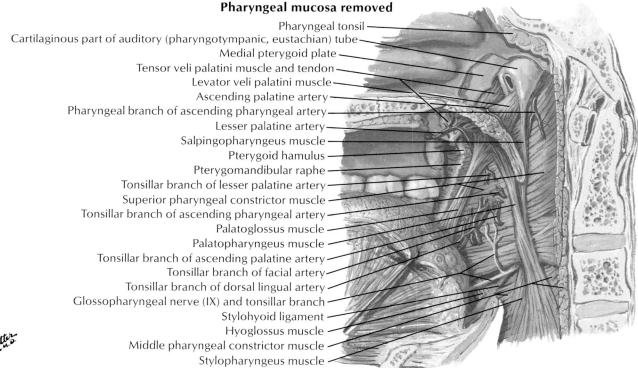

Pharyngeal tonsil
Cartilaginous part of auditory (pharyngotympanic, eustachian) tube
Medial pterygoid plate
Tensor veli palatini muscle and tendon
Levator veli palatini muscle
Ascending palatine artery
Pharyngeal branch of ascending pharyngeal artery
Lesser palatine artery
Salpingopharyngeus muscle
Pterygoid hamulus
Pterygomandibular raphe
Tonsillar branch of lesser palatine artery
Superior pharyngeal constrictor muscle
Tonsillar branch of ascending pharyngeal artery
Palatoglossus muscle
Palatopharyngeus muscle
Tonsillar branch of ascending palatine artery
Tonsillar branch of facial artery
Tonsillar branch of dorsal lingual artery
Glossopharyngeal nerve (IX) and tonsillar branch
Stylohyoid ligament
Hyoglossus muscle
Middle pharyngeal constrictor muscle
Stylopharyngeus muscle

Plate 64   **Pharynx**

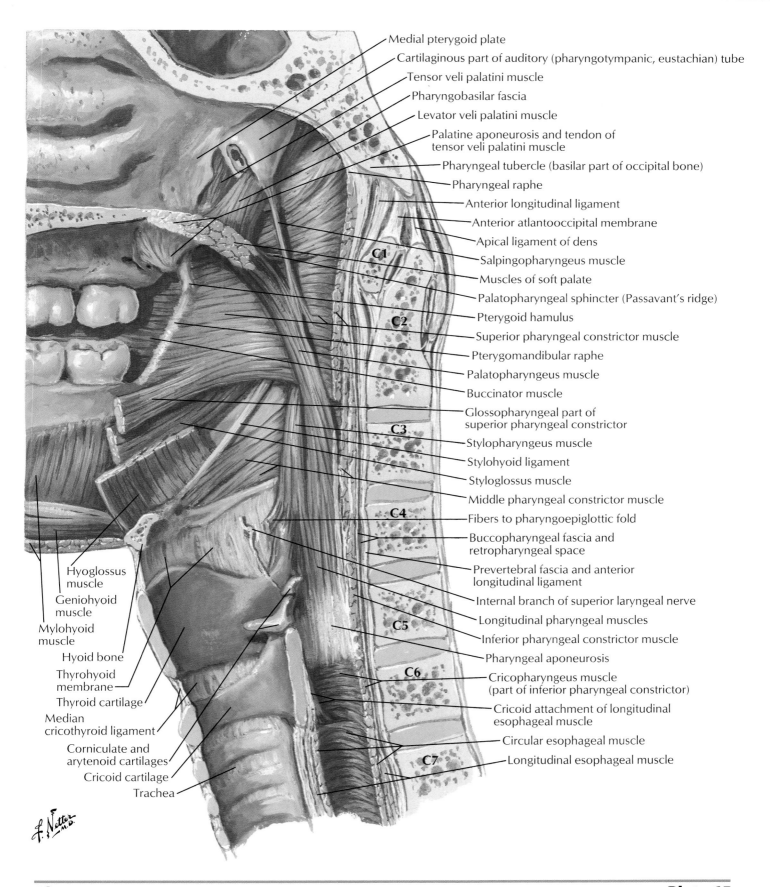

Medial pterygoid plate

Cartilaginous part of auditory (pharyngotympanic, eustachian) tube

Tensor veli palatini muscle

Pharyngobasilar fascia

Levator veli palatini muscle

Palatine aponeurosis and tendon of tensor veli palatini muscle

Pharyngeal tubercle (basilar part of occipital bone)

Pharyngeal raphe

Anterior longitudinal ligament

Anterior atlantooccipital membrane

Apical ligament of dens

Salpingopharyngeus muscle

Muscles of soft palate

Palatopharyngeal sphincter (Passavant's ridge)

Pterygoid hamulus

Superior pharyngeal constrictor muscle

Pterygomandibular raphe

Palatopharyngeus muscle

Buccinator muscle

Glossopharyngeal part of superior pharyngeal constrictor

Stylopharyngeus muscle

Stylohyoid ligament

Styloglossus muscle

Middle pharyngeal constrictor muscle

Fibers to pharyngoepiglottic fold

Buccopharyngeal fascia and retropharyngeal space

Prevertebral fascia and anterior longitudinal ligament

Internal branch of superior laryngeal nerve

Longitudinal pharyngeal muscles

Inferior pharyngeal constrictor muscle

Pharyngeal aponeurosis

Cricopharyngeus muscle (part of inferior pharyngeal constrictor)

Cricoid attachment of longitudinal esophageal muscle

Circular esophageal muscle

Longitudinal esophageal muscle

C1
C2
C3
C4
C5
C6
C7

Hyoglossus muscle

Geniohyoid muscle

Mylohyoid muscle

Hyoid bone

Thyrohyoid membrane

Thyroid cartilage

Median cricothyroid ligament

Corniculate and arytenoid cartilages

Cricoid cartilage

Trachea

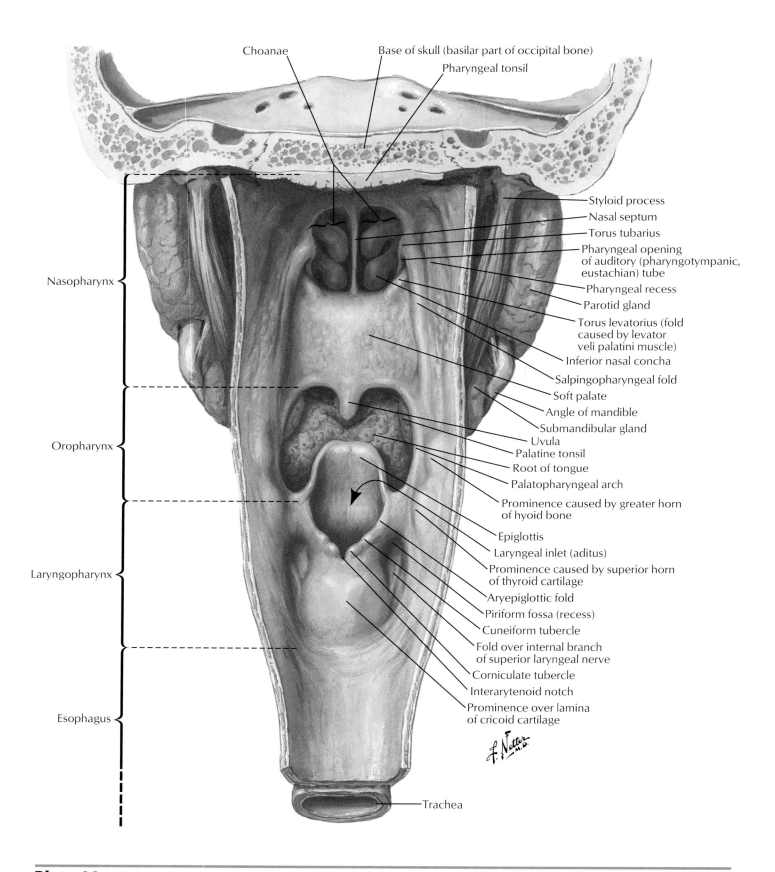

Choanae

Base of skull (basilar part of occipital bone)

Pharyngeal tonsil

Styloid process

Nasal septum

Torus tubarius

Pharyngeal opening of auditory (pharyngotympanic, eustachian) tube

Pharyngeal recess

Parotid gland

Torus levatorius (fold caused by levator veli palatini muscle)

Inferior nasal concha

Salpingopharyngeal fold

Soft palate

Angle of mandible

Submandibular gland

Uvula

Palatine tonsil

Root of tongue

Palatopharyngeal arch

Prominence caused by greater horn of hyoid bone

Epiglottis

Laryngeal inlet (aditus)

Prominence caused by superior horn of thyroid cartilage

Aryepiglottic fold

Piriform fossa (recess)

Cuneiform tubercle

Fold over internal branch of superior laryngeal nerve

Corniculate tubercle

Interarytenoid notch

Prominence over lamina of cricoid cartilage

Nasopharynx

Oropharynx

Laryngopharynx

Esophagus

Trachea

Plate 66

Pharynx

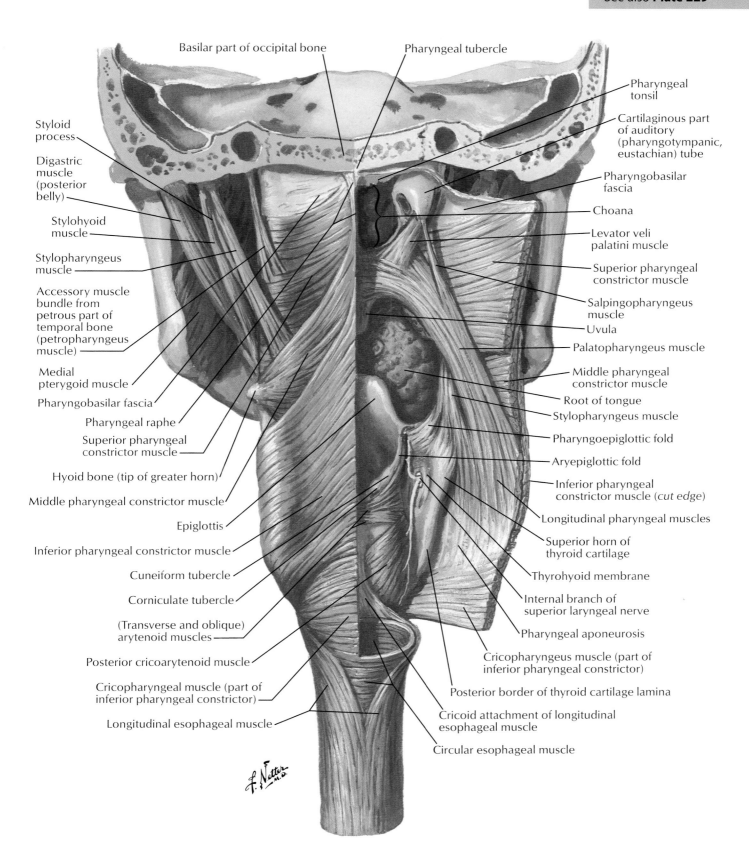

Basilar part of occipital bone

Pharyngeal tubercle

Pharyngeal tonsil

Cartilaginous part of auditory (pharyngotympanic, eustachian) tube

Pharyngobasilar fascia

Choana

Levator veli palatini muscle

Superior pharyngeal constrictor muscle

Salpingopharyngeus muscle

Uvula

Palatopharyngeus muscle

Middle pharyngeal constrictor muscle

Root of tongue

Stylopharyngeus muscle

Pharyngoepiglottic fold

Aryepiglottic fold

Inferior pharyngeal constrictor muscle (*cut edge*)

Longitudinal pharyngeal muscles

Superior horn of thyroid cartilage

Thyrohyoid membrane

Internal branch of superior laryngeal nerve

Pharyngeal aponeurosis

Cricopharyngeus muscle (part of inferior pharyngeal constrictor)

Posterior border of thyroid cartilage lamina

Cricoid attachment of longitudinal esophageal muscle

Circular esophageal muscle

Styloid process

Digastric muscle (posterior belly)

Stylohyoid muscle

Stylopharyngeus muscle

Accessory muscle bundle from petrous part of temporal bone (petropharyngeus muscle)

Medial pterygoid muscle

Pharyngobasilar fascia

Pharyngeal raphe

Superior pharyngeal constrictor muscle

Hyoid bone (tip of greater horn)

Middle pharyngeal constrictor muscle

Epiglottis

Inferior pharyngeal constrictor muscle

Cuneiform tubercle

Corniculate tubercle

(Transverse and oblique) arytenoid muscles

Posterior cricoarytenoid muscle

Cricopharyngeal muscle (part of inferior pharyngeal constrictor)

Longitudinal esophageal muscle

Muscles of Pharynx: Lateral View

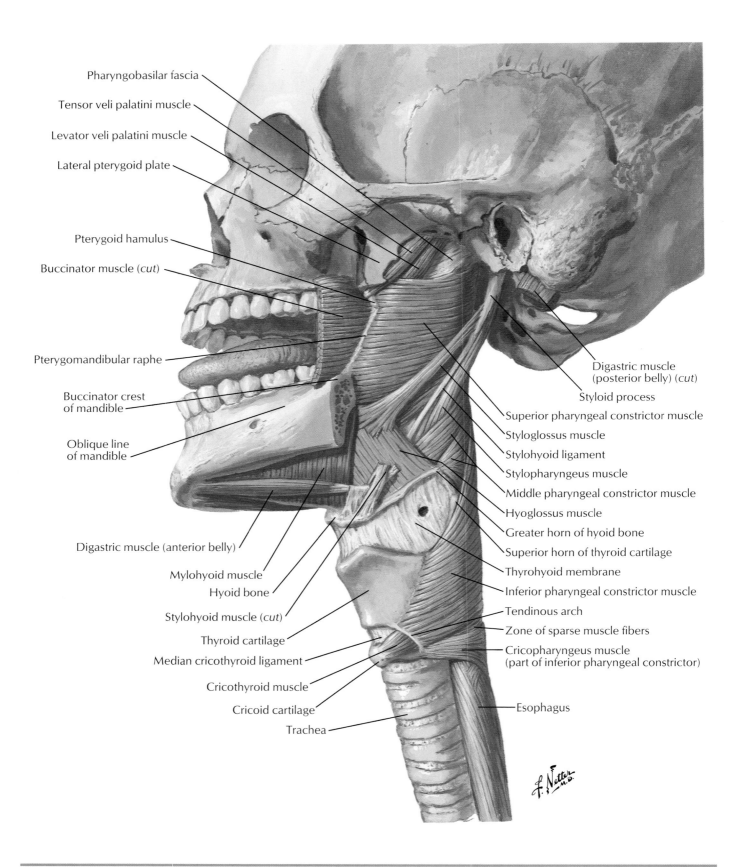

Pharyngobasilar fascia

Tensor veli palatini muscle

Levator veli palatini muscle

Lateral pterygoid plate

Pterygoid hamulus

Buccinator muscle (*cut*)

Pterygomandibular raphe

Buccinator crest
of mandible

Oblique line
of mandible

Digastric muscle (anterior belly)

Mylohyoid muscle

Hyoid bone

Stylohyoid muscle (*cut*)

Thyroid cartilage

Median cricothyroid ligament

Cricothyroid muscle

Cricoid cartilage

Trachea

Digastric muscle
(posterior belly) (*cut*)

Styloid process

Superior pharyngeal constrictor muscle

Styloglossus muscle

Stylohyoid ligament

Stylopharyngeus muscle

Middle pharyngeal constrictor muscle

Hyoglossus muscle

Greater horn of hyoid bone

Superior horn of thyroid cartilage

Thyrohyoid membrane

Inferior pharyngeal constrictor muscle

Tendinous arch

Zone of sparse muscle fibers

Cricopharyngeus muscle
(part of inferior pharyngeal constrictor)

Esophagus

Plate 68   **Pharynx**

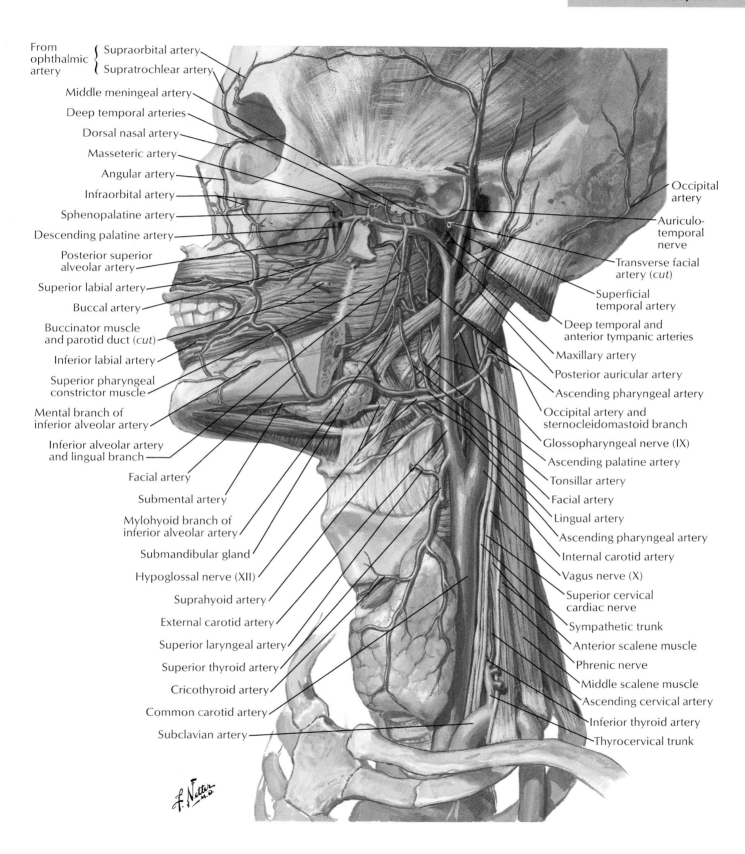

From ophthalmic artery
- Supraorbital artery
- Supratrochlear artery

Middle meningeal artery

Deep temporal arteries

Dorsal nasal artery

Masseteric artery

Angular artery

Infraorbital artery

Sphenopalatine artery

Descending palatine artery

Posterior superior alveolar artery

Superior labial artery

Buccal artery

Buccinator muscle and parotid duct (cut)

Inferior labial artery

Superior pharyngeal constrictor muscle

Mental branch of inferior alveolar artery

Inferior alveolar artery and lingual branch

Facial artery

Submental artery

Mylohyoid branch of inferior alveolar artery

Submandibular gland

Hypoglossal nerve (XII)

Suprahyoid artery

External carotid artery

Superior laryngeal artery

Superior thyroid artery

Cricothyroid artery

Common carotid artery

Subclavian artery

Occipital artery

Auriculo-temporal nerve

Transverse facial artery (cut)

Superficial temporal artery

Deep temporal and anterior tympanic arteries

Maxillary artery

Posterior auricular artery

Ascending pharyngeal artery

Occipital artery and sternocleidomastoid branch

Glossopharyngeal nerve (IX)

Ascending palatine artery

Tonsillar artery

Facial artery

Lingual artery

Ascending pharyngeal artery

Internal carotid artery

Vagus nerve (X)

Superior cervical cardiac nerve

Sympathetic trunk

Anterior scalene muscle

Phrenic nerve

Middle scalene muscle

Ascending cervical artery

Inferior thyroid artery

Thyrocervical trunk

Veins of Oral and Pharyngeal Regions

See also **Plates 3, 30, 103**

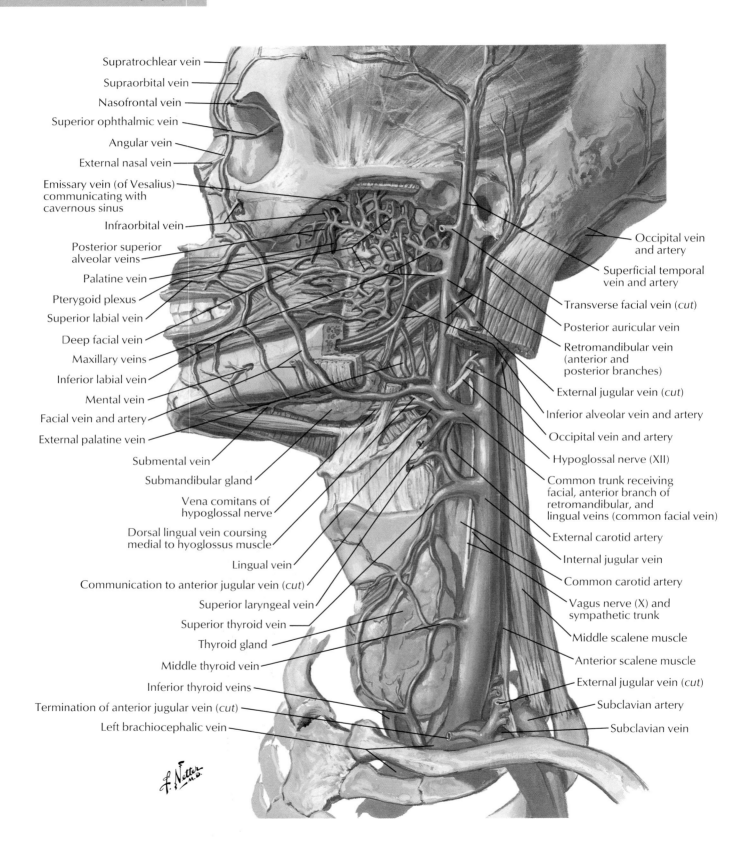

Supratrochlear vein

Supraorbital vein

Nasofrontal vein

Superior ophthalmic vein

Angular vein

External nasal vein

Emissary vein (of Vesalius) communicating with cavernous sinus

Infraorbital vein

Posterior superior alveolar veins

Palatine vein

Pterygoid plexus

Superior labial vein

Deep facial vein

Maxillary veins

Inferior labial vein

Mental vein

Facial vein and artery

External palatine vein

Submental vein

Submandibular gland

Vena comitans of hypoglossal nerve

Dorsal lingual vein coursing medial to hyoglossus muscle

Lingual vein

Communication to anterior jugular vein (cut)

Superior laryngeal vein

Superior thyroid vein

Thyroid gland

Middle thyroid vein

Inferior thyroid veins

Termination of anterior jugular vein (cut)

Left brachiocephalic vein

Occipital vein and artery

Superficial temporal vein and artery

Transverse facial vein (cut)

Posterior auricular vein

Retromandibular vein (anterior and posterior branches)

External jugular vein (cut)

Inferior alveolar vein and artery

Occipital vein and artery

Hypoglossal nerve (XII)

Common trunk receiving facial, anterior branch of retromandibular, and lingual veins (common facial vein)

External carotid artery

Internal jugular vein

Common carotid artery

Vagus nerve (X) and sympathetic trunk

Middle scalene muscle

Anterior scalene muscle

External jugular vein (cut)

Subclavian artery

Subclavian vein

F. Netter M.D.

Plate 70

See also **Plates 24, 44, 45, 121, 124, 125**

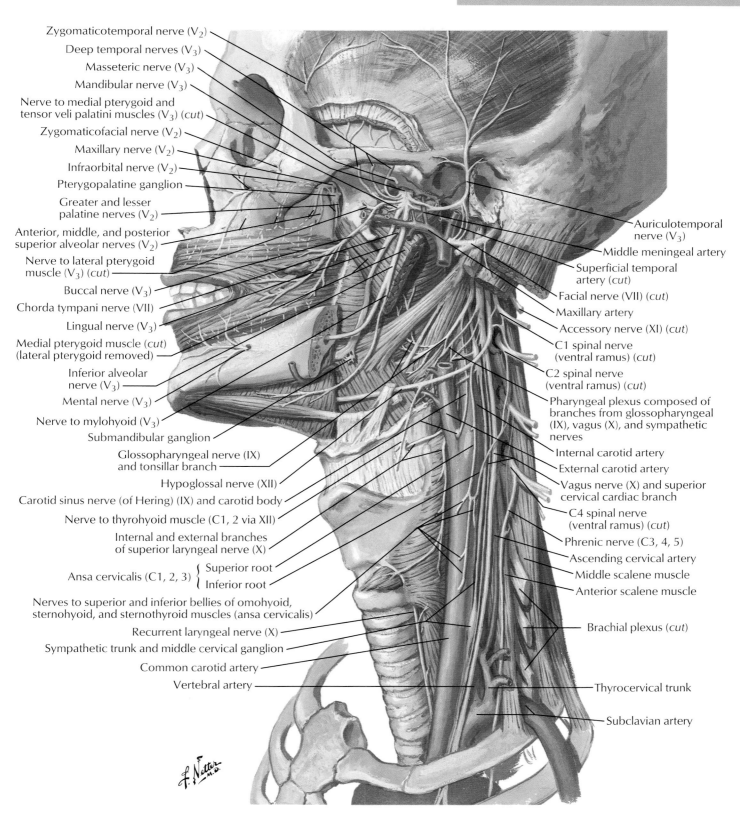

Zygomaticotemporal nerve (V₂)

Deep temporal nerves (V₃)

Masseteric nerve (V₃)

Mandibular nerve (V₃)

Nerve to medial pterygoid and tensor veli palatini muscles (V₃) (cut)

Zygomaticofacial nerve (V₂)

Maxillary nerve (V₂)

Infraorbital nerve (V₂)

Pterygopalatine ganglion

Greater and lesser palatine nerves (V₂)

Anterior, middle, and posterior superior alveolar nerves (V₂)

Nerve to lateral pterygoid muscle (V₃) (cut)

Buccal nerve (V₃)

Chorda tympani nerve (VII)

Lingual nerve (V₃)

Medial pterygoid muscle (cut) (lateral pterygoid removed)

Inferior alveolar nerve (V₃)

Mental nerve (V₃)

Nerve to mylohyoid (V₃)

Submandibular ganglion

Glossopharyngeal nerve (IX) and tonsillar branch

Hypoglossal nerve (XII)

Carotid sinus nerve (of Hering) (IX) and carotid body

Nerve to thyrohyoid muscle (C1, 2 via XII)

Internal and external branches of superior laryngeal nerve (X)

Ansa cervicalis (C1, 2, 3) { Superior root / Inferior root

Nerves to superior and inferior bellies of omohyoid, sternohyoid, and sternothyroid muscles (ansa cervicalis)

Recurrent laryngeal nerve (X)

Sympathetic trunk and middle cervical ganglion

Common carotid artery

Vertebral artery

Auriculotemporal nerve (V₃)

Middle meningeal artery

Superficial temporal artery (cut)

Facial nerve (VII) (cut)

Maxillary artery

Accessory nerve (XI) (cut)

C1 spinal nerve (ventral ramus) (cut)

C2 spinal nerve (ventral ramus) (cut)

Pharyngeal plexus composed of branches from glossopharyngeal (IX), vagus (X), and sympathetic nerves

Internal carotid artery

External carotid artery

Vagus nerve (X) and superior cervical cardiac branch

C4 spinal nerve (ventral ramus) (cut)

Phrenic nerve (C3, 4, 5)

Ascending cervical artery

Middle scalene muscle

Anterior scalene muscle

Brachial plexus (cut)

Thyrocervical trunk

Subclavian artery

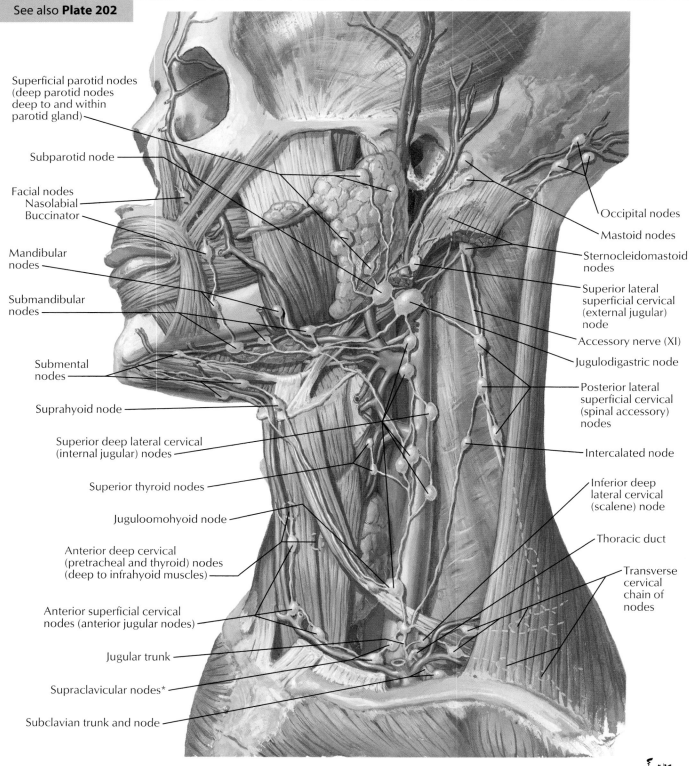

Superficial parotid nodes (deep parotid nodes deep to and within parotid gland)

Subparotid node

Facial nodes
Nasolabial
Buccinator

Mandibular nodes

Submandibular nodes

Submental nodes

Suprahyoid node

Superior deep lateral cervical (internal jugular) nodes

Superior thyroid nodes

Juguloomohyoid node

Anterior deep cervical (pretracheal and thyroid) nodes (deep to infrahyoid muscles)

Anterior superficial cervical nodes (anterior jugular nodes)

Jugular trunk

Supraclavicular nodes*

Subclavian trunk and node

Occipital nodes

Mastoid nodes

Sternocleidomastoid nodes

Superior lateral superficial cervical (external jugular) node

Accessory nerve (XI)

Jugulodigastric node

Posterior lateral superficial cervical (spinal accessory) nodes

Intercalated node

Inferior deep lateral cervical (scalene) node

Thoracic duct

Transverse cervical chain of nodes

*The supraclavicular group of nodes (also known as the lower deep cervical group), especially on the left, are also sometimes referred to as the signal or sentinel lymph nodes of Virchow or Troisier, especially when sufficiently enlarged and palpable. These nodes (or a single node) are so termed because they may be the first recognized presumptive evidence of malignant disease in the viscera.

Plate 72

Pharynx

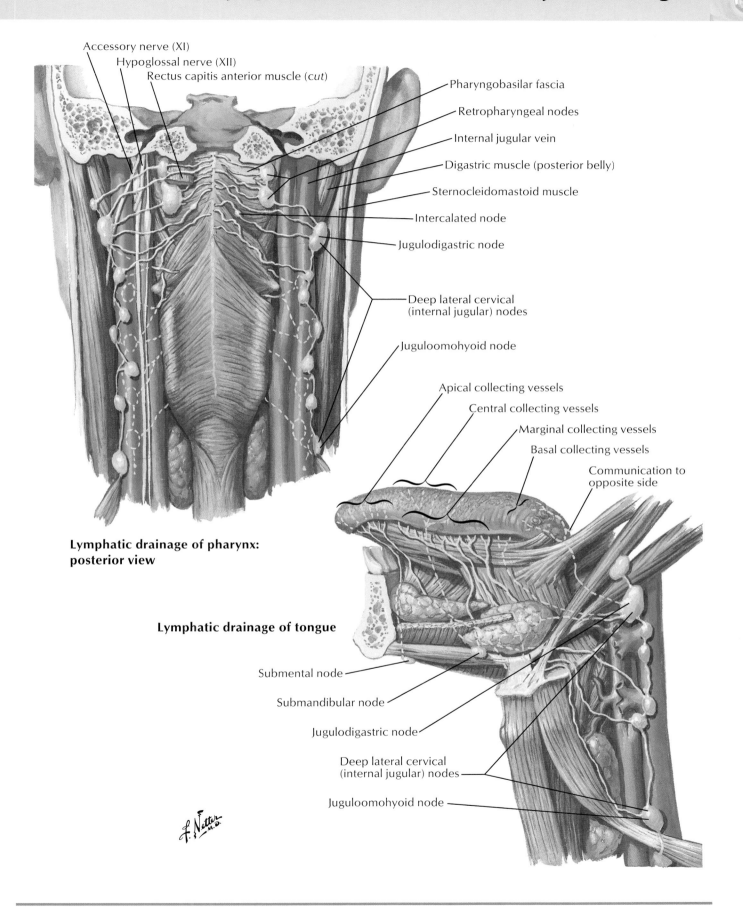

Accessory nerve (XI)

Hypoglossal nerve (XII)

Rectus capitis anterior muscle (*cut*)

Pharyngobasilar fascia

Retropharyngeal nodes

Internal jugular vein

Digastric muscle (posterior belly)

Sternocleidomastoid muscle

Intercalated node

Jugulodigastric node

Deep lateral cervical
(internal jugular) nodes

Juguloomohyoid node

Apical collecting vessels

Central collecting vessels

Marginal collecting vessels

Basal collecting vessels

Communication to
opposite side

**Lymphatic drainage of pharynx:
posterior view**

Lymphatic drainage of tongue

Submental node

Submandibular node

Jugulodigastric node

Deep lateral cervical
(internal jugular) nodes

Juguloomohyoid node

Thyroid Gland: Anterior View

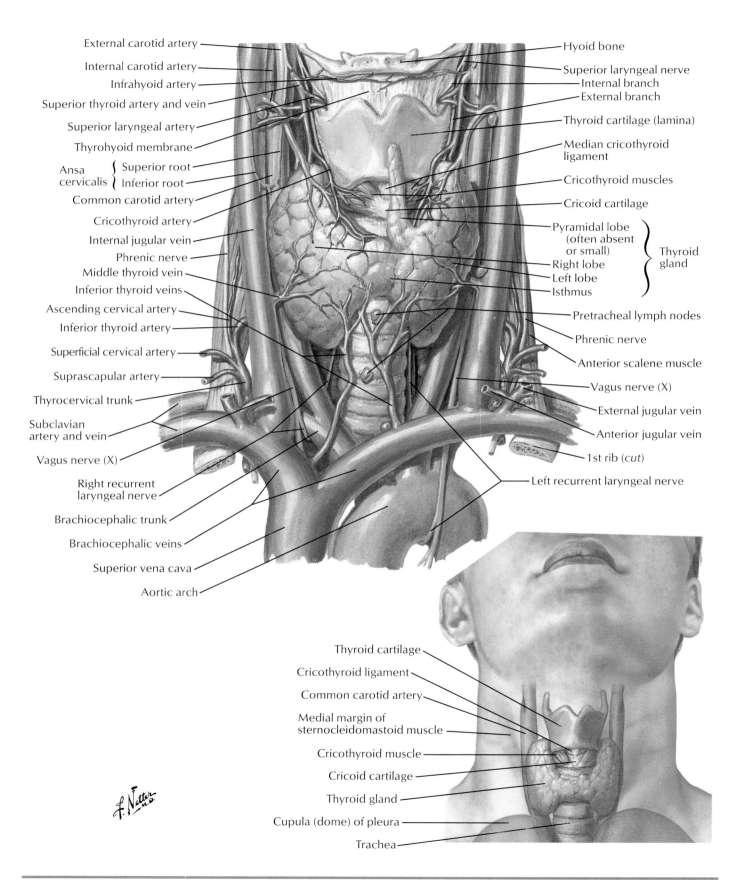

External carotid artery
Internal carotid artery
Infrahyoid artery
Superior thyroid artery and vein
Superior laryngeal artery
Thyrohyoid membrane
Ansa cervicalis { Superior root
{ Inferior root
Common carotid artery
Cricothyroid artery
Internal jugular vein
Phrenic nerve
Middle thyroid vein
Inferior thyroid veins
Ascending cervical artery
Inferior thyroid artery
Superficial cervical artery
Suprascapular artery
Thyrocervical trunk
Subclavian artery and vein
Vagus nerve (X)
Right recurrent laryngeal nerve
Brachiocephalic trunk
Brachiocephalic veins
Superior vena cava
Aortic arch

Hyoid bone
Superior laryngeal nerve
Internal branch
External branch
Thyroid cartilage (lamina)
Median cricothyroid ligament
Cricothyroid muscles
Cricoid cartilage
Pyramidal lobe (often absent or small)
Right lobe
Left lobe
Isthmus
Thyroid gland
Pretracheal lymph nodes
Phrenic nerve
Anterior scalene muscle
Vagus nerve (X)
External jugular vein
Anterior jugular vein
1st rib (cut)
Left recurrent laryngeal nerve

Thyroid cartilage
Cricothyroid ligament
Common carotid artery
Medial margin of sternocleidomastoid muscle
Cricothyroid muscle
Cricoid cartilage
Thyroid gland
Cupula (dome) of pleura
Trachea

f. Netter
_m.d._

Plate 74

Thyroid Gland and Larynx

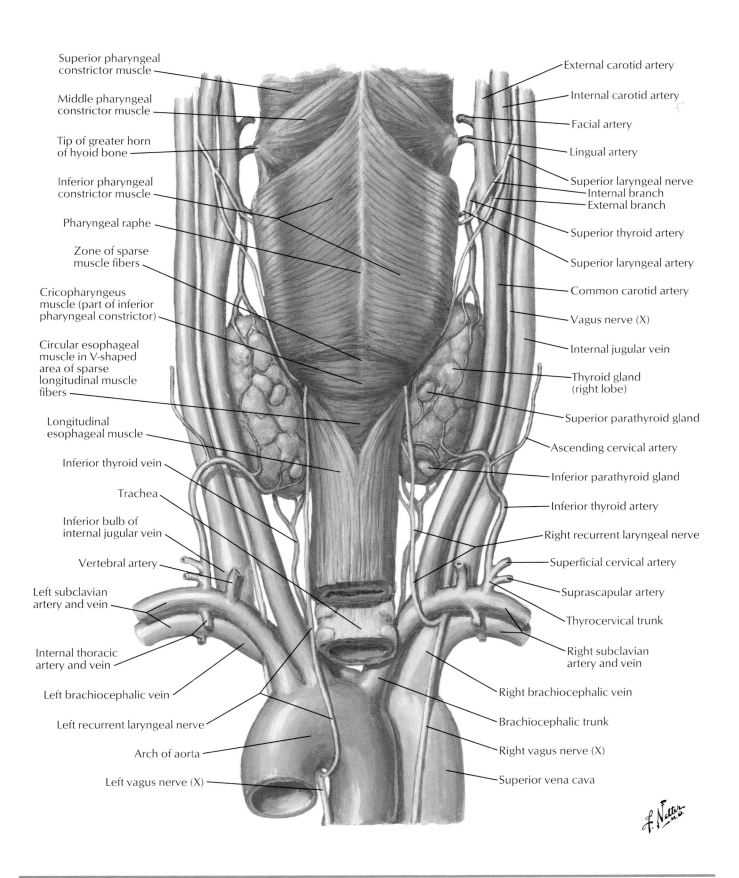

Superior pharyngeal constrictor muscle

Middle pharyngeal constrictor muscle

Tip of greater horn of hyoid bone

Inferior pharyngeal constrictor muscle

Pharyngeal raphe

Zone of sparse muscle fibers

Cricopharyngeus muscle (part of inferior pharyngeal constrictor)

Circular esophageal muscle in V-shaped area of sparse longitudinal muscle fibers

Longitudinal esophageal muscle

Inferior thyroid vein

Trachea

Inferior bulb of internal jugular vein

Vertebral artery

Left subclavian artery and vein

Internal thoracic artery and vein

Left brachiocephalic vein

Left recurrent laryngeal nerve

Arch of aorta

Left vagus nerve (X)

External carotid artery

Internal carotid artery

Facial artery

Lingual artery

Superior laryngeal nerve
Internal branch
External branch

Superior thyroid artery

Superior laryngeal artery

Common carotid artery

Vagus nerve (X)

Internal jugular vein

Thyroid gland (right lobe)

Superior parathyroid gland

Ascending cervical artery

Inferior parathyroid gland

Inferior thyroid artery

Right recurrent laryngeal nerve

Superficial cervical artery

Suprascapular artery

Thyrocervical trunk

Right subclavian artery and vein

Right brachiocephalic vein

Brachiocephalic trunk

Right vagus nerve (X)

Superior vena cava

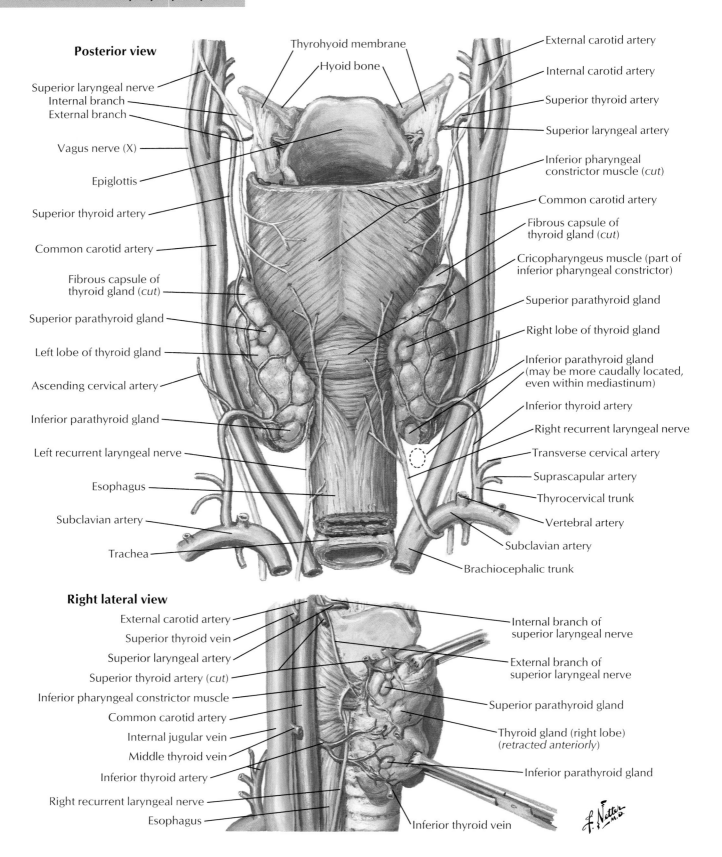

Posterior view

Thyrohyoid membrane

Hyoid bone

Superior laryngeal nerve
Internal branch
External branch

Vagus nerve (X)

Epiglottis

Superior thyroid artery

Common carotid artery

Fibrous capsule of
thyroid gland (*cut*)

Superior parathyroid gland

Left lobe of thyroid gland

Ascending cervical artery

Inferior parathyroid gland

Left recurrent laryngeal nerve

Esophagus

Subclavian artery

Trachea

External carotid artery

Internal carotid artery

Superior thyroid artery

Superior laryngeal artery

Inferior pharyngeal
constrictor muscle (*cut*)

Common carotid artery

Fibrous capsule of
thyroid gland (*cut*)

Cricopharyngeus muscle (part of
inferior pharyngeal constrictor)

Superior parathyroid gland

Right lobe of thyroid gland

Inferior parathyroid gland
(may be more caudally located,
even within mediastinum)

Inferior thyroid artery

Right recurrent laryngeal nerve

Transverse cervical artery

Suprascapular artery

Thyrocervical trunk

Vertebral artery

Subclavian artery

Brachiocephalic trunk

Right lateral view

External carotid artery

Superior thyroid vein

Superior laryngeal artery

Superior thyroid artery (*cut*)

Inferior pharyngeal constrictor muscle

Common carotid artery

Internal jugular vein

Middle thyroid vein

Inferior thyroid artery

Right recurrent laryngeal nerve

Esophagus

Internal branch of
superior laryngeal nerve

External branch of
superior laryngeal nerve

Superior parathyroid gland

Thyroid gland (right lobe)
(*retracted anteriorly*)

Inferior parathyroid gland

Inferior thyroid vein

f. Netter

Plate 76

Thyroid Gland and Larynx

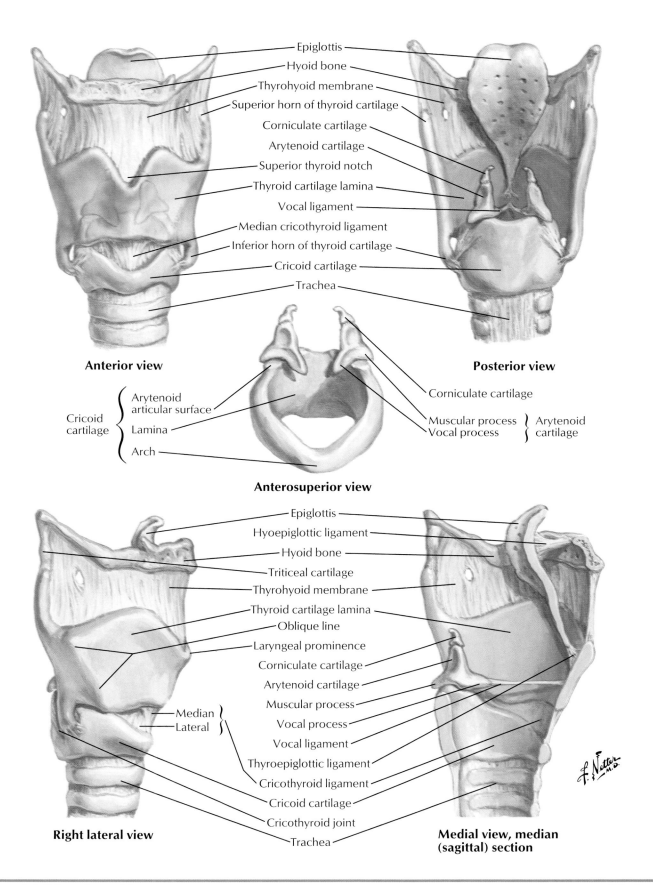

Epiglottis

Hyoid bone

Thyrohyoid membrane

Superior horn of thyroid cartilage

Corniculate cartilage

Arytenoid cartilage

Superior thyroid notch

Thyroid cartilage lamina

Vocal ligament

Median cricothyroid ligament

Inferior horn of thyroid cartilage

Cricoid cartilage

Trachea

Anterior view

Posterior view

Corniculate cartilage

Muscular process ⎫ Arytenoid
Vocal process ⎭ cartilage

Cricoid cartilage ⎧ Arytenoid articular surface

Lamina

Arch

Anterosuperior view

Epiglottis

Hyoepiglottic ligament

Hyoid bone

Triticeal cartilage

Thyrohyoid membrane

Thyroid cartilage lamina

Oblique line

Laryngeal prominence

Corniculate cartilage

Arytenoid cartilage

Muscular process

Vocal process

Vocal ligament

Thyroepiglottic ligament

Cricothyroid ligament ⎰ Median ⎱ Lateral

Cricoid cartilage

Cricothyroid joint

Trachea

Right lateral view

Medial view, median (sagittal) section

F. Netter M.D.

Intrinsic Muscles of Larynx

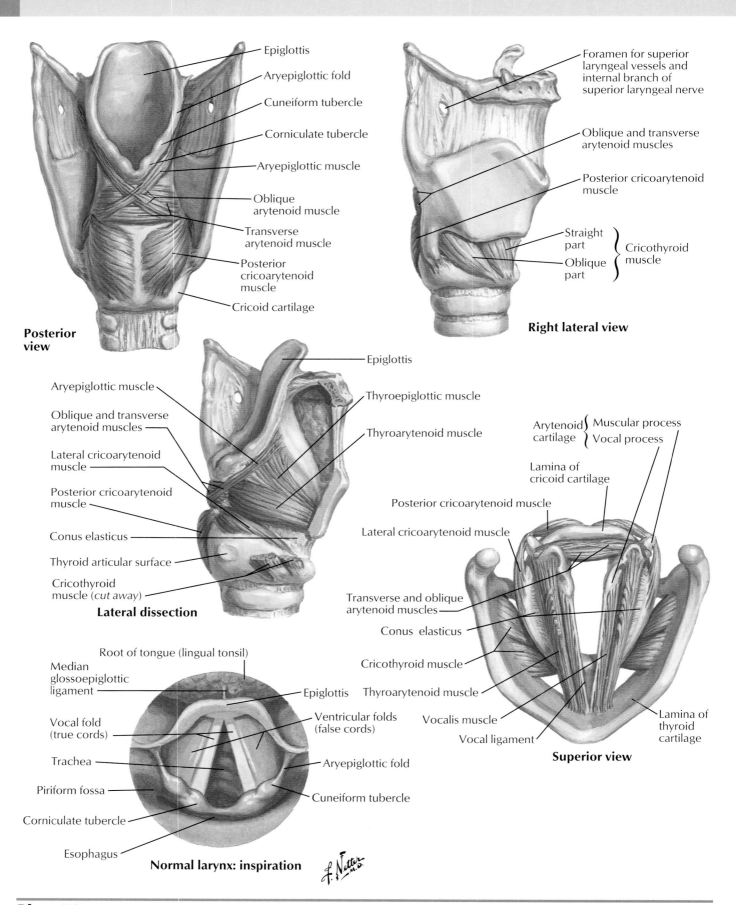

Epiglottis

Aryepiglottic fold

Cuneiform tubercle

Corniculate tubercle

Aryepiglottic muscle

Oblique arytenoid muscle

Transverse arytenoid muscle

Posterior cricoarytenoid muscle

Cricoid cartilage

Posterior view

Foramen for superior laryngeal vessels and internal branch of superior laryngeal nerve

Oblique and transverse arytenoid muscles

Posterior cricoarytenoid muscle

Straight part

Oblique part

Cricothyroid muscle

Right lateral view

Aryepiglottic muscle

Oblique and transverse arytenoid muscles

Lateral cricoarytenoid muscle

Posterior cricoarytenoid muscle

Conus elasticus

Thyroid articular surface

Cricothyroid muscle (*cut away*)

Lateral dissection

Epiglottis

Thyroepiglottic muscle

Thyroarytenoid muscle

Arytenoid cartilage

Muscular process

Vocal process

Lamina of cricoid cartilage

Posterior cricoarytenoid muscle

Lateral cricoarytenoid muscle

Transverse and oblique arytenoid muscles

Conus elasticus

Cricothyroid muscle

Thyroarytenoid muscle

Vocalis muscle

Vocal ligament

Lamina of thyroid cartilage

Superior view

Root of tongue (lingual tonsil)

Median glossoepiglottic ligament

Vocal fold (true cords)

Trachea

Piriform fossa

Corniculate tubercle

Esophagus

Epiglottis

Ventricular folds (false cords)

Aryepiglottic fold

Cuneiform tubercle

Normal larynx: inspiration

f. Netter M.D.

Plate 78

Thyroid Gland and Larynx

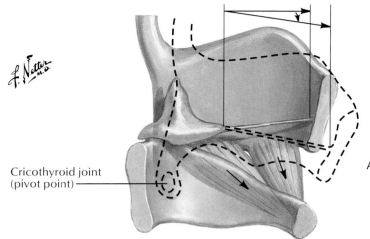

Cricothyroid joint (pivot point)

Action of cricothyroid muscles

Lengthening (increasing tension) of vocal ligaments

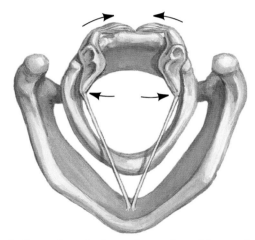

Action of posterior cricoarytenoid muscles

Abduction of vocal ligaments

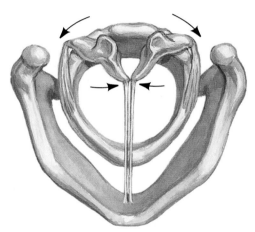

Action of lateral cricoarytenoid muscles

Adduction of vocal ligaments

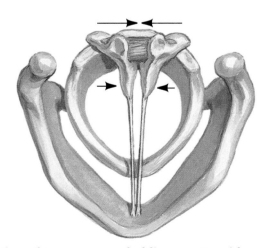

Action of transverse and oblique arytenoid muscles

Adduction of vocal ligaments

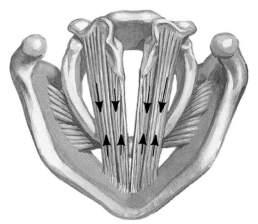

Action of vocalis and thyroarytenoid muscles

Shortening (relaxation) of vocal ligaments

Nerves of Larynx

See also **Plates 74, 76, 229**

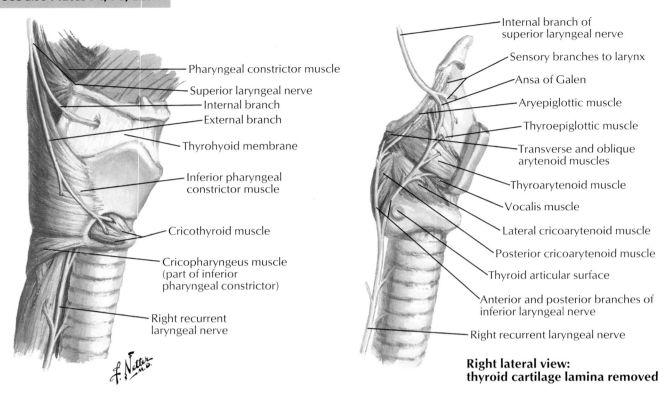

Pharyngeal constrictor muscle

Superior laryngeal nerve

Internal branch

External branch

Thyrohyoid membrane

Inferior pharyngeal constrictor muscle

Cricothyroid muscle

Cricopharyngeus muscle (part of inferior pharyngeal constrictor)

Right recurrent laryngeal nerve

Internal branch of superior laryngeal nerve

Sensory branches to larynx

Ansa of Galen

Aryepiglottic muscle

Thyroepiglottic muscle

Transverse and oblique arytenoid muscles

Thyroarytenoid muscle

Vocalis muscle

Lateral cricoarytenoid muscle

Posterior cricoarytenoid muscle

Thyroid articular surface

Anterior and posterior branches of inferior laryngeal nerve

Right recurrent laryngeal nerve

**Right lateral view:
thyroid cartilage lamina removed**

Coronal section through larynx

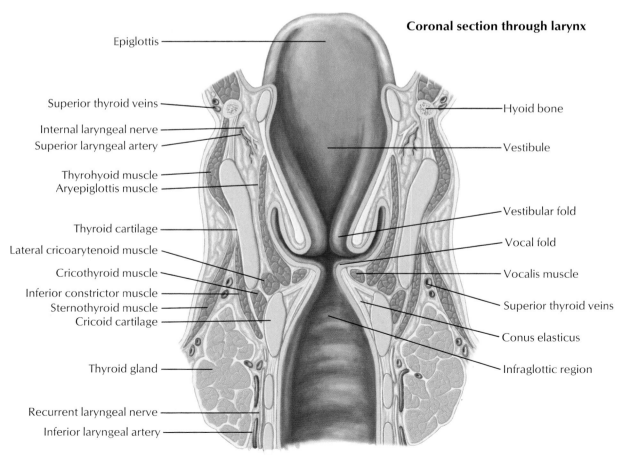

Epiglottis

Superior thyroid veins

Internal laryngeal nerve

Superior laryngeal artery

Thyrohyoid muscle

Aryepiglottis muscle

Thyroid cartilage

Lateral cricoarytenoid muscle

Cricothyroid muscle

Inferior constrictor muscle

Sternothyroid muscle

Cricoid cartilage

Thyroid gland

Recurrent laryngeal nerve

Inferior laryngeal artery

Hyoid bone

Vestibule

Vestibular fold

Vocal fold

Vocalis muscle

Superior thyroid veins

Conus elasticus

Infraglottic region

Plate 80

Thyroid Gland and Larynx

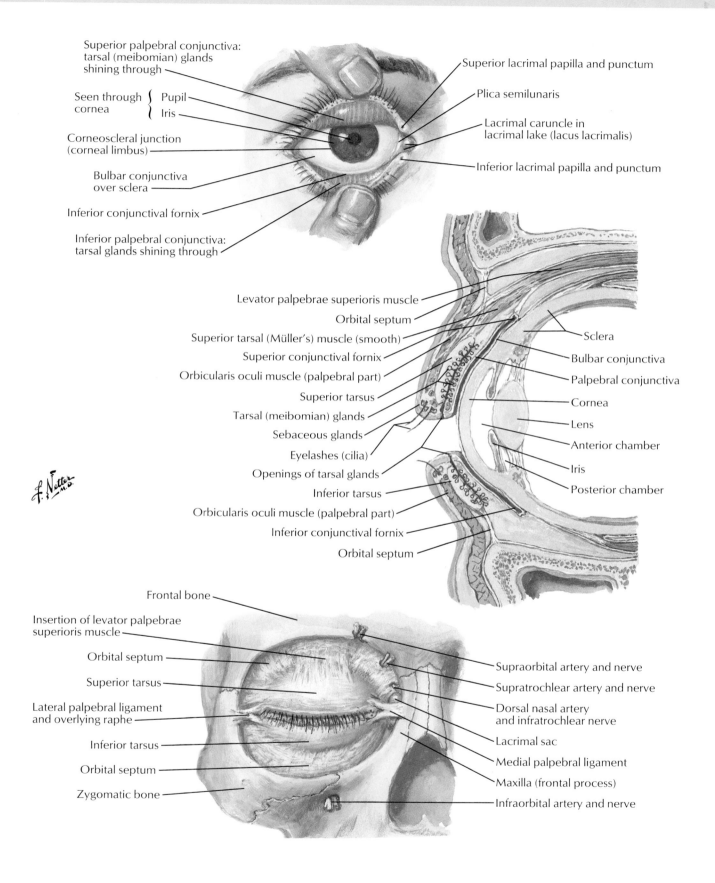

Superior palpebral conjunctiva: tarsal (meibomian) glands shining through

Seen through cornea { Pupil, Iris }

Corneoscleral junction (corneal limbus)

Bulbar conjunctiva over sclera

Inferior conjunctival fornix

Inferior palpebral conjunctiva: tarsal glands shining through

Superior lacrimal papilla and punctum

Plica semilunaris

Lacrimal caruncle in lacrimal lake (lacus lacrimalis)

Inferior lacrimal papilla and punctum

Levator palpebrae superioris muscle

Orbital septum

Superior tarsal (Müller's) muscle (smooth)

Superior conjunctival fornix

Orbicularis oculi muscle (palpebral part)

Superior tarsus

Tarsal (meibomian) glands

Sebaceous glands

Eyelashes (cilia)

Openings of tarsal glands

Inferior tarsus

Orbicularis oculi muscle (palpebral part)

Inferior conjunctival fornix

Orbital septum

Sclera

Bulbar conjunctiva

Palpebral conjunctiva

Cornea

Lens

Anterior chamber

Iris

Posterior chamber

Frontal bone

Insertion of levator palpebrae superioris muscle

Orbital septum

Superior tarsus

Lateral palpebral ligament and overlying raphe

Inferior tarsus

Orbital septum

Zygomatic bone

Supraorbital artery and nerve

Supratrochlear artery and nerve

Dorsal nasal artery and infratrochlear nerve

Lacrimal sac

Medial palpebral ligament

Maxilla (frontal process)

Infraorbital artery and nerve

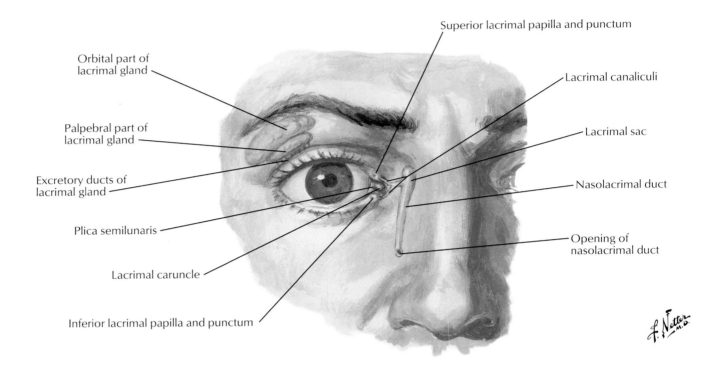

Superior lacrimal papilla and punctum

Orbital part of
lacrimal gland

Lacrimal canaliculi

Palpebral part of
lacrimal gland

Lacrimal sac

Excretory ducts of
lacrimal gland

Nasolacrimal duct

Plica semilunaris

Opening of
nasolacrimal duct

Lacrimal caruncle

Inferior lacrimal papilla and punctum

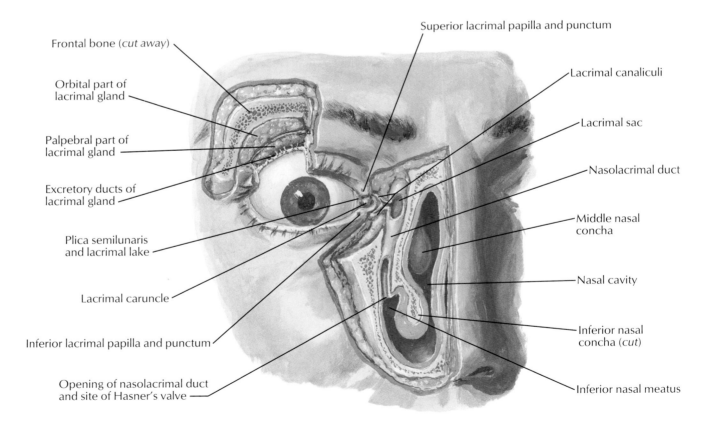

Superior lacrimal papilla and punctum

Frontal bone (*cut away*)

Lacrimal canaliculi

Orbital part of
lacrimal gland

Lacrimal sac

Palpebral part of
lacrimal gland

Nasolacrimal duct

Excretory ducts of
lacrimal gland

Middle nasal
concha

Plica semilunaris
and lacrimal lake

Nasal cavity

Lacrimal caruncle

Inferior nasal
concha (*cut*)

Inferior lacrimal papilla and punctum

Opening of nasolacrimal duct
and site of Hasner's valve

Inferior nasal meatus

Plate 82

Orbit and Contents

Horizontal section

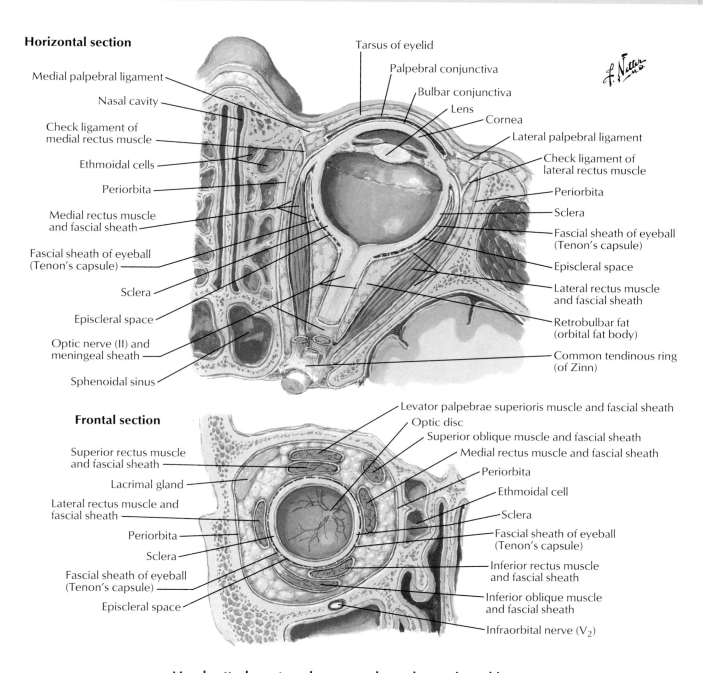

Medial palpebral ligament

Nasal cavity

Check ligament of medial rectus muscle

Ethmoidal cells

Periorbita

Medial rectus muscle and fascial sheath

Fascial sheath of eyeball (Tenon's capsule)

Sclera

Episcleral space

Optic nerve (II) and meningeal sheath

Sphenoidal sinus

Tarsus of eyelid

Palpebral conjunctiva

Bulbar conjunctiva

Lens

Cornea

Lateral palpebral ligament

Check ligament of lateral rectus muscle

Periorbita

Sclera

Fascial sheath of eyeball (Tenon's capsule)

Episcleral space

Lateral rectus muscle and fascial sheath

Retrobulbar fat (orbital fat body)

Common tendinous ring (of Zinn)

Frontal section

Superior rectus muscle and fascial sheath

Lacrimal gland

Lateral rectus muscle and fascial sheath

Periorbita

Sclera

Fascial sheath of eyeball (Tenon's capsule)

Episcleral space

Levator palpebrae superioris muscle and fascial sheath

Optic disc

Superior oblique muscle and fascial sheath

Medial rectus muscle and fascial sheath

Periorbita

Ethmoidal cell

Sclera

Fascial sheath of eyeball (Tenon's capsule)

Inferior rectus muscle and fascial sheath

Inferior oblique muscle and fascial sheath

Infraorbital nerve (V_2)

Muscle attachments and nerves and vessels entering orbit

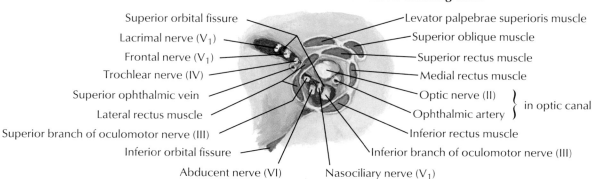

Superior orbital fissure

Lacrimal nerve (V_1)

Frontal nerve (V_1)

Trochlear nerve (IV)

Superior ophthalmic vein

Lateral rectus muscle

Superior branch of oculomotor nerve (III)

Inferior orbital fissure

Abducent nerve (VI)

Levator palpebrae superioris muscle

Superior oblique muscle

Superior rectus muscle

Medial rectus muscle

Optic nerve (II)

Ophthalmic artery

} in optic canal

Inferior rectus muscle

Inferior branch of oculomotor nerve (III)

Nasociliary nerve (V_1)

Extrinsic Eye Muscles

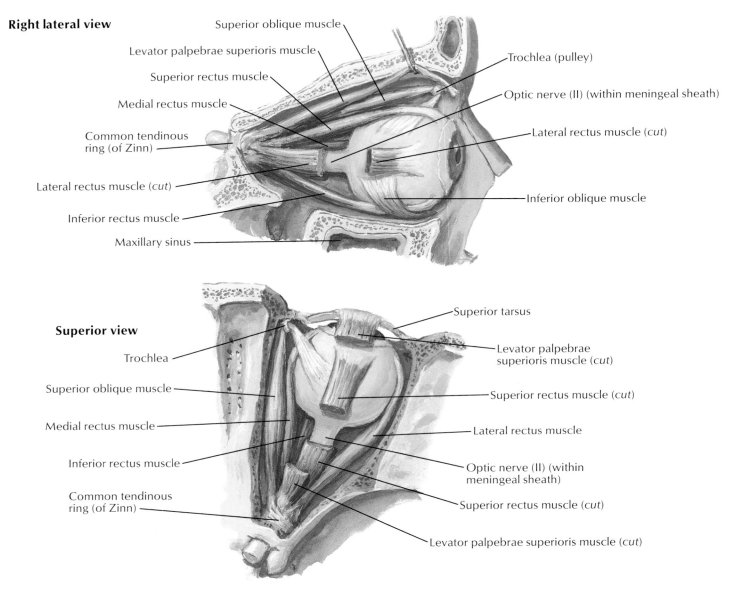

Right lateral view

- Superior oblique muscle
- Levator palpebrae superioris muscle
- Superior rectus muscle
- Medial rectus muscle
- Common tendinous ring (of Zinn)
- Lateral rectus muscle (*cut*)
- Inferior rectus muscle
- Maxillary sinus
- Trochlea (pulley)
- Optic nerve (II) (within meningeal sheath)
- Lateral rectus muscle (*cut*)
- Inferior oblique muscle

Superior view

- Trochlea
- Superior oblique muscle
- Medial rectus muscle
- Inferior rectus muscle
- Common tendinous ring (of Zinn)
- Superior tarsus
- Levator palpebrae superioris muscle (*cut*)
- Superior rectus muscle (*cut*)
- Lateral rectus muscle
- Optic nerve (II) (within meningeal sheath)
- Superior rectus muscle (*cut*)
- Levator palpebrae superioris muscle (*cut*)

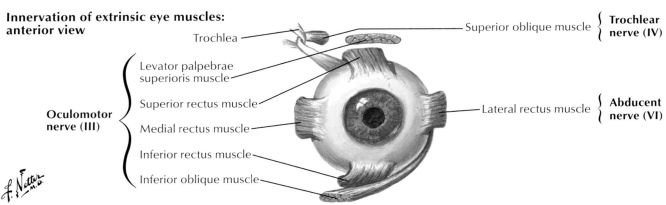

Innervation of extrinsic eye muscles: anterior view

- Trochlea
- Superior oblique muscle } **Trochlear nerve (IV)**
- Oculomotor nerve (III) {
  - Levator palpebrae superioris muscle
  - Superior rectus muscle
  - Medial rectus muscle
  - Inferior rectus muscle
  - Inferior oblique muscle
- Lateral rectus muscle } **Abducent nerve (VI)**

f. Netter M.D.

Plate 84   **Orbit and Contents**

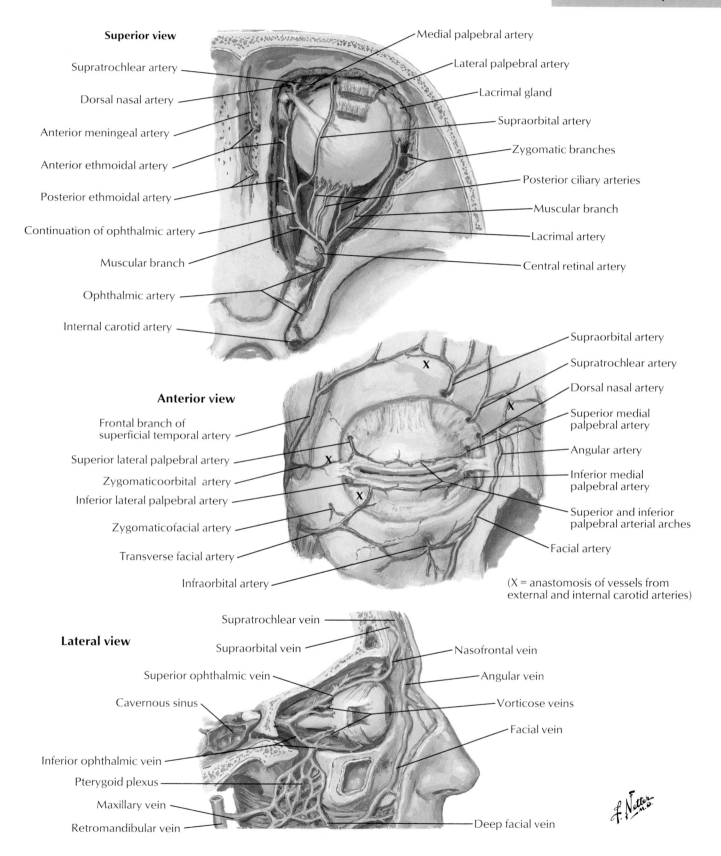

Superior view

Supratrochlear artery

Dorsal nasal artery

Anterior meningeal artery

Anterior ethmoidal artery

Posterior ethmoidal artery

Continuation of ophthalmic artery

Muscular branch

Ophthalmic artery

Internal carotid artery

Medial palpebral artery

Lateral palpebral artery

Lacrimal gland

Supraorbital artery

Zygomatic branches

Posterior ciliary arteries

Muscular branch

Lacrimal artery

Central retinal artery

Anterior view

Frontal branch of superficial temporal artery

Superior lateral palpebral artery

Zygomaticoorbital artery

Inferior lateral palpebral artery

Zygomaticofacial artery

Transverse facial artery

Infraorbital artery

Supraorbital artery

Supratrochlear artery

Dorsal nasal artery

Superior medial palpebral artery

Angular artery

Inferior medial palpebral artery

Superior and inferior palpebral arterial arches

Facial artery

(X = anastomosis of vessels from external and internal carotid arteries)

Lateral view

Supratrochlear vein

Supraorbital vein

Superior ophthalmic vein

Cavernous sinus

Inferior ophthalmic vein

Pterygoid plexus

Maxillary vein

Retromandibular vein

Nasofrontal vein

Angular vein

Vorticose veins

Facial vein

Deep facial vein

Superior view

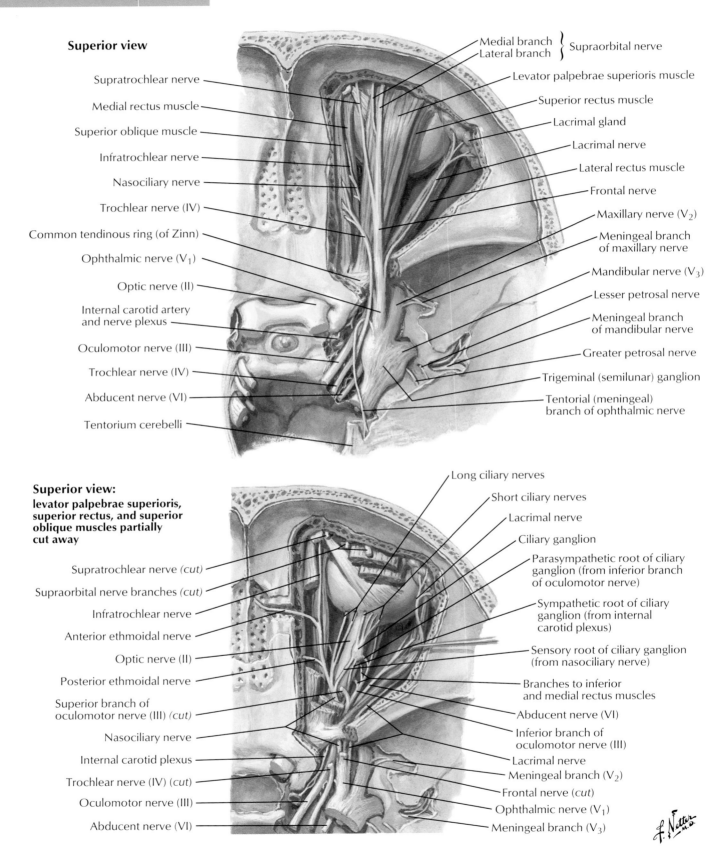

Supratrochlear nerve

Medial rectus muscle

Superior oblique muscle

Infratrochlear nerve

Nasociliary nerve

Trochlear nerve (IV)

Common tendinous ring (of Zinn)

Ophthalmic nerve (V₁)

Optic nerve (II)

Internal carotid artery and nerve plexus

Oculomotor nerve (III)

Trochlear nerve (IV)

Abducent nerve (VI)

Tentorium cerebelli

Medial branch } Supraorbital nerve
Lateral branch

Levator palpebrae superioris muscle

Superior rectus muscle

Lacrimal gland

Lacrimal nerve

Lateral rectus muscle

Frontal nerve

Maxillary nerve (V₂)

Meningeal branch of maxillary nerve

Mandibular nerve (V₃)

Lesser petrosal nerve

Meningeal branch of mandibular nerve

Greater petrosal nerve

Trigeminal (semilunar) ganglion

Tentorial (meningeal) branch of ophthalmic nerve

Superior view:
levator palpebrae superioris, superior rectus, and superior oblique muscles partially cut away

Supratrochlear nerve (cut)

Supraorbital nerve branches (cut)

Infratrochlear nerve

Anterior ethmoidal nerve

Optic nerve (II)

Posterior ethmoidal nerve

Superior branch of oculomotor nerve (III) (cut)

Nasociliary nerve

Internal carotid plexus

Trochlear nerve (IV) (cut)

Oculomotor nerve (III)

Abducent nerve (VI)

Long ciliary nerves

Short ciliary nerves

Lacrimal nerve

Ciliary ganglion

Parasympathetic root of ciliary ganglion (from inferior branch of oculomotor nerve)

Sympathetic root of ciliary ganglion (from internal carotid plexus)

Sensory root of ciliary ganglion (from nasociliary nerve)

Branches to inferior and medial rectus muscles

Abducent nerve (VI)

Inferior branch of oculomotor nerve (III)

Lacrimal nerve

Meningeal branch (V₂)

Frontal nerve (cut)

Ophthalmic nerve (V₁)

Meningeal branch (V₃)

Plate 86

Orbit and Contents

Horizontal section

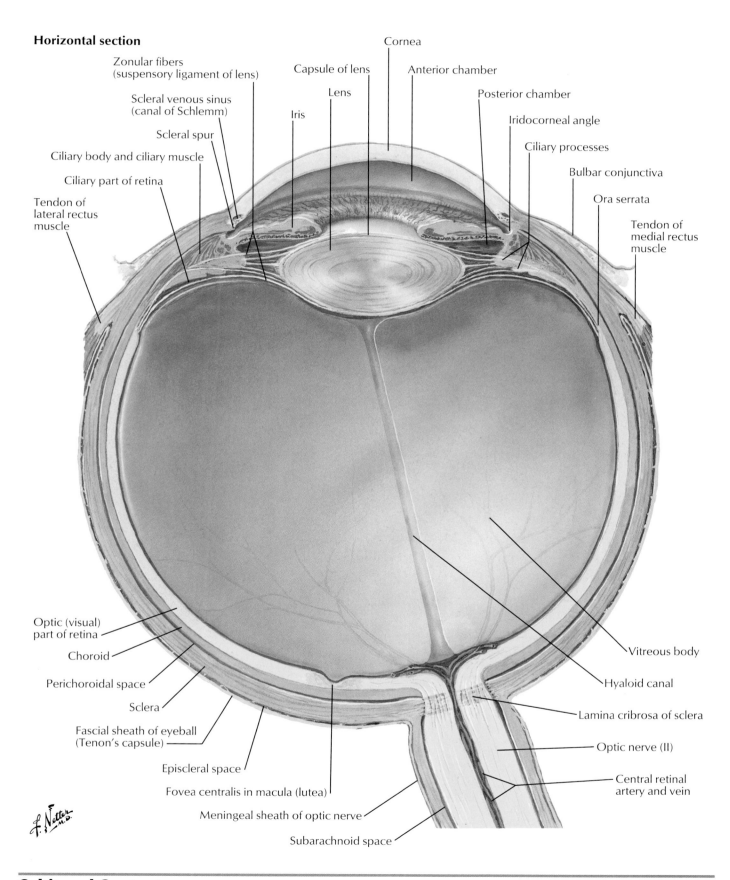

Zonular fibers
(suspensory ligament of lens)

Scleral venous sinus
(canal of Schlemm)

Scleral spur

Ciliary body and ciliary muscle

Ciliary part of retina

Tendon of
lateral rectus
muscle

Iris

Lens

Capsule of lens

Cornea

Anterior chamber

Posterior chamber

Iridocorneal angle

Ciliary processes

Bulbar conjunctiva

Ora serrata

Tendon of
medial rectus
muscle

Optic (visual)
part of retina

Choroid

Perichoroidal space

Sclera

Fascial sheath of eyeball
(Tenon's capsule)

Episcleral space

Fovea centralis in macula (lutea)

Meningeal sheath of optic nerve

Subarachnoid space

Vitreous body

Hyaloid canal

Lamina cribrosa of sclera

Optic nerve (II)

Central retinal
artery and vein

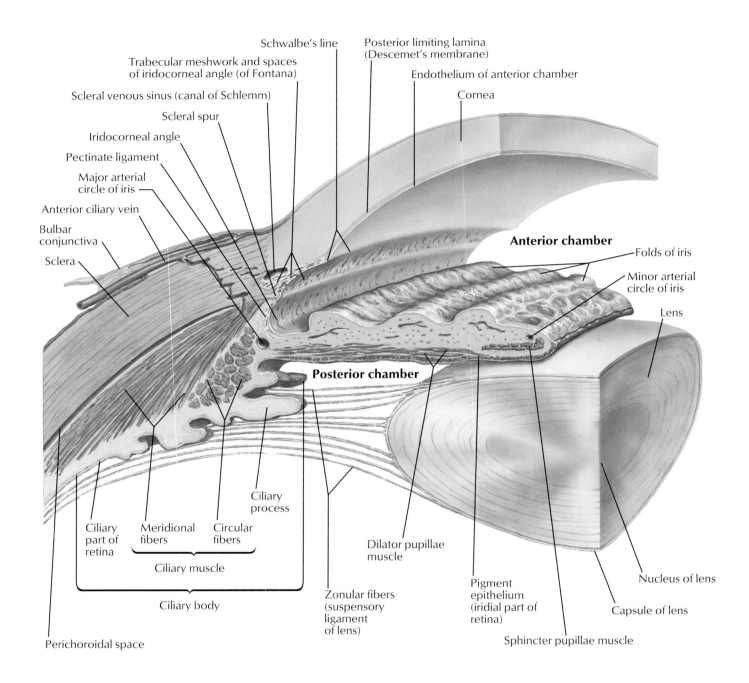

Schwalbe's line

Trabecular meshwork and spaces
of iridocorneal angle (of Fontana)

Scleral venous sinus (canal of Schlemm)

Scleral spur

Iridocorneal angle

Pectinate ligament

Major arterial
circle of iris

Anterior ciliary vein

Bulbar
conjunctiva

Sclera

Posterior limiting lamina
(Descemet's membrane)

Endothelium of anterior chamber

Cornea

Anterior chamber

Folds of iris

Minor arterial
circle of iris

Lens

Posterior chamber

Ciliary
process

Ciliary
part of
retina

Meridional
fibers

Circular
fibers

Ciliary muscle

Ciliary body

Perichoroidal space

Dilator pupillae
muscle

Zonular fibers
(suspensory
ligament
of lens)

Pigment
epithelium
(iridial part of
retina)

Sphincter pupillae muscle

Nucleus of lens

Capsule of lens

Note: For clarity, only single plane of zonular fibers shown;
actually, fibers surround entire circumference of lens.

Plate 88   **Orbit and Contents**

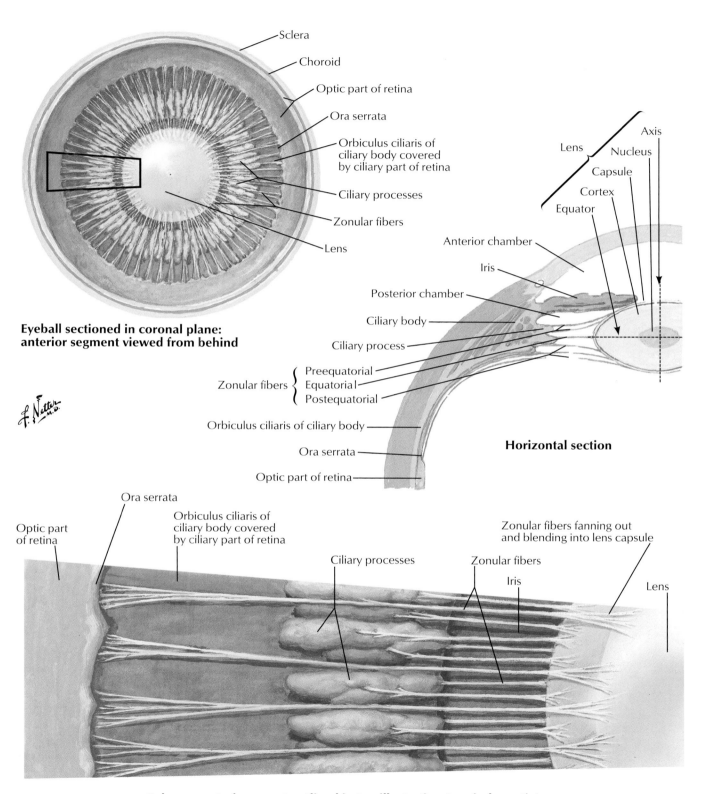

Eyeball sectioned in coronal plane: anterior segment viewed from behind

Sclera

Choroid

Optic part of retina

Ora serrata

Orbiculus ciliaris of ciliary body covered by ciliary part of retina

Ciliary processes

Zonular fibers

Lens

Axis

Lens

Nucleus

Capsule

Cortex

Equator

Anterior chamber

Iris

Posterior chamber

Ciliary body

Ciliary process

Zonular fibers { Preequatorial — Equatorial — Postequatorial

Orbiculus ciliaris of ciliary body

Ora serrata

Optic part of retina

Horizontal section

Ora serrata

Optic part of retina

Orbiculus ciliaris of ciliary body covered by ciliary part of retina

Ciliary processes

Zonular fibers fanning out and blending into lens capsule

Zonular fibers

Iris

Lens

Enlargement of segment outlined in top illustration (semischematic)

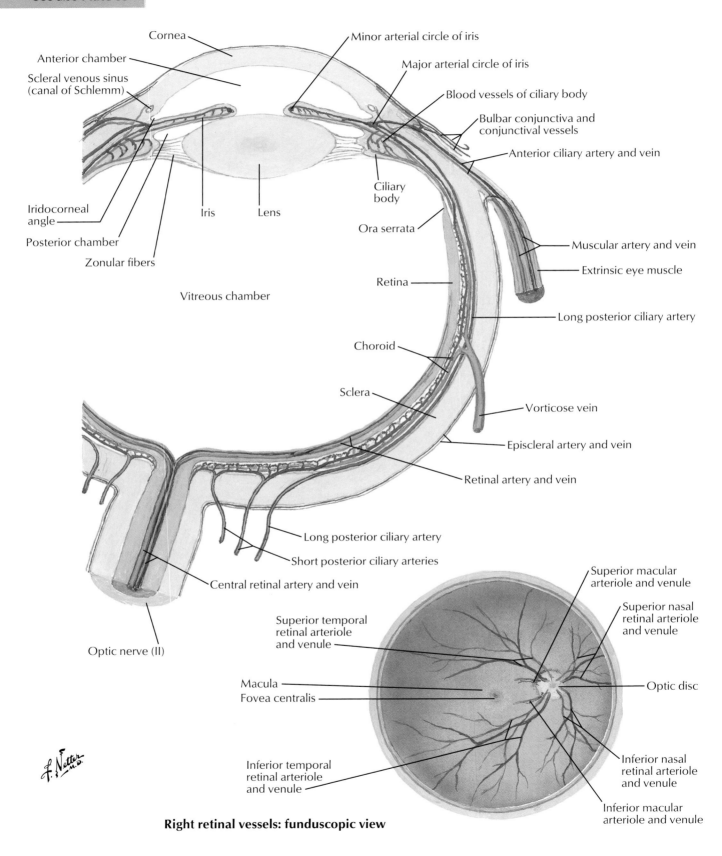

Cornea

Anterior chamber

Scleral venous sinus
(canal of Schlemm)

Minor arterial circle of iris

Major arterial circle of iris

Blood vessels of ciliary body

Bulbar conjunctiva and
conjunctival vessels

Anterior ciliary artery and vein

Ciliary
body

Iridocorneal
angle

Iris   Lens

Posterior chamber

Zonular fibers

Ora serrata

Muscular artery and vein

Extrinsic eye muscle

Retina

Vitreous chamber

Long posterior ciliary artery

Choroid

Sclera

Vorticose vein

Episcleral artery and vein

Retinal artery and vein

Long posterior ciliary artery

Short posterior ciliary arteries

Central retinal artery and vein

Optic nerve (II)

Superior macular
arteriole and venule

Superior temporal
retinal arteriole
and venule

Superior nasal
retinal arteriole
and venule

Macula

Fovea centralis

Optic disc

Inferior nasal
retinal arteriole
and venule

Inferior temporal
retinal arteriole
and venule

Inferior macular
arteriole and venule

Right retinal vessels: funduscopic view

Plate 90   **Orbit and Contents**

Vascular arrangements within the choroid (vascular tunic) of the eyeball

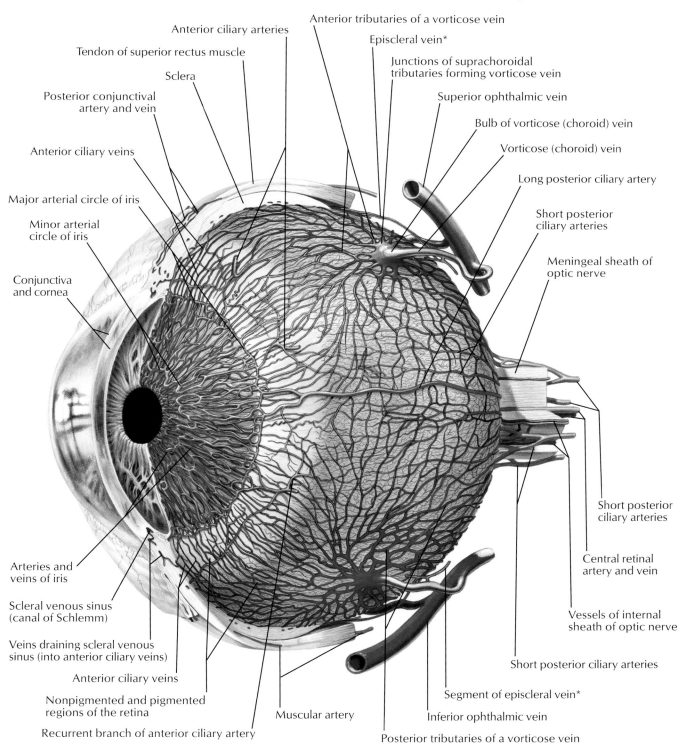

Anterior ciliary arteries

Tendon of superior rectus muscle

Sclera

Posterior conjunctival artery and vein

Anterior ciliary veins

Major arterial circle of iris

Minor arterial circle of iris

Conjunctiva and cornea

Anterior tributaries of a vorticose vein

Episcleral vein*

Junctions of suprachoroidal tributaries forming vorticose vein

Superior ophthalmic vein

Bulb of vorticose (choroid) vein

Vorticose (choroid) vein

Long posterior ciliary artery

Short posterior ciliary arteries

Meningeal sheath of optic nerve

Short posterior ciliary arteries

Central retinal artery and vein

Vessels of internal sheath of optic nerve

Short posterior ciliary arteries

Arteries and veins of iris

Scleral venous sinus (canal of Schlemm)

Veins draining scleral venous sinus (into anterior ciliary veins)

Anterior ciliary veins

Nonpigmented and pigmented regions of the retina

Recurrent branch of anterior ciliary artery

Muscular artery

Segment of episcleral vein*

Inferior ophthalmic vein

Posterior tributaries of a vorticose vein

The episcleral veins are shown here anastomosing with the vorticose veins, which they do; however, they also drain into the anterior ciliary veins.

C. Machado, M.D.

Frontal section

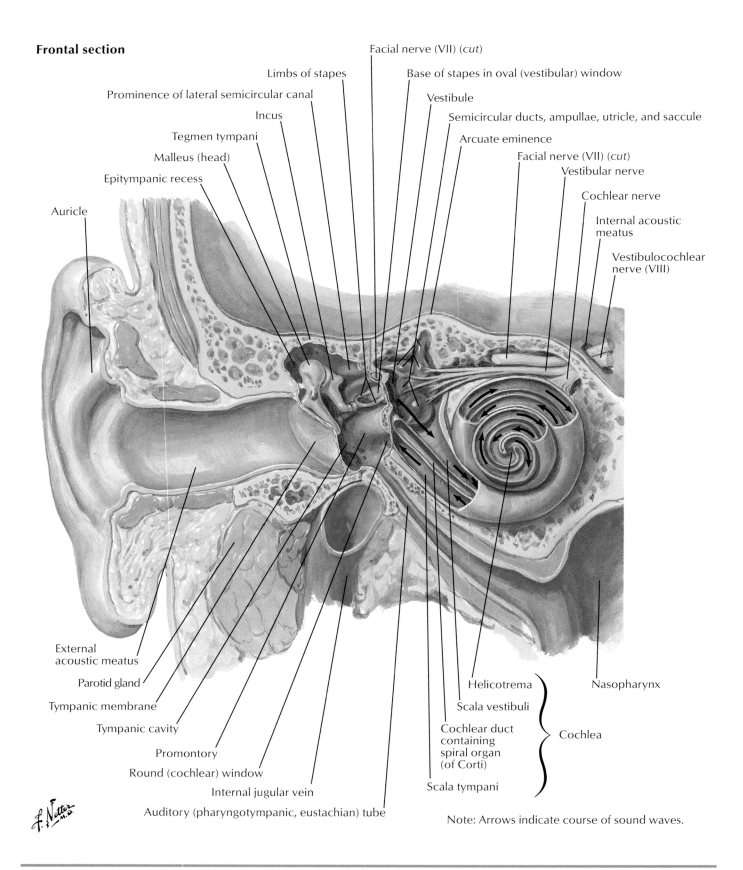

Facial nerve (VII) (*cut*)

Limbs of stapes

Base of stapes in oval (vestibular) window

Prominence of lateral semicircular canal

Vestibule

Incus

Semicircular ducts, ampullae, utricle, and saccule

Tegmen tympani

Arcuate eminence

Malleus (head)

Facial nerve (VII) (*cut*)

Epitympanic recess

Vestibular nerve

Auricle

Cochlear nerve

Internal acoustic meatus

Vestibulocochlear nerve (VIII)

External acoustic meatus

Parotid gland

Tympanic membrane

Tympanic cavity

Promontory

Helicotrema

Nasopharynx

Round (cochlear) window

Scala vestibuli

Internal jugular vein

Cochlear duct containing spiral organ (of Corti)

Cochlea

Auditory (pharyngotympanic, eustachian) tube

Scala tympani

Note: Arrows indicate course of sound waves.

Plate 92

Ear

Right auricle (pinna)

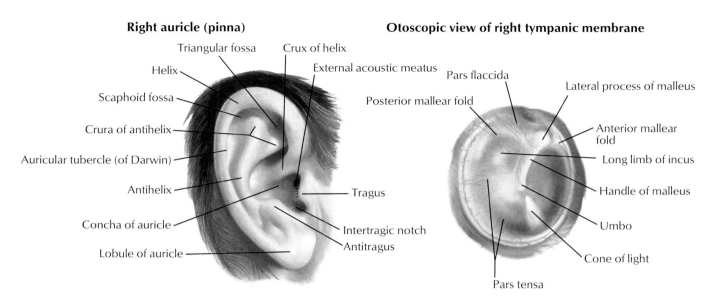

Triangular fossa
Crux of helix
Helix
External acoustic meatus
Scaphoid fossa
Crura of antihelix
Auricular tubercle (of Darwin)
Antihelix
Tragus
Concha of auricle
Intertragic notch
Lobule of auricle
Antitragus

Otoscopic view of right tympanic membrane

Pars flaccida
Posterior mallear fold
Lateral process of malleus
Anterior mallear fold
Long limb of incus
Handle of malleus
Umbo
Cone of light
Pars tensa

Coronal oblique section of external acoustic meatus and middle ear (tympanic cavity)

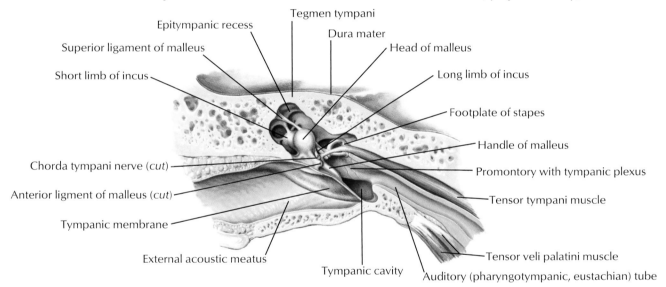

Tegmen tympani
Epitympanic recess
Dura mater
Superior ligament of malleus
Head of malleus
Short limb of incus
Long limb of incus
Footplate of stapes
Handle of malleus
Chorda tympani nerve (*cut*)
Promontory with tympanic plexus
Anterior ligament of malleus (*cut*)
Tensor tympani muscle
Tympanic membrane
External acoustic meatus
Tensor veli palatini muscle
Tympanic cavity
Auditory (pharyngotympanic, eustachian) tube

Right tympanic cavity after removal of tympanic membrane (lateral view)

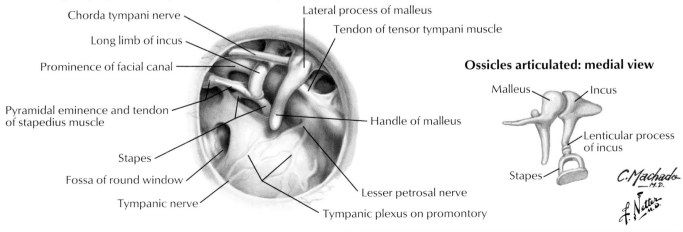

Chorda tympani nerve
Lateral process of malleus
Tendon of tensor tympani muscle
Long limb of incus
Prominence of facial canal
Pyramidal eminence and tendon of stapedius muscle
Handle of malleus
Stapes
Fossa of round window
Tympanic nerve
Lesser petrosal nerve
Tympanic plexus on promontory

Ossicles articulated: medial view

Malleus
Incus
Lenticular process of incus
Stapes

C. Machado M.D.

F. Netter M.D.

Lateral wall of tympanic cavity: medial (internal) view

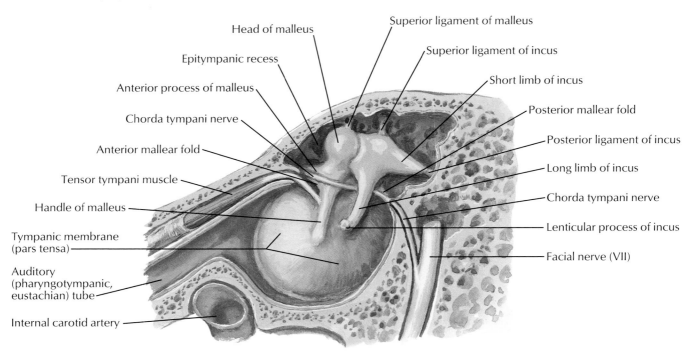

Head of malleus

Epitympanic recess

Anterior process of malleus

Chorda tympani nerve

Anterior mallear fold

Tensor tympani muscle

Handle of malleus

Tympanic membrane (pars tensa)

Auditory (pharyngotympanic, eustachian) tube

Internal carotid artery

Superior ligament of malleus

Superior ligament of incus

Short limb of incus

Posterior mallear fold

Posterior ligament of incus

Long limb of incus

Chorda tympani nerve

Lenticular process of incus

Facial nerve (VII)

Medial wall of tympanic cavity: lateral view

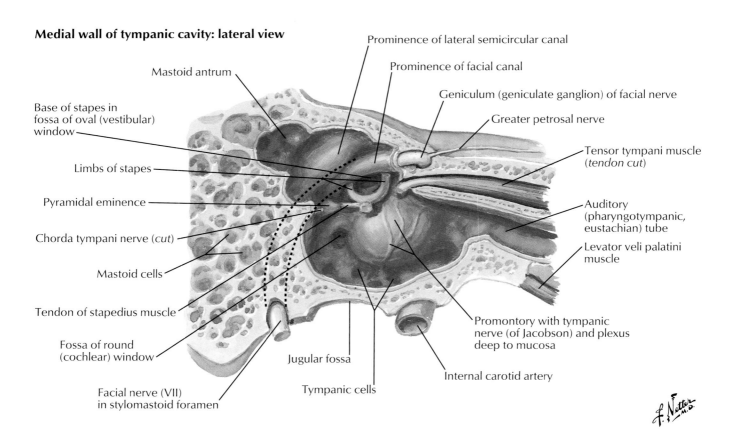

Mastoid antrum

Base of stapes in fossa of oval (vestibular) window

Limbs of stapes

Pyramidal eminence

Chorda tympani nerve (cut)

Mastoid cells

Tendon of stapedius muscle

Fossa of round (cochlear) window

Facial nerve (VII) in stylomastoid foramen

Jugular fossa

Tympanic cells

Prominence of lateral semicircular canal

Prominence of facial canal

Geniculum (geniculate ganglion) of facial nerve

Greater petrosal nerve

Tensor tympani muscle (tendon cut)

Auditory (pharyngotympanic, eustachian) tube

Levator veli palatini muscle

Promontory with tympanic nerve (of Jacobson) and plexus deep to mucosa

Internal carotid artery

Plate 94

Ear

Right bony labyrinth (otic capsule), anterolateral view: surrounding cancellous bone removed

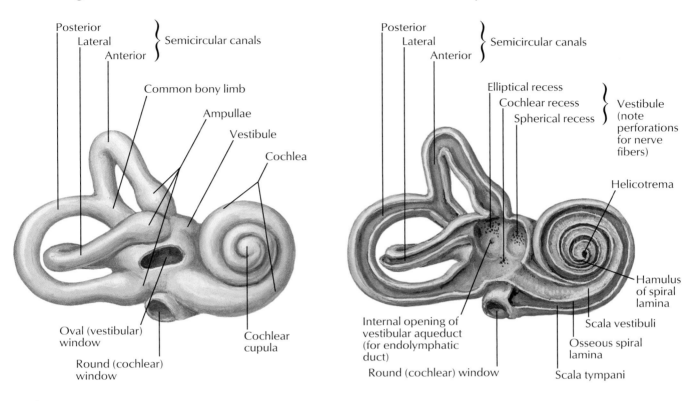

Posterior
Lateral } Semicircular canals
Anterior }

Common bony limb

Ampullae

Vestibule

Cochlea

Oval (vestibular) window

Round (cochlear) window

Cochlear cupula

Dissected right bony labyrinth (otic capsule): membranous labyrinth removed

Posterior
Lateral } Semicircular canals
Anterior }

Elliptical recess
Cochlear recess } Vestibule (note perforations for nerve fibers)
Spherical recess

Helicotrema

Hamulus of spiral lamina

Scala vestibuli

Osseous spiral lamina

Scala tympani

Internal opening of vestibular aqueduct (for endolymphatic duct)

Round (cochlear) window

Right membranous labyrinth with nerves: medial view

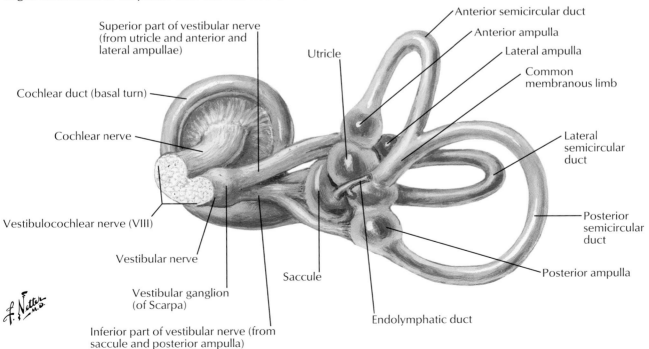

Superior part of vestibular nerve (from utricle and anterior and lateral ampullae)

Utricle

Anterior semicircular duct

Anterior ampulla

Lateral ampulla

Common membranous limb

Cochlear duct (basal turn)

Cochlear nerve

Lateral semicircular duct

Vestibulocochlear nerve (VIII)

Vestibular nerve

Vestibular ganglion (of Scarpa)

Saccule

Posterior semicircular duct

Posterior ampulla

Inferior part of vestibular nerve (from saccule and posterior ampulla)

Endolymphatic duct

Bony and membranous labyrinths: schema

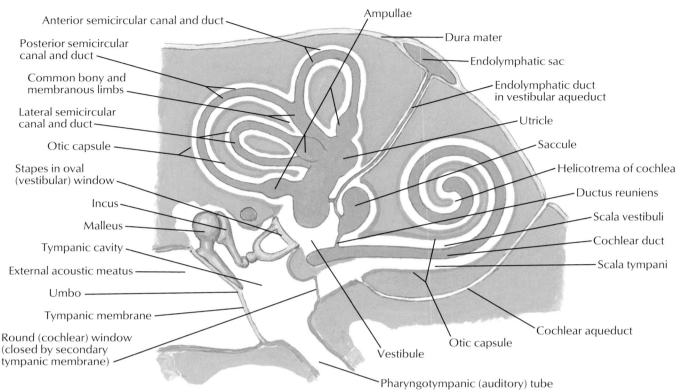

Anterior semicircular canal and duct

Posterior semicircular canal and duct

Common bony and membranous limbs

Lateral semicircular canal and duct

Otic capsule

Stapes in oval (vestibular) window

Incus

Malleus

Tympanic cavity

External acoustic meatus

Umbo

Tympanic membrane

Round (cochlear) window (closed by secondary tympanic membrane)

Ampullae

Dura mater

Endolymphatic sac

Endolymphatic duct in vestibular aqueduct

Utricle

Saccule

Helicotrema of cochlea

Ductus reuniens

Scala vestibuli

Cochlear duct

Scala tympani

Cochlear aqueduct

Otic capsule

Vestibule

Pharyngotympanic (auditory) tube

Section through turn of cochlea

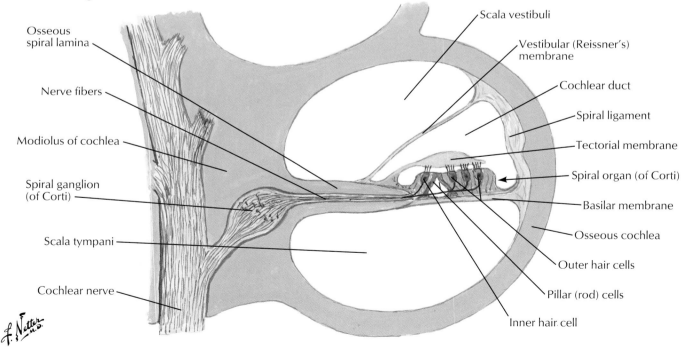

Osseous spiral lamina

Nerve fibers

Modiolus of cochlea

Spiral ganglion (of Corti)

Scala tympani

Cochlear nerve

Scala vestibuli

Vestibular (Reissner's) membrane

Cochlear duct

Spiral ligament

Tectorial membrane

Spiral organ (of Corti)

Basilar membrane

Osseous cochlea

Outer hair cells

Pillar (rod) cells

Inner hair cell

Plate 96

Ear

Superior projection of right bony labyrinth on floor of skull

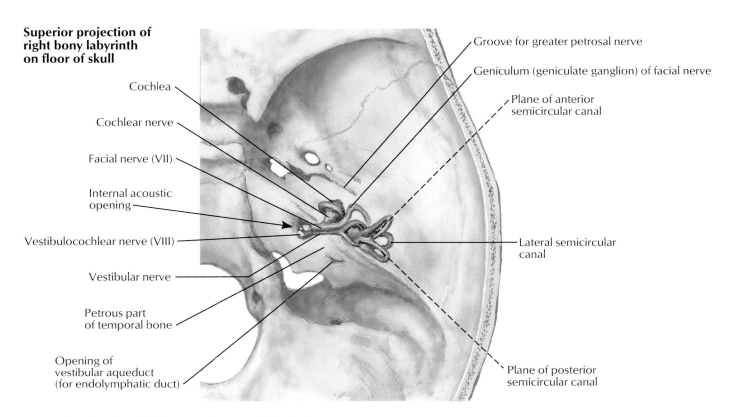

Groove for greater petrosal nerve

Geniculum (geniculate ganglion) of facial nerve

Plane of anterior semicircular canal

Cochlea

Cochlear nerve

Facial nerve (VII)

Internal acoustic opening

Vestibulocochlear nerve (VIII)

Vestibular nerve

Petrous part of temporal bone

Opening of vestibular aqueduct (for endolymphatic duct)

Lateral semicircular canal

Plane of posterior semicircular canal

Lateral projection of right membranous labyrinth

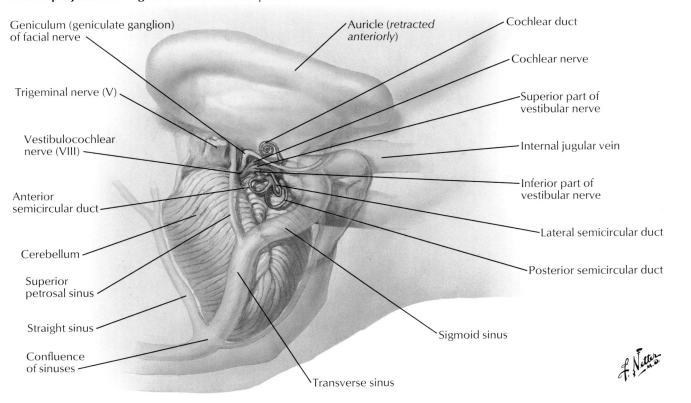

Geniculum (geniculate ganglion) of facial nerve

Auricle (*retracted anteriorly*)

Cochlear duct

Cochlear nerve

Trigeminal nerve (V)

Superior part of vestibular nerve

Vestibulocochlear nerve (VIII)

Internal jugular vein

Anterior semicircular duct

Inferior part of vestibular nerve

Cerebellum

Lateral semicircular duct

Superior petrosal sinus

Posterior semicircular duct

Straight sinus

Confluence of sinuses

Sigmoid sinus

Transverse sinus

Cartilaginous part of auditory (pharyngotympanic, eustachian) tube at base of skull: inferior view

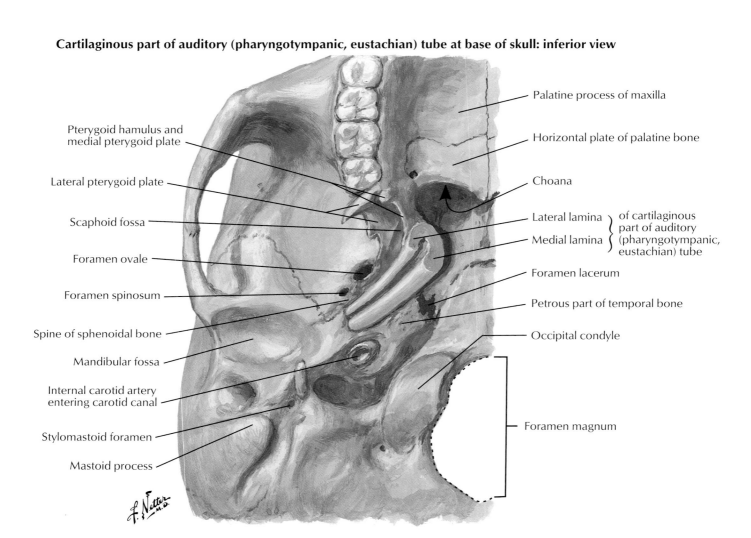

Pterygoid hamulus and medial pterygoid plate

Lateral pterygoid plate

Scaphoid fossa

Foramen ovale

Foramen spinosum

Spine of sphenoidal bone

Mandibular fossa

Internal carotid artery entering carotid canal

Stylomastoid foramen

Mastoid process

Palatine process of maxilla

Horizontal plate of palatine bone

Choana

Lateral lamina ⎱ of cartilaginous
⎰ part of auditory
Medial lamina ⎱ (pharyngotympanic,
⎰ eustachian) tube

Foramen lacerum

Petrous part of temporal bone

Occipital condyle

Foramen magnum

f. Netter M.D.

Plate 98

Ear

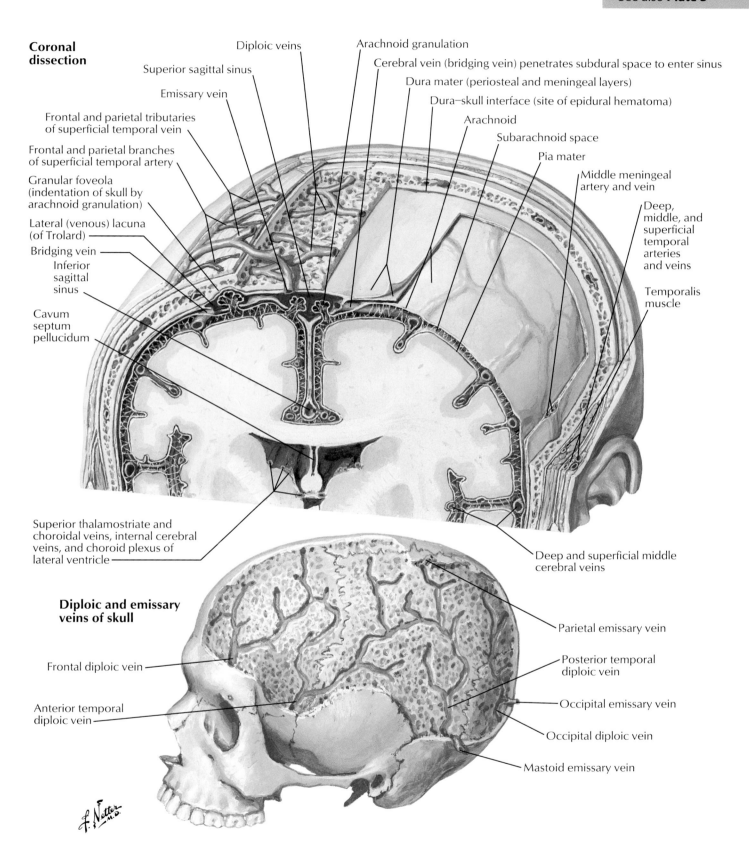

Coronal dissection

Diploic veins

Superior sagittal sinus

Emissary vein

Frontal and parietal tributaries of superficial temporal vein

Frontal and parietal branches of superficial temporal artery

Granular foveola (indentation of skull by arachnoid granulation)

Lateral (venous) lacuna (of Trolard)

Bridging vein

Inferior sagittal sinus

Cavum septum pellucidum

Arachnoid granulation

Cerebral vein (bridging vein) penetrates subdural space to enter sinus

Dura mater (periosteal and meningeal layers)

Dura–skull interface (site of epidural hematoma)

Arachnoid

Subarachnoid space

Pia mater

Middle meningeal artery and vein

Deep, middle, and superficial temporal arteries and veins

Temporalis muscle

Superior thalamostriate and choroidal veins, internal cerebral veins, and choroid plexus of lateral ventricle

Deep and superficial middle cerebral veins

Diploic and emissary veins of skull

Frontal diploic vein

Anterior temporal diploic vein

Parietal emissary vein

Posterior temporal diploic vein

Occipital emissary vein

Occipital diploic vein

Mastoid emissary vein

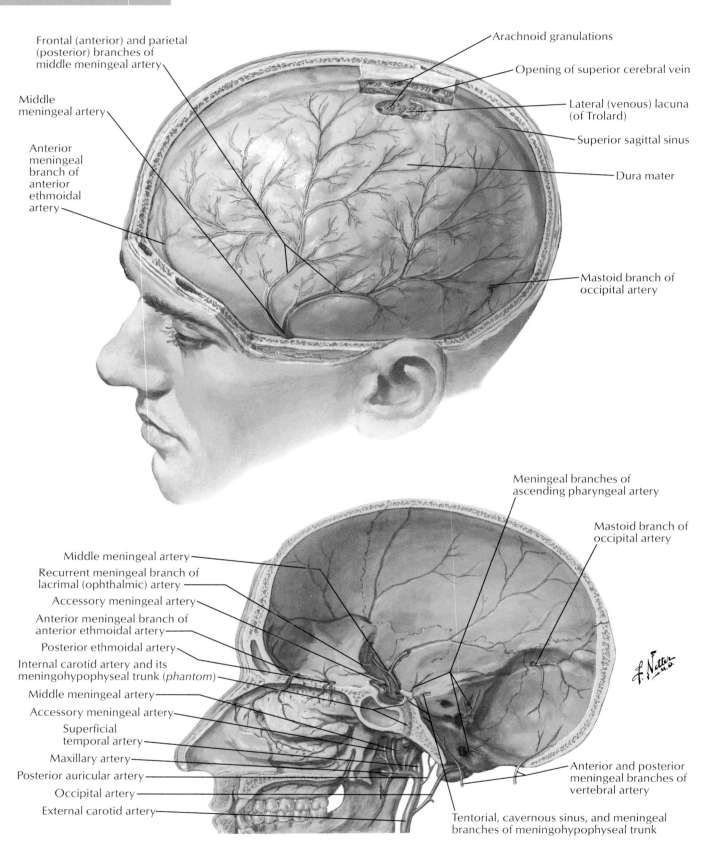

Frontal (anterior) and parietal (posterior) branches of middle meningeal artery

Middle meningeal artery

Anterior meningeal branch of anterior ethmoidal artery

Arachnoid granulations

Opening of superior cerebral vein

Lateral (venous) lacuna (of Trolard)

Superior sagittal sinus

Dura mater

Mastoid branch of occipital artery

Meningeal branches of ascending pharyngeal artery

Mastoid branch of occipital artery

Middle meningeal artery

Recurrent meningeal branch of lacrimal (ophthalmic) artery

Accessory meningeal artery

Anterior meningeal branch of anterior ethmoidal artery

Posterior ethmoidal artery

Internal carotid artery and its meningohypophyseal trunk (*phantom*)

Middle meningeal artery

Accessory meningeal artery

Superficial temporal artery

Maxillary artery

Posterior auricular artery

Occipital artery

External carotid artery

Anterior and posterior meningeal branches of vertebral artery

Tentorial, cavernous sinus, and meningeal branches of meningohypophyseal trunk

Plate 100   **Meninges and Brain**

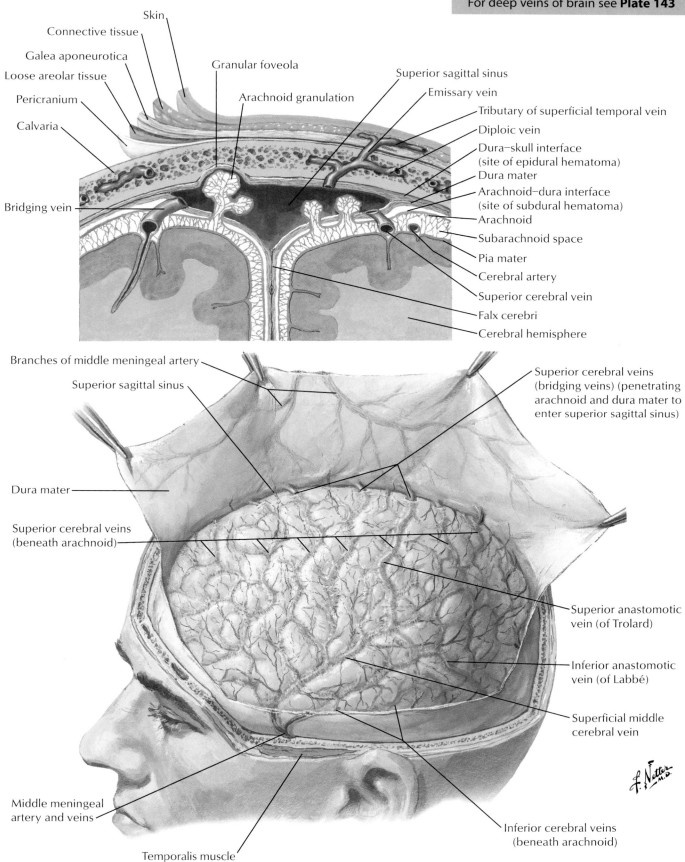

Skin

Connective tissue

Galea aponeurotica

Loose areolar tissue

Pericranium

Calvaria

Granular foveola

Arachnoid granulation

Superior sagittal sinus

Emissary vein

Tributary of superficial temporal vein

Diploic vein

Dura–skull interface (site of epidural hematoma)

Dura mater

Arachnoid–dura interface (site of subdural hematoma)

Arachnoid

Subarachnoid space

Pia mater

Cerebral artery

Superior cerebral vein

Falx cerebri

Cerebral hemisphere

Bridging vein

Branches of middle meningeal artery

Superior sagittal sinus

Dura mater

Superior cerebral veins (beneath arachnoid)

Middle meningeal artery and veins

Temporalis muscle

Superior cerebral veins (bridging veins) (penetrating arachnoid and dura mater to enter superior sagittal sinus)

Superior anastomotic vein (of Trolard)

Inferior anastomotic vein (of Labbé)

Superficial middle cerebral vein

Inferior cerebral veins (beneath arachnoid)

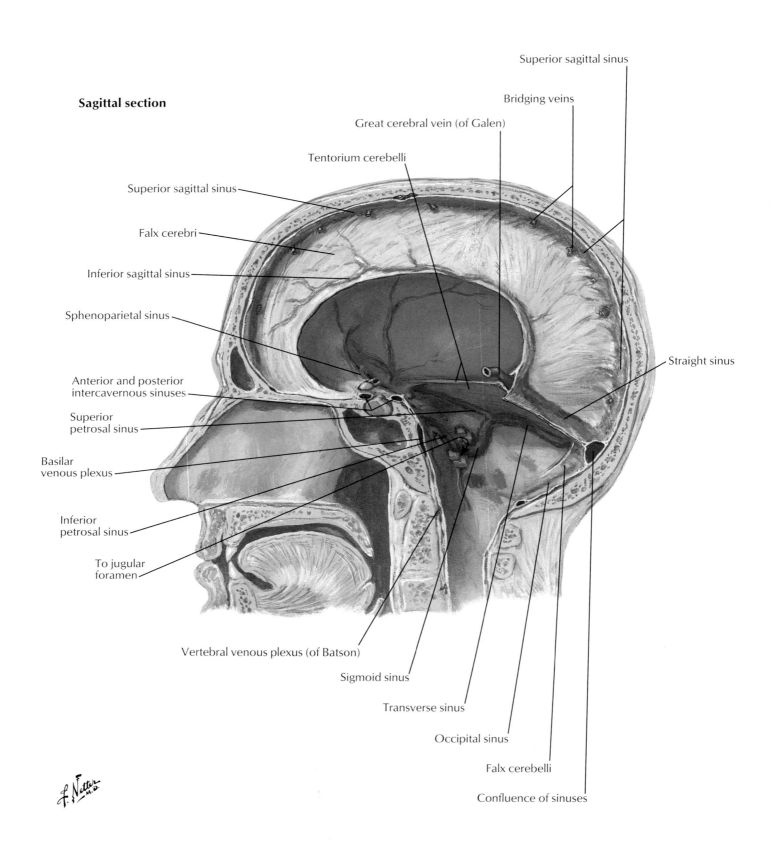

Sagittal section

Superior sagittal sinus

Bridging veins

Great cerebral vein (of Galen)

Tentorium cerebelli

Superior sagittal sinus

Falx cerebri

Inferior sagittal sinus

Sphenoparietal sinus

Straight sinus

Anterior and posterior intercavernous sinuses

Superior petrosal sinus

Basilar venous plexus

Inferior petrosal sinus

To jugular foramen

Vertebral venous plexus (of Batson)

Sigmoid sinus

Transverse sinus

Occipital sinus

Falx cerebelli

Confluence of sinuses

f. Netter.

Plate 102 **Meninges and Brain**

See also **Plate 85**

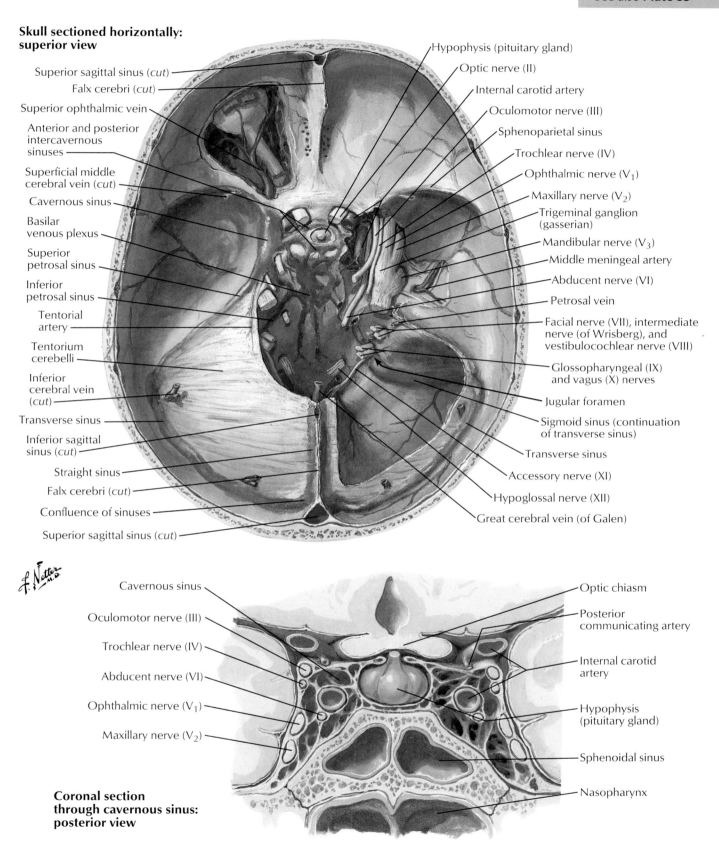

Skull sectioned horizontally: superior view

Superior sagittal sinus (*cut*)

Falx cerebri (*cut*)

Superior ophthalmic vein

Anterior and posterior intercavernous sinuses

Superficial middle cerebral vein (*cut*)

Cavernous sinus

Basilar venous plexus

Superior petrosal sinus

Inferior petrosal sinus

Tentorial artery

Tentorium cerebelli

Inferior cerebral vein (*cut*)

Transverse sinus

Inferior sagittal sinus (*cut*)

Straight sinus

Falx cerebri (*cut*)

Confluence of sinuses

Superior sagittal sinus (*cut*)

Hypophysis (pituitary gland)

Optic nerve (II)

Internal carotid artery

Oculomotor nerve (III)

Sphenoparietal sinus

Trochlear nerve (IV)

Ophthalmic nerve (V$_1$)

Maxillary nerve (V$_2$)

Trigeminal ganglion (gasserian)

Mandibular nerve (V$_3$)

Middle meningeal artery

Abducent nerve (VI)

Petrosal vein

Facial nerve (VII), intermediate nerve (of Wrisberg), and vestibulocochlear nerve (VIII)

Glossopharyngeal (IX) and vagus (X) nerves

Jugular foramen

Sigmoid sinus (continuation of transverse sinus)

Transverse sinus

Accessory nerve (XI)

Hypoglossal nerve (XII)

Great cerebral vein (of Galen)

Cavernous sinus

Oculomotor nerve (III)

Trochlear nerve (IV)

Abducent nerve (VI)

Ophthalmic nerve (V$_1$)

Maxillary nerve (V$_2$)

Optic chiasm

Posterior communicating artery

Internal carotid artery

Hypophysis (pituitary gland)

Sphenoidal sinus

Nasopharynx

Coronal section through cavernous sinus: posterior view

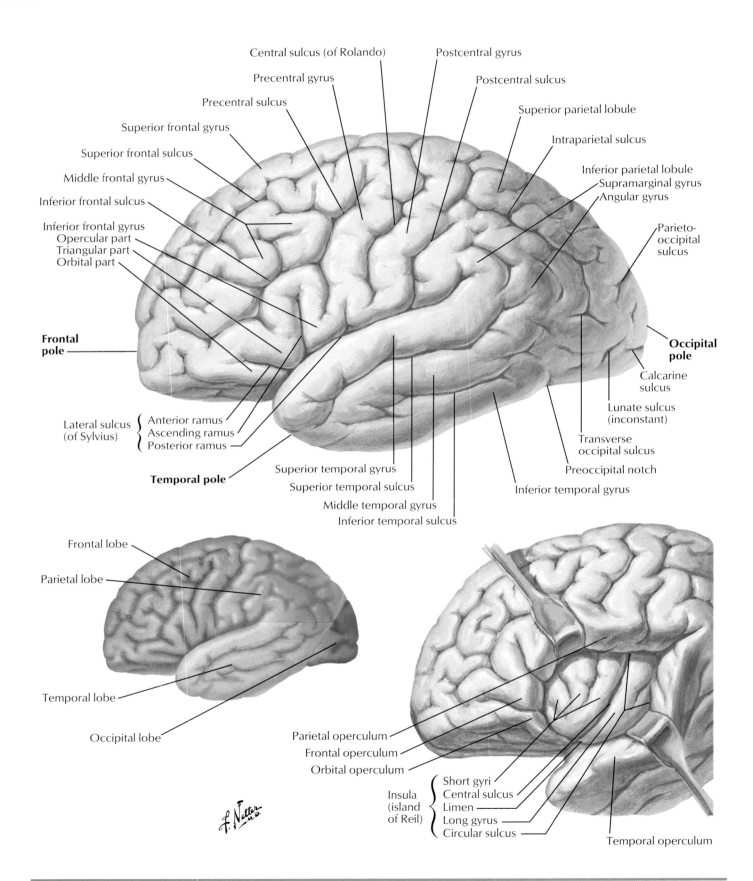

Central sulcus (of Rolando)

Precentral gyrus

Precentral sulcus

Superior frontal gyrus

Superior frontal sulcus

Middle frontal gyrus

Inferior frontal sulcus

Inferior frontal gyrus
Opercular part
Triangular part
Orbital part

Frontal pole

Lateral sulcus
(of Sylvius)
{ Anterior ramus
Ascending ramus
Posterior ramus

Temporal pole

Postcentral gyrus

Postcentral sulcus

Superior parietal lobule

Intraparietal sulcus

Inferior parietal lobule
Supramarginal gyrus
Angular gyrus

Parieto-occipital sulcus

Occipital pole

Calcarine sulcus

Lunate sulcus (inconstant)

Transverse occipital sulcus

Preoccipital notch

Inferior temporal gyrus

Superior temporal gyrus

Superior temporal sulcus

Middle temporal gyrus

Inferior temporal sulcus

Frontal lobe

Parietal lobe

Temporal lobe

Occipital lobe

Parietal operculum

Frontal operculum

Orbital operculum

Insula
(island
of Reil)
{ Short gyri
Central sulcus
Limen
Long gyrus
Circular sulcus

Temporal operculum

Plate 104

Meninges and Brain

Sagittal section of brain in situ

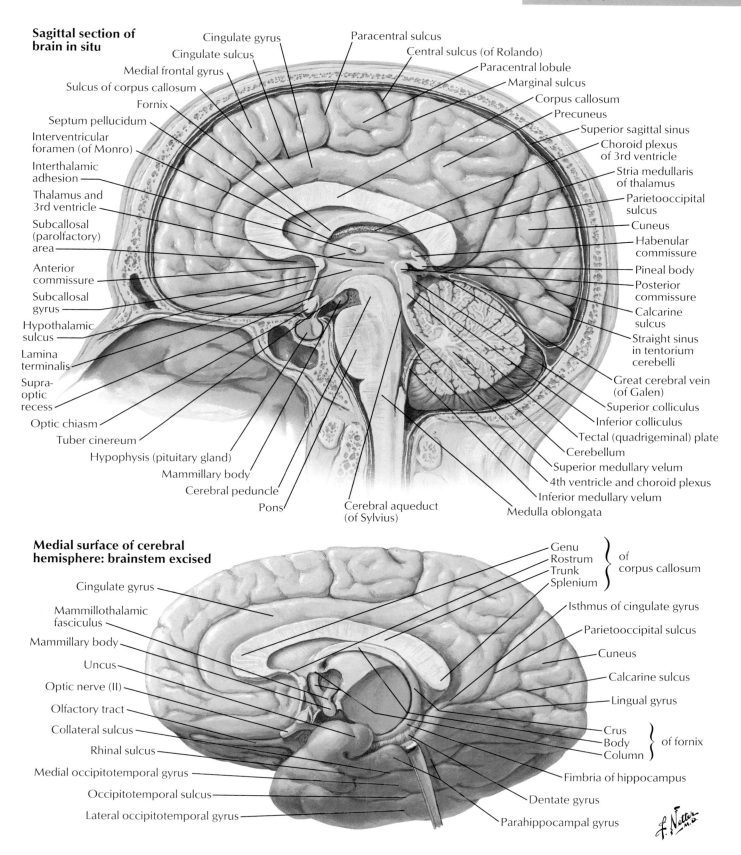

Cinqulate gyrus
Cingulate sulcus
Medial frontal gyrus
Sulcus of corpus callosum
Fornix
Septum pellucidum
Interventricular foramen (of Monro)
Interthalamic adhesion
Thalamus and 3rd ventricle
Subcallosal (parolfactory) area
Anterior commissure
Subcallosal gyrus
Hypothalamic sulcus
Lamina terminalis
Supra-optic recess
Optic chiasm
Tuber cinereum
Hypophysis (pituitary gland)
Mammillary body
Cerebral peduncle
Pons
Cerebral aqueduct (of Sylvius)

Paracentral sulcus
Central sulcus (of Rolando)
Paracentral lobule
Marginal sulcus
Corpus callosum
Precuneus
Superior sagittal sinus
Choroid plexus of 3rd ventricle
Stria medullaris of thalamus
Parietooccipital sulcus
Cuneus
Habenular commissure
Pineal body
Posterior commissure
Calcarine sulcus
Straight sinus in tentorium cerebelli
Great cerebral vein (of Galen)
Superior colliculus
Inferior colliculus
Tectal (quadrigeminal) plate
Cerebellum
Superior medullary velum
4th ventricle and choroid plexus
Inferior medullary velum
Medulla oblongata

Medial surface of cerebral hemisphere: brainstem excised

Cingulate gyrus
Mammillothalamic fasciculus
Mammillary body
Uncus
Optic nerve (II)
Olfactory tract
Collateral sulcus
Rhinal sulcus
Medial occipitotemporal gyrus
Occipitotemporal sulcus
Lateral occipitotemporal gyrus

Genu
Rostrum
Trunk
Splenium
} of corpus callosum
Isthmus of cingulate gyrus
Parietooccipital sulcus
Cuneus
Calcarine sulcus
Lingual gyrus
Crus
Body
Column
} of fornix
Fimbria of hippocampus
Dentate gyrus
Parahippocampal gyrus

Sectioned brainstem

Frontal pole of cerebrum

Straight gyrus

Olfactory sulcus

Orbital sulci

Orbital gyri

Temporal pole of cerebrum

Lateral sulcus (of Sylvius)

Inferior temporal sulcus

Inferior temporal gyrus

Inferior (infero-lateral) margin of cerebrum

Rhinal sulcus

Uncus

Inferior temporal gyrus

Occipitotemporal sulcus

Lateral occipito-temporal gyrus

Collateral sulcus

Parahippocampal gyrus

Medial occipitotemporal gyrus

Calcarine sulcus

Isthmus of cingulate gyrus

Longitudinal cerebral fissure

Genu of corpus callosum

Lamina terminalis

Olfactory bulb

Olfactory tract

Optic chiasm

Optic nerve (II) (cut)

Hypophysis (pituitary gland)

Anterior perforated substance

Optic tract

Tuber cinereum

Mammillary body

Posterior perforated substance (in interpeduncular fossa)

Cerebral crus

Lateral geniculate body

Substantia nigra

Medial geniculate body

Red nucleus

Pulvinar of thalamus

Superior colliculus (of corpora quadrigemina)

Cerebral aqueduct

Splenium of corpus callosum

Apex of cuneus

Occipital pole of cerebrum

Longitudinal cerebral fissure

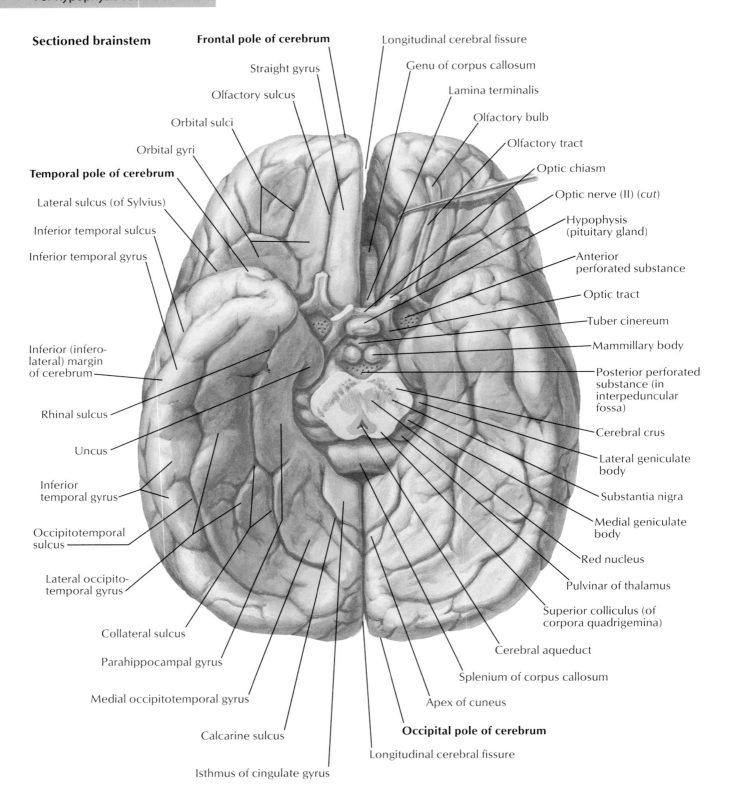

Plate 106

Meninges and Brain

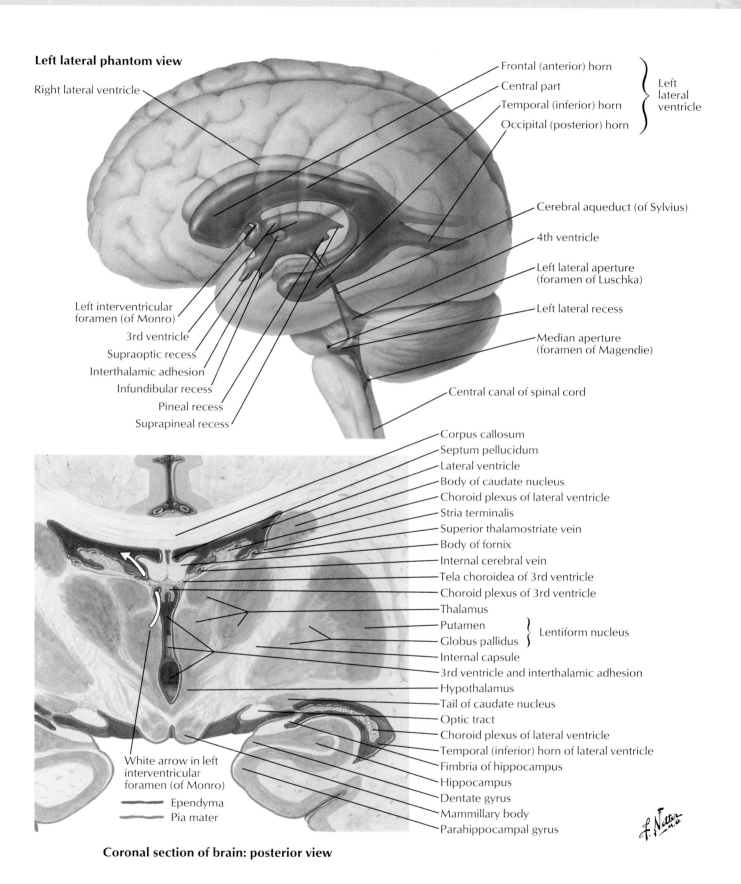

Left lateral phantom view

Right lateral ventricle

Frontal (anterior) horn
Central part
Temporal (inferior) horn
Occipital (posterior) horn
} Left lateral ventricle

Cerebral aqueduct (of Sylvius)

4th ventricle

Left lateral aperture (foramen of Luschka)

Left lateral recess

Left interventricular foramen (of Monro)
3rd ventricle
Supraoptic recess
Interthalamic adhesion
Infundibular recess
Pineal recess
Suprapineal recess

Median aperture (foramen of Magendie)

Central canal of spinal cord

Corpus callosum
Septum pellucidum
Lateral ventricle
Body of caudate nucleus
Choroid plexus of lateral ventricle
Stria terminalis
Superior thalamostriate vein
Body of fornix
Internal cerebral vein
Tela choroidea of 3rd ventricle
Choroid plexus of 3rd ventricle
Thalamus
Putamen
Globus pallidus
} Lentiform nucleus
Internal capsule
3rd ventricle and interthalamic adhesion
Hypothalamus
Tail of caudate nucleus
Optic tract
Choroid plexus of lateral ventricle
Temporal (inferior) horn of lateral ventricle
Fimbria of hippocampus
Hippocampus
Dentate gyrus
Mammillary body
Parahippocampal gyrus

White arrow in left interventricular foramen (of Monro)
Ependyma
Pia mater

Coronal section of brain: posterior view

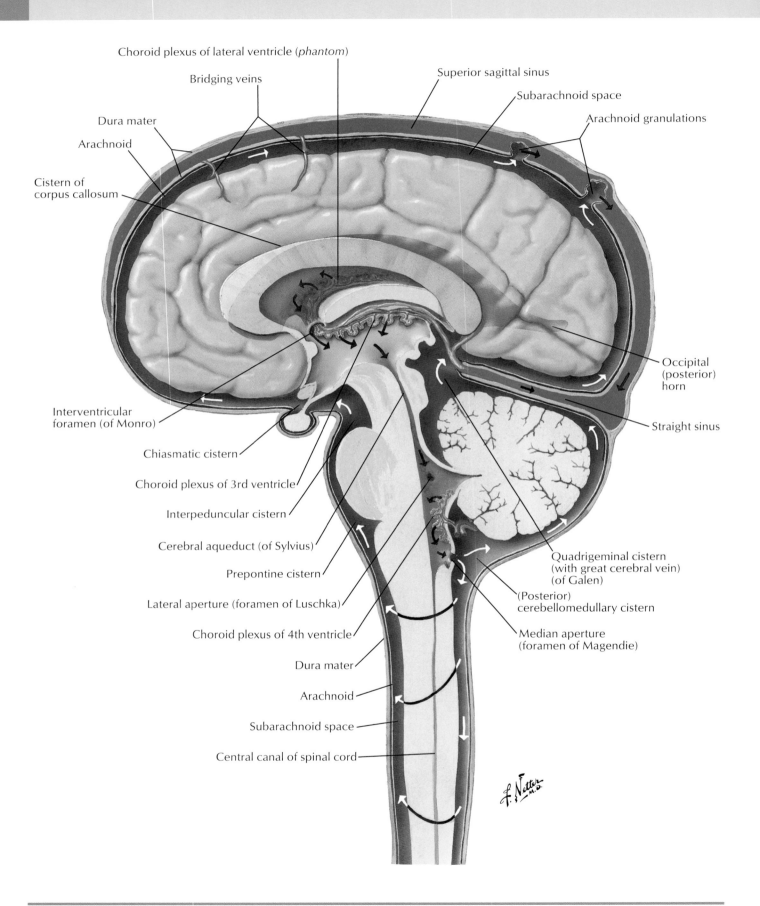

Choroid plexus of lateral ventricle (*phantom*)

Bridging veins

Dura mater

Arachnoid

Cistern of corpus callosum

Superior sagittal sinus

Subarachnoid space

Arachnoid granulations

Occipital (posterior) horn

Straight sinus

Interventricular foramen (of Monro)

Chiasmatic cistern

Choroid plexus of 3rd ventricle

Interpeduncular cistern

Cerebral aqueduct (of Sylvius)

Prepontine cistern

Lateral aperture (foramen of Luschka)

Choroid plexus of 4th ventricle

Dura mater

Arachnoid

Subarachnoid space

Central canal of spinal cord

Quadrigeminal cistern (with great cerebral vein) (of Galen)

(Posterior) cerebellomedullary cistern

Median aperture (foramen of Magendie)

Plate 108

Meninges and Brain

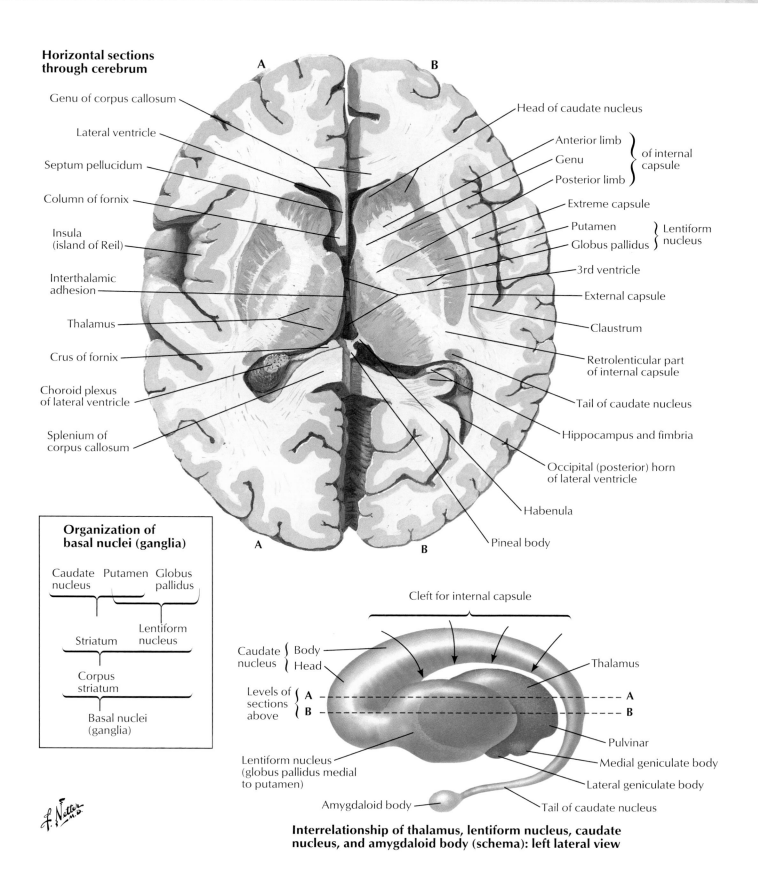

Horizontal sections through cerebrum

Genu of corpus callosum

Lateral ventricle

Septum pellucidum

Column of fornix

Insula (island of Reil)

Interthalamic adhesion

Thalamus

Crus of fornix

Choroid plexus of lateral ventricle

Splenium of corpus callosum

A

B

Head of caudate nucleus

Anterior limb

Genu

Posterior limb

} of internal capsule

Extreme capsule

Putamen

Globus pallidus

} Lentiform nucleus

3rd ventricle

External capsule

Claustrum

Retrolenticular part of internal capsule

Tail of caudate nucleus

Hippocampus and fimbria

Occipital (posterior) horn of lateral ventricle

Habenula

Pineal body

A

B

Organization of basal nuclei (ganglia)

Caudate nucleus   Putamen   Globus pallidus

Lentiform nucleus

Striatum

Corpus striatum

Basal nuclei (ganglia)

Cleft for internal capsule

Caudate nucleus { Body / Head

Thalamus

Levels of sections above { A / B

A

B

Pulvinar

Medial geniculate body

Lateral geniculate body

Tail of caudate nucleus

Lentiform nucleus (globus pallidus medial to putamen)

Amygdaloid body

Interrelationship of thalamus, lentiform nucleus, caudate nucleus, and amygdaloid body (schema): left lateral view

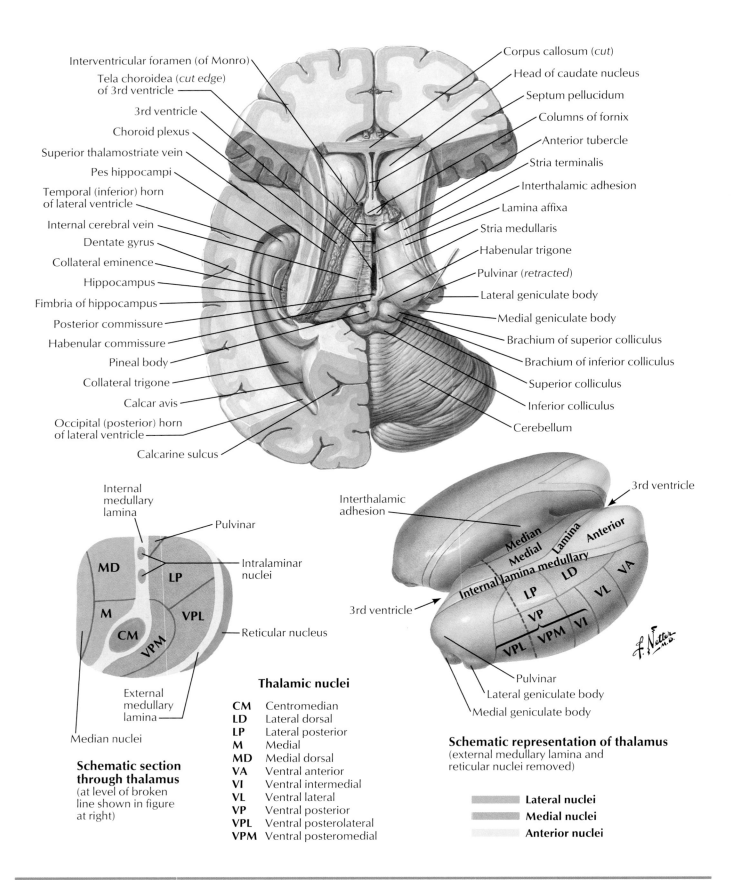

Interventricular foramen (of Monro)

Tela choroidea (*cut edge*) of 3rd ventricle

3rd ventricle

Choroid plexus

Superior thalamostriate vein

Pes hippocampi

Temporal (inferior) horn of lateral ventricle

Internal cerebral vein

Dentate gyrus

Collateral eminence

Hippocampus

Fimbria of hippocampus

Posterior commissure

Habenular commissure

Pineal body

Collateral trigone

Calcar avis

Occipital (posterior) horn of lateral ventricle

Calcarine sulcus

Corpus callosum (*cut*)

Head of caudate nucleus

Septum pellucidum

Columns of fornix

Anterior tubercle

Stria terminalis

Interthalamic adhesion

Lamina affixa

Stria medullaris

Habenular trigone

Pulvinar (*retracted*)

Lateral geniculate body

Medial geniculate body

Brachium of superior colliculus

Brachium of inferior colliculus

Superior colliculus

Inferior colliculus

Cerebellum

Internal medullary lamina

Pulvinar

Intralaminar nuclei

Reticular nucleus

MD

LP

M

CM

VPM

VPL

External medullary lamina

Median nuclei

Schematic section through thalamus (at level of broken line shown in figure at right)

Interthalamic adhesion

3rd ventricle

3rd ventricle

Median

Medial

Lamina

Anterior

Internal lamina medullary

LD

VA

LP

VL

VP

VI

VPL

VPM

Pulvinar

Lateral geniculate body

Medial geniculate body

Schematic representation of thalamus (external medullary lamina and reticular nuclei removed)

Thalamic nuclei

CM	Centromedian
LD	Lateral dorsal
LP	Lateral posterior
M	Medial
MD	Medial dorsal
VA	Ventral anterior
VI	Ventral intermedial
VL	Ventral lateral
VP	Ventral posterior
VPL	Ventral posterolateral
VPM	Ventral posteromedial

Lateral nuclei
Medial nuclei
Anterior nuclei

Plate 110
Meninges and Brain

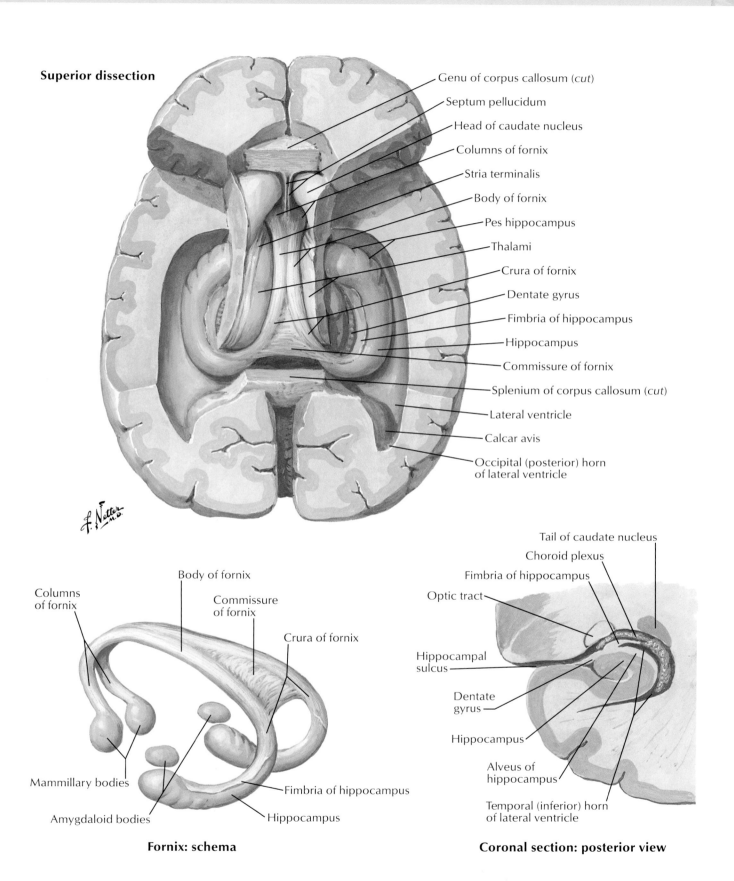

Superior dissection

Genu of corpus callosum (*cut*)

Septum pellucidum

Head of caudate nucleus

Columns of fornix

Stria terminalis

Body of fornix

Pes hippocampus

Thalami

Crura of fornix

Dentate gyrus

Fimbria of hippocampus

Hippocampus

Commissure of fornix

Splenium of corpus callosum (*cut*)

Lateral ventricle

Calcar avis

Occipital (posterior) horn of lateral ventricle

Columns of fornix

Body of fornix

Commissure of fornix

Crura of fornix

Mammillary bodies

Amygdaloid bodies

Fimbria of hippocampus

Hippocampus

Fornix: schema

Tail of caudate nucleus

Choroid plexus

Fimbria of hippocampus

Optic tract

Hippocampal sulcus

Dentate gyrus

Hippocampus

Alveus of hippocampus

Temporal (inferior) horn of lateral ventricle

Coronal section: posterior view

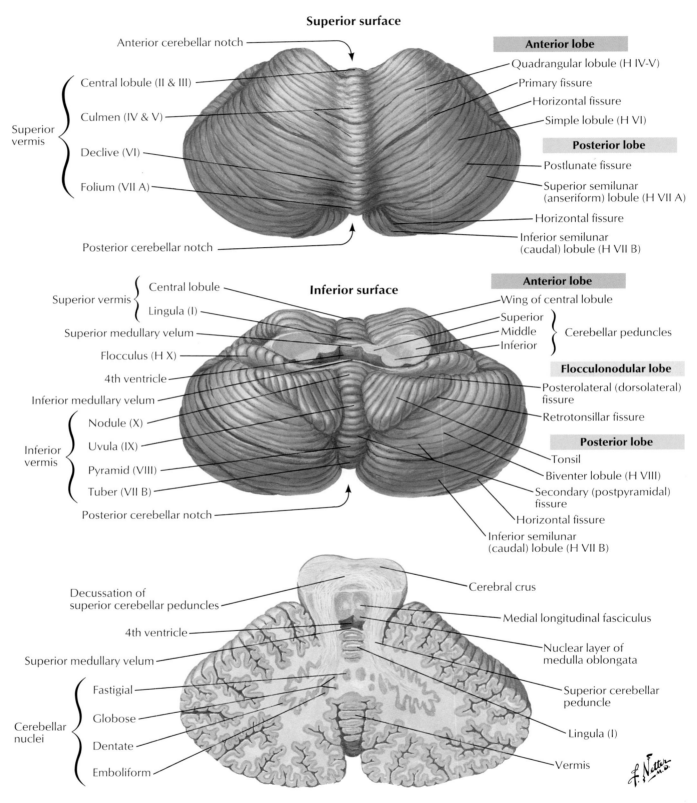

Superior surface

Anterior cerebellar notch

Anterior lobe

Quadrangular lobule (H IV-V)

Primary fissure

Horizontal fissure

Simple lobule (H VI)

Posterior lobe

Postlunate fissure

Superior semilunar (anseriform) lobule (H VII A)

Horizontal fissure

Inferior semilunar (caudal) lobule (H VII B)

Central lobule (II & III)

Culmen (IV & V)

Declive (VI)

Folium (VII A)

Superior vermis

Posterior cerebellar notch

Inferior surface

Superior vermis

Central lobule

Lingula (I)

Superior medullary velum

Flocculus (H X)

4th ventricle

Inferior medullary velum

Nodule (X)

Uvula (IX)

Pyramid (VIII)

Tuber (VII B)

Inferior vermis

Posterior cerebellar notch

Anterior lobe

Wing of central lobule

Superior

Middle

Inferior

Cerebellar peduncles

Flocculonodular lobe

Posterolateral (dorsolateral) fissure

Retrotonsillar fissure

Posterior lobe

Tonsil

Biventer lobule (H VIII)

Secondary (postpyramidal) fissure

Horizontal fissure

Inferior semilunar (caudal) lobule (H VII B)

Decussation of superior cerebellar peduncles

4th ventricle

Superior medullary velum

Fastigial

Globose

Dentate

Emboliform

Cerebellar nuclei

Cerebral crus

Medial longitudinal fasciculus

Nuclear layer of medulla oblongata

Superior cerebellar peduncle

Lingula (I)

Vermis

Section in plane of superior cerebellar peduncle

Plate 112 **Meninges and Brain**

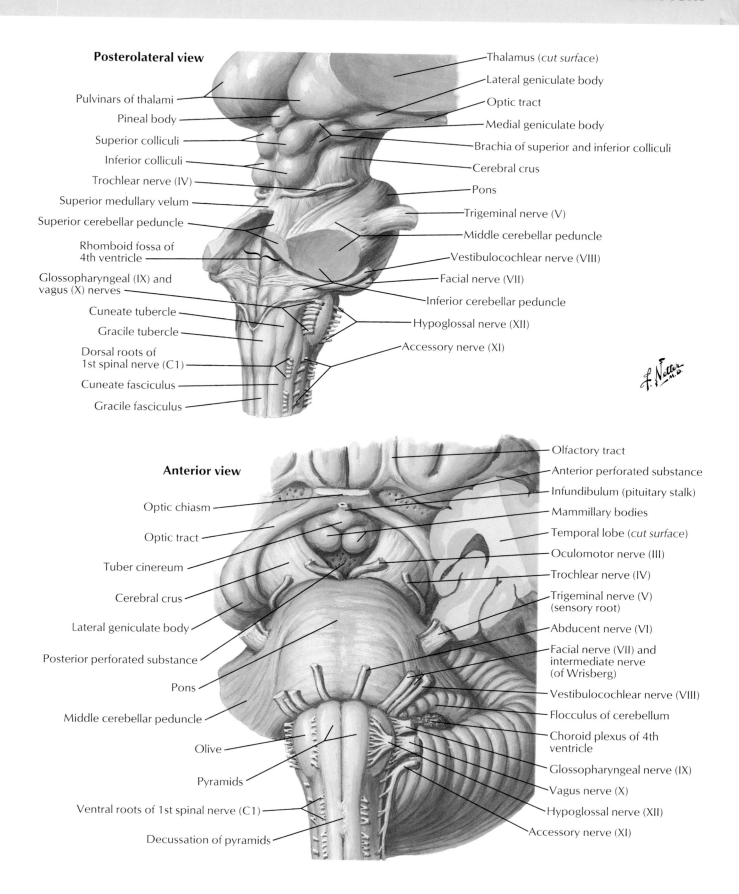

Posterolateral view

Pulvinars of thalami
Pineal body
Superior colliculi
Inferior colliculi
Trochlear nerve (IV)
Superior medullary velum
Superior cerebellar peduncle
Rhomboid fossa of 4th ventricle
Glossopharyngeal (IX) and vagus (X) nerves
Cuneate tubercle
Gracile tubercle
Dorsal roots of 1st spinal nerve (C1)
Cuneate fasciculus
Gracile fasciculus

Thalamus (*cut surface*)
Lateral geniculate body
Optic tract
Medial geniculate body
Brachia of superior and inferior colliculi
Cerebral crus
Pons
Trigeminal nerve (V)
Middle cerebellar peduncle
Vestibulocochlear nerve (VIII)
Facial nerve (VII)
Inferior cerebellar peduncle
Hypoglossal nerve (XII)
Accessory nerve (XI)

F. Netter M.D.

Anterior view

Optic chiasm
Optic tract
Tuber cinereum
Cerebral crus
Lateral geniculate body
Posterior perforated substance
Pons
Middle cerebellar peduncle
Olive
Pyramids
Ventral roots of 1st spinal nerve (C1)
Decussation of pyramids

Olfactory tract
Anterior perforated substance
Infundibulum (pituitary stalk)
Mammillary bodies
Temporal lobe (*cut surface*)
Oculomotor nerve (III)
Trochlear nerve (IV)
Trigeminal nerve (V) (sensory root)
Abducent nerve (VI)
Facial nerve (VII) and intermediate nerve (of Wrisberg)
Vestibulocochlear nerve (VIII)
Flocculus of cerebellum
Choroid plexus of 4th ventricle
Glossopharyngeal nerve (IX)
Vagus nerve (X)
Hypoglossal nerve (XII)
Accessory nerve (XI)

Fourth Ventricle and Cerebellum

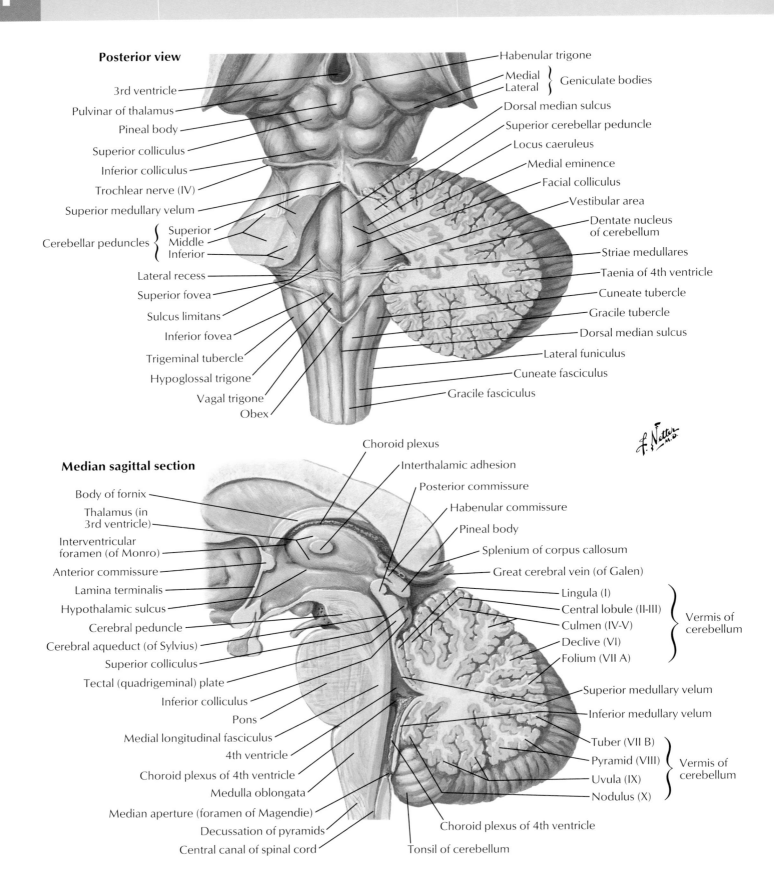

Posterior view

- Habenular trigone
- 3rd ventricle
- Pulvinar of thalamus
- Pineal body
- Superior colliculus
- Inferior colliculus
- Trochlear nerve (IV)
- Superior medullary velum
- Cerebellar peduncles { Superior / Middle / Inferior }
- Lateral recess
- Superior fovea
- Sulcus limitans
- Inferior fovea
- Trigeminal tubercle
- Hypoglossal trigone
- Vagal trigone
- Obex
- Medial / Lateral } Geniculate bodies
- Dorsal median sulcus
- Superior cerebellar peduncle
- Locus caeruleus
- Medial eminence
- Facial colliculus
- Vestibular area
- Dentate nucleus of cerebellum
- Striae medullares
- Taenia of 4th ventricle
- Cuneate tubercle
- Gracile tubercle
- Dorsal median sulcus
- Lateral funiculus
- Cuneate fasciculus
- Gracile fasciculus

f. Netter m.d.

Median sagittal section

- Choroid plexus
- Interthalamic adhesion
- Posterior commissure
- Habenular commissure
- Pineal body
- Splenium of corpus callosum
- Great cerebral vein (of Galen)
- Body of fornix
- Thalamus (in 3rd ventricle)
- Interventricular foramen (of Monro)
- Anterior commissure
- Lamina terminalis
- Hypothalamic sulcus
- Cerebral peduncle
- Cerebral aqueduct (of Sylvius)
- Superior colliculus
- Tectal (quadrigeminal) plate
- Inferior colliculus
- Pons
- Medial longitudinal fasciculus
- 4th ventricle
- Choroid plexus of 4th ventricle
- Medulla oblongata
- Median aperture (foramen of Magendie)
- Decussation of pyramids
- Central canal of spinal cord
- Lingula (I)
- Central lobule (II-III)
- Culmen (IV-V)
- Declive (VI)
- Folium (VII A)
  } Vermis of cerebellum
- Superior medullary velum
- Inferior medullary velum
- Tuber (VII B)
- Pyramid (VIII)
- Uvula (IX)
- Nodulus (X)
  } Vermis of cerebellum
- Choroid plexus of 4th ventricle
- Tonsil of cerebellum

Plate 114 **Meninges and Brain**

Posterior phantom view

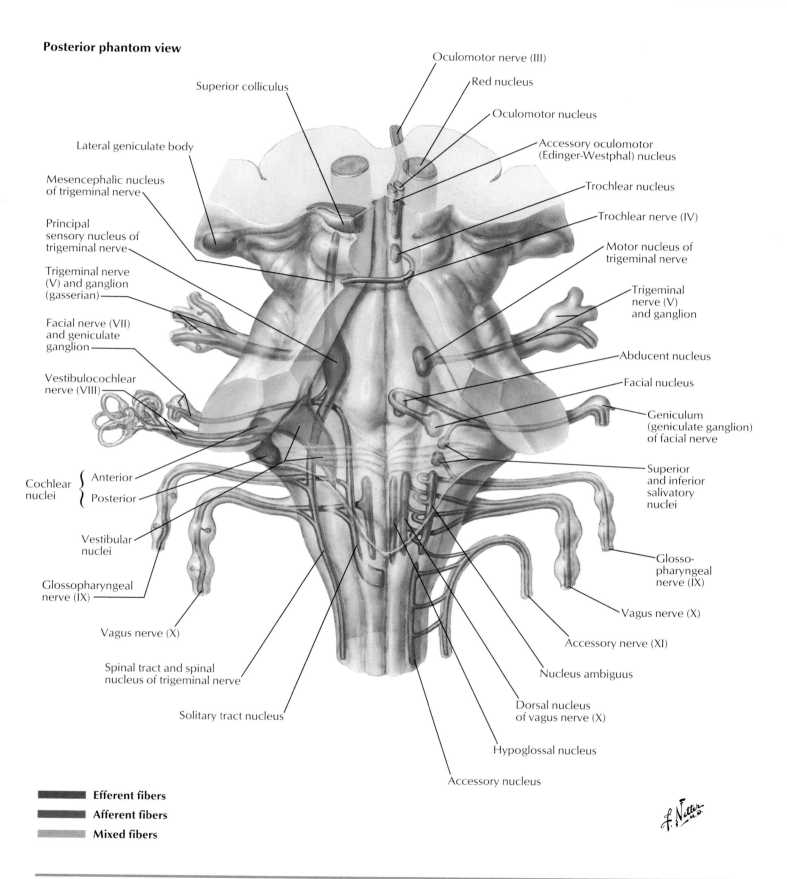

Superior colliculus

Oculomotor nerve (III)

Red nucleus

Oculomotor nucleus

Accessory oculomotor
(Edinger-Westphal) nucleus

Lateral geniculate body

Trochlear nucleus

Mesencephalic nucleus
of trigeminal nerve

Trochlear nerve (IV)

Principal
sensory nucleus of
trigeminal nerve

Motor nucleus of
trigeminal nerve

Trigeminal nerve
(V) and ganglion
(gasserian)

Trigeminal
nerve (V)
and ganglion

Facial nerve (VII)
and geniculate
ganglion

Abducent nucleus

Facial nucleus

Vestibulocochlear
nerve (VIII)

Geniculum
(geniculate ganglion)
of facial nerve

Cochlear
nuclei { Anterior

Posterior

Superior
and inferior
salivatory
nuclei

Vestibular
nuclei

Glosso-
pharyngeal
nerve (IX)

Glossopharyngeal
nerve (IX)

Vagus nerve (X)

Vagus nerve (X)

Spinal tract and spinal
nucleus of trigeminal nerve

Accessory nerve (XI)

Nucleus ambiguus

Solitary tract nucleus

Dorsal nucleus
of vagus nerve (X)

Hypoglossal nucleus

Accessory nucleus

▬▬▬ **Efferent fibers**

▬▬▬ **Afferent fibers**

▬▬▬ **Mixed fibers**

Cranial Nerve Nuclei in Brainstem: Schema (continued)

Medial dissection

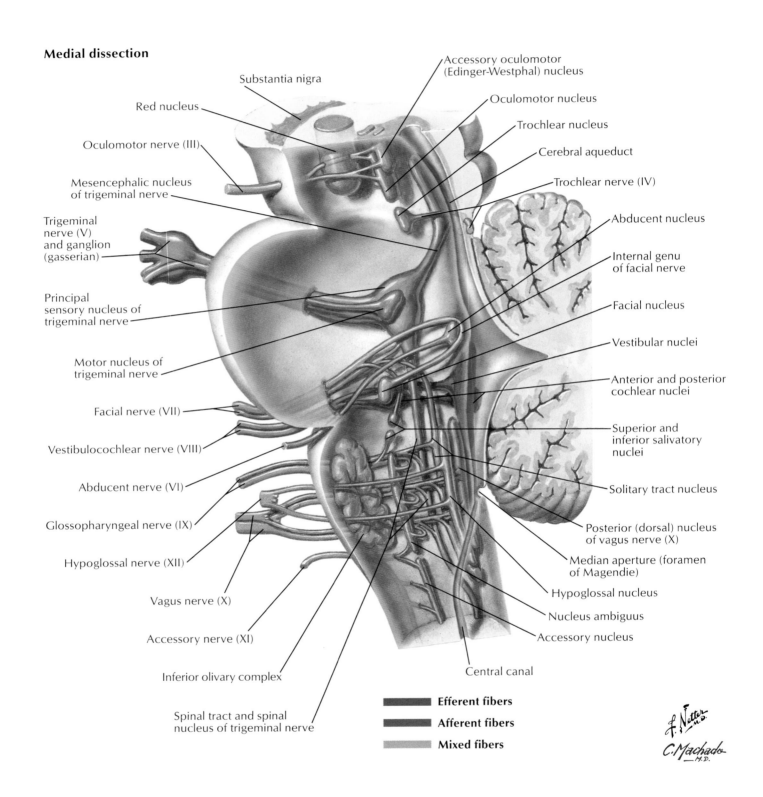

Substantia nigra

Red nucleus

Oculomotor nerve (III)

Mesencephalic nucleus of trigeminal nerve

Trigeminal nerve (V) and ganglion (gasserian)

Principal sensory nucleus of trigeminal nerve

Motor nucleus of trigeminal nerve

Facial nerve (VII)

Vestibulocochlear nerve (VIII)

Abducent nerve (VI)

Glossopharyngeal nerve (IX)

Hypoglossal nerve (XII)

Vagus nerve (X)

Accessory nerve (XI)

Inferior olivary complex

Spinal tract and spinal nucleus of trigeminal nerve

Accessory oculomotor (Edinger-Westphal) nucleus

Oculomotor nucleus

Trochlear nucleus

Cerebral aqueduct

Trochlear nerve (IV)

Abducent nucleus

Internal genu of facial nerve

Facial nucleus

Vestibular nuclei

Anterior and posterior cochlear nuclei

Superior and inferior salivatory nuclei

Solitary tract nucleus

Posterior (dorsal) nucleus of vagus nerve (X)

Median aperture (foramen of Magendie)

Hypoglossal nucleus

Nucleus ambiguus

Accessory nucleus

Central canal

Efferent fibers
Afferent fibers
Mixed fibers

Plate 116   **Cranial and Cervical Nerves**

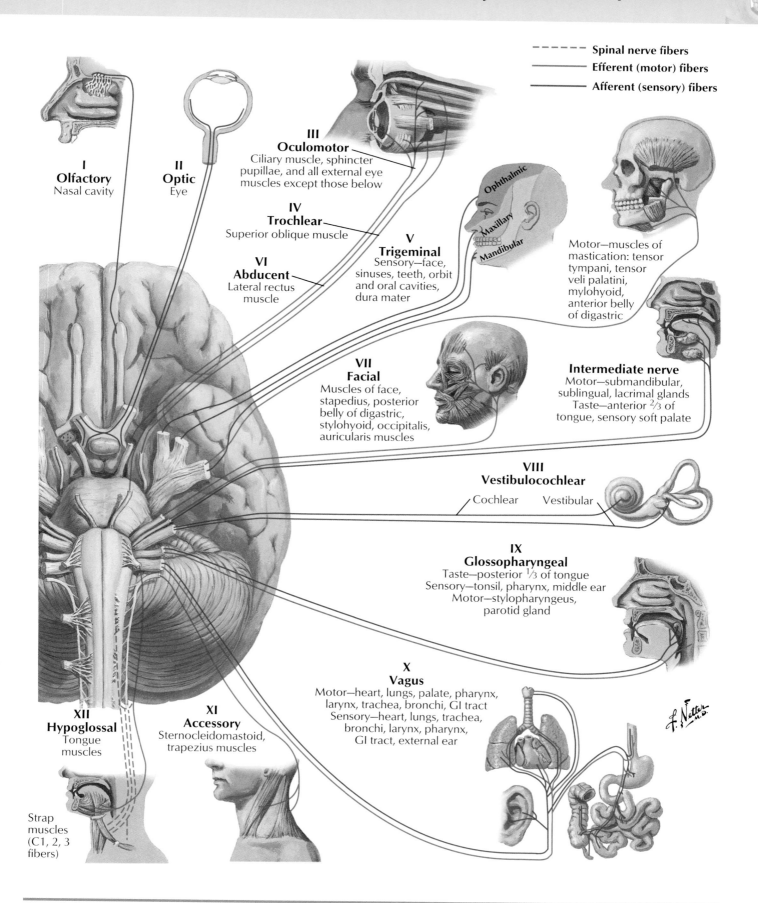

- - - - - Spinal nerve fibers
——— Efferent (motor) fibers
——— Afferent (sensory) fibers

I Olfactory
Nasal cavity

II Optic
Eye

III Oculomotor
Ciliary muscle, sphincter pupillae, and all external eye muscles except those below

IV Trochlear
Superior oblique muscle

VI Abducent
Lateral rectus muscle

V Trigeminal
Sensory—face, sinuses, teeth, orbit and oral cavities, dura mater

Ophthalmic
Maxillary
Mandibular

Motor—muscles of mastication: tensor tympani, tensor veli palatini, mylohyoid, anterior belly of digastric

VII Facial
Muscles of face, stapedius, posterior belly of digastric, stylohyoid, occipitalis, auricularis muscles

Intermediate nerve
Motor—submandibular, sublingual, lacrimal glands
Taste—anterior 2/3 of tongue, sensory soft palate

VIII Vestibulocochlear
Cochlear   Vestibular

IX Glossopharyngeal
Taste—posterior 1/3 of tongue
Sensory—tonsil, pharynx, middle ear
Motor—stylopharyngeus, parotid gland

X Vagus
Motor—heart, lungs, palate, pharynx, larynx, trachea, bronchi, GI tract
Sensory—heart, lungs, trachea, bronchi, larynx, pharynx, GI tract, external ear

XII Hypoglossal
Tongue muscles

XI Accessory
Sternocleidomastoid, trapezius muscles

Strap muscles (C1, 2, 3 fibers)

F. Netter M.D.

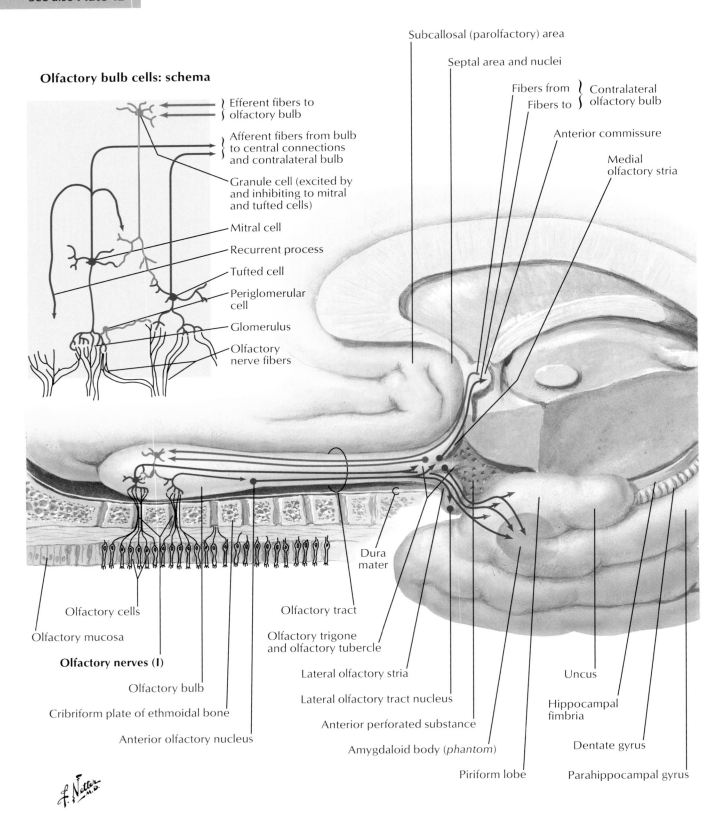

Olfactory bulb cells: schema

Efferent fibers to olfactory bulb

Afferent fibers from bulb to central connections and contralateral bulb

Granule cell (excited by and inhibiting to mitral and tufted cells)

Mitral cell

Recurrent process

Tufted cell

Periglomerular cell

Glomerulus

Olfactory nerve fibers

Subcallosal (parolfactory) area

Septal area and nuclei

Fibers from } Contralateral
Fibers to } olfactory bulb

Anterior commissure

Medial olfactory stria

Dura mater

Olfactory cells

Olfactory mucosa

Olfactory nerves (I)

Olfactory bulb

Cribriform plate of ethmoidal bone

Anterior olfactory nucleus

Olfactory tract

Olfactory trigone and olfactory tubercle

Lateral olfactory stria

Lateral olfactory tract nucleus

Anterior perforated substance

Amygdaloid body (*phantom*)

Piriform lobe

Uncus

Hippocampal fimbria

Dentate gyrus

Parahippocampal gyrus

Plate 118　　　　　　　　　　　　　　　　　　　　**Cranial and Cervical Nerves**

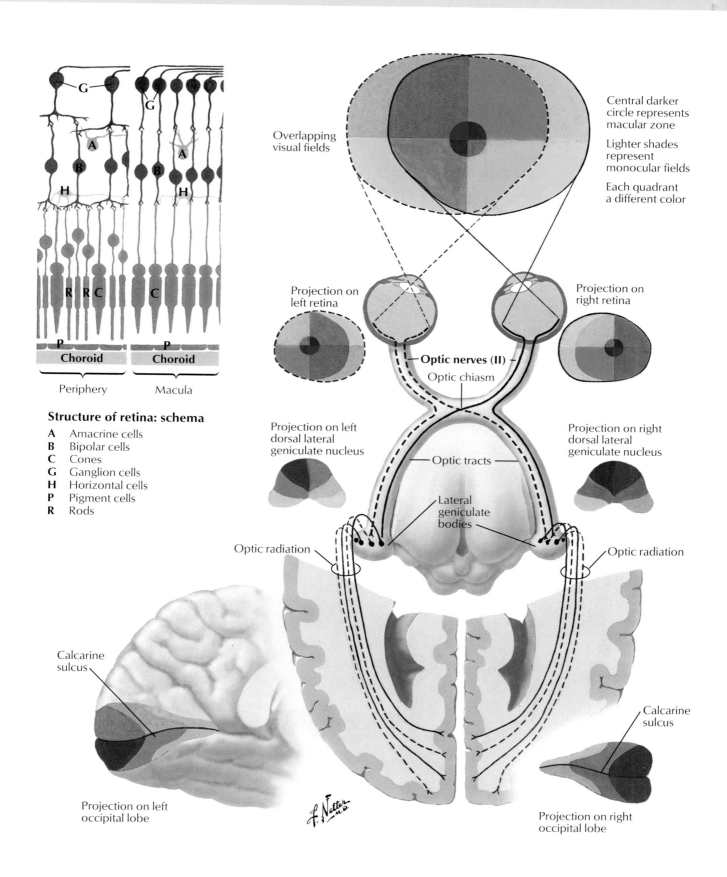

Overlapping visual fields

Central darker circle represents macular zone

Lighter shades represent monocular fields

Each quadrant a different color

Projection on left retina

Projection on right retina

Optic nerves (II)

Optic chiasm

Projection on left dorsal lateral geniculate nucleus

Projection on right dorsal lateral geniculate nucleus

Optic tracts

Lateral geniculate bodies

Optic radiation

Optic radiation

Calcarine sulcus

Calcarine sulcus

Projection on left occipital lobe

Projection on right occipital lobe

Choroid

Choroid

Periphery

Macula

Structure of retina: schema

A   Amacrine cells
B   Bipolar cells
C   Cones
G   Ganglion cells
H   Horizontal cells
P   Pigment cells
R   Rods

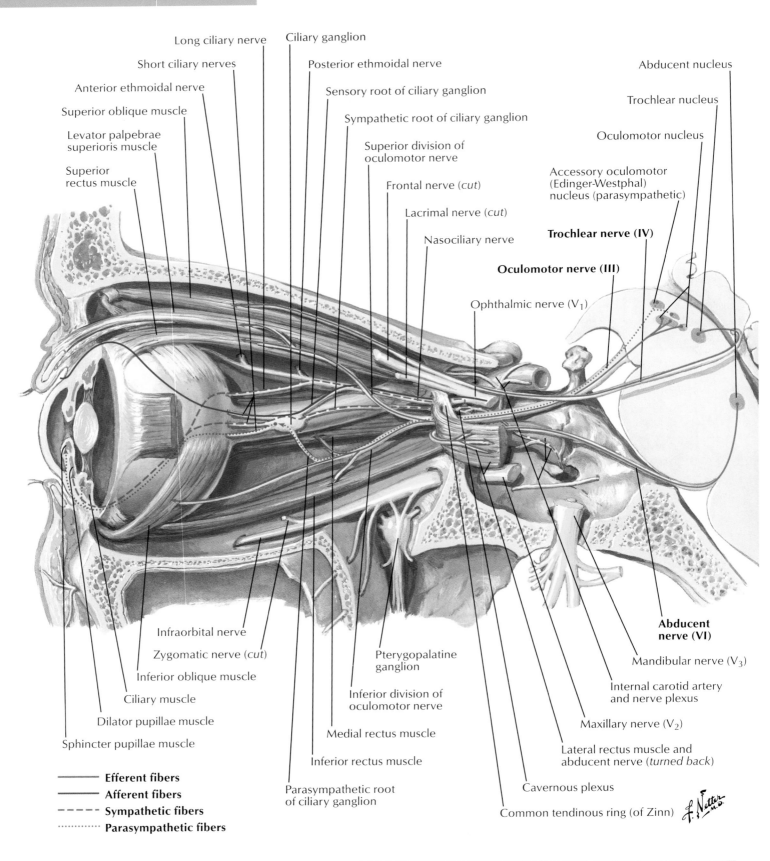

Long ciliary nerve

Short ciliary nerves

Anterior ethmoidal nerve

Superior oblique muscle

Levator palpebrae superioris muscle

Superior rectus muscle

Ciliary ganglion

Posterior ethmoidal nerve

Sensory root of ciliary ganglion

Sympathetic root of ciliary ganglion

Superior division of oculomotor nerve

Frontal nerve (*cut*)

Lacrimal nerve (*cut*)

Nasociliary nerve

Abducent nucleus

Trochlear nucleus

Oculomotor nucleus

Accessory oculomotor (Edinger-Westphal) nucleus (parasympathetic)

Trochlear nerve (IV)

Oculomotor nerve (III)

Ophthalmic nerve (V₁)

Infraorbital nerve

Zygomatic nerve (*cut*)

Inferior oblique muscle

Ciliary muscle

Dilator pupillae muscle

Sphincter pupillae muscle

Pterygopalatine ganglion

Inferior division of oculomotor nerve

Medial rectus muscle

Inferior rectus muscle

Parasympathetic root of ciliary ganglion

Abducent nerve (VI)

Mandibular nerve (V₃)

Internal carotid artery and nerve plexus

Maxillary nerve (V₂)

Lateral rectus muscle and abducent nerve (*turned back*)

Cavernous plexus

Common tendinous ring (of Zinn)

——— **Efferent fibers**
——— **Afferent fibers**
- - - - **Sympathetic fibers**
········· **Parasympathetic fibers**

Plate 120

Cranial and Cervical Nerves

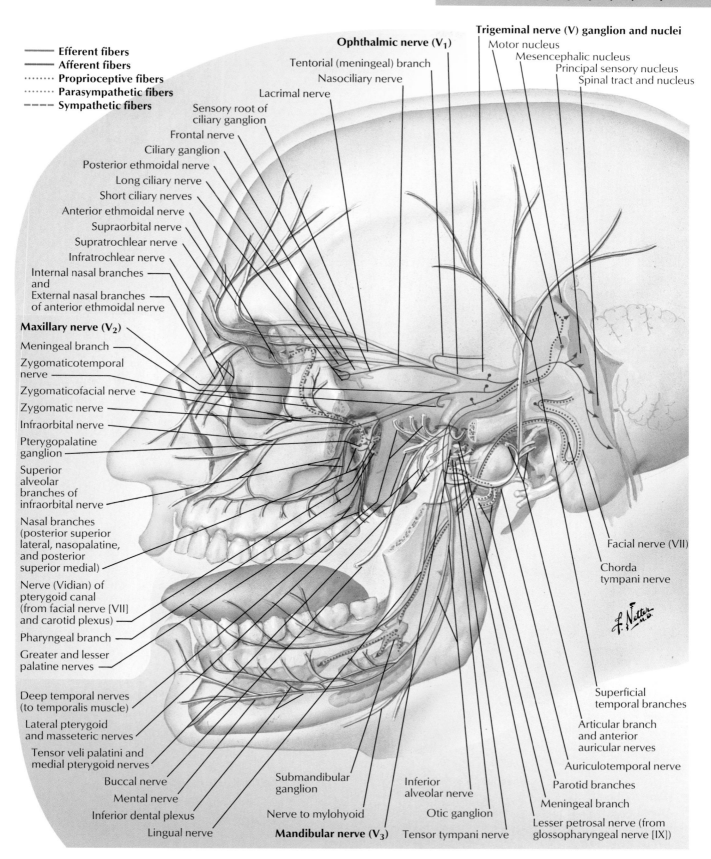

Efferent fibers
Afferent fibers
Proprioceptive fibers
Parasympathetic fibers
Sympathetic fibers

Ophthalmic nerve (V₁)
Tentorial (meningeal) branch
Nasociliary nerve
Lacrimal nerve
Sensory root of ciliary ganglion
Frontal nerve
Ciliary ganglion
Posterior ethmoidal nerve
Long ciliary nerve
Short ciliary nerves
Anterior ethmoidal nerve
Supraorbital nerve
Supratrochlear nerve
Infratrochlear nerve
Internal nasal branches and
External nasal branches of anterior ethmoidal nerve

Trigeminal nerve (V) ganglion and nuclei
Motor nucleus
Mesencephalic nucleus
Principal sensory nucleus
Spinal tract and nucleus

Maxillary nerve (V₂)
Meningeal branch
Zygomaticotemporal nerve
Zygomaticofacial nerve
Zygomatic nerve
Infraorbital nerve
Pterygopalatine ganglion
Superior alveolar branches of infraorbital nerve
Nasal branches (posterior superior lateral, nasopalatine, and posterior superior medial)
Nerve (Vidian) of pterygoid canal (from facial nerve [VII] and carotid plexus)
Pharyngeal branch
Greater and lesser palatine nerves
Deep temporal nerves (to temporalis muscle)
Lateral pterygoid and masseteric nerves
Tensor veli palatini and medial pterygoid nerves
Buccal nerve
Mental nerve
Inferior dental plexus
Lingual nerve

Submandibular ganglion
Nerve to mylohyoid
Mandibular nerve (V₃)

Inferior alveolar nerve
Otic ganglion
Tensor tympani nerve

Facial nerve (VII)
Chorda tympani nerve

Superficial temporal branches
Articular branch and anterior auricular nerves
Auriculotemporal nerve
Parotid branches
Meningeal branch
Lesser petrosal nerve (from glossopharyngeal nerve [IX])

F. Netter M.D.

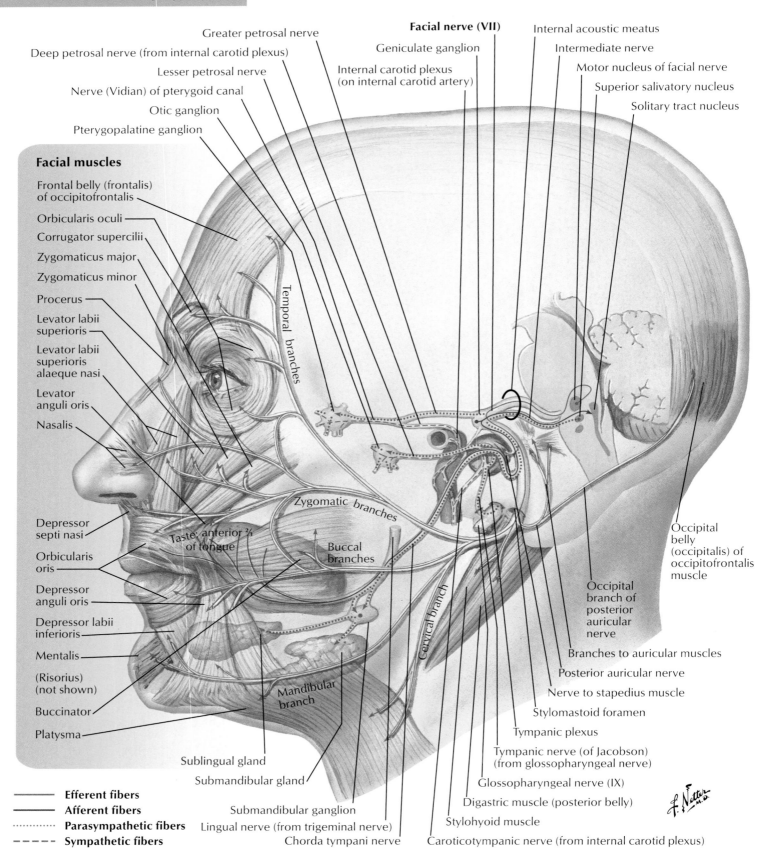

Greater petrosal nerve

Deep petrosal nerve (from internal carotid plexus)

Lesser petrosal nerve

Nerve (Vidian) of pterygoid canal

Otic ganglion

Pterygopalatine ganglion

Facial nerve (VII)

Geniculate ganglion

Internal carotid plexus (on internal carotid artery)

Internal acoustic meatus

Intermediate nerve

Motor nucleus of facial nerve

Superior salivatory nucleus

Solitary tract nucleus

Facial muscles

Frontal belly (frontalis) of occipitofrontalis

Orbicularis oculi

Corrugator supercilii

Zygomaticus major

Zygomaticus minor

Procerus

Levator labii superioris

Levator labii superioris alaeque nasi

Levator anguli oris

Nasalis

Depressor septi nasi

Orbicularis oris

Depressor anguli oris

Depressor labii inferioris

Mentalis

(Risorius) (not shown)

Buccinator

Platysma

Temporal branches

Zygomatic branches

Taste: anterior ⅔ of tongue

Buccal branches

Mandibular branch

Cervical branch

Sublingual gland

Submandibular gland

Submandibular ganglion

Lingual nerve (from trigeminal nerve)

Chorda tympani nerve

Occipital belly (occipitalis) of occipitofrontalis muscle

Occipital branch of posterior auricular nerve

Branches to auricular muscles

Posterior auricular nerve

Nerve to stapedius muscle

Stylomastoid foramen

Tympanic plexus

Tympanic nerve (of Jacobson) (from glossopharyngeal nerve)

Glossopharyngeal nerve (IX)

Digastric muscle (posterior belly)

Stylohyoid muscle

Caroticotympanic nerve (from internal carotid plexus)

———— **Efferent fibers**

———— **Afferent fibers**

············ **Parasympathetic fibers**

- - - - **Sympathetic fibers**

Plate 122

Cranial and Cervical Nerves

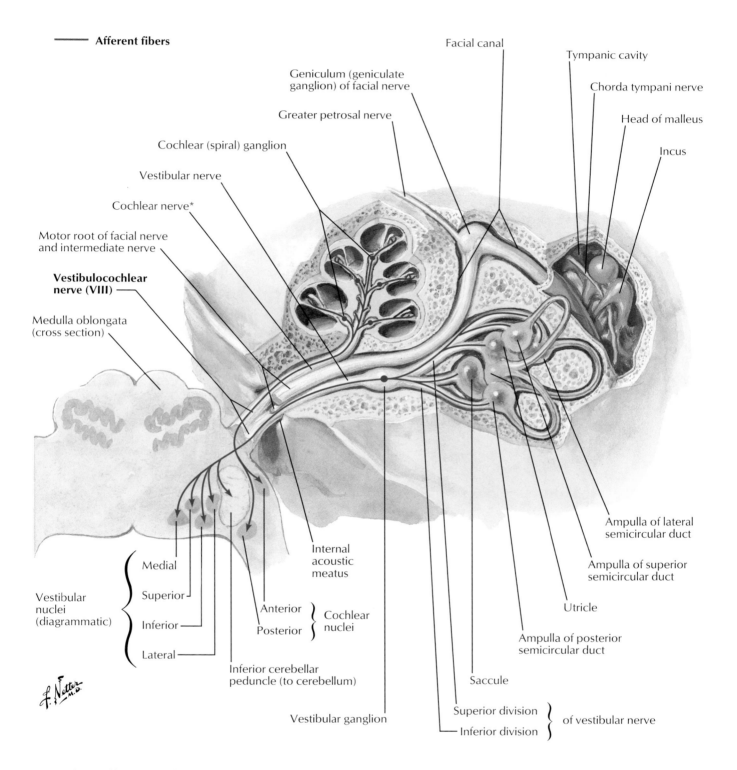

Afferent fibers

Geniculum (geniculate ganglion) of facial nerve

Greater petrosal nerve

Cochlear (spiral) ganglion

Vestibular nerve

Cochlear nerve*

Motor root of facial nerve and intermediate nerve

Vestibulocochlear nerve (VIII)

Medulla oblongata (cross section)

Facial canal

Tympanic cavity

Chorda tympani nerve

Head of malleus

Incus

Internal acoustic meatus

Ampulla of lateral semicircular duct

Ampulla of superior semicircular duct

Utricle

Ampulla of posterior semicircular duct

Saccule

Vestibular nuclei (diagrammatic)

Medial

Superior

Inferior

Lateral

Anterior

Posterior

} Cochlear nuclei

Inferior cerebellar peduncle (to cerebellum)

Vestibular ganglion

Superior division

Inferior division

} of vestibular nerve

*Note: The cochlear nerve also contains efferent fibers to the sensory epithelium. These fibers are derived from the vestibular nerve while in the internal auditory meatus.

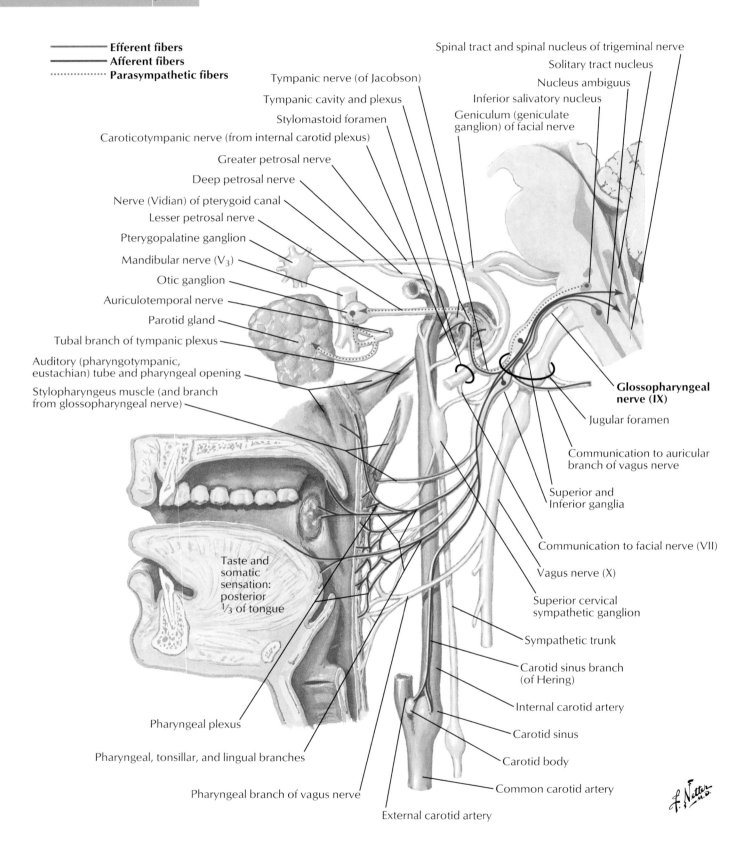

Efferent fibers
Afferent fibers
Parasympathetic fibers

Tympanic nerve (of Jacobson)
Tympanic cavity and plexus
Stylomastoid foramen
Caroticotympanic nerve (from internal carotid plexus)
Greater petrosal nerve
Deep petrosal nerve
Nerve (Vidian) of pterygoid canal
Lesser petrosal nerve
Pterygopalatine ganglion
Mandibular nerve (V₃)
Otic ganglion
Auriculotemporal nerve
Parotid gland
Tubal branch of tympanic plexus
Auditory (pharyngotympanic, eustachian) tube and pharyngeal opening
Stylopharyngeus muscle (and branch from glossopharyngeal nerve)

Taste and somatic sensation: posterior ⅓ of tongue

Pharyngeal plexus

Pharyngeal, tonsillar, and lingual branches

Pharyngeal branch of vagus nerve

External carotid artery

Spinal tract and spinal nucleus of trigeminal nerve
Solitary tract nucleus
Nucleus ambiguus
Inferior salivatory nucleus
Geniculum (geniculate ganglion) of facial nerve

Glossopharyngeal nerve (IX)
Jugular foramen
Communication to auricular branch of vagus nerve
Superior and Inferior ganglia
Communication to facial nerve (VII)
Vagus nerve (X)
Superior cervical sympathetic ganglion
Sympathetic trunk
Carotid sinus branch (of Hering)
Internal carotid artery
Carotid sinus
Carotid body
Common carotid artery

Plate 124

Cranial and Cervical Nerves

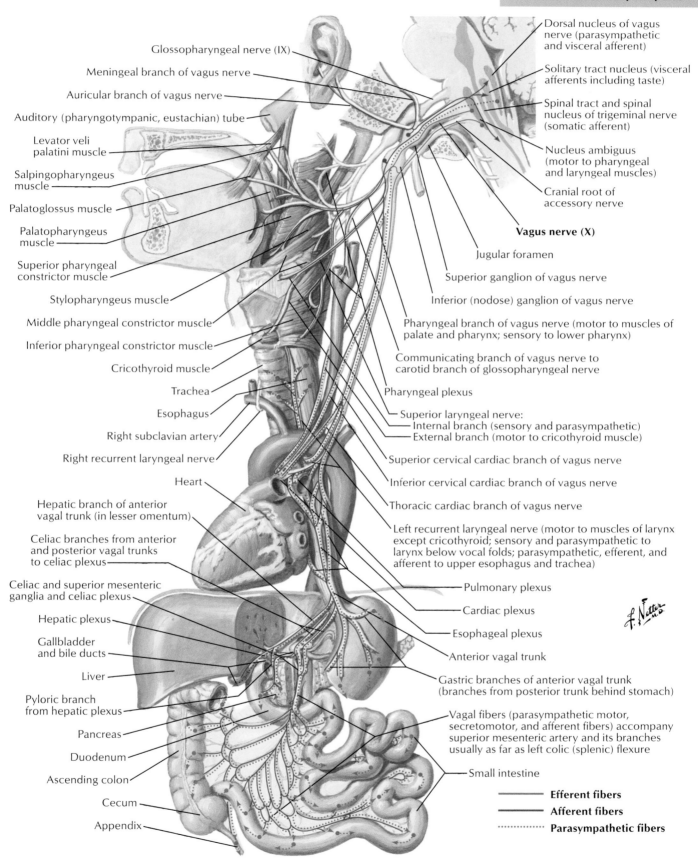

Glossopharyngeal nerve (IX)

Meningeal branch of vagus nerve

Auricular branch of vagus nerve

Auditory (pharyngotympanic, eustachian) tube

Levator veli palatini muscle

Salpingopharyngeus muscle

Palatoglossus muscle

Palatopharyngeus muscle

Superior pharyngeal constrictor muscle

Stylopharyngeus muscle

Middle pharyngeal constrictor muscle

Inferior pharyngeal constrictor muscle

Cricothyroid muscle

Trachea

Esophagus

Right subclavian artery

Right recurrent laryngeal nerve

Heart

Hepatic branch of anterior vagal trunk (in lesser omentum)

Celiac branches from anterior and posterior vagal trunks to celiac plexus

Celiac and superior mesenteric ganglia and celiac plexus

Hepatic plexus

Gallbladder and bile ducts

Liver

Pyloric branch from hepatic plexus

Pancreas

Duodenum

Ascending colon

Cecum

Appendix

Dorsal nucleus of vagus nerve (parasympathetic and visceral afferent)

Solitary tract nucleus (visceral afferents including taste)

Spinal tract and spinal nucleus of trigeminal nerve (somatic afferent)

Nucleus ambiguus (motor to pharyngeal and laryngeal muscles)

Cranial root of accessory nerve

Vagus nerve (X)

Jugular foramen

Superior ganglion of vagus nerve

Inferior (nodose) ganglion of vagus nerve

Pharyngeal branch of vagus nerve (motor to muscles of palate and pharynx; sensory to lower pharynx)

Communicating branch of vagus nerve to carotid branch of glossopharyngeal nerve

Pharyngeal plexus

Superior laryngeal nerve:
Internal branch (sensory and parasympathetic)
External branch (motor to cricothyroid muscle)

Superior cervical cardiac branch of vagus nerve

Inferior cervical cardiac branch of vagus nerve

Thoracic cardiac branch of vagus nerve

Left recurrent laryngeal nerve (motor to muscles of larynx except cricothyroid; sensory and parasympathetic to larynx below vocal folds; parasympathetic, efferent, and afferent to upper esophagus and trachea)

Pulmonary plexus

Cardiac plexus

Esophageal plexus

Anterior vagal trunk

Gastric branches of anterior vagal trunk (branches from posterior trunk behind stomach)

Vagal fibers (parasympathetic motor, secretomotor, and afferent fibers) accompany superior mesenteric artery and its branches usually as far as left colic (splenic) flexure

Small intestine

⎯⎯⎯ **Efferent fibers**
⎯⎯⎯ **Afferent fibers**
············ **Parasympathetic fibers**

f. Netter M.D.

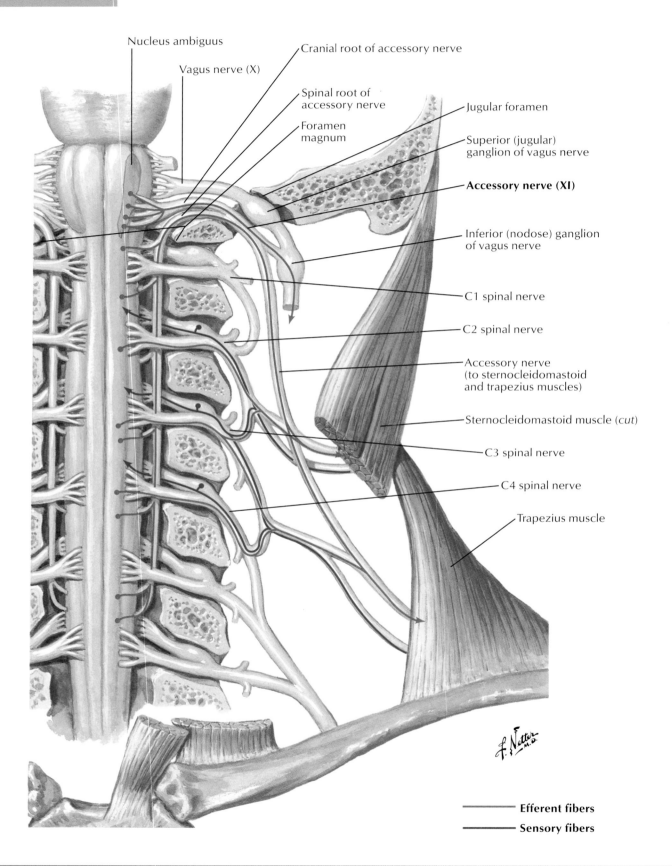

Nucleus ambiguus

Vagus nerve (X)

Cranial root of accessory nerve

Spinal root of accessory nerve

Foramen magnum

Jugular foramen

Superior (jugular) ganglion of vagus nerve

Accessory nerve (XI)

Inferior (nodose) ganglion of vagus nerve

C1 spinal nerve

C2 spinal nerve

Accessory nerve (to sternocleidomastoid and trapezius muscles)

Sternocleidomastoid muscle (*cut*)

C3 spinal nerve

C4 spinal nerve

Trapezius muscle

—— **Efferent fibers**

—— **Sensory fibers**

Plate 126

Cranial and Cervical Nerves

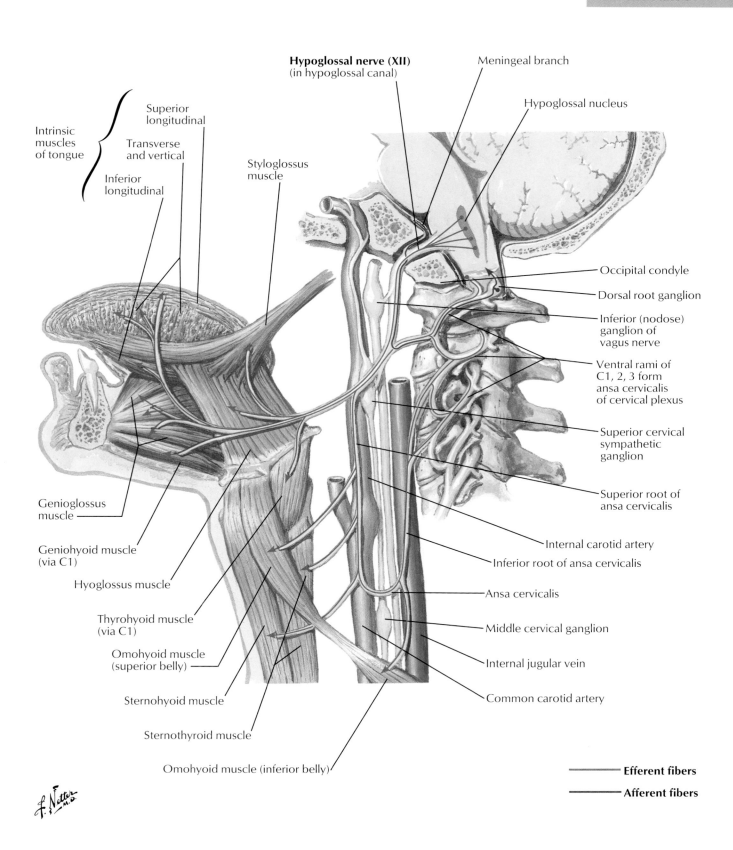

Hypoglossal nerve (XII)
(in hypoglossal canal)

Meningeal branch

Hypoglossal nucleus

Intrinsic muscles of tongue
Superior longitudinal
Transverse and vertical
Inferior longitudinal

Styloglossus muscle

Occipital condyle

Dorsal root ganglion

Inferior (nodose) ganglion of vagus nerve

Ventral rami of C1, 2, 3 form ansa cervicalis of cervical plexus

Superior cervical sympathetic ganglion

Superior root of ansa cervicalis

Genioglossus muscle

Geniohyoid muscle (via C1)

Hyoglossus muscle

Thyrohyoid muscle (via C1)

Omohyoid muscle (superior belly)

Sternohyoid muscle

Sternothyroid muscle

Omohyoid muscle (inferior belly)

Internal carotid artery

Inferior root of ansa cervicalis

Ansa cervicalis

Middle cervical ganglion

Internal jugular vein

Common carotid artery

———— Efferent fibers

———— Afferent fibers

Cervical Plexus: Schema

See also **Plate 31**

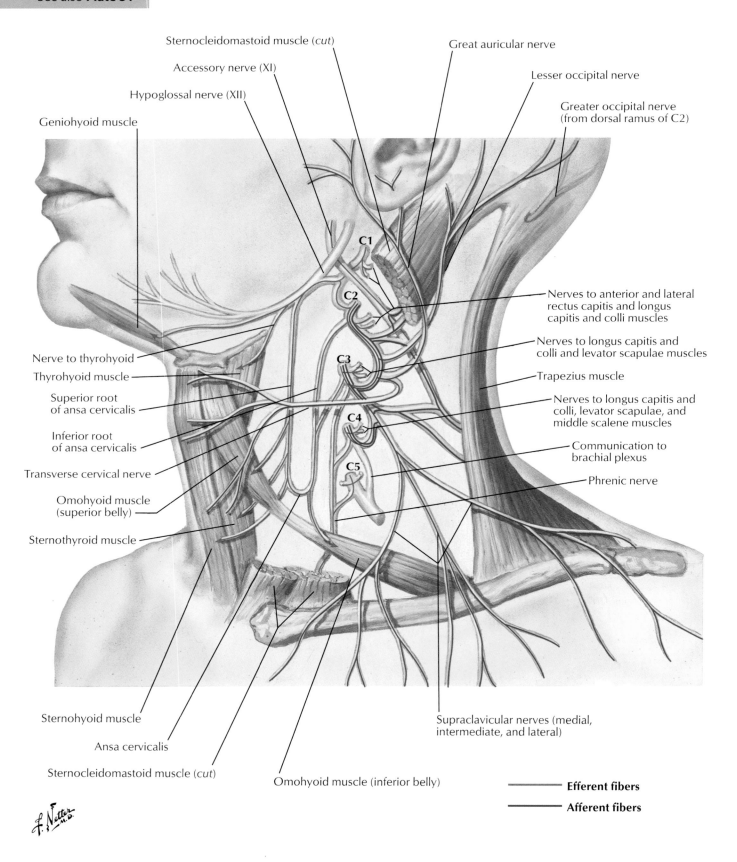

Sternocleidomastoid muscle (*cut*)

Accessory nerve (XI)

Hypoglossal nerve (XII)

Geniohyoid muscle

Great auricular nerve

Lesser occipital nerve

Greater occipital nerve (from dorsal ramus of C2)

C1

C2

C3

C4

C5

Nerve to thyrohyoid

Thyrohyoid muscle

Superior root of ansa cervicalis

Inferior root of ansa cervicalis

Transverse cervical nerve

Omohyoid muscle (superior belly)

Sternothyroid muscle

Nerves to anterior and lateral rectus capitis and longus capitis and colli muscles

Nerves to longus capitis and colli and levator scapulae muscles

Trapezius muscle

Nerves to longus capitis and colli, levator scapulae, and middle scalene muscles

Communication to brachial plexus

Phrenic nerve

Sternohyoid muscle

Ansa cervicalis

Sternocleidomastoid muscle (*cut*)

Omohyoid muscle (inferior belly)

Supraclavicular nerves (medial, intermediate, and lateral)

Efferent fibers

Afferent fibers

Plate 128   **Cranial and Cervical Nerves**

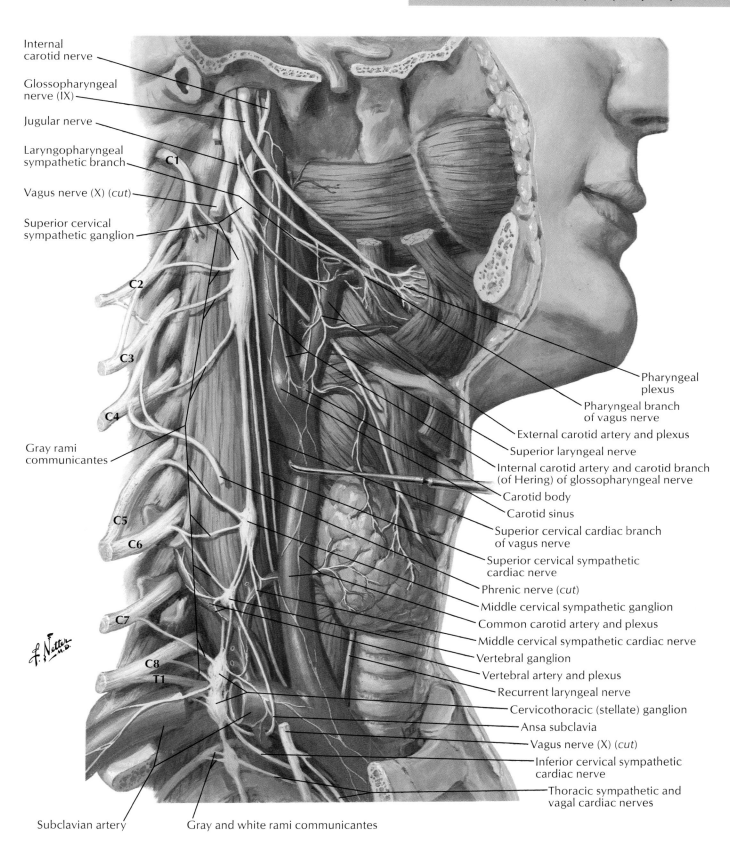

Internal carotid nerve

Glossopharyngeal nerve (IX)

Jugular nerve

Laryngopharyngeal sympathetic branch

Vagus nerve (X) (*cut*)

Superior cervical sympathetic ganglion

Gray rami communicantes

C1

C2

C3

C4

C5

C6

C7

C8
T1

Subclavian artery

Gray and white rami communicantes

Pharyngeal plexus

Pharyngeal branch of vagus nerve

External carotid artery and plexus

Superior laryngeal nerve

Internal carotid artery and carotid branch (of Hering) of glossopharyngeal nerve

Carotid body

Carotid sinus

Superior cervical cardiac branch of vagus nerve

Superior cervical sympathetic cardiac nerve

Phrenic nerve (*cut*)

Middle cervical sympathetic ganglion

Common carotid artery and plexus

Middle cervical sympathetic cardiac nerve

Vertebral ganglion

Vertebral artery and plexus

Recurrent laryngeal nerve

Cervicothoracic (stellate) ganglion

Ansa subclavia

Vagus nerve (X) (*cut*)

Inferior cervical sympathetic cardiac nerve

Thoracic sympathetic and vagal cardiac nerves

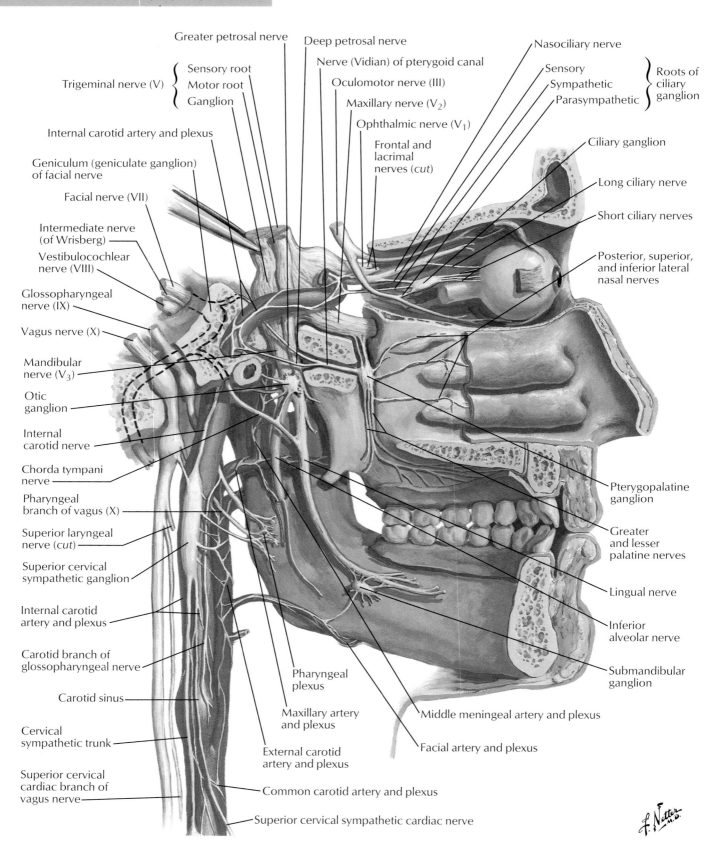

Greater petrosal nerve

Deep petrosal nerve

Nasociliary nerve

Trigeminal nerve (V) { Sensory root / Motor root / Ganglion

Nerve (Vidian) of pterygoid canal

Sensory
Sympathetic
Parasympathetic } Roots of ciliary ganglion

Oculomotor nerve (III)

Maxillary nerve (V₂)

Ophthalmic nerve (V₁)

Internal carotid artery and plexus

Frontal and lacrimal nerves (*cut*)

Ciliary ganglion

Geniculum (geniculate ganglion) of facial nerve

Long ciliary nerve

Facial nerve (VII)

Short ciliary nerves

Intermediate nerve (of Wrisberg)

Posterior, superior, and inferior lateral nasal nerves

Vestibulocochlear nerve (VIII)

Glossopharyngeal nerve (IX)

Vagus nerve (X)

Mandibular nerve (V₃)

Otic ganglion

Internal carotid nerve

Chorda tympani nerve

Pterygopalatine ganglion

Pharyngeal branch of vagus (X)

Superior laryngeal nerve (*cut*)

Superior cervical sympathetic ganglion

Greater and lesser palatine nerves

Internal carotid artery and plexus

Lingual nerve

Carotid branch of glossopharyngeal nerve

Inferior alveolar nerve

Carotid sinus

Pharyngeal plexus

Submandibular ganglion

Cervical sympathetic trunk

Maxillary artery and plexus

Middle meningeal artery and plexus

Superior cervical cardiac branch of vagus nerve

External carotid artery and plexus

Facial artery and plexus

Common carotid artery and plexus

Superior cervical sympathetic cardiac nerve

Plate 130

Cranial and Cervical Nerves

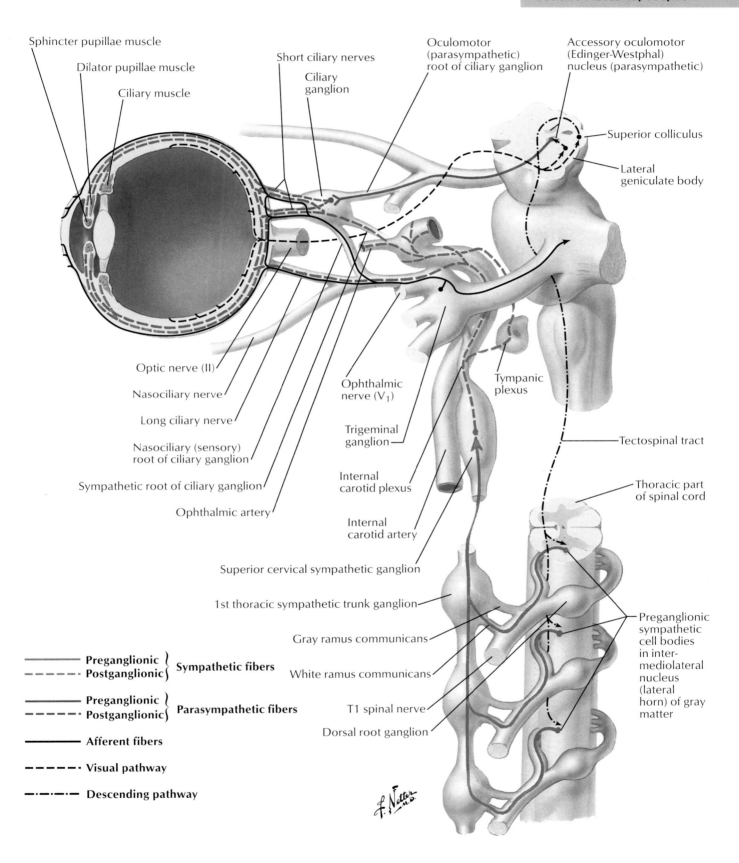

Sphincter pupillae muscle

Dilator pupillae muscle

Ciliary muscle

Short ciliary nerves

Ciliary ganglion

Oculomotor (parasympathetic) root of ciliary ganglion

Accessory oculomotor (Edinger-Westphal) nucleus (parasympathetic)

Superior colliculus

Lateral geniculate body

Optic nerve (II)

Nasociliary nerve

Long ciliary nerve

Nasociliary (sensory) root of ciliary ganglion

Sympathetic root of ciliary ganglion

Ophthalmic artery

Ophthalmic nerve (V_1)

Trigeminal ganglion

Internal carotid plexus

Internal carotid artery

Superior cervical sympathetic ganglion

1st thoracic sympathetic trunk ganglion

Gray ramus communicans

White ramus communicans

T1 spinal nerve

Dorsal root ganglion

Tympanic plexus

Tectospinal tract

Thoracic part of spinal cord

Preganglionic sympathetic cell bodies in intermediolateral nucleus (lateral horn) of gray matter

——————— **Preganglionic** } **Sympathetic fibers**
– – – – – – **Postganglionic**

——————— **Preganglionic** } **Parasympathetic fibers**
– – – – – – **Postganglionic**

——————— **Afferent fibers**

– – – – – – **Visual pathway**

–··–··– **Descending pathway**

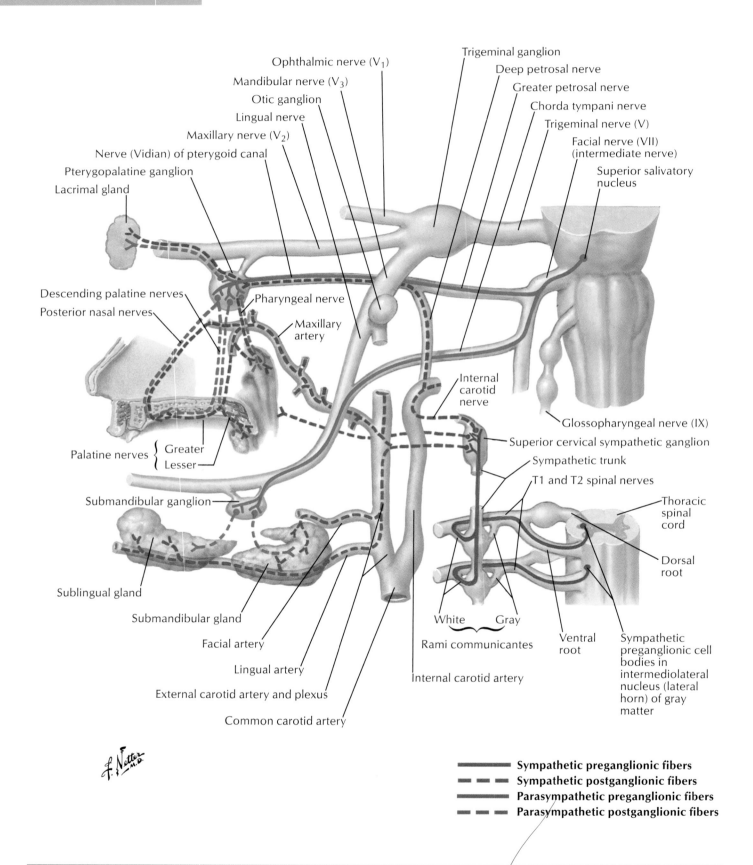

Ophthalmic nerve (V₁)

Mandibular nerve (V₃)

Otic ganglion

Lingual nerve

Maxillary nerve (V₂)

Nerve (Vidian) of pterygoid canal

Pterygopalatine ganglion

Lacrimal gland

Trigeminal ganglion

Deep petrosal nerve

Greater petrosal nerve

Chorda tympani nerve

Trigeminal nerve (V)

Facial nerve (VII) (intermediate nerve)

Superior salivatory nucleus

Descending palatine nerves

Posterior nasal nerves

Pharyngeal nerve

Maxillary artery

Internal carotid nerve

Palatine nerves { Greater / Lesser

Glossopharyngeal nerve (IX)

Superior cervical sympathetic ganglion

Sympathetic trunk

T1 and T2 spinal nerves

Submandibular ganglion

Thoracic spinal cord

Dorsal root

Sublingual gland

Submandibular gland

Facial artery

Lingual artery

External carotid artery and plexus

Common carotid artery

White   Gray

Rami communicantes

Internal carotid artery

Ventral root

Sympathetic preganglionic cell bodies in intermediolateral nucleus (lateral horn) of gray matter

f. Netter

▬▬▬▬ **Sympathetic preganglionic fibers**
▬ ▬ ▬ **Sympathetic postganglionic fibers**
▬▬▬▬ **Parasympathetic preganglionic fibers**
▬ ▬ ▬ **Parasympathetic postganglionic fibers**

Plate 132   *Cranial and Cervical Nerves*

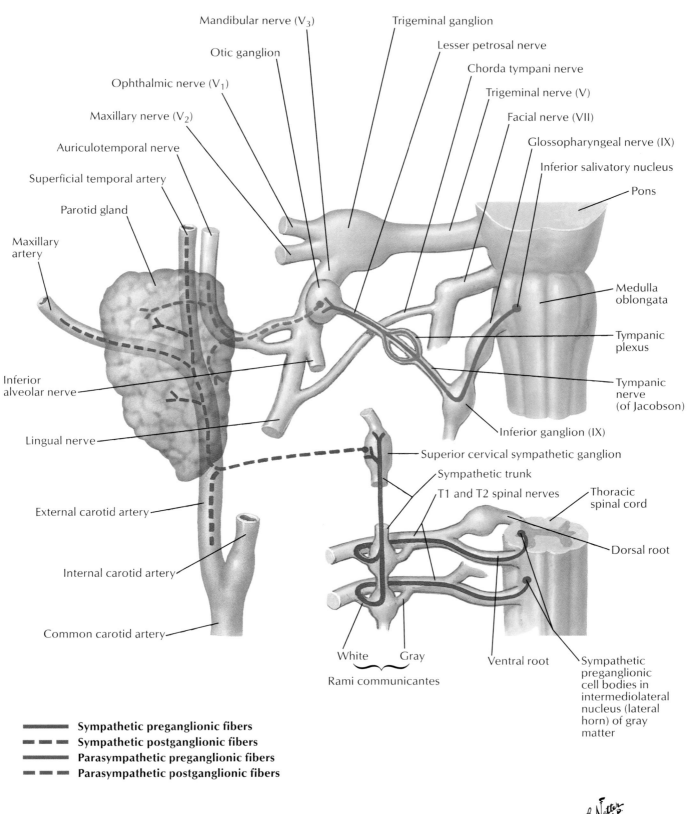

Mandibular nerve (V₃)

Otic ganglion

Ophthalmic nerve (V₁)

Maxillary nerve (V₂)

Auriculotemporal nerve

Superficial temporal artery

Parotid gland

Maxillary artery

Inferior alveolar nerve

Lingual nerve

External carotid artery

Internal carotid artery

Common carotid artery

Trigeminal ganglion

Lesser petrosal nerve

Chorda tympani nerve

Trigeminal nerve (V)

Facial nerve (VII)

Glossopharyngeal nerve (IX)

Inferior salivatory nucleus

Pons

Medulla oblongata

Tympanic plexus

Tympanic nerve (of Jacobson)

Inferior ganglion (IX)

Superior cervical sympathetic ganglion

Sympathetic trunk

T1 and T2 spinal nerves

Thoracic spinal cord

Dorsal root

Ventral root

Sympathetic preganglionic cell bodies in intermediolateral nucleus (lateral horn) of gray matter

White   Gray
Rami communicantes

———— **Sympathetic preganglionic fibers**
– – – – **Sympathetic postganglionic fibers**
———— **Parasympathetic preganglionic fibers**
– – – – **Parasympathetic postganglionic fibers**

Cranial and Cervical Nerves

Plate 133

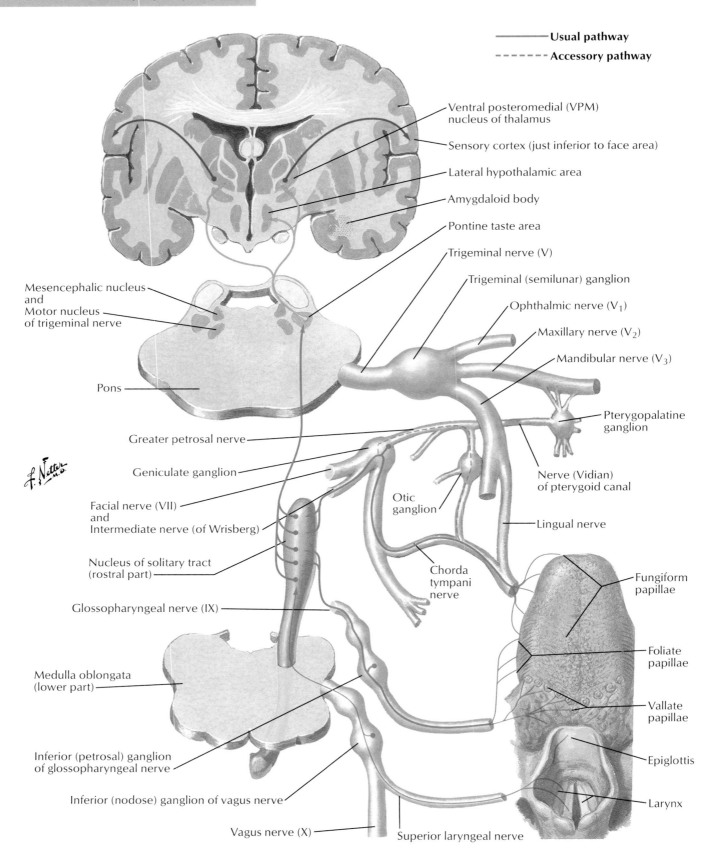

Usual pathway
Accessory pathway

Ventral posteromedial (VPM) nucleus of thalamus

Sensory cortex (just inferior to face area)

Lateral hypothalamic area

Amygdaloid body

Pontine taste area

Trigeminal nerve (V)

Trigeminal (semilunar) ganglion

Ophthalmic nerve (V₁)

Maxillary nerve (V₂)

Mandibular nerve (V₃)

Pterygopalatine ganglion

Nerve (Vidian) of pterygoid canal

Lingual nerve

Fungiform papillae

Foliate papillae

Vallate papillae

Epiglottis

Larynx

Mesencephalic nucleus and Motor nucleus of trigeminal nerve

Pons

Greater petrosal nerve

Geniculate ganglion

Facial nerve (VII) and Intermediate nerve (of Wrisberg)

Nucleus of solitary tract (rostral part)

Glossopharyngeal nerve (IX)

Otic ganglion

Chorda tympani nerve

Medulla oblongata (lower part)

Inferior (petrosal) ganglion of glossopharyngeal nerve

Inferior (nodose) ganglion of vagus nerve

Vagus nerve (X)

Superior laryngeal nerve

Plate 134

Cranial and Cervical Nerves

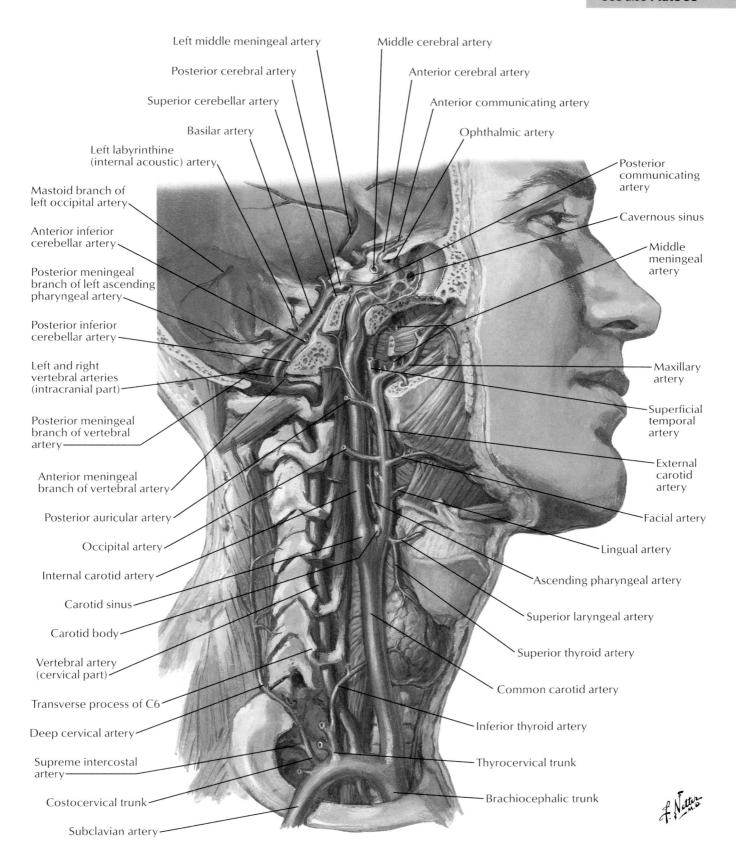

Left middle meningeal artery

Posterior cerebral artery

Superior cerebellar artery

Basilar artery

Left labyrinthine (internal acoustic) artery

Mastoid branch of left occipital artery

Anterior inferior cerebellar artery

Posterior meningeal branch of left ascending pharyngeal artery

Posterior inferior cerebellar artery

Left and right vertebral arteries (intracranial part)

Posterior meningeal branch of vertebral artery

Anterior meningeal branch of vertebral artery

Posterior auricular artery

Occipital artery

Internal carotid artery

Carotid sinus

Carotid body

Vertebral artery (cervical part)

Transverse process of C6

Deep cervical artery

Supreme intercostal artery

Costocervical trunk

Subclavian artery

Middle cerebral artery

Anterior cerebral artery

Anterior communicating artery

Ophthalmic artery

Posterior communicating artery

Cavernous sinus

Middle meningeal artery

Maxillary artery

Superficial temporal artery

External carotid artery

Facial artery

Lingual artery

Ascending pharyngeal artery

Superior laryngeal artery

Superior thyroid artery

Common carotid artery

Inferior thyroid artery

Thyrocervical trunk

Brachiocephalic trunk

Cerebral Vasculature

Plate 135

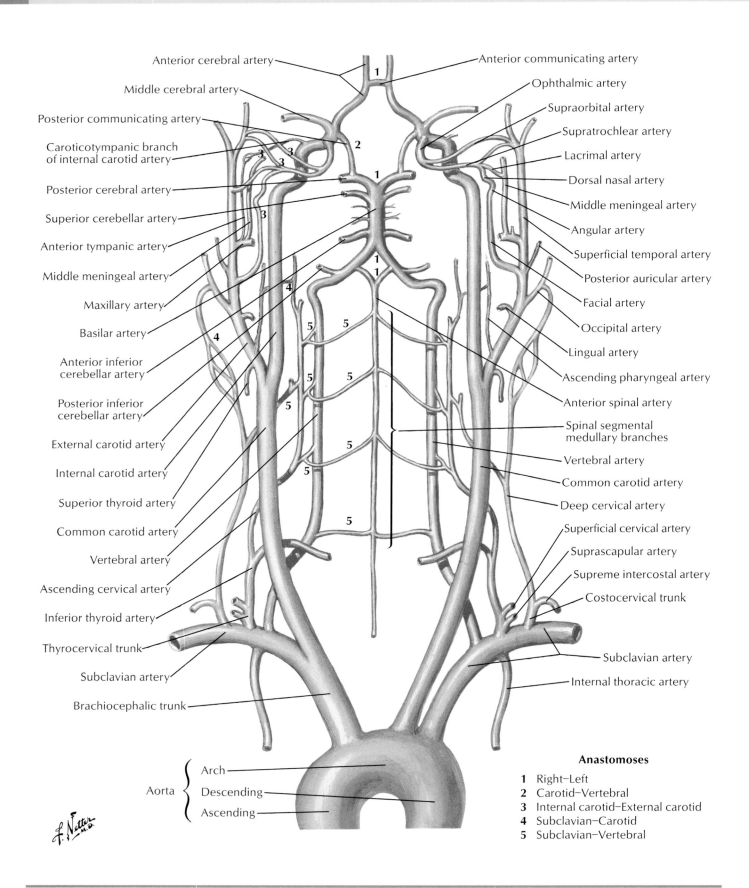

Anterior cerebral artery

Middle cerebral artery

Posterior communicating artery

Caroticotympanic branch
of internal carotid artery

Posterior cerebral artery

Superior cerebellar artery

Anterior tympanic artery

Middle meningeal artery

Maxillary artery

Basilar artery

Anterior inferior
cerebellar artery

Posterior inferior
cerebellar artery

External carotid artery

Internal carotid artery

Superior thyroid artery

Common carotid artery

Vertebral artery

Ascending cervical artery

Inferior thyroid artery

Thyrocervical trunk

Subclavian artery

Brachiocephalic trunk

Aorta
{ Arch
Descending
Ascending

Anterior communicating artery

Ophthalmic artery

Supraorbital artery

Supratrochlear artery

Lacrimal artery

Dorsal nasal artery

Middle meningeal artery

Angular artery

Superficial temporal artery

Posterior auricular artery

Facial artery

Occipital artery

Lingual artery

Ascending pharyngeal artery

Anterior spinal artery

Spinal segmental
medullary branches

Vertebral artery

Common carotid artery

Deep cervical artery

Superficial cervical artery

Suprascapular artery

Supreme intercostal artery

Costocervical trunk

Subclavian artery

Internal thoracic artery

Anastomoses

1 Right–Left
2 Carotid–Vertebral
3 Internal carotid–External carotid
4 Subclavian–Carotid
5 Subclavian–Vertebral

Plate 136 **Cerebral Vasculature**

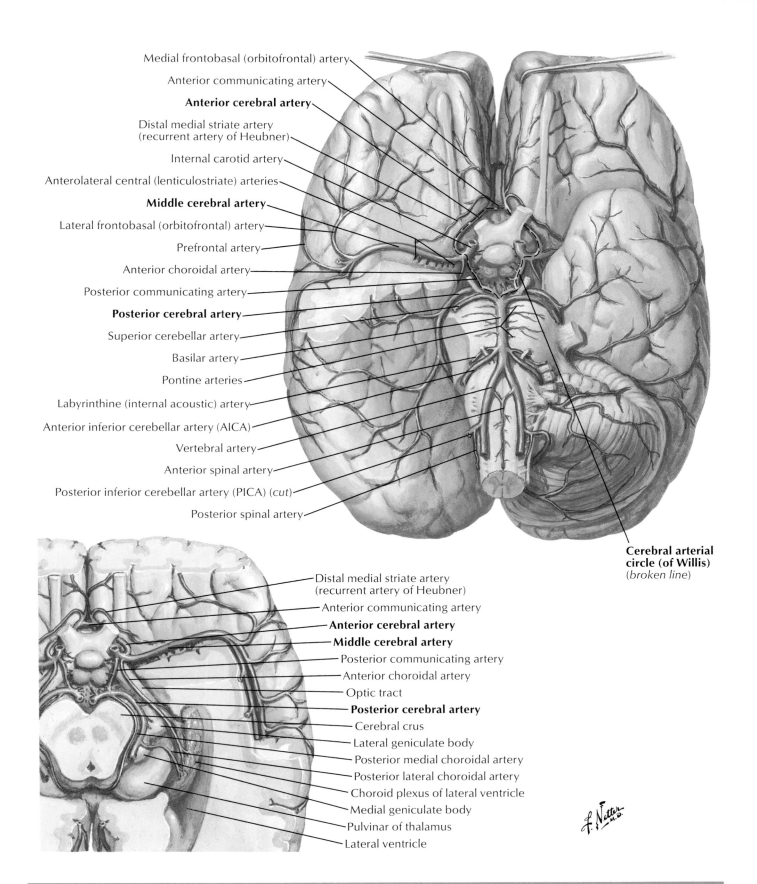

Medial frontobasal (orbitofrontal) artery

Anterior communicating artery

Anterior cerebral artery

Distal medial striate artery
(recurrent artery of Heubner)

Internal carotid artery

Anterolateral central (lenticulostriate) arteries

Middle cerebral artery

Lateral frontobasal (orbitofrontal) artery

Prefrontal artery

Anterior choroidal artery

Posterior communicating artery

Posterior cerebral artery

Superior cerebellar artery

Basilar artery

Pontine arteries

Labyrinthine (internal acoustic) artery

Anterior inferior cerebellar artery (AICA)

Vertebral artery

Anterior spinal artery

Posterior inferior cerebellar artery (PICA) (*cut*)

Posterior spinal artery

Cerebral arterial circle (of Willis)
(*broken line*)

Distal medial striate artery
(recurrent artery of Heubner)

Anterior communicating artery

Anterior cerebral artery

Middle cerebral artery

Posterior communicating artery

Anterior choroidal artery

Optic tract

Posterior cerebral artery

Cerebral crus

Lateral geniculate body

Posterior medial choroidal artery

Posterior lateral choroidal artery

Choroid plexus of lateral ventricle

Medial geniculate body

Pulvinar of thalamus

Lateral ventricle

Cerebral Vasculature

Plate 137

Vessels dissected out: inferior view

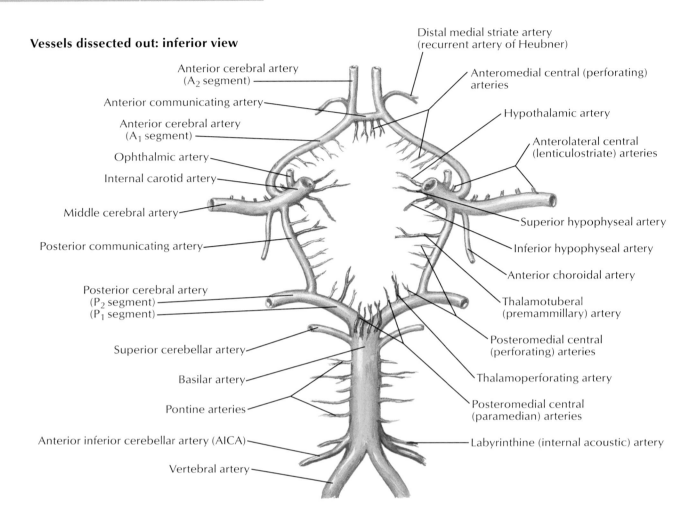

Distal medial striate artery
(recurrent artery of Heubner)

Anterior cerebral artery
(A₂ segment)

Anteromedial central (perforating)
arteries

Anterior communicating artery

Hypothalamic artery

Anterior cerebral artery
(A₁ segment)

Anterolateral central
(lenticulostriate) arteries

Ophthalmic artery

Internal carotid artery

Middle cerebral artery

Superior hypophyseal artery

Posterior communicating artery

Inferior hypophyseal artery

Anterior choroidal artery

Posterior cerebral artery
(P₂ segment)
(P₁ segment)

Thalamotuberal
(premammillary) artery

Superior cerebellar artery

Posteromedial central
(perforating) arteries

Basilar artery

Thalamoperforating artery

Pontine arteries

Posteromedial central
(paramedian) arteries

Anterior inferior cerebellar artery (AICA)

Labyrinthine (internal acoustic) artery

Vertebral artery

Vessels in situ: inferior view

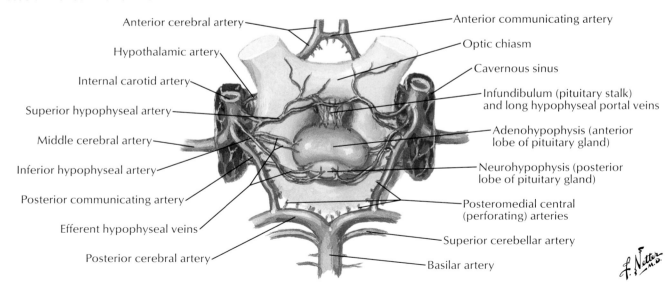

Anterior cerebral artery

Anterior communicating artery

Hypothalamic artery

Optic chiasm

Internal carotid artery

Cavernous sinus

Superior hypophyseal artery

Infundibulum (pituitary stalk)
and long hypophyseal portal veins

Middle cerebral artery

Adenohypophysis (anterior
lobe of pituitary gland)

Inferior hypophyseal artery

Neurohypophysis (posterior
lobe of pituitary gland)

Posterior communicating artery

Posteromedial central
(perforating) arteries

Efferent hypophyseal veins

Superior cerebellar artery

Posterior cerebral artery

Basilar artery

Plate 138   **Cerebral Vasculature**

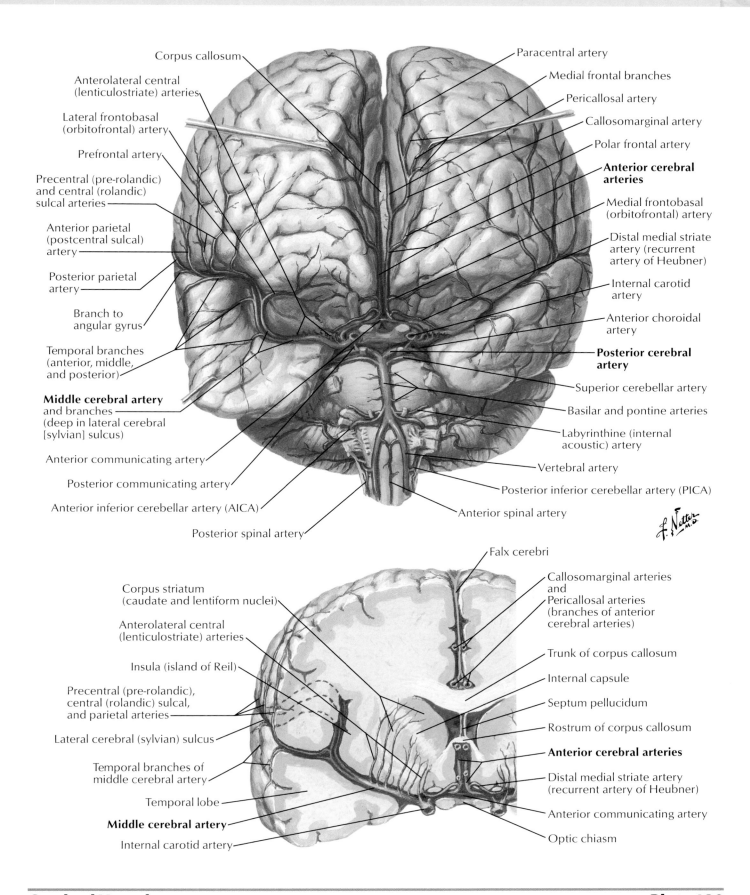

Corpus callosum

Anterolateral central (lenticulostriate) arteries

Lateral frontobasal (orbitofrontal) artery

Prefrontal artery

Precentral (pre-rolandic) and central (rolandic) sulcal arteries

Anterior parietal (postcentral sulcal) artery

Posterior parietal artery

Branch to angular gyrus

Temporal branches (anterior, middle, and posterior)

Middle cerebral artery and branches (deep in lateral cerebral [sylvian] sulcus)

Anterior communicating artery

Posterior communicating artery

Anterior inferior cerebellar artery (AICA)

Posterior spinal artery

Paracentral artery

Medial frontal branches

Pericallosal artery

Callosomarginal artery

Polar frontal artery

Anterior cerebral arteries

Medial frontobasal (orbitofrontal) artery

Distal medial striate artery (recurrent artery of Heubner)

Internal carotid artery

Anterior choroidal artery

Posterior cerebral artery

Superior cerebellar artery

Basilar and pontine arteries

Labyrinthine (internal acoustic) artery

Vertebral artery

Posterior inferior cerebellar artery (PICA)

Anterior spinal artery

Falx cerebri

Corpus striatum (caudate and lentiform nuclei)

Anterolateral central (lenticulostriate) arteries

Insula (island of Reil)

Precentral (pre-rolandic), central (rolandic) sulcal, and parietal arteries

Lateral cerebral (sylvian) sulcus

Temporal branches of middle cerebral artery

Temporal lobe

Middle cerebral artery

Internal carotid artery

Callosomarginal arteries and Pericallosal arteries (branches of anterior cerebral arteries)

Trunk of corpus callosum

Internal capsule

Septum pellucidum

Rostrum of corpus callosum

Anterior cerebral arteries

Distal medial striate artery (recurrent artery of Heubner)

Anterior communicating artery

Optic chiasm

Arteries of Brain: Lateral and Medial Views

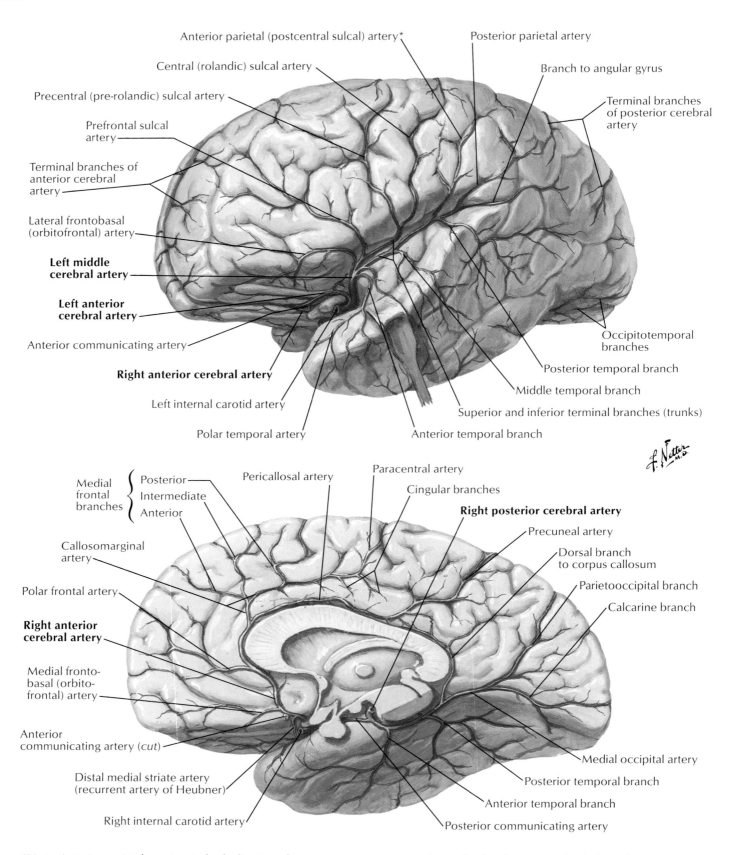

Anterior parietal (postcentral sulcal) artery*

Central (rolandic) sulcal artery

Precentral (pre-rolandic) sulcal artery

Prefrontal sulcal artery

Terminal branches of anterior cerebral artery

Lateral frontobasal (orbitofrontal) artery

Left middle cerebral artery

Left anterior cerebral artery

Anterior communicating artery

Right anterior cerebral artery

Left internal carotid artery

Polar temporal artery

Posterior parietal artery

Branch to angular gyrus

Terminal branches of posterior cerebral artery

Occipitotemporal branches

Posterior temporal branch

Middle temporal branch

Superior and inferior terminal branches (trunks)

Anterior temporal branch

Medial frontal branches { Posterior / Intermediate / Anterior

Pericallosal artery

Paracentral artery

Cingular branches

Right posterior cerebral artery

Precuneal artery

Dorsal branch to corpus callosum

Parietooccipital branch

Calcarine branch

Callosomarginal artery

Polar frontal artery

Right anterior cerebral artery

Medial fronto-basal (orbito-frontal) artery

Anterior communicating artery (*cut*)

Distal medial striate artery (recurrent artery of Heubner)

Right internal carotid artery

Medial occipital artery

Posterior temporal branch

Anterior temporal branch

Posterior communicating artery

*Note: Anterior parietal (postcentral sulcal) artery also occurs as separate anterior parietal and postcentral sulcal arteries.

Plate 140

Cerebral Vasculature

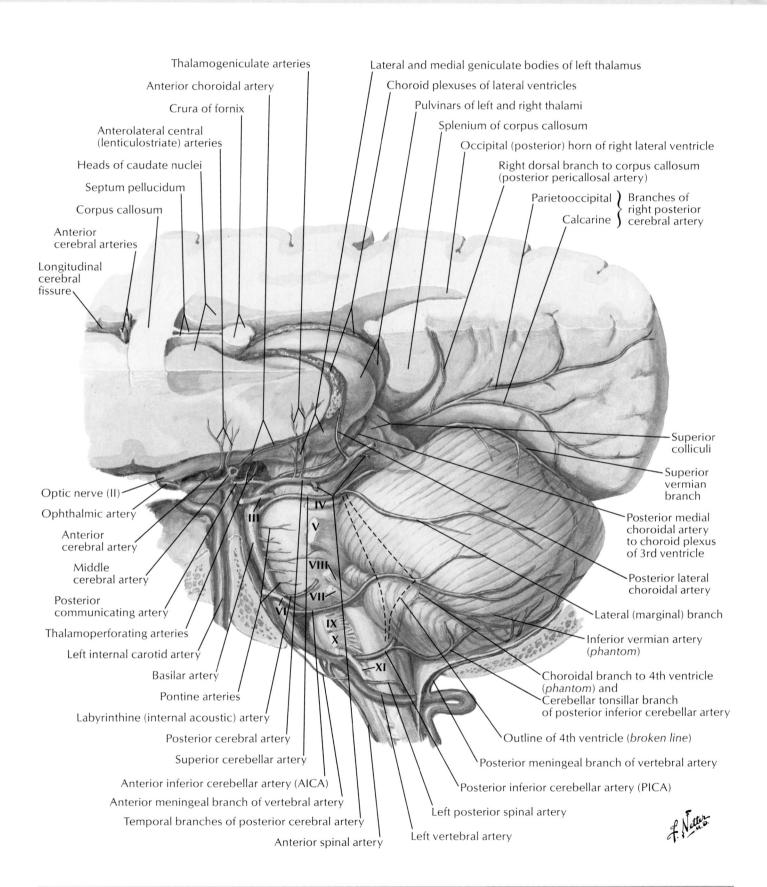

Thalamogeniculate arteries

Anterior choroidal artery

Crura of fornix

Anterolateral central (lenticulostriate) arteries

Heads of caudate nuclei

Septum pellucidum

Corpus callosum

Anterior cerebral arteries

Longitudinal cerebral fissure

Lateral and medial geniculate bodies of left thalamus

Choroid plexuses of lateral ventricles

Pulvinars of left and right thalami

Splenium of corpus callosum

Occipital (posterior) horn of right lateral ventricle

Right dorsal branch to corpus callosum (posterior pericallosal artery)

Parietooccipital ⎫ Branches of
            ⎬ right posterior
Calcarine ⎭ cerebral artery

Superior colliculi

Superior vermian branch

Posterior medial choroidal artery to choroid plexus of 3rd ventricle

Posterior lateral choroidal artery

Lateral (marginal) branch

Inferior vermian artery (phantom)

Choroidal branch to 4th ventricle (phantom) and Cerebellar tonsillar branch of posterior inferior cerebellar artery

Optic nerve (II)

Ophthalmic artery

Anterior cerebral artery

Middle cerebral artery

Posterior communicating artery

Thalamoperforating arteries

Left internal carotid artery

Basilar artery

Pontine arteries

Labyrinthine (internal acoustic) artery

Posterior cerebral artery

Superior cerebellar artery

Anterior inferior cerebellar artery (AICA)

Anterior meningeal branch of vertebral artery

Temporal branches of posterior cerebral artery

Anterior spinal artery

III

IV

V

VIII

VII

VI

IX

X

XI

Outline of 4th ventricle (broken line)

Posterior meningeal branch of vertebral artery

Posterior inferior cerebellar artery (PICA)

Left posterior spinal artery

Left vertebral artery

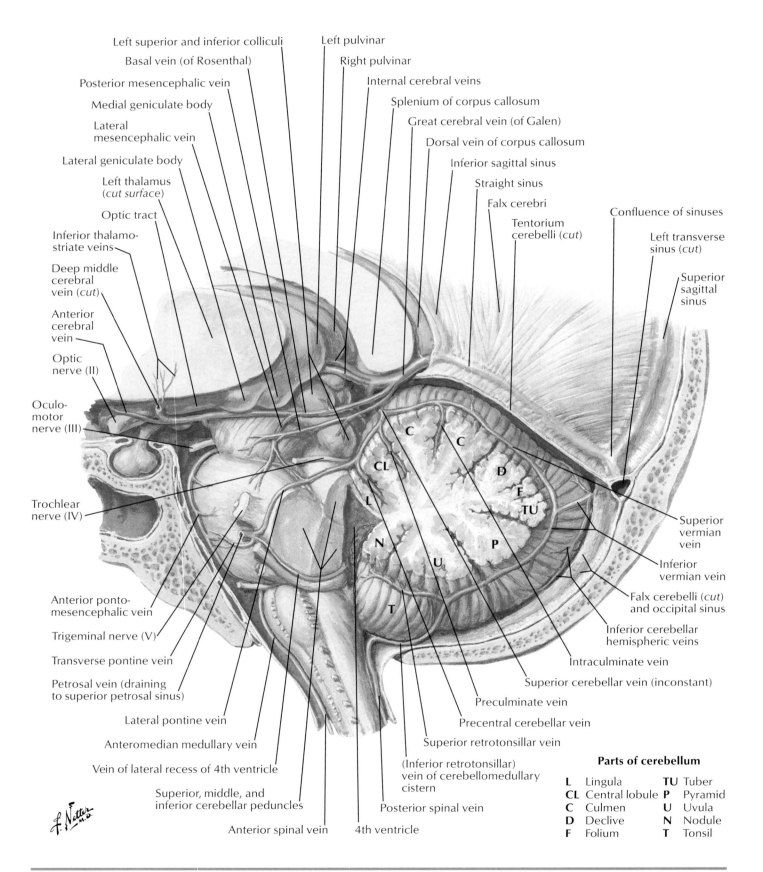

Left superior and inferior colliculi

Basal vein (of Rosenthal)

Posterior mesencephalic vein

Medial geniculate body

Lateral mesencephalic vein

Lateral geniculate body

Left thalamus (*cut surface*)

Optic tract

Inferior thalamo-striate veins

Deep middle cerebral vein (*cut*)

Anterior cerebral vein

Optic nerve (II)

Oculo-motor nerve (III)

Trochlear nerve (IV)

Anterior ponto-mesencephalic vein

Trigeminal nerve (V)

Transverse pontine vein

Petrosal vein (draining to superior petrosal sinus)

Lateral pontine vein

Anteromedian medullary vein

Vein of lateral recess of 4th ventricle

Superior, middle, and inferior cerebellar peduncles

Anterior spinal vein

Left pulvinar

Right pulvinar

Internal cerebral veins

Splenium of corpus callosum

Great cerebral vein (of Galen)

Dorsal vein of corpus callosum

Inferior sagittal sinus

Straight sinus

Falx cerebri

Tentorium cerebelli (*cut*)

Confluence of sinuses

Left transverse sinus (*cut*)

Superior sagittal sinus

Superior vermian vein

Inferior vermian vein

Falx cerebelli (*cut*) and occipital sinus

Inferior cerebellar hemispheric veins

Intraculminate vein

Superior cerebellar vein (inconstant)

Precentral cerebellar vein

Preculminate vein

Superior retrotonsillar vein

(Inferior retrotonsillar) vein of cerebellomedullary cistern

Posterior spinal vein

4th ventricle

Parts of cerebellum

L	Lingula	**TU**	Tuber
CL	Central lobule	**P**	Pyramid
C	Culmen	**U**	Uvula
D	Declive	**N**	Nodule
F	Folium	**T**	Tonsil

Plate 142   **Cerebral Vasculature**

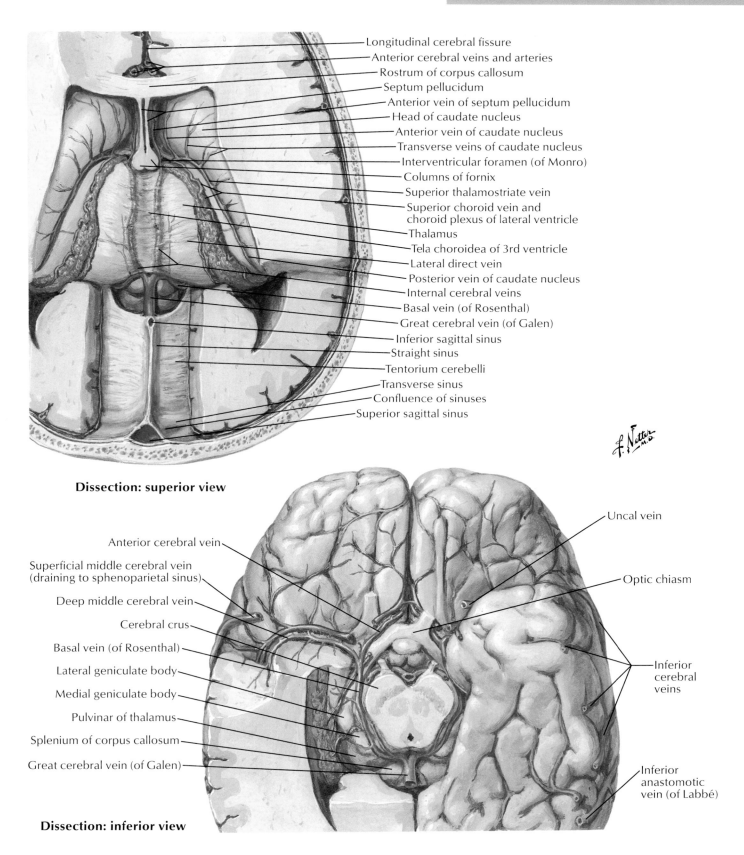

Longitudinal cerebral fissure
Anterior cerebral veins and arteries
Rostrum of corpus callosum
Septum pellucidum
Anterior vein of septum pellucidum
Head of caudate nucleus
Anterior vein of caudate nucleus
Transverse veins of caudate nucleus
Interventricular foramen (of Monro)
Columns of fornix
Superior thalamostriate vein
Superior choroid vein and choroid plexus of lateral ventricle
Thalamus
Tela choroidea of 3rd ventricle
Lateral direct vein
Posterior vein of caudate nucleus
Internal cerebral veins
Basal vein (of Rosenthal)
Great cerebral vein (of Galen)
Inferior sagittal sinus
Straight sinus
Tentorium cerebelli
Transverse sinus
Confluence of sinuses
Superior sagittal sinus

Dissection: superior view

Anterior cerebral vein
Superficial middle cerebral vein (draining to sphenoparietal sinus)
Deep middle cerebral vein
Cerebral crus
Basal vein (of Rosenthal)
Lateral geniculate body
Medial geniculate body
Pulvinar of thalamus
Splenium of corpus callosum
Great cerebral vein (of Galen)

Uncal vein
Optic chiasm
Inferior cerebral veins
Inferior anastomotic vein (of Labbé)

Dissection: inferior view

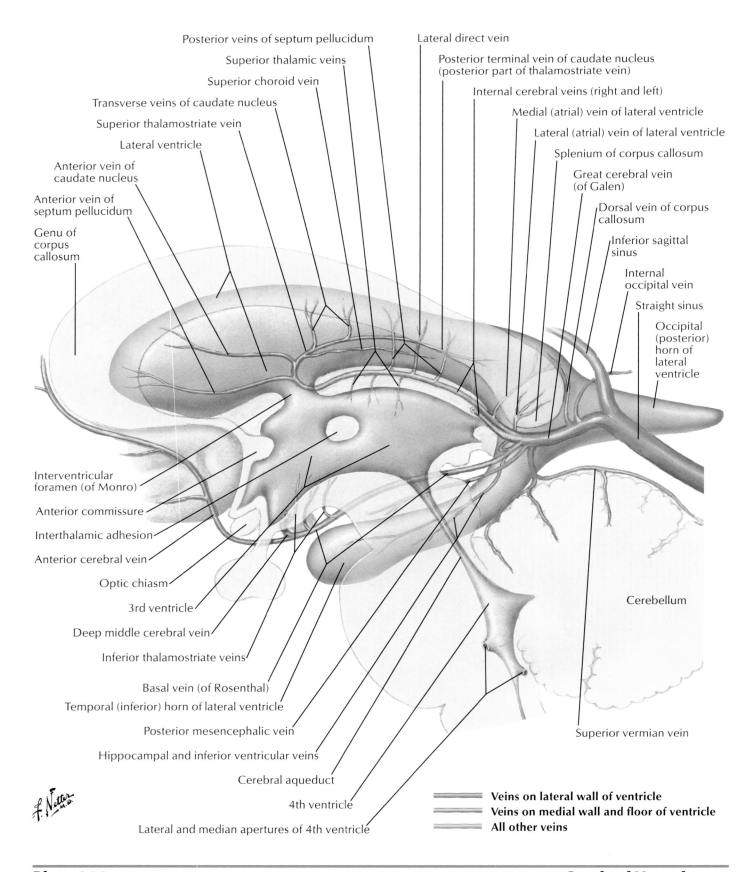

Posterior veins of septum pellucidum

Superior thalamic veins

Superior choroid vein

Transverse veins of caudate nucleus

Superior thalamostriate vein

Lateral ventricle

Anterior vein of caudate nucleus

Anterior vein of septum pellucidum

Genu of corpus callosum

Lateral direct vein

Posterior terminal vein of caudate nucleus (posterior part of thalamostriate vein)

Internal cerebral veins (right and left)

Medial (atrial) vein of lateral ventricle

Lateral (atrial) vein of lateral ventricle

Splenium of corpus callosum

Great cerebral vein (of Galen)

Dorsal vein of corpus callosum

Inferior sagittal sinus

Internal occipital vein

Straight sinus

Occipital (posterior) horn of lateral ventricle

Cerebellum

Interventricular foramen (of Monro)

Anterior commissure

Interthalamic adhesion

Anterior cerebral vein

Optic chiasm

3rd ventricle

Deep middle cerebral vein

Inferior thalamostriate veins

Basal vein (of Rosenthal)

Temporal (inferior) horn of lateral ventricle

Posterior mesencephalic vein

Hippocampal and inferior ventricular veins

Cerebral aqueduct

4th ventricle

Lateral and median apertures of 4th ventricle

Superior vermian vein

Veins on lateral wall of ventricle
Veins on medial wall and floor of ventricle
All other veins

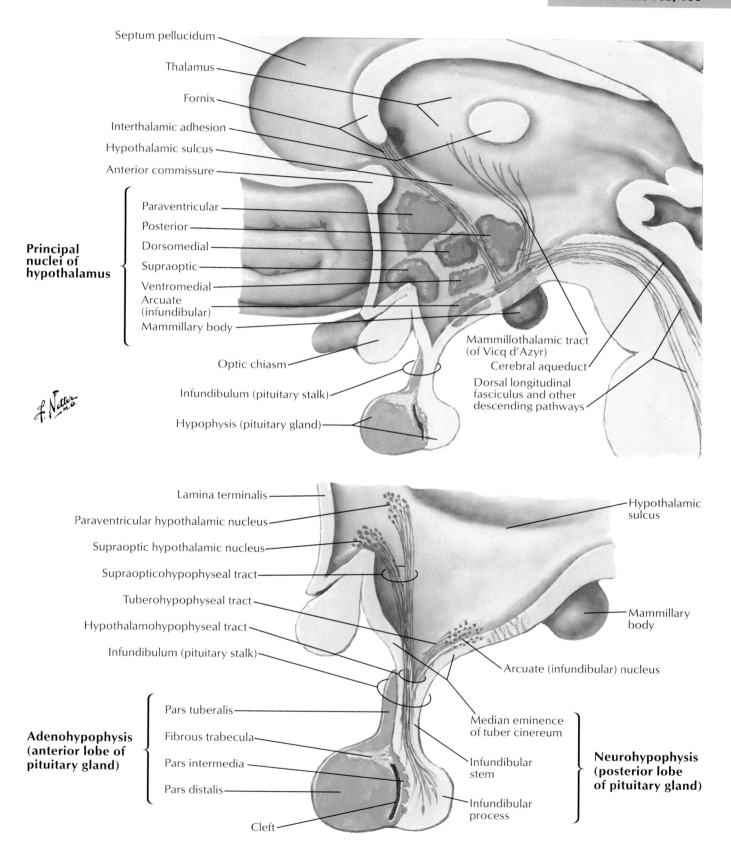

Septum pellucidum

Thalamus

Fornix

Interthalamic adhesion

Hypothalamic sulcus

Anterior commissure

Principal nuclei of hypothalamus

Paraventricular

Posterior

Dorsomedial

Supraoptic

Ventromedial

Arcuate (infundibular)

Mammillary body

Optic chiasm

Infundibulum (pituitary stalk)

Hypophysis (pituitary gland)

Mammillothalamic tract (of Vicq d'Azyr)

Cerebral aqueduct

Dorsal longitudinal fasciculus and other descending pathways

Lamina terminalis

Paraventricular hypothalamic nucleus

Supraoptic hypothalamic nucleus

Supraopticohypophyseal tract

Tuberohypophyseal tract

Hypothalamohypophyseal tract

Infundibulum (pituitary stalk)

Adenohypophysis (anterior lobe of pituitary gland)

Pars tuberalis

Fibrous trabecula

Pars intermedia

Pars distalis

Cleft

Hypothalamic sulcus

Mammillary body

Arcuate (infundibular) nucleus

Median eminence of tuber cinereum

Infundibular stem

Infundibular process

Neurohypophysis (posterior lobe of pituitary gland)

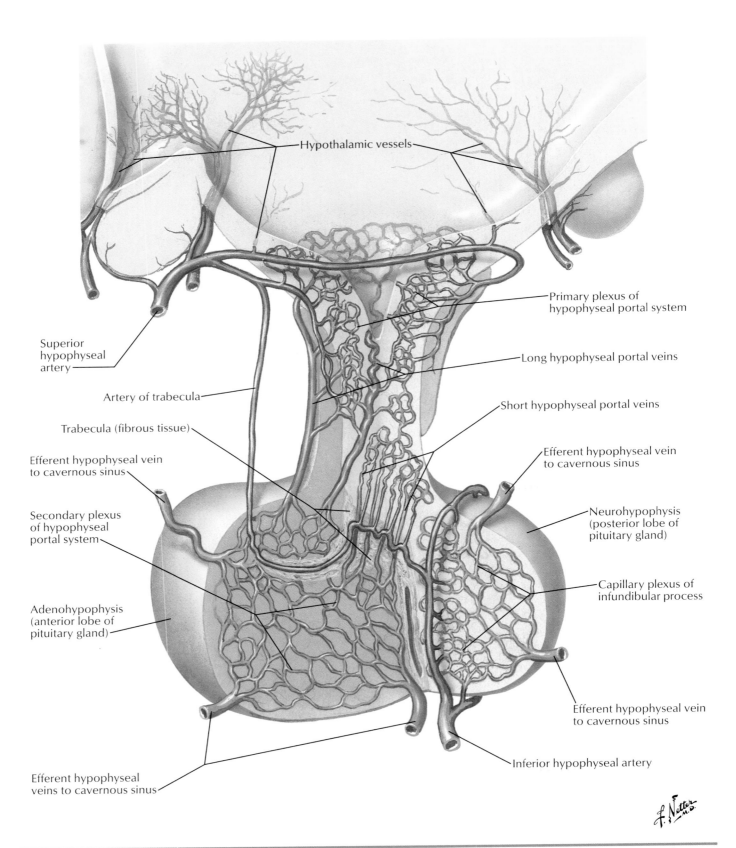

Hypothalamic vessels

Primary plexus of hypophyseal portal system

Superior hypophyseal artery

Long hypophyseal portal veins

Artery of trabecula

Short hypophyseal portal veins

Trabecula (fibrous tissue)

Efferent hypophyseal vein to cavernous sinus

Efferent hypophyseal vein to cavernous sinus

Neurohypophysis (posterior lobe of pituitary gland)

Secondary plexus of hypophyseal portal system

Adenohypophysis (anterior lobe of pituitary gland)

Capillary plexus of infundibular process

Efferent hypophyseal vein to cavernous sinus

Efferent hypophyseal veins to cavernous sinus

Inferior hypophyseal artery

Plate 146

Cerebral Vasculature

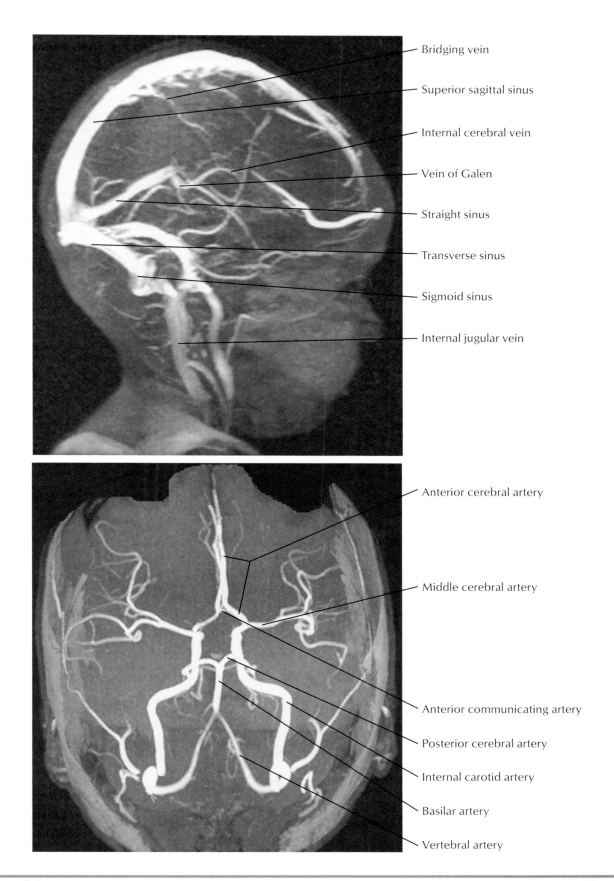

Bridging vein

Superior sagittal sinus

Internal cerebral vein

Vein of Galen

Straight sinus

Transverse sinus

Sigmoid sinus

Internal jugular vein

Anterior cerebral artery

Middle cerebral artery

Anterior communicating artery

Posterior cerebral artery

Internal carotid artery

Basilar artery

Vertebral artery

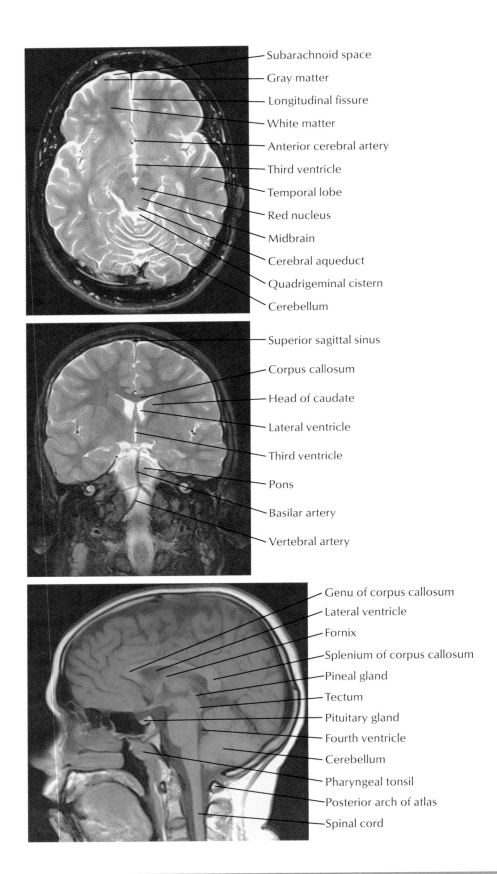

- Subarachnoid space
- Gray matter
- Longitudinal fissure
- White matter
- Anterior cerebral artery
- Third ventricle
- Temporal lobe
- Red nucleus
- Midbrain
- Cerebral aqueduct
- Quadrigeminal cistern
- Cerebellum

- Superior sagittal sinus
- Corpus callosum
- Head of caudate
- Lateral ventricle
- Third ventricle
- Pons
- Basilar artery
- Vertebral artery

- Genu of corpus callosum
- Lateral ventricle
- Fornix
- Splenium of corpus callosum
- Pineal gland
- Tectum
- Pituitary gland
- Fourth ventricle
- Cerebellum
- Pharyngeal tonsil
- Posterior arch of atlas
- Spinal cord

Plate 148

Regional Scans

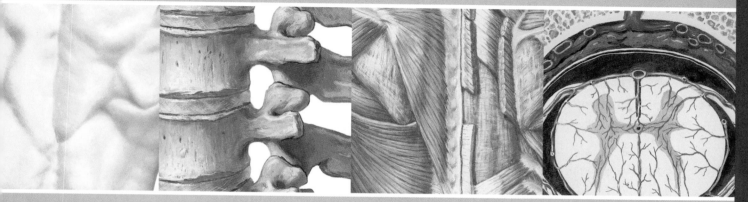

Section 2 BACK AND SPINAL CORD

Topographic Anatomy
Plate 149

149 Back

Bones and Ligaments
Plates 150-156

150 Vertebral Column

151 Thoracic Vertebrae

152 Lumbar Vertebrae

153 Lumbar Vertebrae: Radiographs

154 Sacrum and Coccyx

155 Vertebral Ligaments: Lumbosacral Region

156 Vertebral Ligaments: Lumbar Region

Spinal Cord
Plates 157-167

157 Spinal Cord and Ventral Rami in Situ

158 Relation of Spinal Nerve Roots to Vertebrae

159 Dermatomes

160 Sympathetic Nervous System: Schema

161 Parasympathetic Nervous System: Schema

162 Spinal Membranes and Nerve Roots

163 Spinal Nerve Origin: Cross Sections

164 Arteries of Spinal Cord: Schema

165 Arteries of Spinal Cord: Intrinsic Distribution

166 Veins of Spinal Cord and Vertebral Column

167 Veins of the Vertebral Column: Vertebral Veins

2 BACK AND SPINAL CORD

Muscles and Nerves

Plates 168-172

168 Muscles of Back: Superficial Layers

169 Muscles of Back: Intermediate Layers

170 Muscles of Back: Deep Layers

171 Nerves of Back

172 Suboccipital Triangle

Cross-sectional Anatomy

Plates 173-174

173 Lumbar Region of Back: Cross Section

174 Typical Thoracic Spinal Nerve

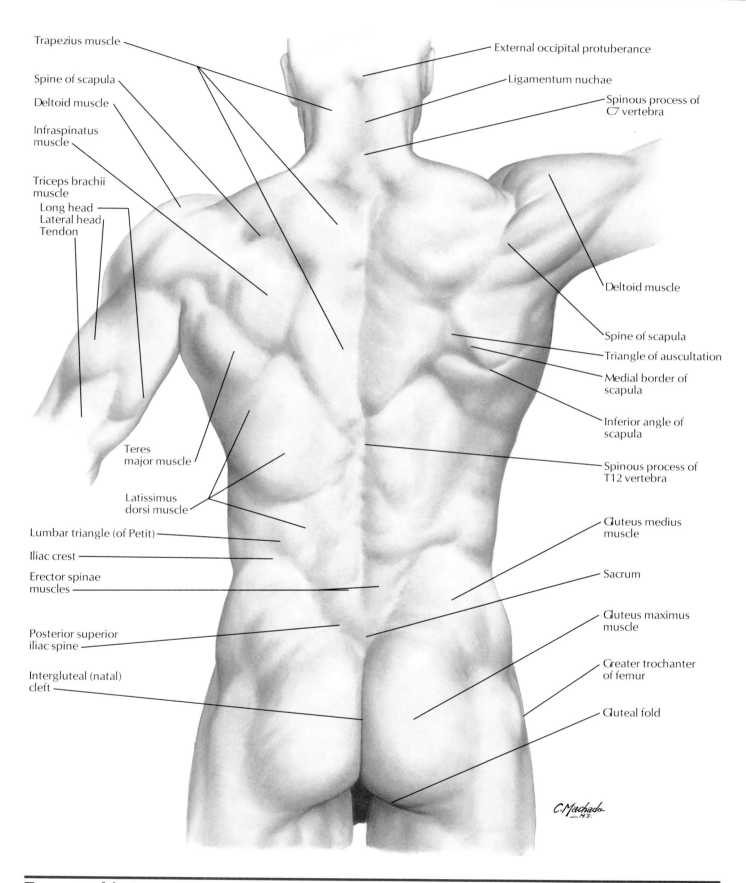

Trapezius muscle

Spine of scapula

Deltoid muscle

Infraspinatus
muscle

Triceps brachii
muscle
Long head
Lateral head
Tendon

Teres
major muscle

Latissimus
dorsi muscle

Lumbar triangle (of Petit)

Iliac crest

Erector spinae
muscles

Posterior superior
iliac spine

Intergluteal (natal)
cleft

External occipital protuberance

Ligamentum nuchae

Spinous process of
C7 vertebra

Deltoid muscle

Spine of scapula

Triangle of auscultation

Medial border of
scapula

Inferior angle of
scapula

Spinous process of
T12 vertebra

Gluteus medius
muscle

Sacrum

Gluteus maximus
muscle

Greater trochanter
of femur

Gluteal fold

C.Machado
—M.D.

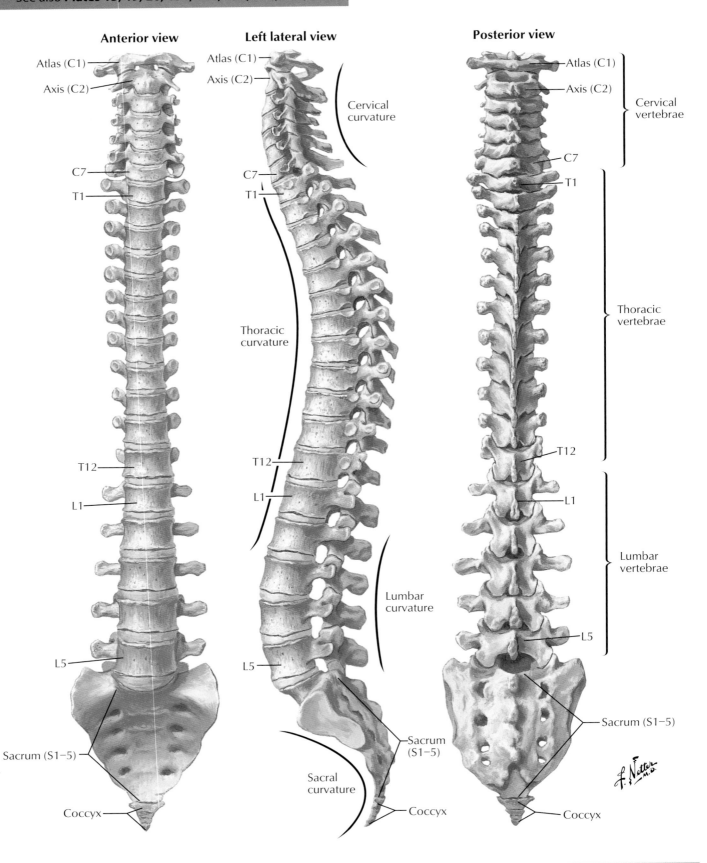

Anterior view

Atlas (C1)
Axis (C2)
C7
T1
T12
L1
L5
Sacrum (S1–5)
Coccyx

Left lateral view

Atlas (C1)
Axis (C2)
Cervical curvature
C7
T1
Thoracic curvature
T12
L1
Lumbar curvature
L5
Sacrum (S1–5)
Sacral curvature
Coccyx

Posterior view

Atlas (C1)
Axis (C2)
Cervical vertebrae
C7
T1
Thoracic vertebrae
T12
L1
Lumbar vertebrae
L5
Sacrum (S1–5)
Coccyx

f. Netter M.D.

Plate 150

Bones and Ligaments

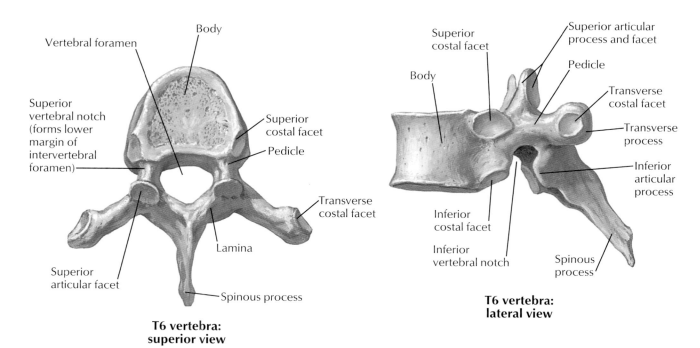

Body

Vertebral foramen

Superior
vertebral notch
(forms lower
margin of
intervertebral
foramen)

Superior
costal facet

Pedicle

Transverse
costal facet

Lamina

Superior
articular facet

Spinous process

**T6 vertebra:
superior view**

Superior
costal facet

Body

Superior articular
process and facet

Pedicle

Transverse
costal facet

Transverse
process

Inferior
articular
process

Inferior
costal facet

Inferior
vertebral notch

Spinous
process

**T6 vertebra:
lateral view**

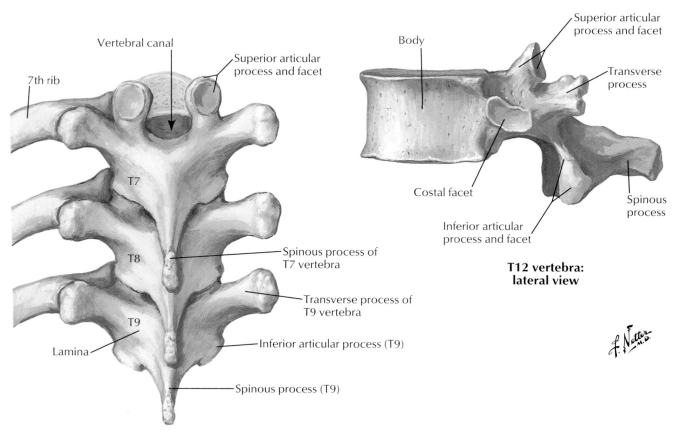

Vertebral canal

Superior articular
process and facet

7th rib

T7

T8

T9

Lamina

Spinous process of
T7 vertebra

Transverse process of
T9 vertebra

Inferior articular process (T9)

Spinous process (T9)

**T7, T8, and T9 vertebrae:
posterior view**

Body

Superior articular
process and facet

Transverse
process

Costal facet

Inferior articular
process and facet

Spinous
process

**T12 vertebra:
lateral view**

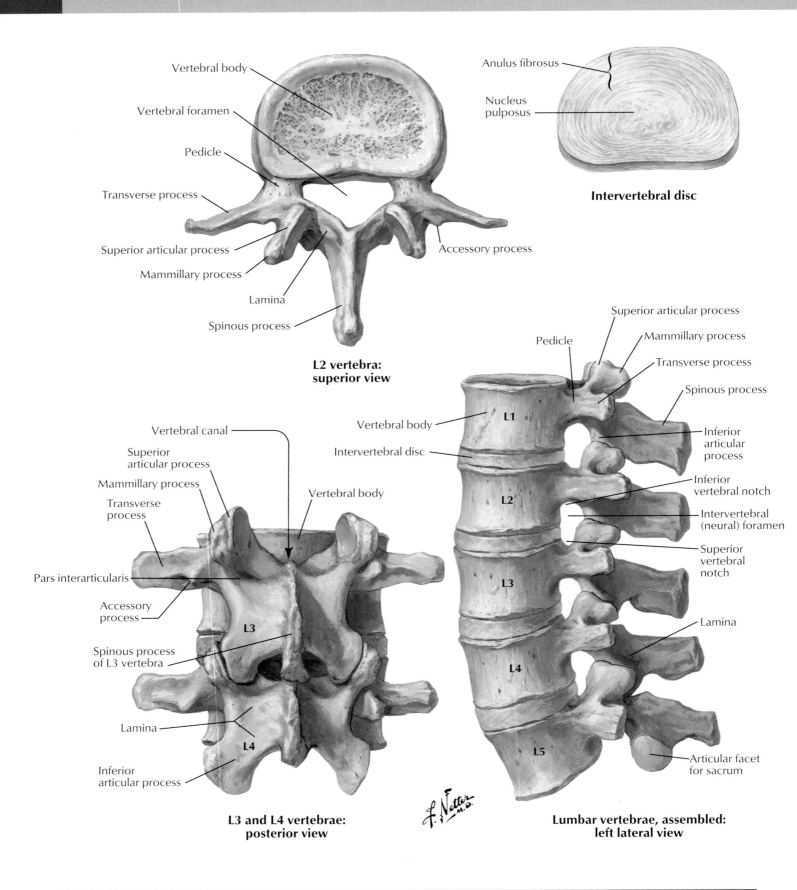

Vertebral body

Vertebral foramen

Pedicle

Transverse process

Superior articular process

Mammillary process

Lamina

Spinous process

**L2 vertebra:
superior view**

Anulus fibrosus

Nucleus
pulposus

Intervertebral disc

Vertebral canal

Superior
articular process

Mammillary process

Transverse
process

Pars interarticularis

Accessory
process

Spinous process
of L3 vertebra

Lamina

Inferior
articular process

Vertebral body

L3

L4

**L3 and L4 vertebrae:
posterior view**

Superior articular process

Pedicle

Mammillary process

Transverse process

Spinous process

Vertebral body

Intervertebral disc

Inferior
articular
process

Inferior
vertebral notch

Intervertebral
(neural) foramen

Superior
vertebral
notch

Lamina

Articular facet
for sacrum

L1

L2

L3

L4

L5

**Lumbar vertebrae, assembled:
left lateral view**

Accessory process

*F. Netter
M.D.*

Plate 152   **Bones and Ligaments**

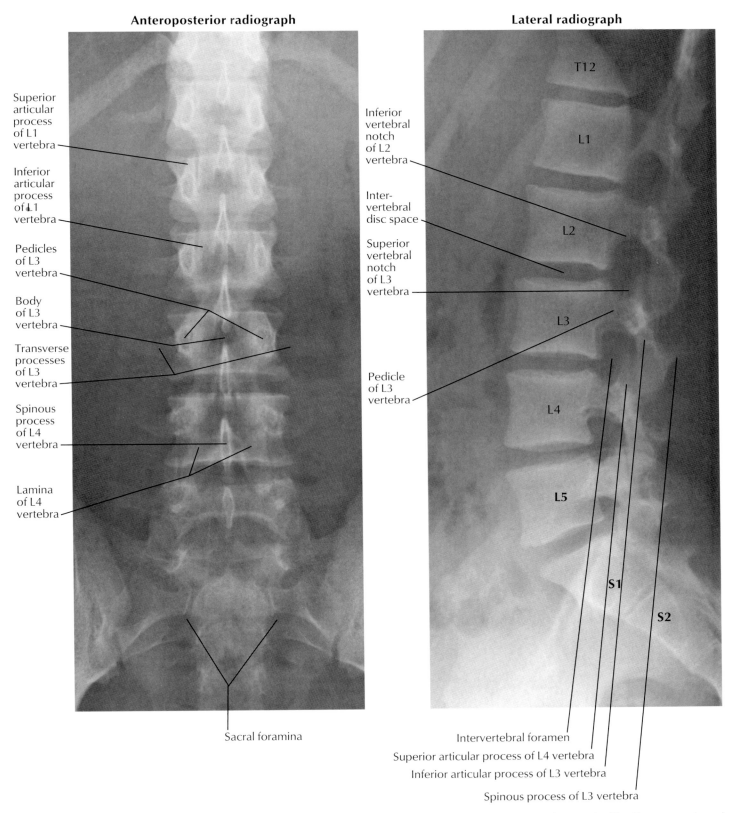

Anteroposterior radiograph

Lateral radiograph

Superior articular process of L1 vertebra

Inferior articular process of L1 vertebra

Pedicles of L3 vertebra

Body of L3 vertebra

Transverse processes of L3 vertebra

Spinous process of L4 vertebra

Lamina of L4 vertebra

Sacral foramina

T12

Inferior vertebral notch of L2 vertebra

Inter-vertebral disc space

Superior vertebral notch of L3 vertebra

Pedicle of L3 vertebra

L1

L2

L3

L4

L5

S1

S2

Intervertebral foramen

Superior articular process of L4 vertebra

Inferior articular process of L3 vertebra

Spinous process of L3 vertebra

Note: The vertebral bodies are numbered

Base of sacrum

Lumbosacral
articular surface

Superior
articular process

Ala (wing)

Promontory

Sacral part
of pelvic brim
(linea terminalis)

Anterior (pelvic)
sacral foramina

Transverse
ridges

Apex of sacrum

Transverse process
of coccyx

Coccyx

**Anterior inferior
view**

Pelvic surface

Superior
articular
process

Sacral
canal

Dorsal surface

Pelvic surface

Sacral hiatus

Median sagittal section

Facets of
superior articular
processes

Auricular surface

Sacral tuberosity

Lateral sacral crest

Median sacral crest

Intermediate sacral crest

Posterior
sacral
foramina

Sacral cornu
(horn)

Coccygeal cornu
(horn)

Transverse process
of coccyx

Sacral hiatus

Dorsal surface

Posterior superior view

Median sacral crest

Sacral canal

Intervertebral
foramen

Posterior
sacral foramen

Anterior (pelvic)
sacral foramen

**Transverse section
through S2 foramina**

Plate 154   **Bones and Ligaments**

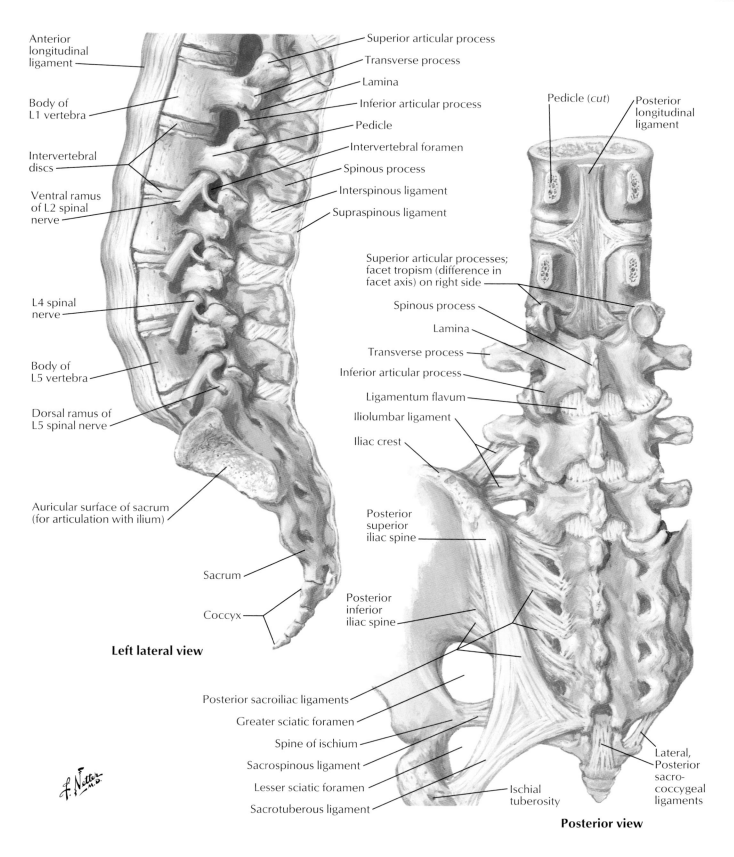

Anterior longitudinal ligament

Body of L1 vertebra

Intervertebral discs

Ventral ramus of L2 spinal nerve

L4 spinal nerve

Body of L5 vertebra

Dorsal ramus of L5 spinal nerve

Superior articular process

Transverse process

Lamina

Inferior articular process

Pedicle

Intervertebral foramen

Spinous process

Interspinous ligament

Supraspinous ligament

Pedicle (*cut*)

Posterior longitudinal ligament

Superior articular processes; facet tropism (difference in facet axis) on right side

Spinous process

Lamina

Transverse process

Inferior articular process

Ligamentum flavum

Iliolumbar ligament

Iliac crest

Auricular surface of sacrum (for articulation with ilium)

Sacrum

Coccyx

Left lateral view

Posterior superior iliac spine

Posterior inferior iliac spine

Posterior sacroiliac ligaments

Greater sciatic foramen

Spine of ischium

Sacrospinous ligament

Lesser sciatic foramen

Sacrotuberous ligament

Ischial tuberosity

Lateral, Posterior sacro-coccygeal ligaments

Posterior view

Left lateral view
(*partially sectioned in median plane*)

Anterior longitudinal ligament

Lumbar vertebral body

Intervertebral disc

Anterior longitudinal ligament

Posterior longitudinal ligament

Inferior articular process

Capsule of zygapophyseal joint (*partially opened*)

Superior articular process

Transverse process

Spinous process

Ligamentum flavum

Interspinous ligament

Supraspinous ligament

Intervertebral foramen

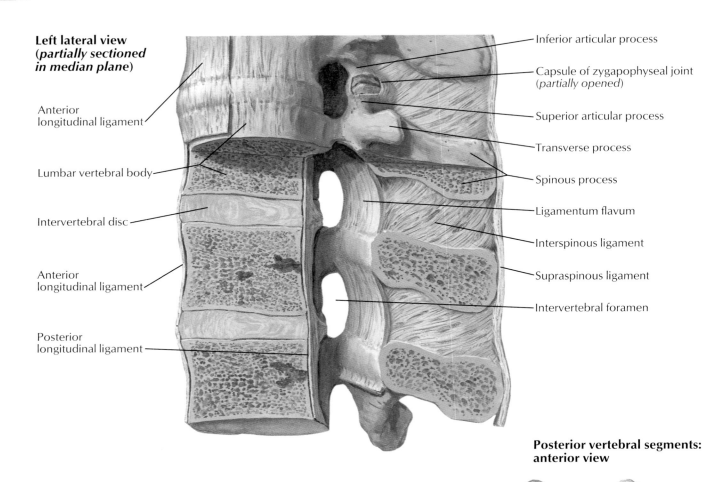

Anterior vertebral segments: posterior view
(*pedicles sectioned*)

Pedicle (*cut surface*)

Posterior surface of vertebral bodies

Posterior longitudinal ligament

Intervertebral disc

Posterior vertebral segments: anterior view

Pedicle (*cut surface*)

Ligamentum flavum

Lamina

Superior articular process

Transverse process

Inferior articular facet

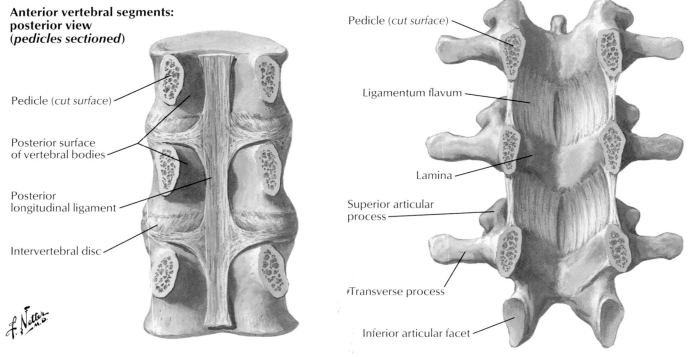

Plate 156   **Bones and Ligaments**

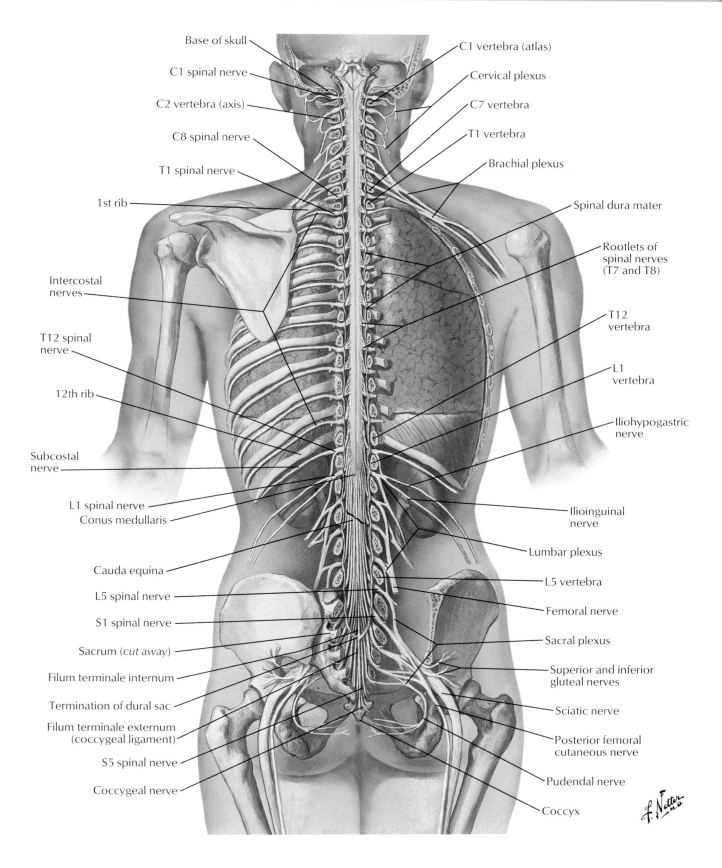

Base of skull

C1 spinal nerve

C2 vertebra (axis)

C8 spinal nerve

T1 spinal nerve

1st rib

Intercostal nerves

T12 spinal nerve

12th rib

Subcostal nerve

L1 spinal nerve

Conus medullaris

Cauda equina

L5 spinal nerve

S1 spinal nerve

Sacrum (cut away)

Filum terminale internum

Termination of dural sac

Filum terminale externum (coccygeal ligament)

S5 spinal nerve

Coccygeal nerve

C1 vertebra (atlas)

Cervical plexus

C7 vertebra

T1 vertebra

Brachial plexus

Spinal dura mater

Rootlets of spinal nerves (T7 and T8)

T12 vertebra

L1 vertebra

Iliohypogastric nerve

Ilioinguinal nerve

Lumbar plexus

L5 vertebra

Femoral nerve

Sacral plexus

Superior and inferior gluteal nerves

Sciatic nerve

Posterior femoral cutaneous nerve

Pudendal nerve

Coccyx

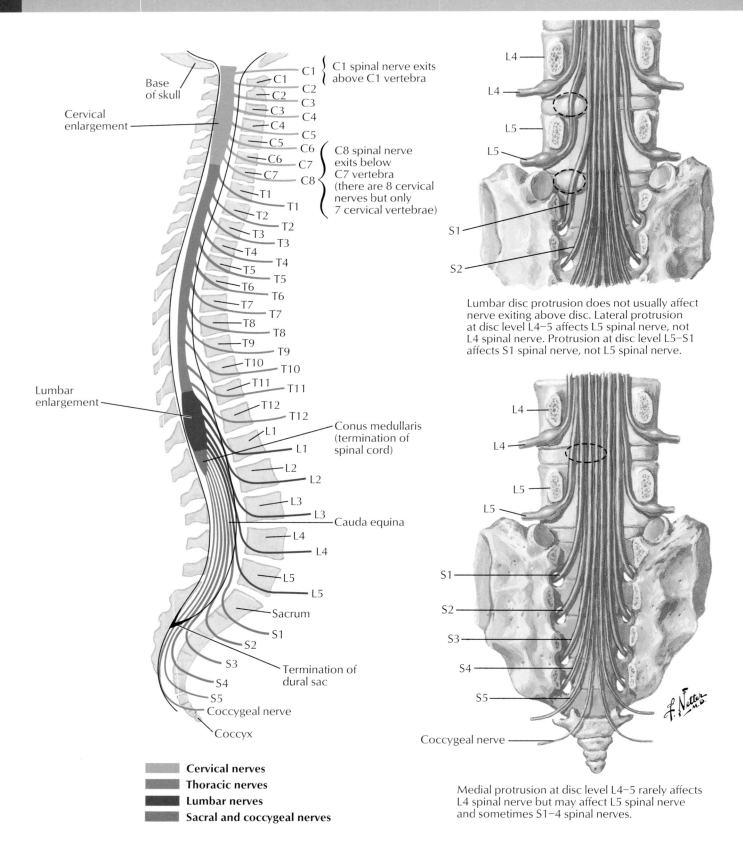

Base of skull

Cervical enlargement

C1
C1
C2
C3
C4
C5
C6
C7

C1
C2
C3
C4
C5
C6
C7
C8

C1 spinal nerve exits above C1 vertebra

C8 spinal nerve exits below C7 vertebra (there are 8 cervical nerves but only 7 cervical vertebrae)

T1
T2
T3
T4
T5
T6
T7
T8
T9
T10
T11
T12

T1
T2
T3
T4
T5
T6
T7
T8
T9
T10
T11
T12

Lumbar enlargement

L1
L2
L3
L4
L5

L1
L2
L3
L4
L5

Conus medullaris (termination of spinal cord)

Cauda equina

Sacrum

S1
S2
S3
S4
S5

Termination of dural sac

Coccygeal nerve

Coccyx

Cervical nerves
Thoracic nerves
Lumbar nerves
Sacral and coccygeal nerves

L4
L4
L5
L5
S1
S2

Lumbar disc protrusion does not usually affect nerve exiting above disc. Lateral protrusion at disc level L4–5 affects L5 spinal nerve, not L4 spinal nerve. Protrusion at disc level L5–S1 affects S1 spinal nerve, not L5 spinal nerve.

L4
L4
L5
L5
S1
S2
S3
S4
S5
Coccygeal nerve

Medial protrusion at disc level L4–5 rarely affects L4 spinal nerve but may affect L5 spinal nerve and sometimes S1–4 spinal nerves.

Plate 158   **Spinal Cord**

See also **Plates 401, 470;** for maps of cutaneous nerves see **Plates 2, 402, 460, 462-464, 466, 467, 526-530**

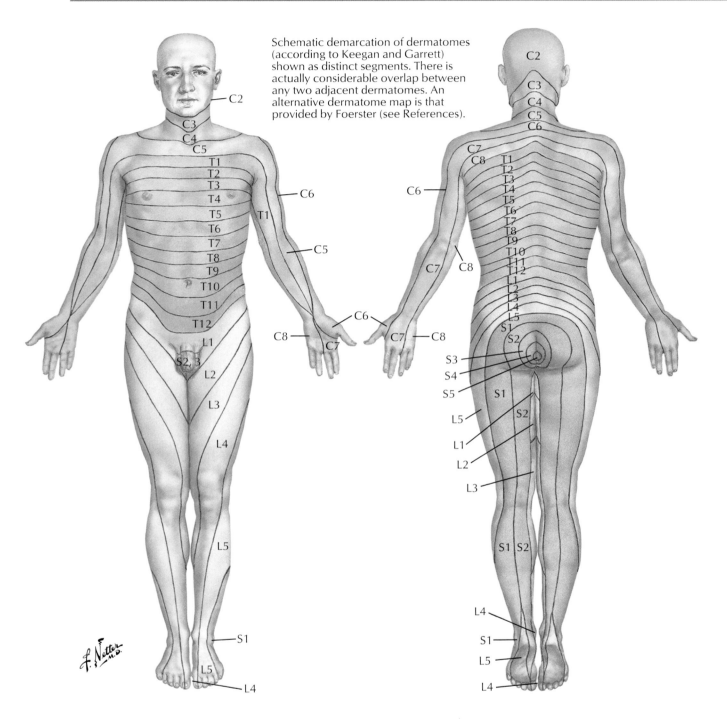

Schematic demarcation of dermatomes (according to Keegan and Garrett) shown as distinct segments. There is actually considerable overlap between any two adjacent dermatomes. An alternative dermatome map is that provided by Foerster (see References).

Levels of principal dermatomes

C5	Clavicles
C5, 6	Lateral sides of upper limbs
C8, T1	Medial sides of upper limbs
C6	Thumb
C6, 7, 8	Hand
C8	Ring and little fingers
T4	Level of nipples

T10	Level of umbilicus
L1	Inguinal or groin regions
L1, 2, 3, 4	Anterior and inner surfaces of lower limbs
L4, 5, S1	Foot
L4	Medial side of great toe
L5, S1, 2	Lateral and posterior surfaces of lower limbs
S1	Lateral margin of foot and little toe
S2, 3, 4	Perineum

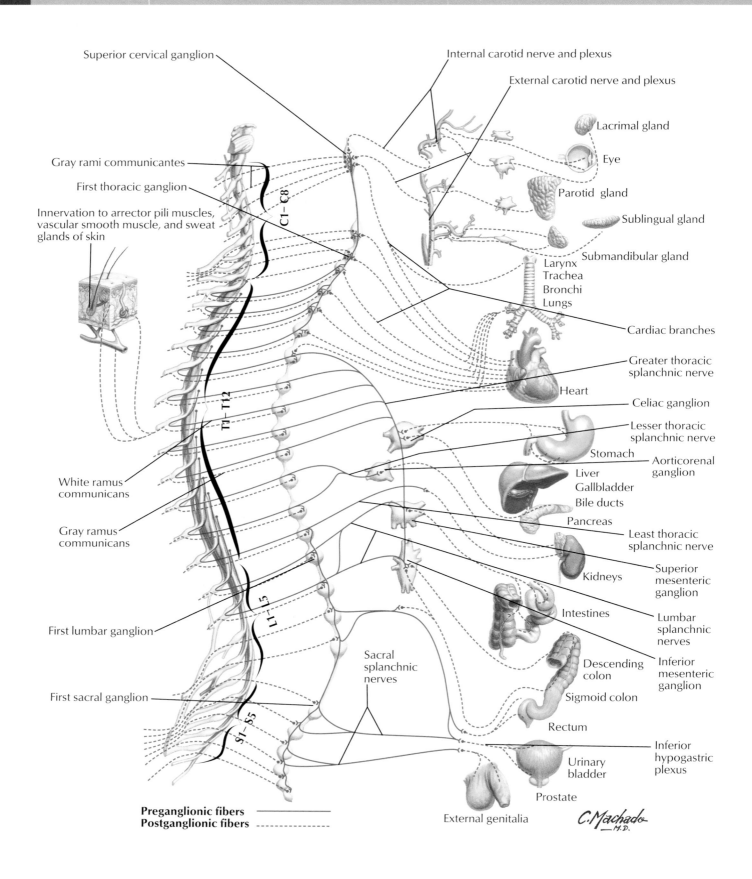

Superior cervical ganglion

Internal carotid nerve and plexus

External carotid nerve and plexus

Lacrimal gland

Eye

Gray rami communicantes

Parotid gland

First thoracic ganglion

Sublingual gland

Innervation to arrector pili muscles, vascular smooth muscle, and sweat glands of skin

Submandibular gland

Larynx
Trachea
Bronchi
Lungs

Cardiac branches

Greater thoracic splanchnic nerve

Heart

Celiac ganglion

Lesser thoracic splanchnic nerve

Stomach

Aorticorenal ganglion

Liver
Gallbladder
Bile ducts

Pancreas

White ramus communicans

Least thoracic splanchnic nerve

Gray ramus communicans

Superior mesenteric ganglion

Kidneys

Intestines

Lumbar splanchnic nerves

First lumbar ganglion

Inferior mesenteric ganglion

Sacral splanchnic nerves

Descending colon

Sigmoid colon

First sacral ganglion

Rectum

Inferior hypogastric plexus

Urinary bladder

Prostate

External genitalia

C1–C8

T1–T12

L1–L5

S1–S5

Preganglionic fibers ——————
Postganglionic fibers - - - - - - -

C. Machado
M.D.

Plate 160 **Spinal Cord**

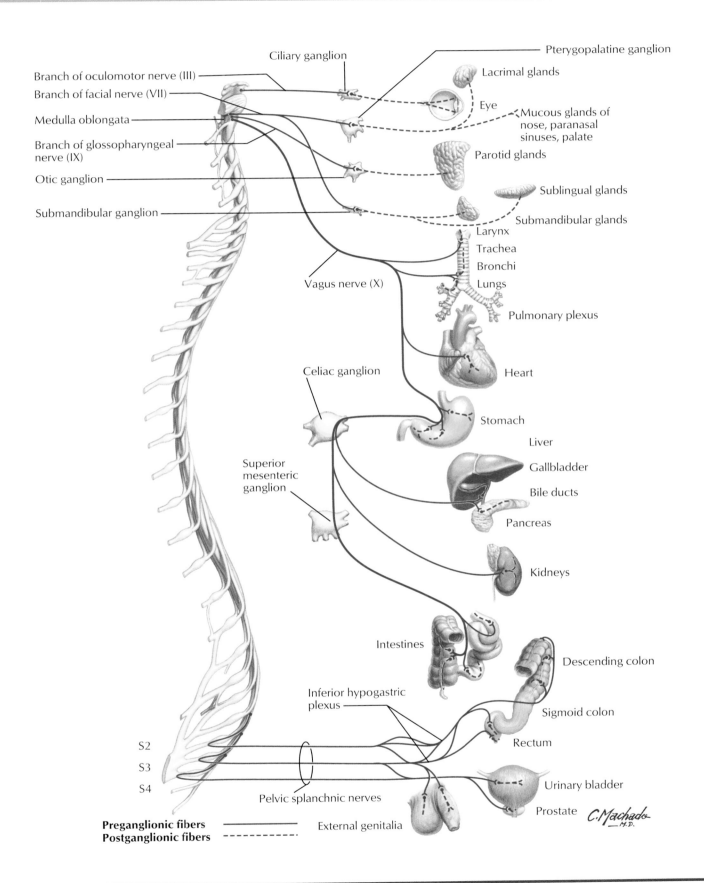

Ciliary ganglion

Pterygopalatine ganglion

Branch of oculomotor nerve (III)

Lacrimal glands

Branch of facial nerve (VII)

Eye

Medulla oblongata

Mucous glands of nose, paranasal sinuses, palate

Branch of glossopharyngeal nerve (IX)

Parotid glands

Otic ganglion

Sublingual glands

Submandibular ganglion

Submandibular glands

Larynx

Trachea

Bronchi

Lungs

Vagus nerve (X)

Pulmonary plexus

Heart

Celiac ganglion

Stomach

Liver

Gallbladder

Superior mesenteric ganglion

Bile ducts

Pancreas

Kidneys

Intestines

Descending colon

Inferior hypogastric plexus

Sigmoid colon

S2

Rectum

S3

S4

Urinary bladder

Pelvic splanchnic nerves

Prostate

Preganglionic fibers ⎯⎯⎯⎯⎯⎯
Postganglionic fibers - - - - - -

External genitalia

C. Machado M.D.

Posterior view

Ventral root of spinal nerve

Dorsal root of spinal nerve

Dorsal root (spinal) ganglion

White and gray rami communicantes to and from sympathetic trunk

Ventral ramus of spinal nerve

Dorsal ramus of spinal nerve

Dura mater

Arachnoid mater

Mesothelial septum in dorsal median sulcus

Pia mater overlying spinal cord

Rootlets of dorsal root

Denticulate ligament

Dorsal horn

Membranes removed: anterior view
(greatly magnified)

Ventral horn

Lateral horn

Gray matter

White matter

Rootlets of dorsal root

Dorsal root of spinal nerve

Rootlets of ventral root

Dorsal root (spinal) ganglion

Dorsal ramus of spinal nerve

Ventral ramus of spinal nerve

Ventral root of spinal nerve

Spinal nerve

Gray and white rami communicantes

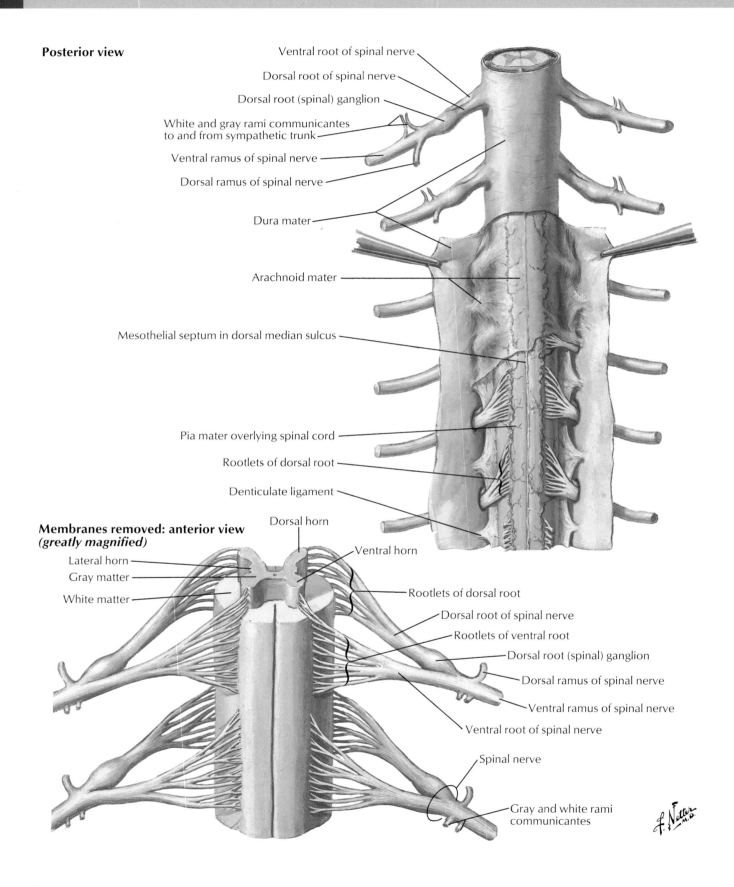

Plate 162

Spinal Cord

Section through thoracic vertebra

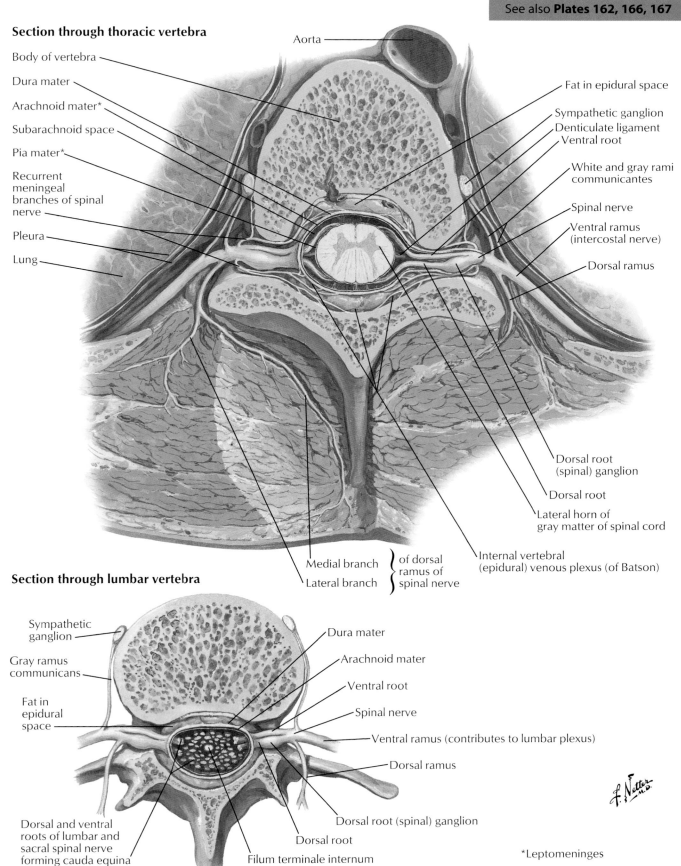

Aorta

Body of vertebra

Dura mater

Arachnoid mater*

Subarachnoid space

Pia mater*

Recurrent meningeal branches of spinal nerve

Pleura

Lung

Fat in epidural space

Sympathetic ganglion

Denticulate ligament

Ventral root

White and gray rami communicantes

Spinal nerve

Ventral ramus (intercostal nerve)

Dorsal ramus

Dorsal root (spinal) ganglion

Dorsal root

Lateral horn of gray matter of spinal cord

Internal vertebral (epidural) venous plexus (of Batson)

Medial branch } of dorsal
Lateral branch } ramus of spinal nerve

Section through lumbar vertebra

Sympathetic ganglion

Gray ramus communicans

Fat in epidural space

Dura mater

Arachnoid mater

Ventral root

Spinal nerve

Ventral ramus (contributes to lumbar plexus)

Dorsal ramus

Dorsal root (spinal) ganglion

Dorsal root

Dorsal and ventral roots of lumbar and sacral spinal nerve forming cauda equina

Filum terminale internum

*Leptomeninges

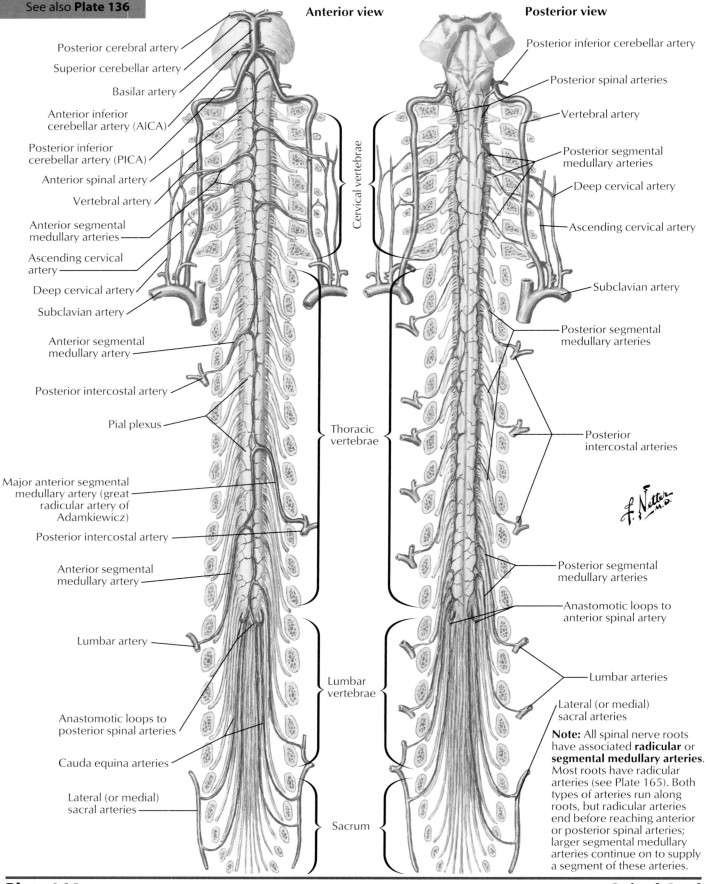

Anterior view

Posterior view

Posterior cerebral artery

Superior cerebellar artery

Basilar artery

Anterior inferior cerebellar artery (AICA)

Posterior inferior cerebellar artery (PICA)

Anterior spinal artery

Vertebral artery

Anterior segmental medullary arteries

Ascending cervical artery

Deep cervical artery

Subclavian artery

Anterior segmental medullary artery

Posterior intercostal artery

Pial plexus

Major anterior segmental medullary artery (great radicular artery of Adamkiewicz)

Posterior intercostal artery

Anterior segmental medullary artery

Lumbar artery

Anastomotic loops to posterior spinal arteries

Cauda equina arteries

Lateral (or medial) sacral arteries

Cervical vertebrae

Thoracic vertebrae

Lumbar vertebrae

Sacrum

Posterior inferior cerebellar artery

Posterior spinal arteries

Vertebral artery

Posterior segmental medullary arteries

Deep cervical artery

Ascending cervical artery

Subclavian artery

Posterior segmental medullary arteries

Posterior intercostal arteries

Posterior segmental medullary arteries

Anastomotic loops to anterior spinal artery

Lumbar arteries

Lateral (or medial) sacral arteries

Note: All spinal nerve roots have associated **radicular** or **segmental medullary arteries.** Most roots have radicular arteries (see Plate 165). Both types of arteries run along roots, but radicular arteries end before reaching anterior or posterior spinal arteries; larger segmental medullary arteries continue on to supply a segment of these arteries.

Plate 164

Spinal Cord

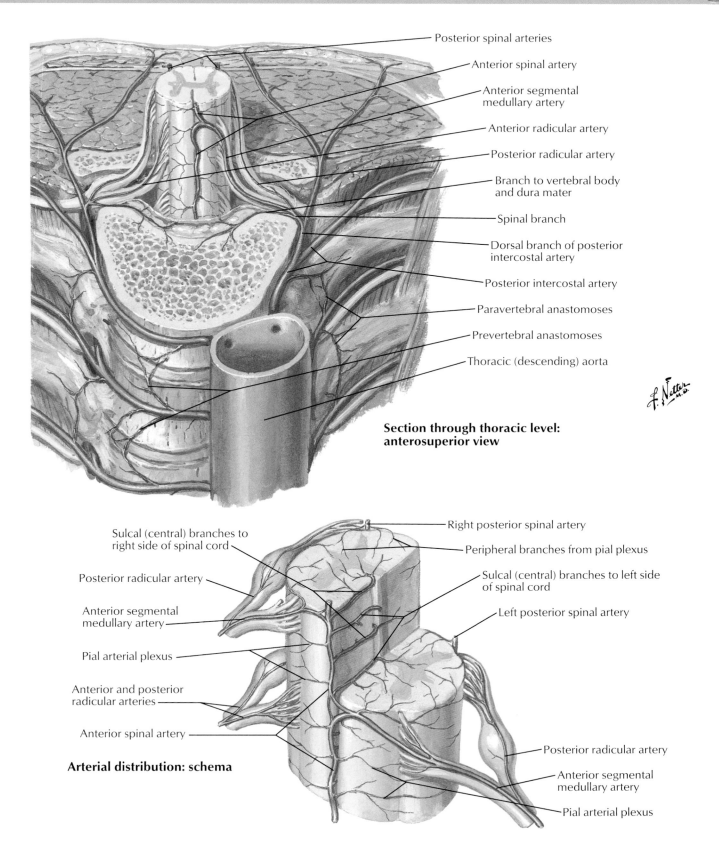

Posterior spinal arteries

Anterior spinal artery

Anterior segmental medullary artery

Anterior radicular artery

Posterior radicular artery

Branch to vertebral body and dura mater

Spinal branch

Dorsal branch of posterior intercostal artery

Posterior intercostal artery

Paravertebral anastomoses

Prevertebral anastomoses

Thoracic (descending) aorta

Section through thoracic level: anterosuperior view

Sulcal (central) branches to right side of spinal cord

Posterior radicular artery

Anterior segmental medullary artery

Pial arterial plexus

Anterior and posterior radicular arteries

Anterior spinal artery

Arterial distribution: schema

Right posterior spinal artery

Peripheral branches from pial plexus

Sulcal (central) branches to left side of spinal cord

Left posterior spinal artery

Posterior radicular artery

Anterior segmental medullary artery

Pial arterial plexus

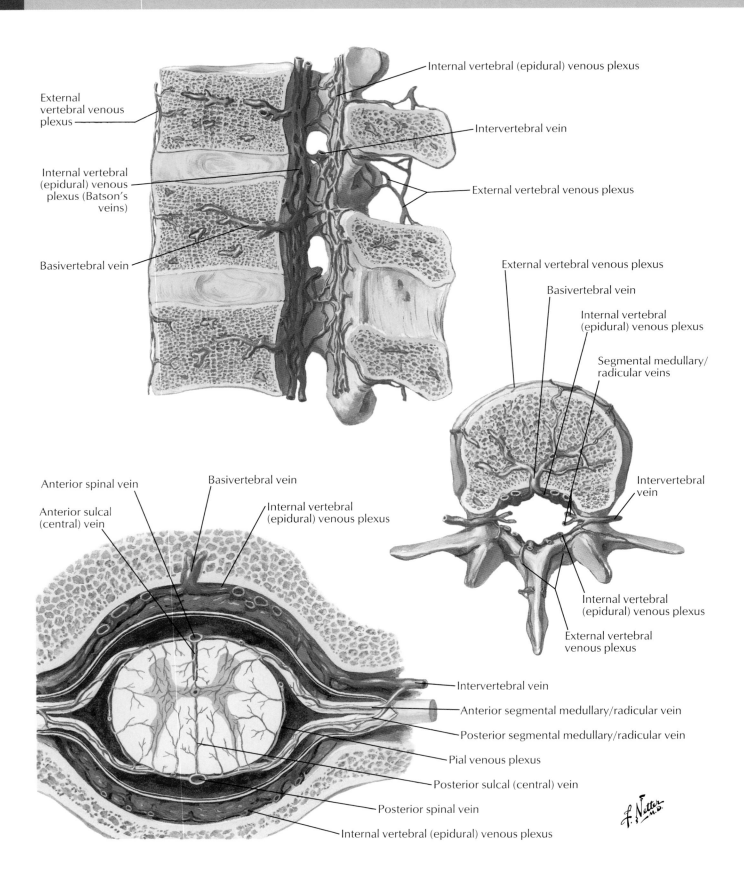

External vertebral venous plexus

Internal vertebral (epidural) venous plexus (Batson's veins)

Basivertebral vein

Internal vertebral (epidural) venous plexus

Intervertebral vein

External vertebral venous plexus

External vertebral venous plexus

Basivertebral vein

Internal vertebral (epidural) venous plexus

Segmental medullary/radicular veins

Intervertebral vein

Internal vertebral (epidural) venous plexus

External vertebral venous plexus

Anterior spinal vein

Anterior sulcal (central) vein

Basivertebral vein

Internal vertebral (epidural) venous plexus

Intervertebral vein

Anterior segmental medullary/radicular vein

Posterior segmental medullary/radicular vein

Pial venous plexus

Posterior sulcal (central) vein

Posterior spinal vein

Internal vertebral (epidural) venous plexus

Plate 166   **Spinal Cord**

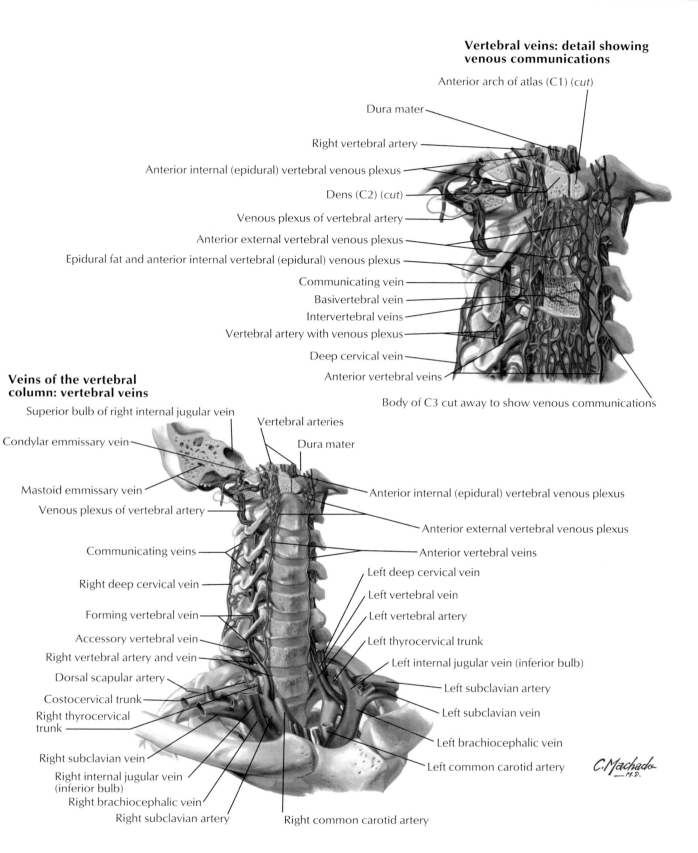

Vertebral veins: detail showing venous communications

Anterior arch of atlas (C1) (cut)

Dura mater

Right vertebral artery

Anterior internal (epidural) vertebral venous plexus

Dens (C2) (cut)

Venous plexus of vertebral artery

Anterior external vertebral venous plexus

Epidural fat and anterior internal vertebral (epidural) venous plexus

Communicating vein

Basivertebral vein

Intervertebral veins

Vertebral artery with venous plexus

Deep cervical vein

Anterior vertebral veins

Body of C3 cut away to show venous communications

Veins of the vertebral column: vertebral veins

Superior bulb of right internal jugular vein

Vertebral arteries

Dura mater

Condylar emmissary vein

Mastoid emmissary vein

Venous plexus of vertebral artery

Anterior internal (epidural) vertebral venous plexus

Anterior external vertebral venous plexus

Communicating veins

Anterior vertebral veins

Left deep cervical vein

Right deep cervical vein

Left vertebral vein

Left vertebral artery

Forming vertebral vein

Left thyrocervical trunk

Accessory vertebral vein

Left internal jugular vein (inferior bulb)

Right vertebral artery and vein

Dorsal scapular artery

Left subclavian artery

Costocervical trunk

Left subclavian vein

Right thyrocervical trunk

Left brachiocephalic vein

Right subclavian vein

Left common carotid artery

Right internal jugular vein (inferior bulb)

Right brachiocephalic vein

Right subclavian artery

Right common carotid artery

C. Machado
M.D.

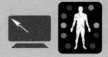

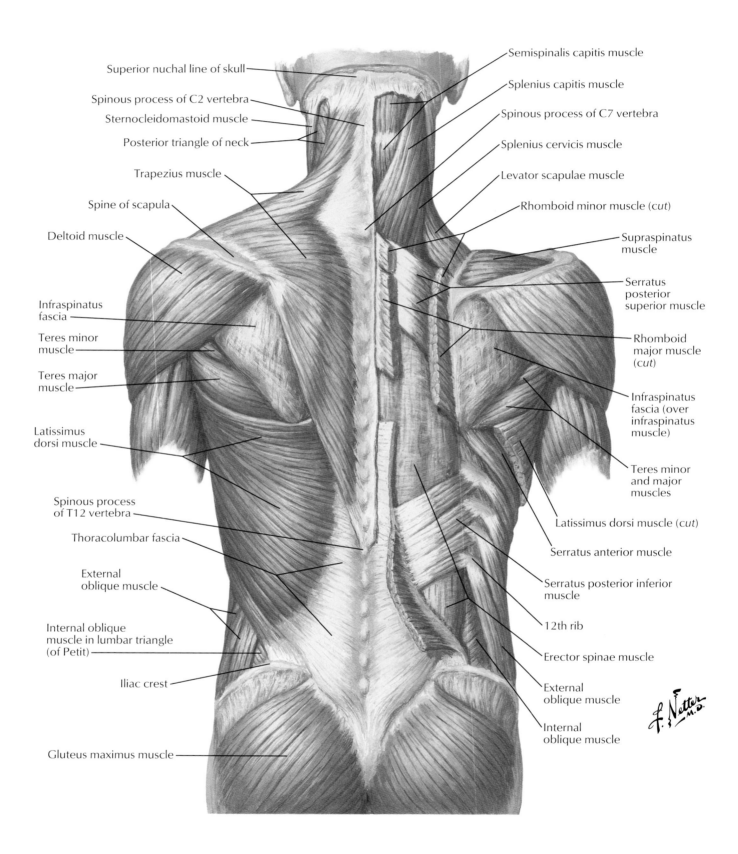

Superior nuchal line of skull

Spinous process of C2 vertebra

Sternocleidomastoid muscle

Posterior triangle of neck

Trapezius muscle

Spine of scapula

Deltoid muscle

Infraspinatus fascia

Teres minor muscle

Teres major muscle

Latissimus dorsi muscle

Spinous process of T12 vertebra

Thoracolumbar fascia

External oblique muscle

Internal oblique muscle in lumbar triangle (of Petit)

Iliac crest

Gluteus maximus muscle

Semispinalis capitis muscle

Splenius capitis muscle

Spinous process of C7 vertebra

Splenius cervicis muscle

Levator scapulae muscle

Rhomboid minor muscle (*cut*)

Supraspinatus muscle

Serratus posterior superior muscle

Rhomboid major muscle (*cut*)

Infraspinatus fascia (over infraspinatus muscle)

Teres minor and major muscles

Latissimus dorsi muscle (*cut*)

Serratus anterior muscle

Serratus posterior inferior muscle

12th rib

Erector spinae muscle

External oblique muscle

Internal oblique muscle

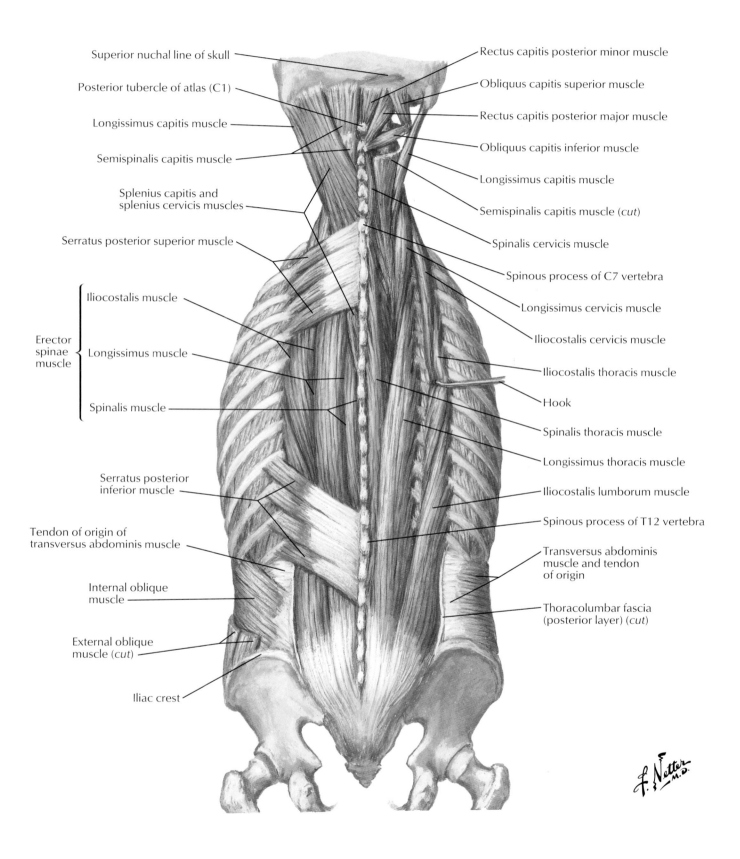

Superior nuchal line of skull

Posterior tubercle of atlas (C1)

Longissimus capitis muscle

Semispinalis capitis muscle

Splenius capitis and splenius cervicis muscles

Serratus posterior superior muscle

Iliocostalis muscle

Erector spinae muscle

Longissimus muscle

Spinalis muscle

Serratus posterior inferior muscle

Tendon of origin of transversus abdominis muscle

Internal oblique muscle

External oblique muscle (cut)

Iliac crest

Rectus capitis posterior minor muscle

Obliquus capitis superior muscle

Rectus capitis posterior major muscle

Obliquus capitis inferior muscle

Longissimus capitis muscle

Semispinalis capitis muscle (cut)

Spinalis cervicis muscle

Spinous process of C7 vertebra

Longissimus cervicis muscle

Iliocostalis cervicis muscle

Iliocostalis thoracis muscle

Hook

Spinalis thoracis muscle

Longissimus thoracis muscle

Iliocostalis lumborum muscle

Spinous process of T12 vertebra

Transversus abdominis muscle and tendon of origin

Thoracolumbar fascia (posterior layer) (cut)

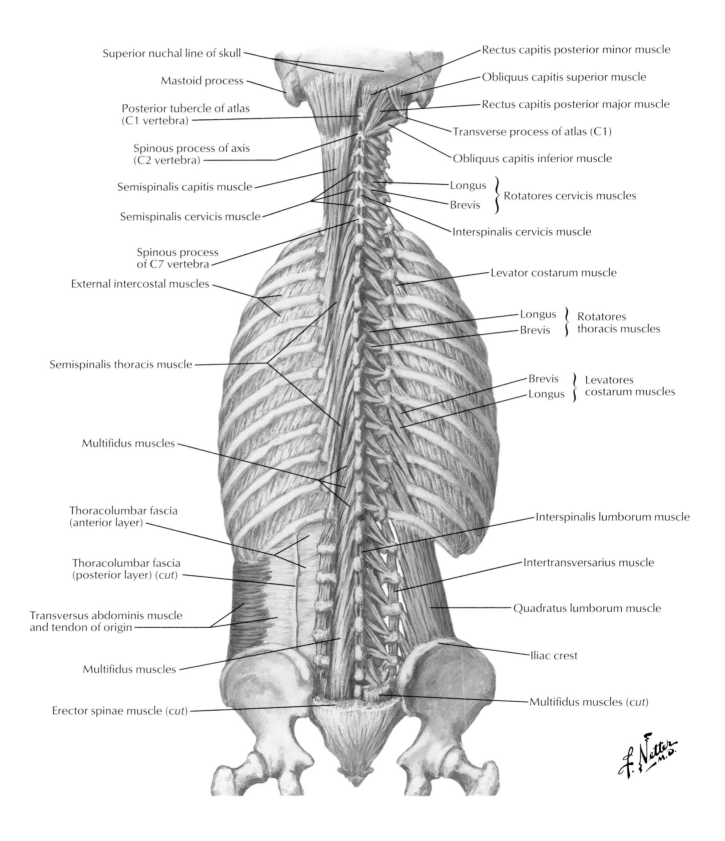

Superior nuchal line of skull

Mastoid process

Posterior tubercle of atlas
(C1 vertebra)

Spinous process of axis
(C2 vertebra)

Semispinalis capitis muscle

Semispinalis cervicis muscle

Spinous process
of C7 vertebra

External intercostal muscles

Semispinalis thoracis muscle

Multifidus muscles

Thoracolumbar fascia
(anterior layer)

Thoracolumbar fascia
(posterior layer) (cut)

Transversus abdominis muscle
and tendon of origin

Multifidus muscles

Erector spinae muscle (cut)

Rectus capitis posterior minor muscle

Obliquus capitis superior muscle

Rectus capitis posterior major muscle

Transverse process of atlas (C1)

Obliquus capitis inferior muscle

Longus
Brevis } Rotatores cervicis muscles

Interspinalis cervicis muscle

Levator costarum muscle

Longus } Rotatores
Brevis } thoracis muscles

Brevis } Levatores
Longus } costarum muscles

Interspinalis lumborum muscle

Intertransversarius muscle

Quadratus lumborum muscle

Iliac crest

Multifidus muscles (cut)

Plate 170

Muscles and Nerves

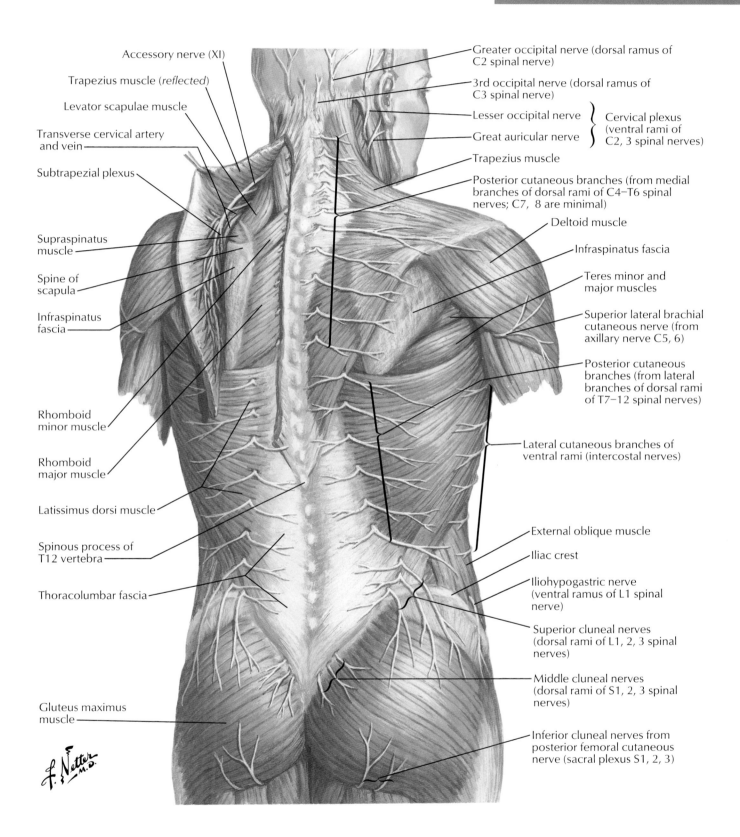

Accessory nerve (XI)

Trapezius muscle (*reflected*)

Levator scapulae muscle

Transverse cervical artery and vein

Subtrapezial plexus

Supraspinatus muscle

Spine of scapula

Infraspinatus fascia

Rhomboid minor muscle

Rhomboid major muscle

Latissimus dorsi muscle

Spinous process of T12 vertebra

Thoracolumbar fascia

Gluteus maximus muscle

Greater occipital nerve (dorsal ramus of C2 spinal nerve)

3rd occipital nerve (dorsal ramus of C3 spinal nerve)

Lesser occipital nerve ⎫ Cervical plexus
Great auricular nerve ⎭ (ventral rami of C2, 3 spinal nerves)

Trapezius muscle

Posterior cutaneous branches (from medial branches of dorsal rami of C4–T6 spinal nerves; C7, 8 are minimal)

Deltoid muscle

Infraspinatus fascia

Teres minor and major muscles

Superior lateral brachial cutaneous nerve (from axillary nerve C5, 6)

Posterior cutaneous branches (from lateral branches of dorsal rami of T7–12 spinal nerves)

Lateral cutaneous branches of ventral rami (intercostal nerves)

External oblique muscle

Iliac crest

Iliohypogastric nerve (ventral ramus of L1 spinal nerve)

Superior cluneal nerves (dorsal rami of L1, 2, 3 spinal nerves)

Middle cluneal nerves (dorsal rami of S1, 2, 3 spinal nerves)

Inferior cluneal nerves from posterior femoral cutaneous nerve (sacral plexus S1, 2, 3)

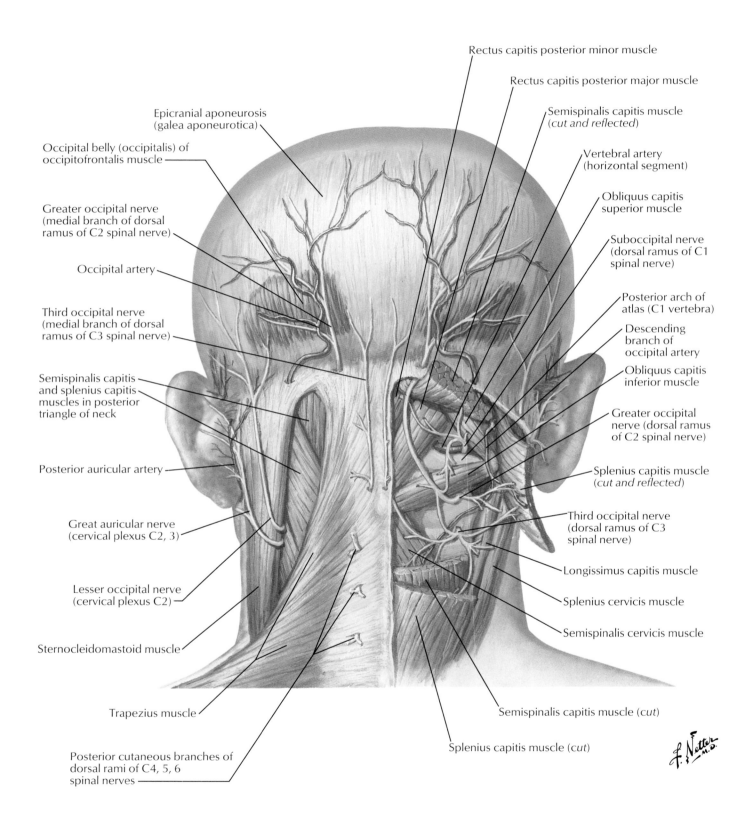

Rectus capitis posterior minor muscle

Rectus capitis posterior major muscle

Semispinalis capitis muscle (*cut and reflected*)

Epicranial aponeurosis (galea aponeurotica)

Vertebral artery (horizontal segment)

Occipital belly (occipitalis) of occipitofrontalis muscle

Obliquus capitis superior muscle

Greater occipital nerve (medial branch of dorsal ramus of C2 spinal nerve)

Suboccipital nerve (dorsal ramus of C1 spinal nerve)

Occipital artery

Posterior arch of atlas (C1 vertebra)

Third occipital nerve (medial branch of dorsal ramus of C3 spinal nerve)

Descending branch of occipital artery

Obliquus capitis inferior muscle

Semispinalis capitis and splenius capitis muscles in posterior triangle of neck

Greater occipital nerve (dorsal ramus of C2 spinal nerve)

Posterior auricular artery

Splenius capitis muscle (*cut and reflected*)

Third occipital nerve (dorsal ramus of C3 spinal nerve)

Great auricular nerve (cervical plexus C2, 3)

Longissimus capitis muscle

Lesser occipital nerve (cervical plexus C2)

Splenius cervicis muscle

Semispinalis cervicis muscle

Sternocleidomastoid muscle

Trapezius muscle

Semispinalis capitis muscle (*cut*)

Splenius capitis muscle (*cut*)

Posterior cutaneous branches of dorsal rami of C4, 5, 6 spinal nerves

f. Netter M.D.

Plate 172 **Muscles and Nerves**

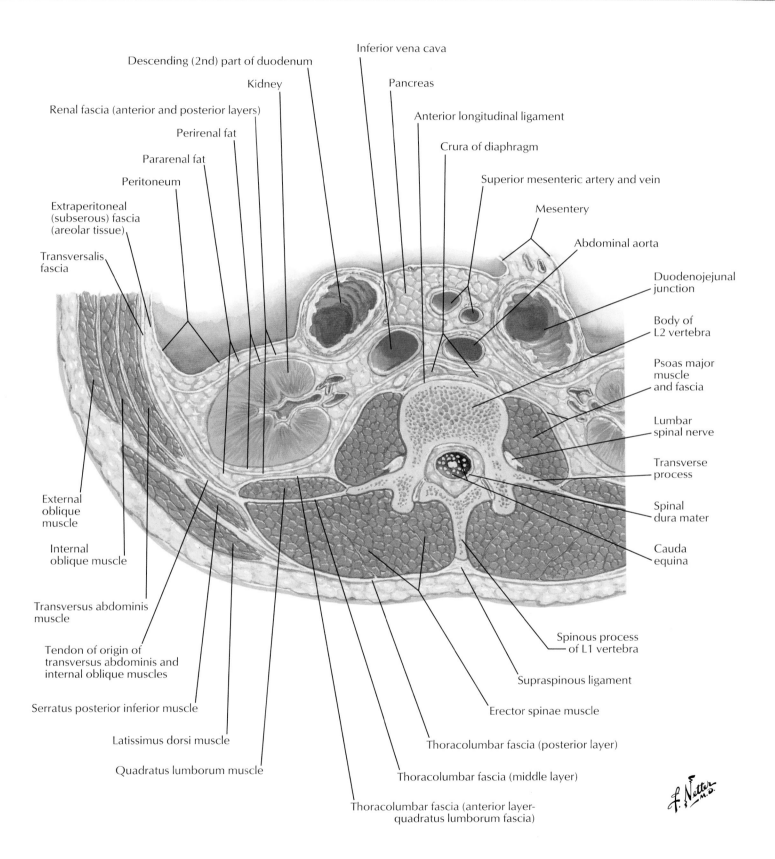

Descending (2nd) part of duodenum

Kidney

Renal fascia (anterior and posterior layers)

Perirenal fat

Pararenal fat

Peritoneum

Extraperitoneal (subserous) fascia (areolar tissue)

Transversalis fascia

External oblique muscle

Internal oblique muscle

Transversus abdominis muscle

Tendon of origin of transversus abdominis and internal oblique muscles

Serratus posterior inferior muscle

Latissimus dorsi muscle

Quadratus lumborum muscle

Inferior vena cava

Pancreas

Anterior longitudinal ligament

Crura of diaphragm

Superior mesenteric artery and vein

Mesentery

Abdominal aorta

Duodenojejunal junction

Body of L2 vertebra

Psoas major muscle and fascia

Lumbar spinal nerve

Transverse process

Spinal dura mater

Cauda equina

Spinous process of L1 vertebra

Supraspinous ligament

Erector spinae muscle

Thoracolumbar fascia (posterior layer)

Thoracolumbar fascia (middle layer)

Thoracolumbar fascia (anterior layer-quadratus lumborum fascia)

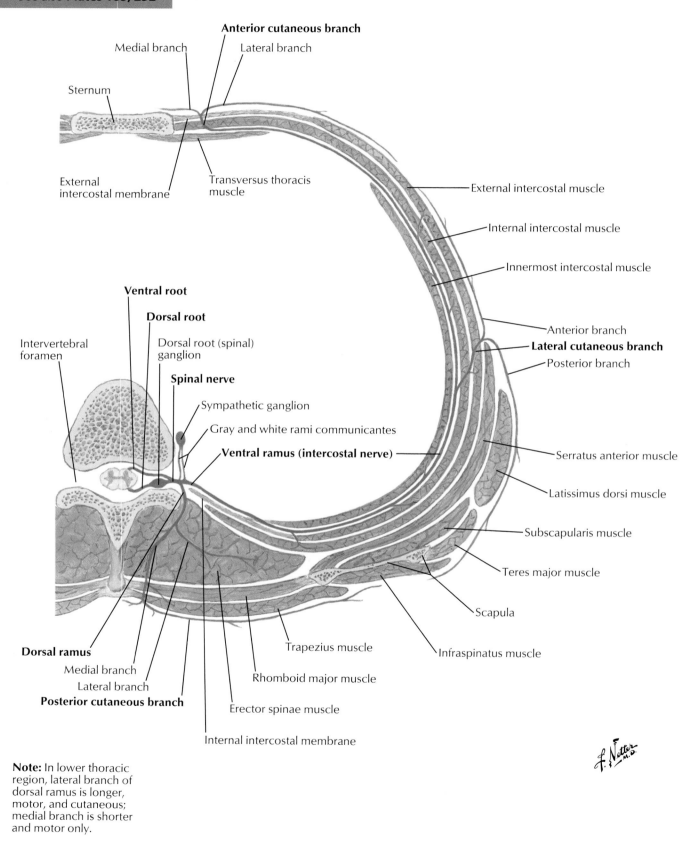

Anterior cutaneous branch

Medial branch

Lateral branch

Sternum

External intercostal membrane

Transversus thoracis muscle

External intercostal muscle

Internal intercostal muscle

Innermost intercostal muscle

Ventral root

Dorsal root

Dorsal root (spinal) ganglion

Intervertebral foramen

Spinal nerve

Sympathetic ganglion

Gray and white rami communicantes

Ventral ramus (intercostal nerve)

Anterior branch

Lateral cutaneous branch

Posterior branch

Serratus anterior muscle

Latissimus dorsi muscle

Subscapularis muscle

Teres major muscle

Scapula

Infraspinatus muscle

Trapezius muscle

Rhomboid major muscle

Erector spinae muscle

Internal intercostal membrane

Dorsal ramus

Medial branch

Lateral branch

Posterior cutaneous branch

Note: In lower thoracic region, lateral branch of dorsal ramus is longer, motor, and cutaneous; medial branch is shorter and motor only.

Plate 174

Cross-sectional Anatomy

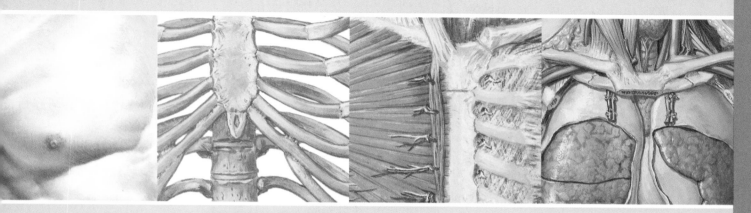

Section 3 **THORAX**

Topographic Anatomy
Plate 175

175   Thorax

Mammary Gland
Plates 176-178

176   Mammary Gland

177   Arteries of Mammary Gland

178   Lymph Vessels and Nodes of Mammary Gland

Body Wall
Plates 179-189

179   Bony Framework of Thorax

180   Ribs and Sternocostal Joints

181   Costovertebral Joints

182   Anterior Thoracic Wall

183   Anterior Thoracic Wall (continued)

184   Anterior Thoracic Wall: Internal View

185   Intercostal Nerves and Arteries

186   Veins of the Internal Thoracic Wall

187   Phrenic Nerve

188   Diaphragm: Thoracic Surface

189   Diaphragm: Abdominal Surface

Lungs
Plates 190-204

190   Topography of Lungs: Anterior View

191   Topography of Lungs: Posterior View

192 Lungs in Situ: Anterior View

193 Lungs: Medial Views

194 Bronchopulmonary Segments

195 Bronchopulmonary Segments (continued)

196 Trachea and Major Bronchi

197 Nomenclature of Bronchi: Schema

198 Intrapulmonary Airways: Schema

199 Intrapulmonary Blood Circulation: Schema

200 Great Vessels of Superior Mediastinum

201 Bronchial Arteries and Veins

202 Lymph Vessels and Nodes of Lung

203 Autonomic Nerves in Thorax

204 Innervation of Tracheobronchial Tree: Schema

Heart
Plates 205-223

205 Heart in Situ

206 Heart: Anterior Exposure

207 Radiograph of Chest

208 Heart: Base and Diaphragmatic Surface

209 Pericardial Sac

210 Mediastinum: Cross Section

211 Coronary Arteries and Cardiac Veins

212 Coronary Arteries: Arteriographic Views

213 Coronary Arteries: Arteriographic Views (continued)

214 Right Atrium and Ventricle

215 Left Atrium and Ventricle

216 Valves and Fibrous Skeleton of Heart

217 Valves and Fibrous Skeleton of Heart (continued)

218 Atria, Ventricles, and Interventricular Septum

219 Conducting System of Heart

220 Nerves of Heart

221 Innervation of Heart: Schema

222 Innervation of Blood Vessels: Schema

223 Prenatal and Postnatal Circulation

Mediastinum
Plates 224-234

224 Mediastinum: Right Lateral View

225 Mediastinum: Left Lateral View

226 Esophagus in Situ

227 Topography and Constrictions of Esophagus

228 Musculature of Esophagus

229 Pharyngoesophageal Junction

230 Esophagogastric Junction

231 Arteries of Esophagus

232 Veins of Esophagus

233 Lymph Vessels and Nodes of Esophagus

234 Nerves of Esophagus

Regional Scans
Plate 235

235 Chest Scans: Axial CT Images

Cross-sectional Anatomy
Plates 236-239

236 Cross Section of Thorax at T3 Level

237 Cross Section of Thorax at T3-4 Disc Level

238 Cross Section of Thorax at T4-5 Disc Level

239 Cross Section of Thorax at T7 Level

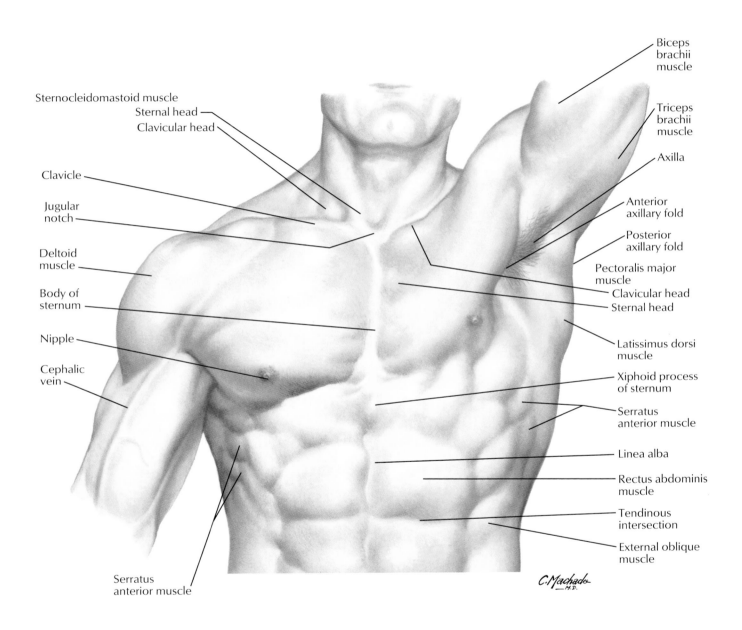

Sternocleidomastoid muscle
Sternal head
Clavicular head

Clavicle

Jugular notch

Deltoid muscle

Body of sternum

Nipple

Cephalic vein

Serratus anterior muscle

Biceps brachii muscle

Triceps brachii muscle

Axilla

Anterior axillary fold

Posterior axillary fold

Pectoralis major muscle
Clavicular head
Sternal head

Latissimus dorsi muscle

Xiphoid process of sternum

Serratus anterior muscle

Linea alba

Rectus abdominis muscle

Tendinous intersection

External oblique muscle

C. Machado
_M.D._

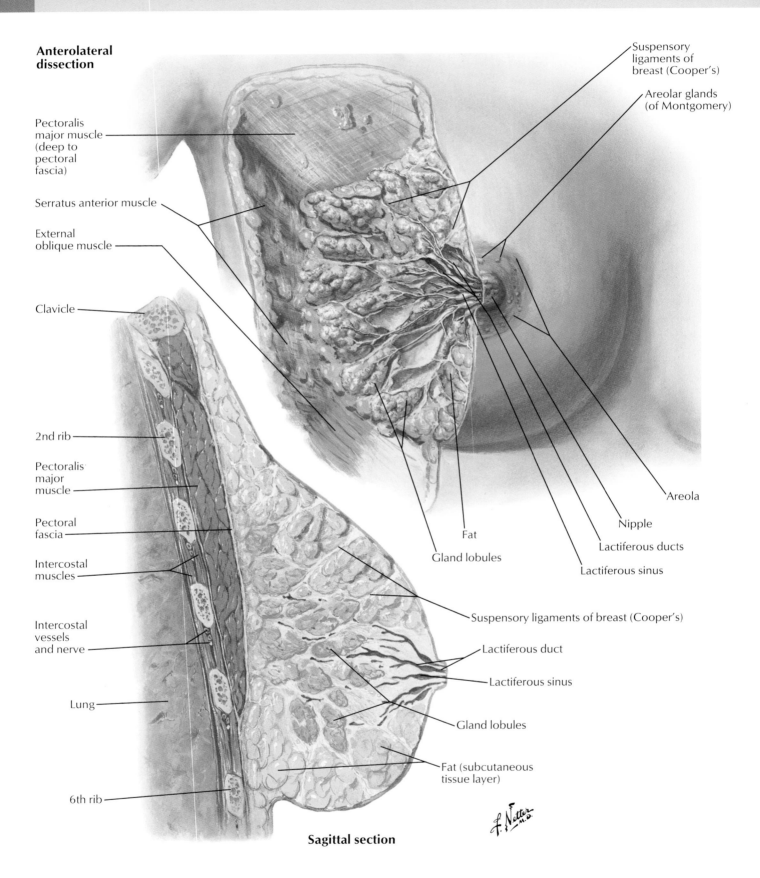

Anterolateral dissection

Pectoralis major muscle (deep to pectoral fascia)

Serratus anterior muscle

External oblique muscle

Clavicle

2nd rib

Pectoralis major muscle

Pectoral fascia

Intercostal muscles

Intercostal vessels and nerve

Lung

6th rib

Suspensory ligaments of breast (Cooper's)

Areolar glands (of Montgomery)

Areola

Nipple

Lactiferous ducts

Lactiferous sinus

Fat

Gland lobules

Suspensory ligaments of breast (Cooper's)

Lactiferous duct

Lactiferous sinus

Gland lobules

Fat (subcutaneous tissue layer)

Sagittal section

Plate 176 **Mammary Gland**

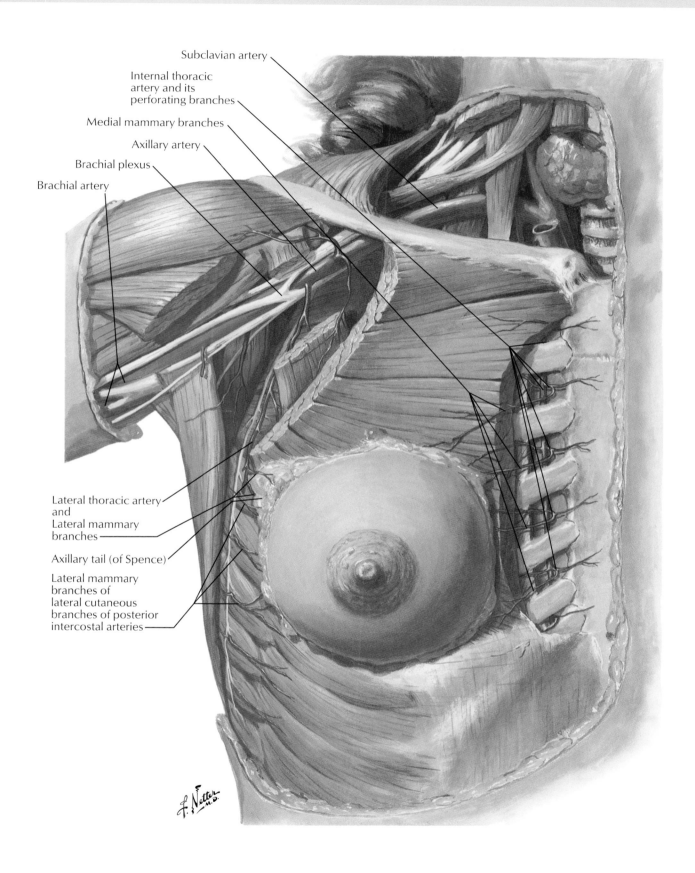

Subclavian artery

Internal thoracic artery and its perforating branches

Medial mammary branches

Axillary artery

Brachial plexus

Brachial artery

Lateral thoracic artery and Lateral mammary branches

Axillary tail (of Spence)

Lateral mammary branches of lateral cutaneous branches of posterior intercostal arteries

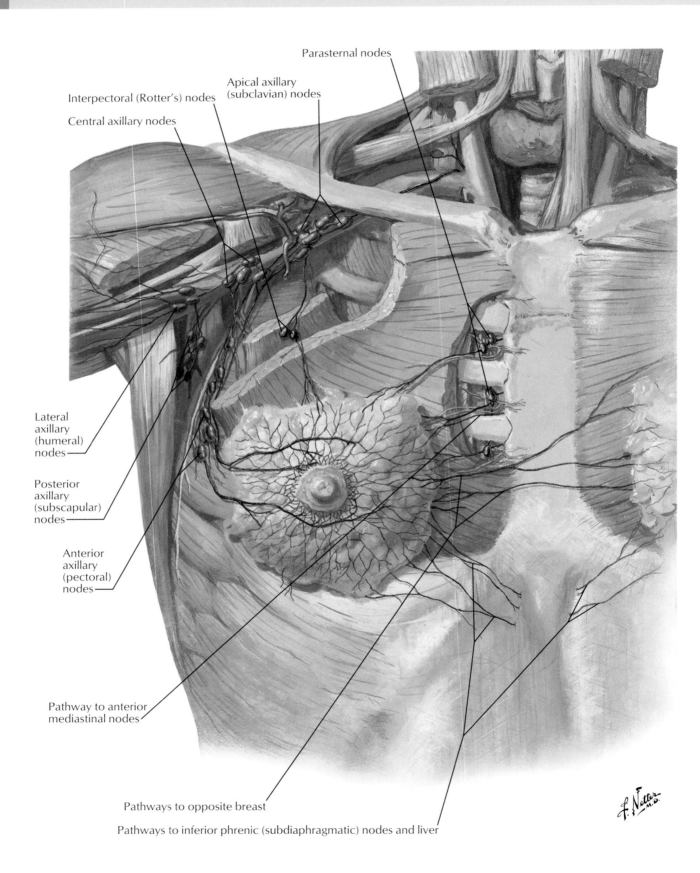

Parasternal nodes

Apical axillary
(subclavian) nodes

Interpectoral (Rotter's) nodes

Central axillary nodes

Lateral
axillary
(humeral)
nodes

Posterior
axillary
(subscapular)
nodes

Anterior
axillary
(pectoral)
nodes

Pathway to anterior
mediastinal nodes

Pathways to opposite breast

Pathways to inferior phrenic (subdiaphragmatic) nodes and liver

Plate 178

Mammary Gland

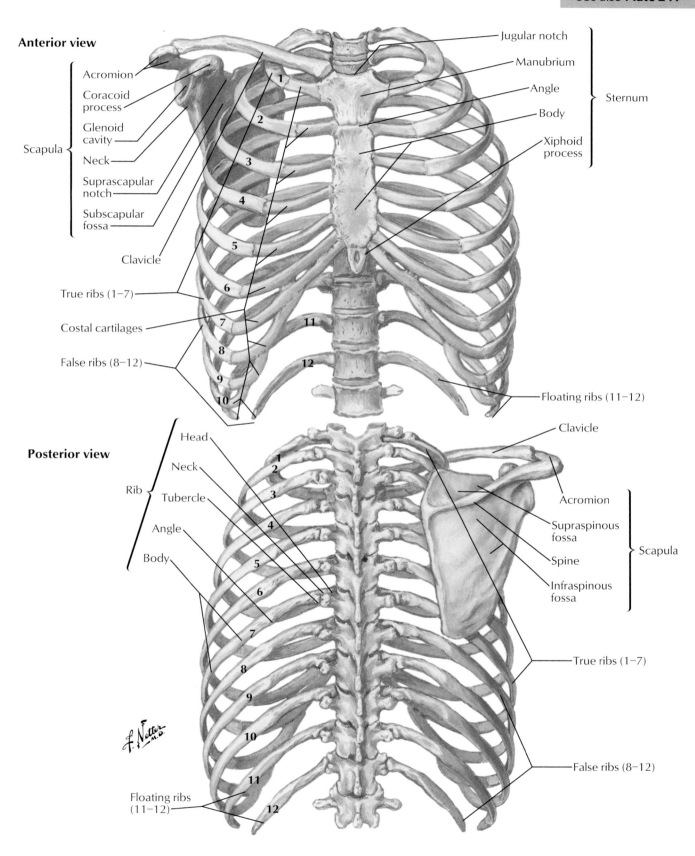

Anterior view

Jugular notch

Manubrium

Angle — Sternum

Body

Xiphoid process

Acromion

Coracoid process

Glenoid cavity

Neck — Scapula

Suprascapular notch

Subscapular fossa

Clavicle

True ribs (1–7)

Costal cartilages

False ribs (8–12)

Floating ribs (11–12)

1
2
3
4
5
6
7
8
9
10
11
12

Posterior view

Head

Neck

Tubercle — Rib

Angle

Body

Clavicle

Acromion

Supraspinous fossa

Spine — Scapula

Infraspinous fossa

True ribs (1–7)

False ribs (8–12)

Floating ribs (11–12)

1
2
3
4
5
6
7
8
9
10
11
12

F. Netter M.D.

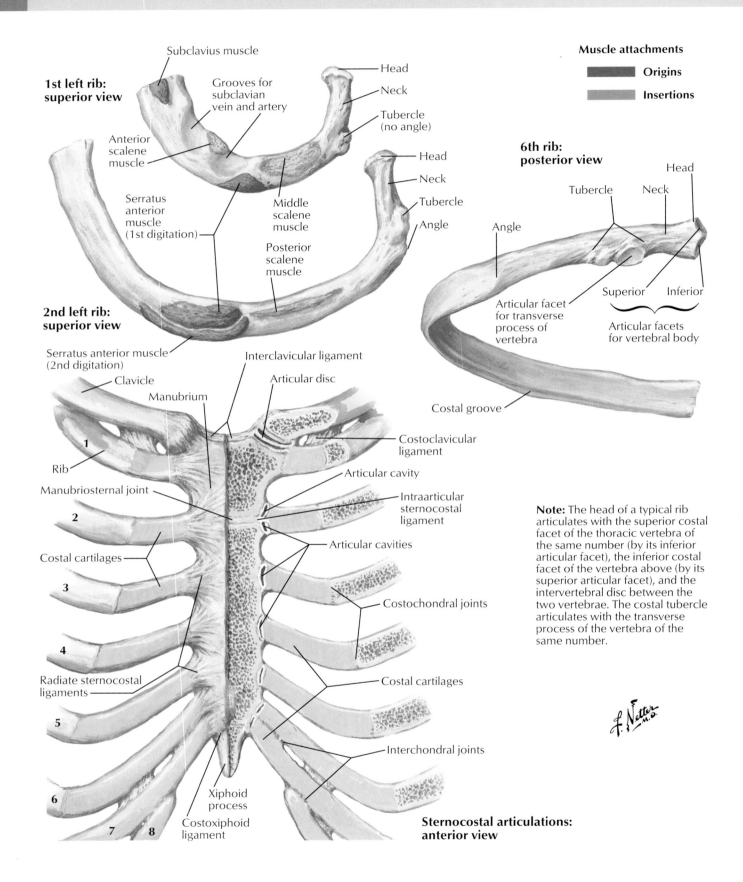

1st left rib: superior view

Subclavius muscle

Grooves for subclavian vein and artery

Anterior scalene muscle

Serratus anterior muscle (1st digitation)

Middle scalene muscle

Posterior scalene muscle

Head

Neck

Tubercle (no angle)

Head

Neck

Tubercle

Angle

Muscle attachments

■ Origins

■ Insertions

6th rib: posterior view

Angle

Tubercle

Neck

Head

Articular facet for transverse process of vertebra

Superior

Inferior

Articular facets for vertebral body

Costal groove

2nd left rib: superior view

Serratus anterior muscle (2nd digitation)

Clavicle

Manubrium

Interclavicular ligament

Articular disc

Rib

1

Manubriosternal joint

Costoclavicular ligament

Articular cavity

Intraarticular sternocostal ligament

2

Costal cartilages

Articular cavities

3

Costochondral joints

4

Radiate sternocostal ligaments

Costal cartilages

5

Interchondral joints

6

7   8

Xiphoid process

Costoxiphoid ligament

Sternocostal articulations: anterior view

Note: The head of a typical rib articulates with the superior costal facet of the thoracic vertebra of the same number (by its inferior articular facet), the inferior costal facet of the vertebra above (by its superior articular facet), and the intervertebral disc between the two vertebrae. The costal tubercle articulates with the transverse process of the vertebra of the same number.

f. Netter M.D.

Plate 180

Body Wall

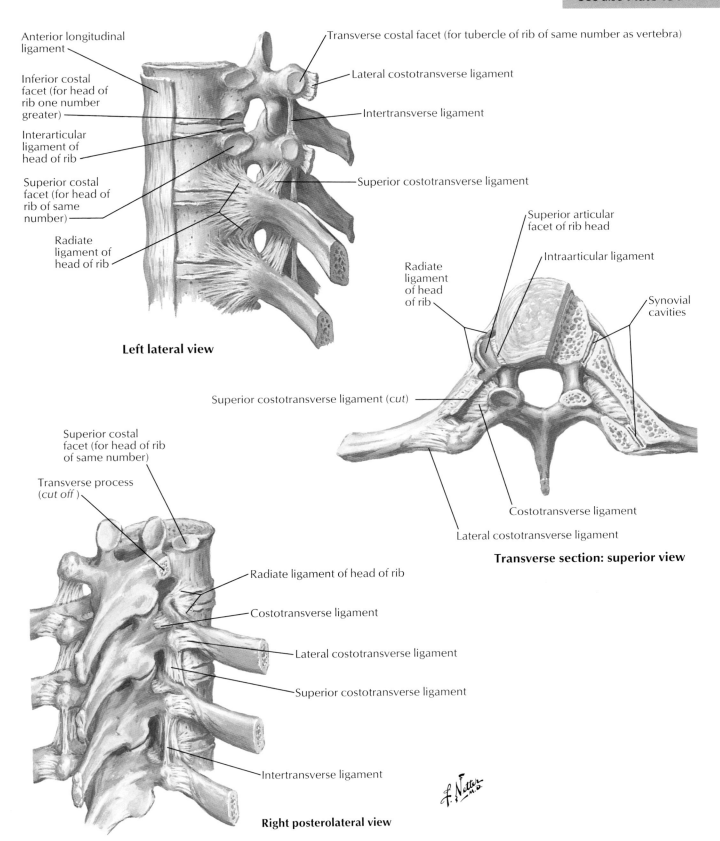

Anterior longitudinal ligament

Inferior costal facet (for head of rib one number greater)

Interarticular ligament of head of rib

Superior costal facet (for head of rib of same number)

Radiate ligament of head of rib

Transverse costal facet (for tubercle of rib of same number as vertebra)

Lateral costotransverse ligament

Intertransverse ligament

Superior costotransverse ligament

Left lateral view

Superior articular facet of rib head

Intraarticular ligament

Radiate ligament of head of rib

Synovial cavities

Superior costotransverse ligament (*cut*)

Costotransverse ligament

Lateral costotransverse ligament

Transverse section: superior view

Superior costal facet (for head of rib of same number)

Transverse process (*cut off*)

Radiate ligament of head of rib

Costotransverse ligament

Lateral costotransverse ligament

Superior costotransverse ligament

Intertransverse ligament

Right posterolateral view

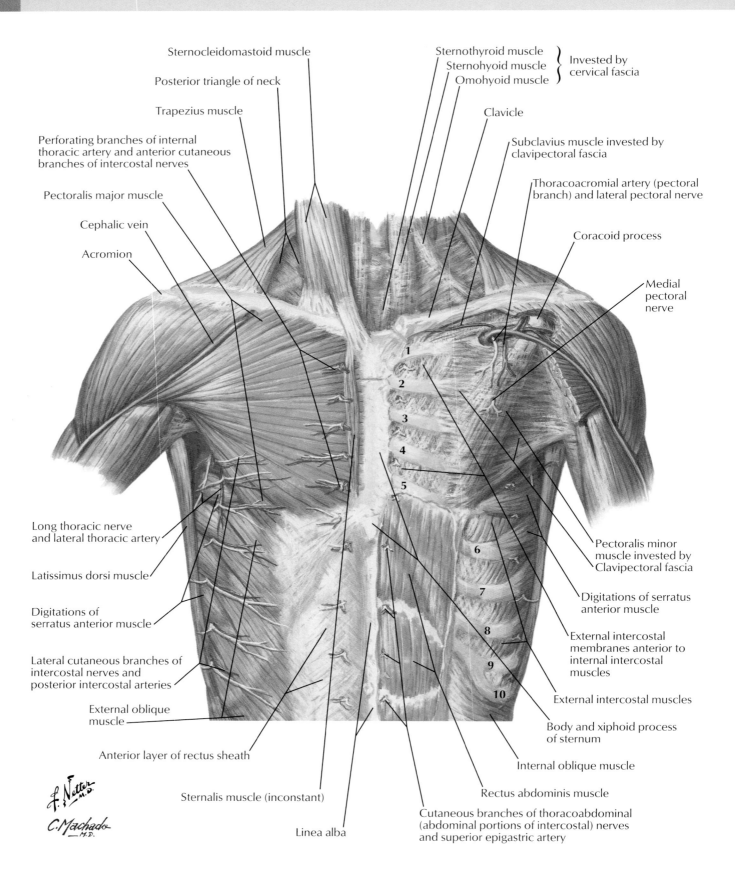

Sternocleidomastoid muscle

Posterior triangle of neck

Trapezius muscle

Perforating branches of internal
thoracic artery and anterior cutaneous
branches of intercostal nerves

Pectoralis major muscle

Cephalic vein

Acromion

Sternothyroid muscle
Sternohyoid muscle   } Invested by
Omohyoid muscle   }   cervical fascia

Clavicle

Subclavius muscle invested by
clavipectoral fascia

Thoracoacromial artery (pectoral
branch) and lateral pectoral nerve

Coracoid process

Medial
pectoral
nerve

Long thoracic nerve
and lateral thoracic artery

Latissimus dorsi muscle

Digitations of
serratus anterior muscle

Lateral cutaneous branches of
intercostal nerves and
posterior intercostal arteries

External oblique
muscle

Anterior layer of rectus sheath

Sternalis muscle (inconstant)

Linea alba

Pectoralis minor
muscle invested by
Clavipectoral fascia

Digitations of serratus
anterior muscle

External intercostal
membranes anterior to
internal intercostal
muscles

External intercostal muscles

Body and xiphoid process
of sternum

Internal oblique muscle

Rectus abdominis muscle

Cutaneous branches of thoracoabdominal
(abdominal portions of intercostal) nerves
and superior epigastric artery

Plate 182   **Body Wall**

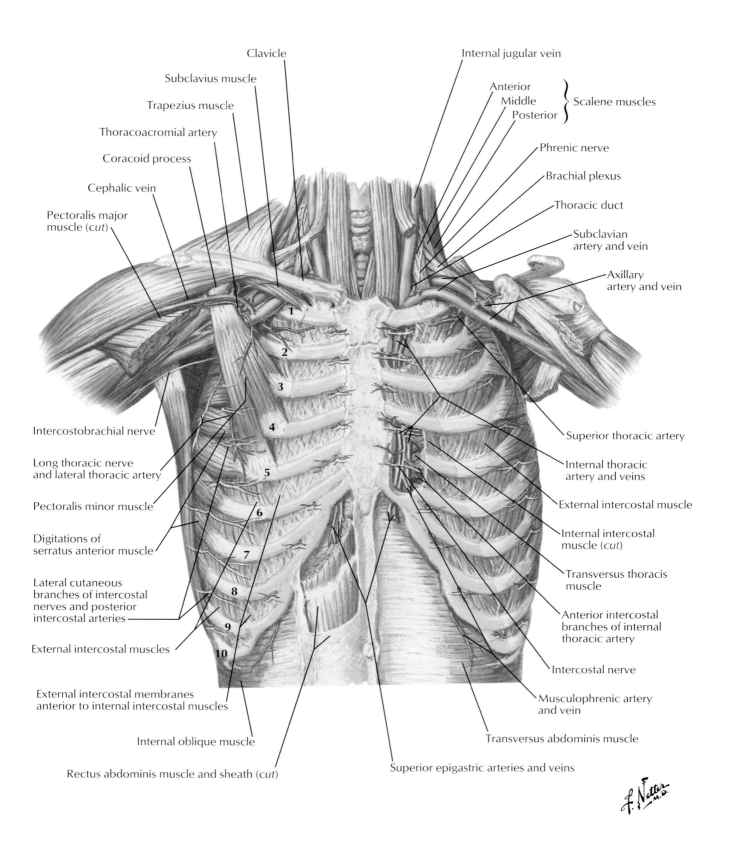

Clavicle

Subclavius muscle

Trapezius muscle

Thoracoacromial artery

Coracoid process

Cephalic vein

Pectoralis major muscle (cut)

Intercostobrachial nerve

Long thoracic nerve and lateral thoracic artery

Pectoralis minor muscle

Digitations of serratus anterior muscle

Lateral cutaneous branches of intercostal nerves and posterior intercostal arteries

External intercostal muscles

External intercostal membranes anterior to internal intercostal muscles

Internal oblique muscle

Rectus abdominis muscle and sheath (cut)

Internal jugular vein

Anterior
Middle
Posterior
} Scalene muscles

Phrenic nerve

Brachial plexus

Thoracic duct

Subclavian artery and vein

Axillary artery and vein

Superior thoracic artery

Internal thoracic artery and veins

External intercostal muscle

Internal intercostal muscle (cut)

Transversus thoracis muscle

Anterior intercostal branches of internal thoracic artery

Intercostal nerve

Musculophrenic artery and vein

Transversus abdominis muscle

Superior epigastric arteries and veins

1
2
3
4
5
6
7
8
9
10

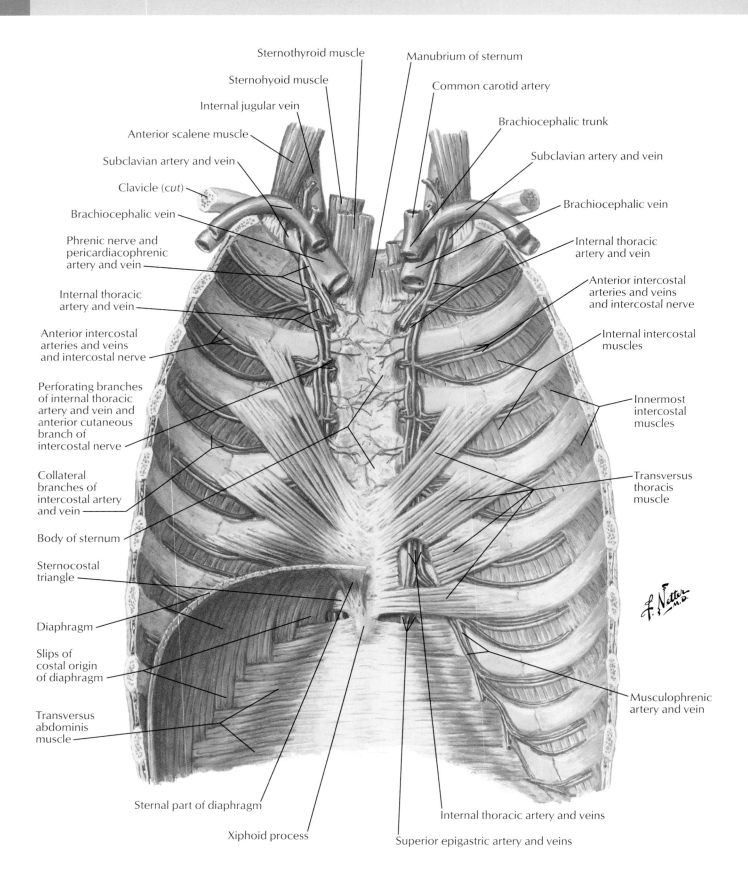

Sternothyroid muscle

Sternohyoid muscle

Internal jugular vein

Anterior scalene muscle

Subclavian artery and vein

Clavicle (*cut*)

Brachiocephalic vein

Phrenic nerve and pericardiacophrenic artery and vein

Internal thoracic artery and vein

Anterior intercostal arteries and veins and intercostal nerve

Perforating branches of internal thoracic artery and vein and anterior cutaneous branch of intercostal nerve

Collateral branches of intercostal artery and vein

Body of sternum

Sternocostal triangle

Diaphragm

Slips of costal origin of diaphragm

Transversus abdominis muscle

Manubrium of sternum

Common carotid artery

Brachiocephalic trunk

Subclavian artery and vein

Brachiocephalic vein

Internal thoracic artery and vein

Anterior intercostal arteries and veins and intercostal nerve

Internal intercostal muscles

Innermost intercostal muscles

Transversus thoracis muscle

Musculophrenic artery and vein

Sternal part of diaphragm

Xiphoid process

Superior epigastric artery and veins

Internal thoracic artery and veins

Plate 184   **Body Wall**

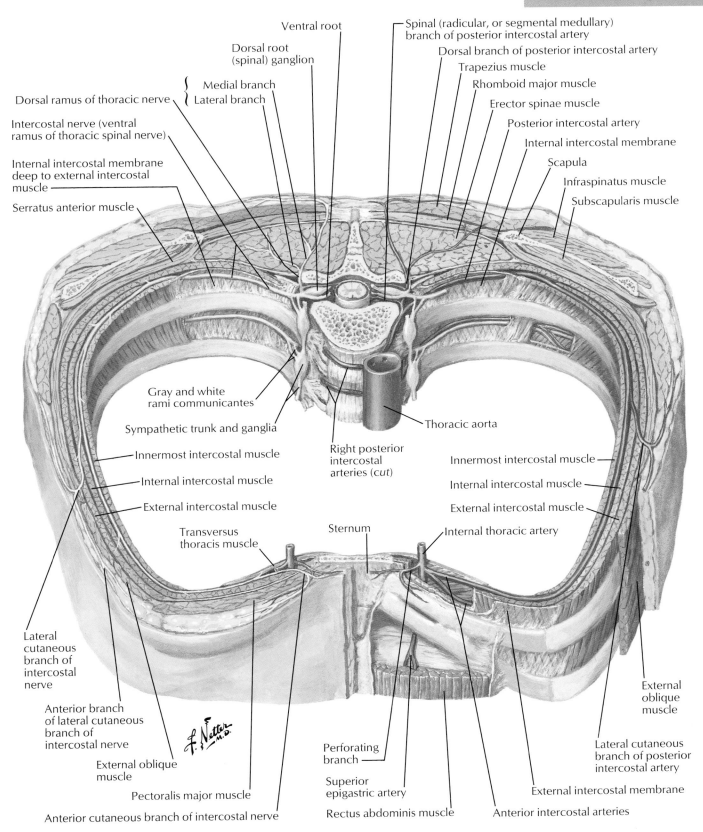

Ventral root

Dorsal root (spinal) ganglion

Medial branch
Lateral branch

Dorsal ramus of thoracic nerve

Intercostal nerve (ventral ramus of thoracic spinal nerve)

Internal intercostal membrane deep to external intercostal muscle

Serratus anterior muscle

Spinal (radicular, or segmental medullary) branch of posterior intercostal artery

Dorsal branch of posterior intercostal artery

Trapezius muscle

Rhomboid major muscle

Erector spinae muscle

Posterior intercostal artery

Internal intercostal membrane

Scapula

Infraspinatus muscle

Subscapularis muscle

Gray and white rami communicantes

Sympathetic trunk and ganglia

Innermost intercostal muscle

Internal intercostal muscle

External intercostal muscle

Right posterior intercostal arteries (cut)

Thoracic aorta

Innermost intercostal muscle

Internal intercostal muscle

External intercostal muscle

Transversus thoracis muscle

Sternum

Internal thoracic artery

Lateral cutaneous branch of intercostal nerve

Anterior branch of lateral cutaneous branch of intercostal nerve

External oblique muscle

Pectoralis major muscle

Anterior cutaneous branch of intercostal nerve

Perforating branch

Superior epigastric artery

Rectus abdominis muscle

External oblique muscle

Lateral cutaneous branch of posterior intercostal artery

External intercostal membrane

Anterior intercostal arteries

F. Netter, M.D.

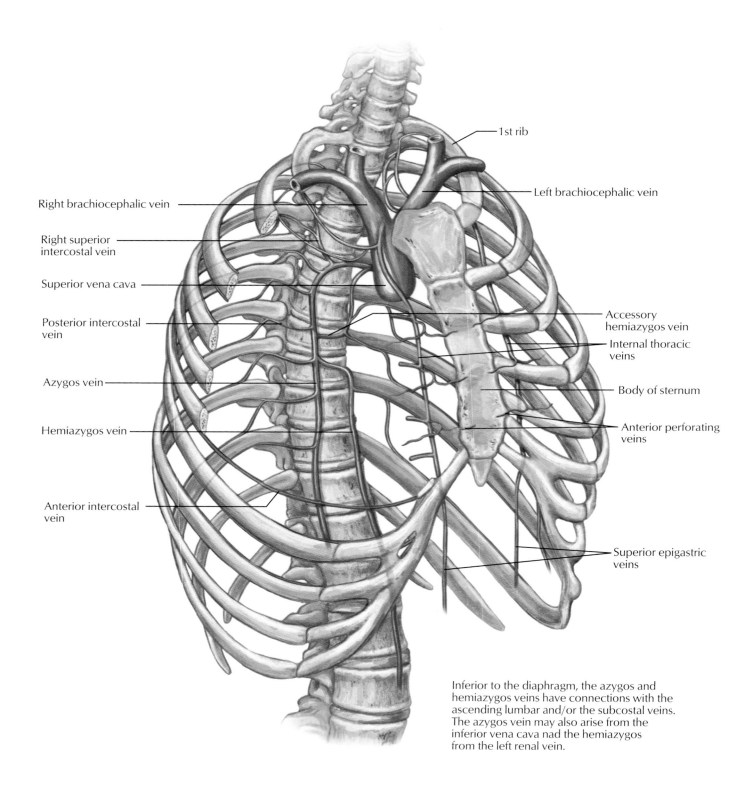

1st rib

Right brachiocephalic vein

Right superior intercostal vein

Superior vena cava

Posterior intercostal vein

Azygos vein

Hemiazygos vein

Anterior intercostal vein

Left brachiocephalic vein

Accessory hemiazygos vein

Internal thoracic veins

Body of sternum

Anterior perforating veins

Superior epigastric veins

Inferior to the diaphragm, the azygos and hemiazygos veins have connections with the ascending lumbar and/or the subcostal veins. The azygos vein may also arise from the inferior vena cava nad the hemiazygos from the left renal vein.

Plate 186   **Body Wall**

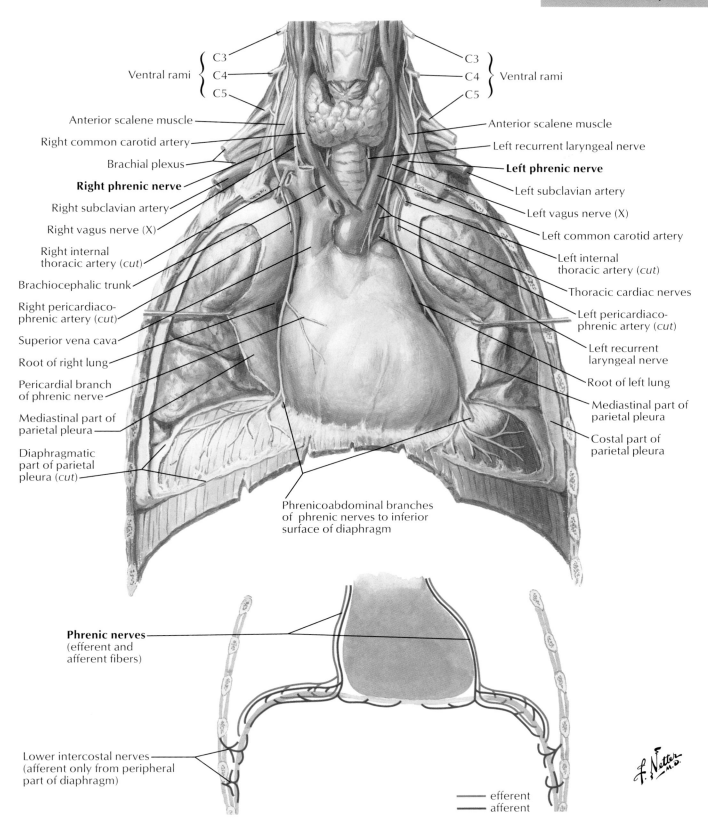

Ventral rami { C3 C4 C5

C3 C4 C5 } Ventral rami

Anterior scalene muscle

Right common carotid artery

Brachial plexus

Right phrenic nerve

Right subclavian artery

Right vagus nerve (X)

Right internal thoracic artery (*cut*)

Brachiocephalic trunk

Right pericardiaco- phrenic artery (*cut*)

Superior vena cava

Root of right lung

Pericardial branch of phrenic nerve

Mediastinal part of parietal pleura

Diaphragmatic part of parietal pleura (*cut*)

Anterior scalene muscle

Left recurrent laryngeal nerve

Left phrenic nerve

Left subclavian artery

Left vagus nerve (X)

Left common carotid artery

Left internal thoracic artery (*cut*)

Thoracic cardiac nerves

Left pericardiaco- phrenic artery (*cut*)

Left recurrent laryngeal nerve

Root of left lung

Mediastinal part of parietal pleura

Costal part of parietal pleura

Phrenicoabdominal branches of phrenic nerves to inferior surface of diaphragm

Phrenic nerves (efferent and afferent fibers)

Lower intercostal nerves (afferent only from peripheral part of diaphragm)

—— efferent —— afferent

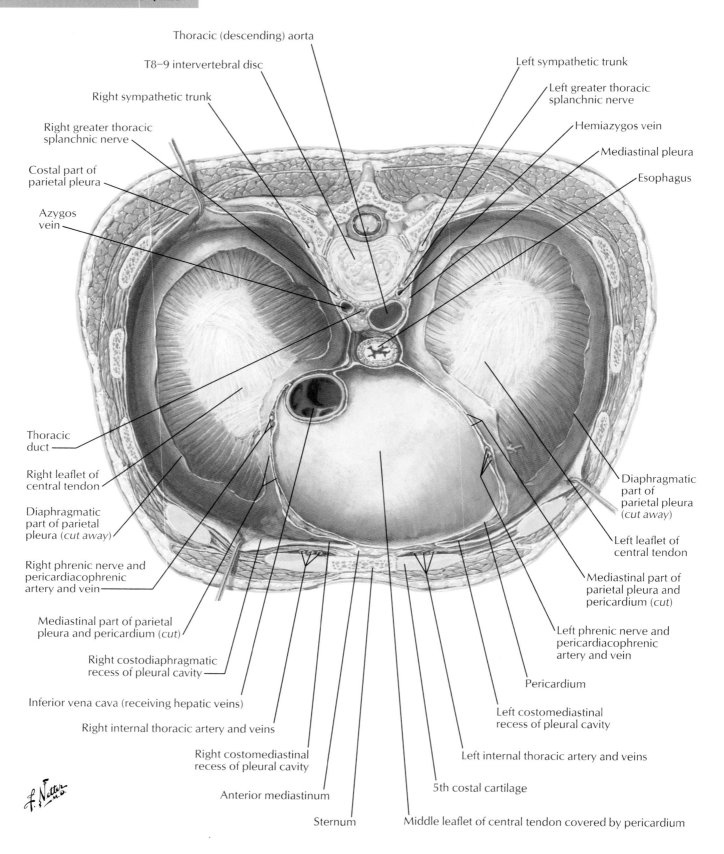

Thoracic (descending) aorta

T8–9 intervertebral disc

Right sympathetic trunk

Right greater thoracic splanchnic nerve

Costal part of parietal pleura

Azygos vein

Thoracic duct

Right leaflet of central tendon

Diaphragmatic part of parietal pleura (cut away)

Right phrenic nerve and pericardiacophrenic artery and vein

Mediastinal part of parietal pleura and pericardium (cut)

Right costodiaphragmatic recess of pleural cavity

Inferior vena cava (receiving hepatic veins)

Right internal thoracic artery and veins

Right costomediastinal recess of pleural cavity

Anterior mediastinum

Sternum

Left sympathetic trunk

Left greater thoracic splanchnic nerve

Hemiazygos vein

Mediastinal pleura

Esophagus

Diaphragmatic part of parietal pleura (cut away)

Left leaflet of central tendon

Mediastinal part of parietal pleura and pericardium (cut)

Left phrenic nerve and pericardiacophrenic artery and vein

Pericardium

Left costomediastinal recess of pleural cavity

Left internal thoracic artery and veins

5th costal cartilage

Middle leaflet of central tendon covered by pericardium

Plate 188

Body Wall

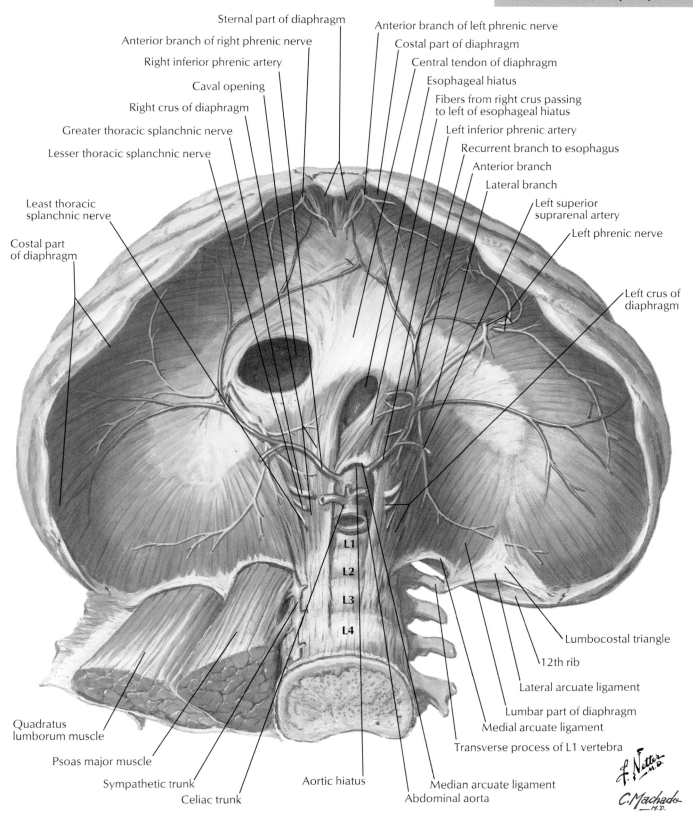

Sternal part of diaphragm

Anterior branch of right phrenic nerve

Right inferior phrenic artery

Caval opening

Right crus of diaphragm

Greater thoracic splanchnic nerve

Lesser thoracic splanchnic nerve

Least thoracic splanchnic nerve

Costal part of diaphragm

Anterior branch of left phrenic nerve

Costal part of diaphragm

Central tendon of diaphragm

Esophageal hiatus

Fibers from right crus passing to left of esophageal hiatus

Left inferior phrenic artery

Recurrent branch to esophagus

Anterior branch

Lateral branch

Left superior suprarenal artery

Left phrenic nerve

Left crus of diaphragm

Lumbocostal triangle

12th rib

Lateral arcuate ligament

Lumbar part of diaphragm

Medial arcuate ligament

Transverse process of L1 vertebra

Median arcuate ligament

Abdominal aorta

Aortic hiatus

Celiac trunk

Sympathetic trunk

Psoas major muscle

Quadratus lumborum muscle

L1

L2

L3

L4

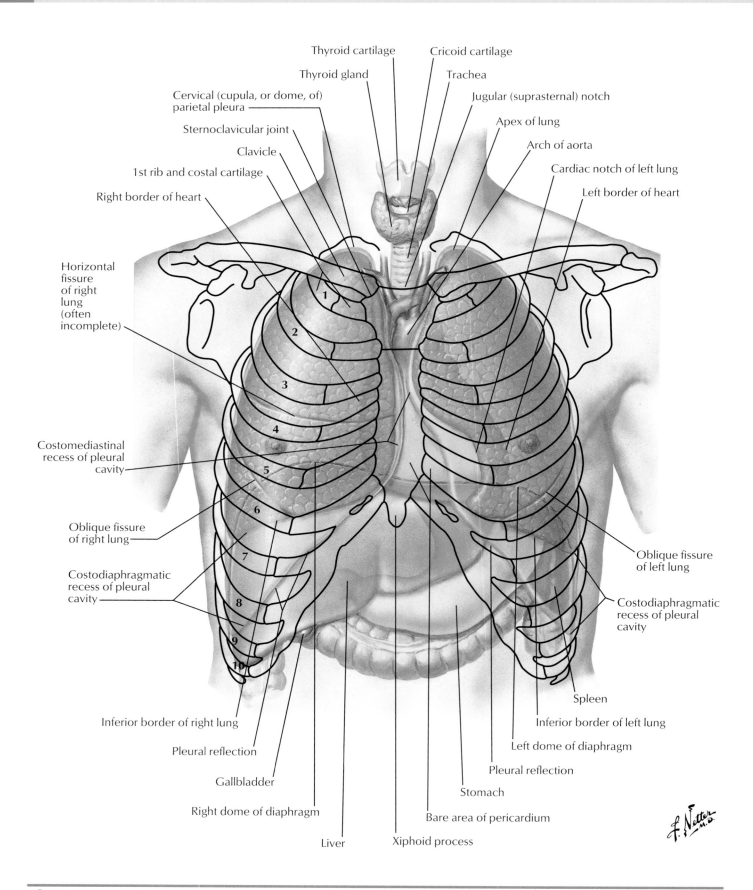

Thyroid cartilage

Cricoid cartilage

Thyroid gland

Trachea

Cervical (cupula, or dome, of) parietal pleura

Jugular (suprasternal) notch

Sternoclavicular joint

Apex of lung

Clavicle

Arch of aorta

1st rib and costal cartilage

Cardiac notch of left lung

Right border of heart

Left border of heart

Horizontal fissure of right lung (often incomplete)

Costomediastinal recess of pleural cavity

Oblique fissure of right lung

Oblique fissure of left lung

Costodiaphragmatic recess of pleural cavity

Costodiaphragmatic recess of pleural cavity

Inferior border of right lung

Spleen

Pleural reflection

Inferior border of left lung

Gallbladder

Left dome of diaphragm

Right dome of diaphragm

Pleural reflection

Liver

Stomach

Xiphoid process

Bare area of pericardium

Plate 190 **Lungs**

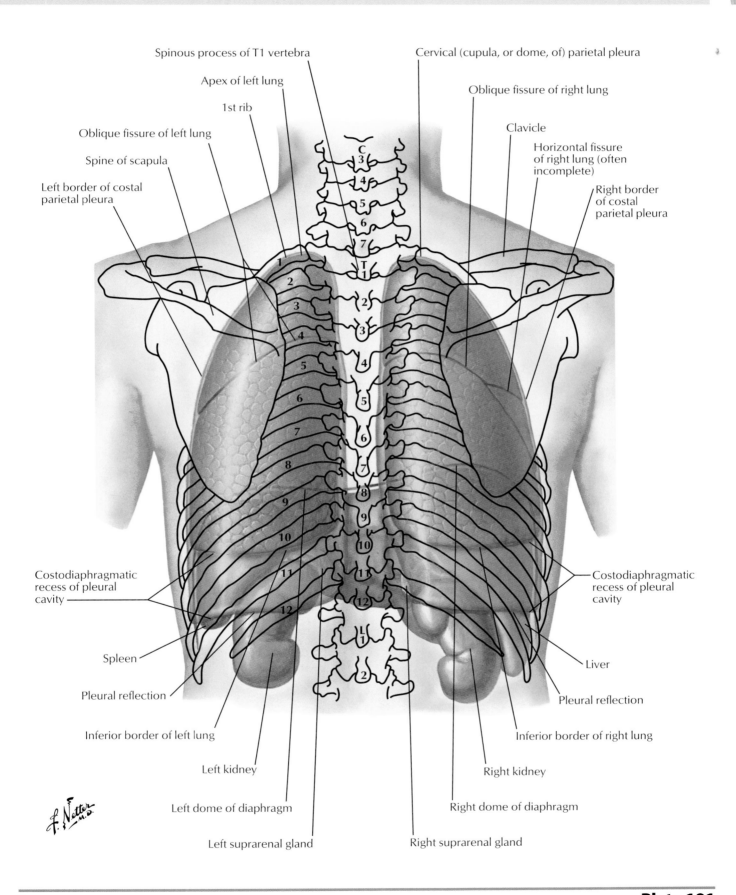

Spinous process of T1 vertebra

Apex of left lung

1st rib

Oblique fissure of left lung

Spine of scapula

Left border of costal parietal pleura

Cervical (cupula, or dome, of) parietal pleura

Oblique fissure of right lung

Clavicle

Horizontal fissure of right lung (often incomplete)

Right border of costal parietal pleura

Costodiaphragmatic recess of pleural cavity

Costodiaphragmatic recess of pleural cavity

Spleen

Pleural reflection

Inferior border of left lung

Left kidney

Left dome of diaphragm

Left suprarenal gland

Liver

Pleural reflection

Inferior border of right lung

Right kidney

Right dome of diaphragm

Right suprarenal gland

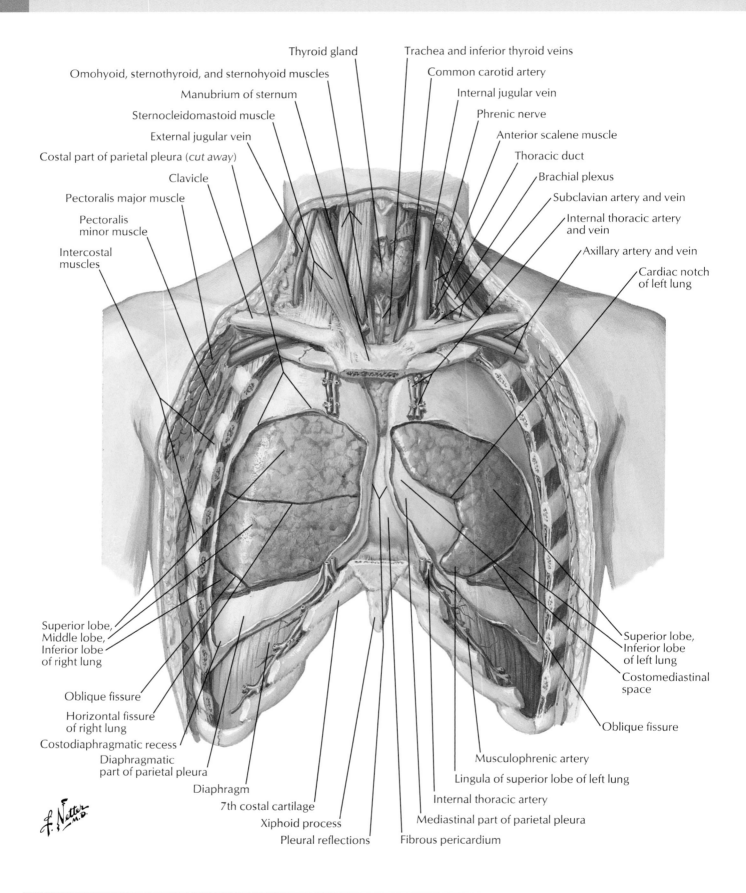

Thyroid gland

Trachea and inferior thyroid veins

Omohyoid, sternothyroid, and sternohyoid muscles

Common carotid artery

Manubrium of sternum

Internal jugular vein

Sternocleidomastoid muscle

Phrenic nerve

External jugular vein

Anterior scalene muscle

Costal part of parietal pleura (cut away)

Thoracic duct

Clavicle

Brachial plexus

Pectoralis major muscle

Subclavian artery and vein

Pectoralis minor muscle

Internal thoracic artery and vein

Intercostal muscles

Axillary artery and vein

Cardiac notch of left lung

Superior lobe,
Middle lobe,
Inferior lobe
of right lung

Superior lobe,
Inferior lobe
of left lung

Oblique fissure

Costomediastinal space

Horizontal fissure of right lung

Oblique fissure

Costodiaphragmatic recess

Diaphragmatic part of parietal pleura

Musculophrenic artery

Diaphragm

Lingula of superior lobe of left lung

7th costal cartilage

Internal thoracic artery

Xiphoid process

Mediastinal part of parietal pleura

Pleural reflections

Fibrous pericardium

Plate 192

Lungs

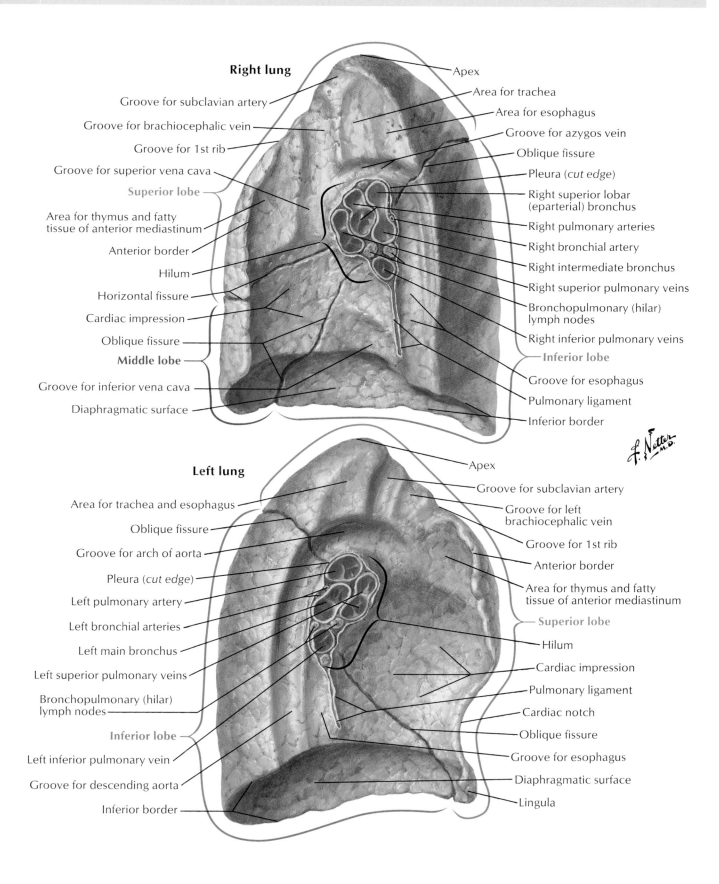

Right lung

Apex

Groove for subclavian artery

Area for trachea

Groove for brachiocephalic vein

Area for esophagus

Groove for 1st rib

Groove for azygos vein

Groove for superior vena cava

Oblique fissure

Superior lobe

Pleura (*cut edge*)

Area for thymus and fatty tissue of anterior mediastinum

Right superior lobar (eparterial) bronchus

Anterior border

Right pulmonary arteries

Hilum

Right bronchial artery

Horizontal fissure

Right intermediate bronchus

Cardiac impression

Right superior pulmonary veins

Oblique fissure

Bronchopulmonary (hilar) lymph nodes

Middle lobe

Right inferior pulmonary veins

Groove for inferior vena cava

Inferior lobe

Diaphragmatic surface

Groove for esophagus

Pulmonary ligament

Inferior border

Left lung

Apex

Area for trachea and esophagus

Groove for subclavian artery

Oblique fissure

Groove for left brachiocephalic vein

Groove for arch of aorta

Groove for 1st rib

Pleura (*cut edge*)

Anterior border

Left pulmonary artery

Area for thymus and fatty tissue of anterior mediastinum

Left bronchial arteries

Superior lobe

Left main bronchus

Hilum

Left superior pulmonary veins

Cardiac impression

Bronchopulmonary (hilar) lymph nodes

Pulmonary ligament

Cardiac notch

Inferior lobe

Oblique fissure

Left inferior pulmonary vein

Groove for esophagus

Groove for descending aorta

Diaphragmatic surface

Inferior border

Lingula

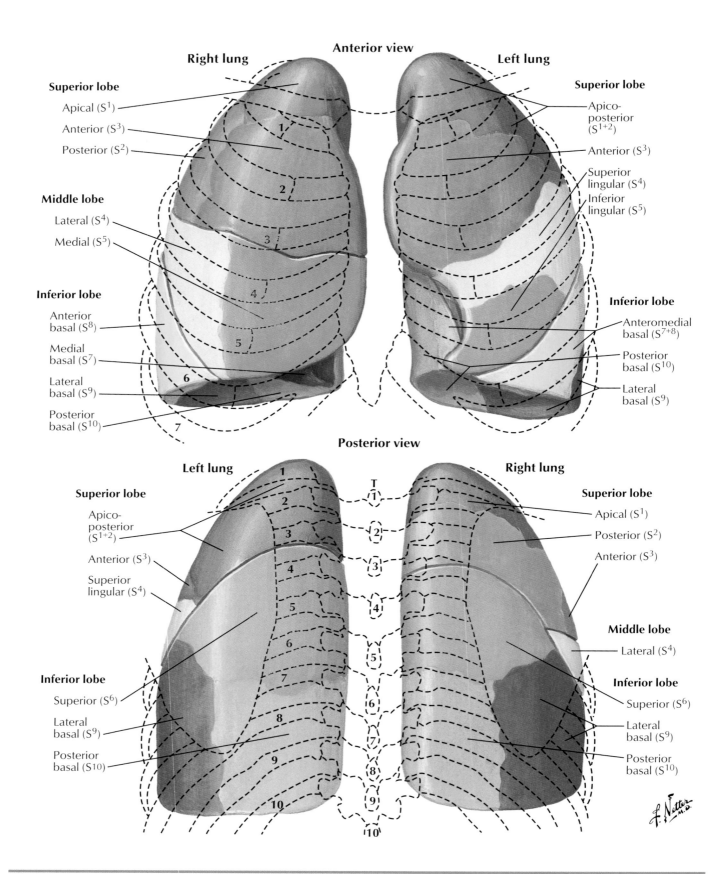

Anterior view

Right lung

Superior lobe
Apical (S^1)
Anterior (S^3)
Posterior (S^2)

Middle lobe
Lateral (S^4)
Medial (S^5)

Inferior lobe
Anterior basal (S^8)
Medial basal (S^7)
Lateral basal (S^9)
Posterior basal (S^{10})

Left lung

Superior lobe
Apico-posterior (S^{1+2})
Anterior (S^3)
Superior lingular (S^4)
Inferior lingular (S^5)

Inferior lobe
Anteromedial basal (S^{7+8})
Posterior basal (S^{10})
Lateral basal (S^9)

Posterior view

Left lung

Superior lobe
Apico-posterior (S^{1+2})
Anterior (S^3)
Superior lingular (S^4)

Inferior lobe
Superior (S^6)
Lateral basal (S^9)
Posterior basal (S^{10})

Right lung

Superior lobe
Apical (S^1)
Posterior (S^2)
Anterior (S^3)

Middle lobe
Lateral (S^4)

Inferior lobe
Superior (S^6)
Lateral basal (S^9)
Posterior basal (S^{10})

Plate 194 **Lungs**

Lateral views

Right lung

Left lung

Superior lobe

Apical (S^1)

Posterior (S^2)

Anterior (S^3)

Middle lobe

Lateral (S^4)

Medial (S^5)

Inferior lobe

Superior (S^6)

Anterior basal (S^8)

Lateral basal (S^9)

Superior lobe

Apico-posterior (S^{1+2})

Anterior (S^3)

Superior lingular (S^4)

Inferior lingular (S^5)

Inferior lobe

Superior (S^6)

Antero-medial basal (S^{7+8})

Lateral basal (S^9)

Medial views

Right lung

Left lung

Superior lobe

Apical (S^1)

Posterior (S^2)

Anterior (S^3)

Middle lobe

Medial (S^5)

Inferior lobe

Superior (S^6)

Medial basal (S^7)

Anterior basal (S^8)

Lateral basal (S^9)

Posterior basal (S^{10})

Superior lobe

Apico-posterior (S^{1+2})

Anterior (S^3)

Superior lingular (S^4)

Inferior lingular (S^5)

Inferior lobe

Superior (S^6)

Anteromedial basal (S^{7+8})

Lateral basal (S^9)

Posterior basal (S^{10})

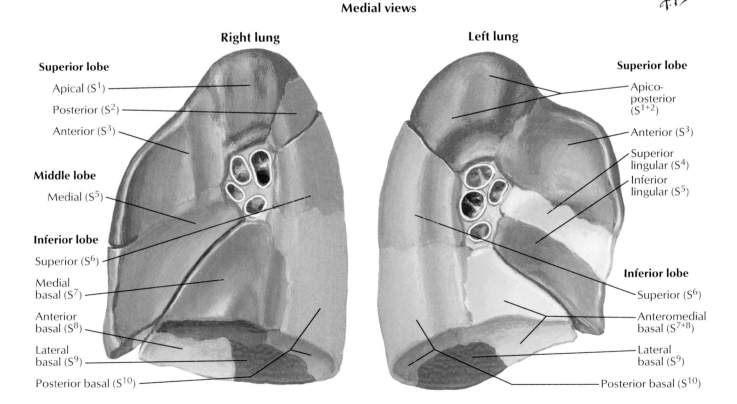

Lungs

Plate 195

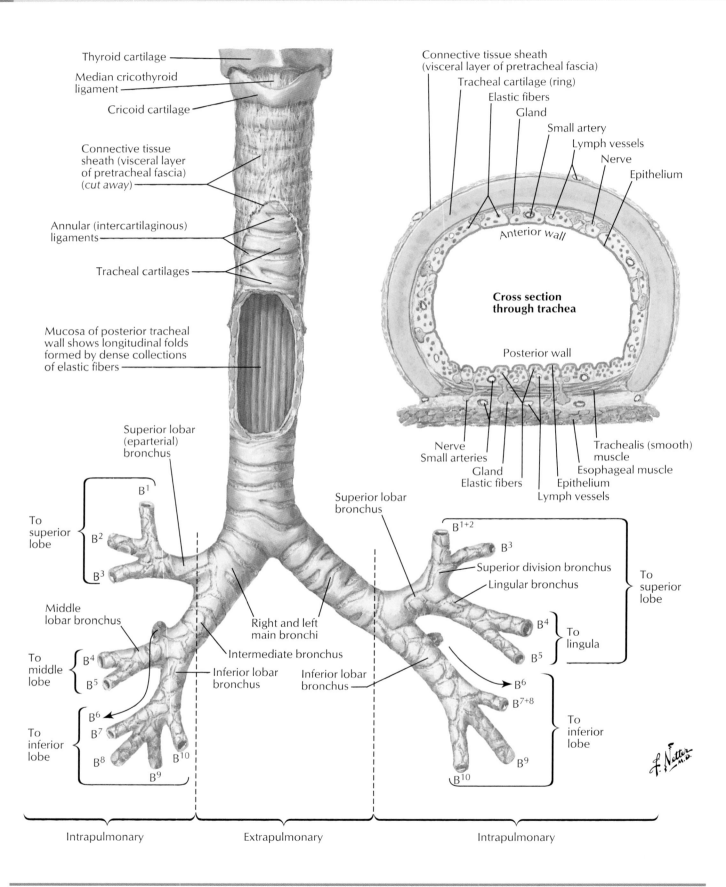

Thyroid cartilage

Median cricothyroid ligament

Cricoid cartilage

Connective tissue sheath (visceral layer of pretracheal fascia) (*cut away*)

Annular (intercartilaginous) ligaments

Tracheal cartilages

Mucosa of posterior tracheal wall shows longitudinal folds formed by dense collections of elastic fibers

Connective tissue sheath (visceral layer of pretracheal fascia)

Tracheal cartilage (ring)

Elastic fibers

Gland

Small artery

Lymph vessels

Nerve

Epithelium

Anterior wall

Cross section through trachea

Posterior wall

Nerve
Small arteries

Gland
Elastic fibers

Trachealis (smooth) muscle

Esophageal muscle

Epithelium

Lymph vessels

Superior lobar (eparterial) bronchus

B^1

To superior lobe

B^2

B^3

Superior lobar bronchus

B^{1+2}

B^3

Superior division bronchus

Lingular bronchus

To superior lobe

Middle lobar bronchus

Right and left main bronchi

Intermediate bronchus

B^4

To lingula

B^5

To middle lobe

B^4

B^5

Inferior lobar bronchus

Inferior lobar bronchus

B^6

B^{7+8}

To inferior lobe

B^6

To inferior lobe

B^7

B^8

B^{10}

B^9

B^9

B^{10}

Intrapulmonary

Extrapulmonary

Intrapulmonary

Plate 196

Lungs

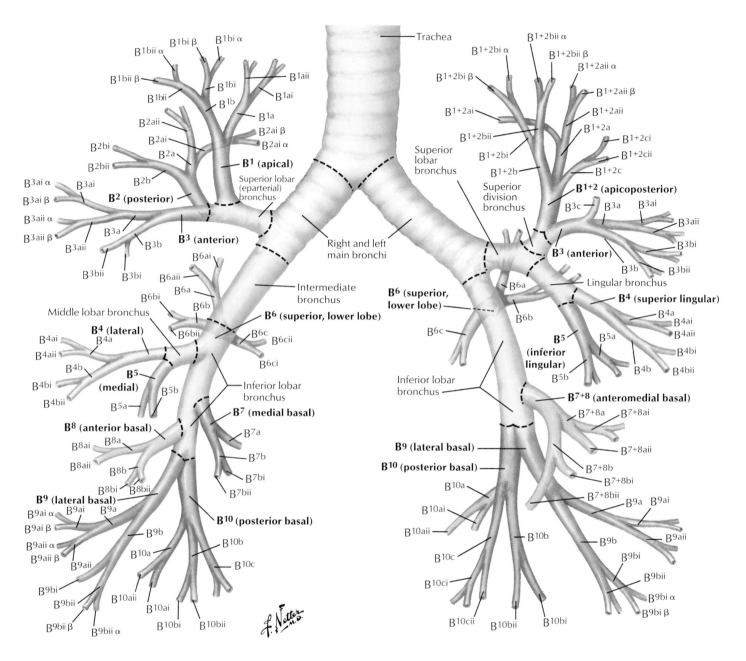

Nomenclature in common usage for bronchopulmonary segments (Plates 194 and 195) is that of Jackson and Huber, and segmental bronchi are named accordingly. Ikeda proposed nomenclature (as demonstrated here) for bronchial subdivisions as far as the 6th generation. For simplification on this illustration, only some bronchial subdivisions are labeled as far as the 5th or 6th generation. Segmental bronchi (B) are numbered from 1 to 10 in each lung, corresponding to pulmonary segments. In the left lung,

B^1 and B^2 are combined as are B^7 and B^8. Subsegmental, or 4th order, bronchi are indicated by the addition of lower-case letters a, b, or c when an additional branch is present. Fifth order bronchi are designated by Roman numerals i (anterior) or ii (posterior) and 6th order bronchi by Greek letters α or β. Several texts use alternate numbers (as proposed by Boyden) for segmental bronchi.

Variations of the standard bronchial pattern shown here are common, especially in peripheral airways.

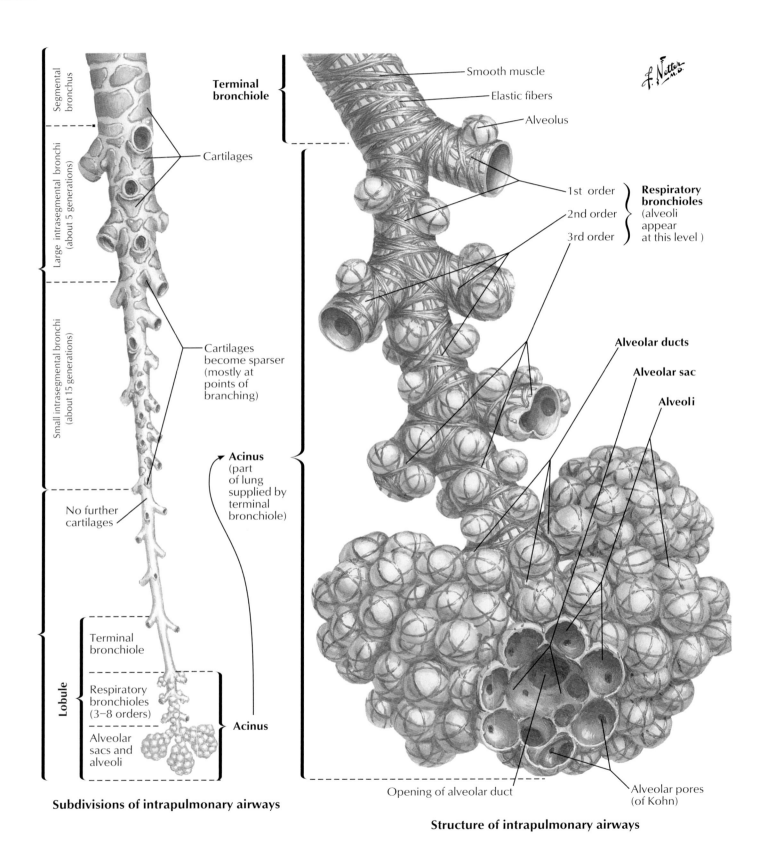

Subdivisions of intrapulmonary airways

Segmental bronchus

Large intrasegmental bronchi (about 5 generations)

Small intrasegmental bronchi (about 15 generations)

Cartilages

Cartilages become sparser (mostly at points of branching)

No further cartilages

Acinus (part of lung supplied by terminal bronchiole)

Lobule

Terminal bronchiole

Respiratory bronchioles (3–8 orders)

Alveolar sacs and alveoli

Acinus

Structure of intrapulmonary airways

Terminal bronchiole

Smooth muscle

Elastic fibers

Alveolus

1st order
2nd order
3rd order

Respiratory bronchioles (alveoli appear at this level)

Alveolar ducts

Alveolar sac

Alveoli

Opening of alveolar duct

Alveolar pores (of Kohn)

F. Netter M.D.

Plate 198   **Lungs**

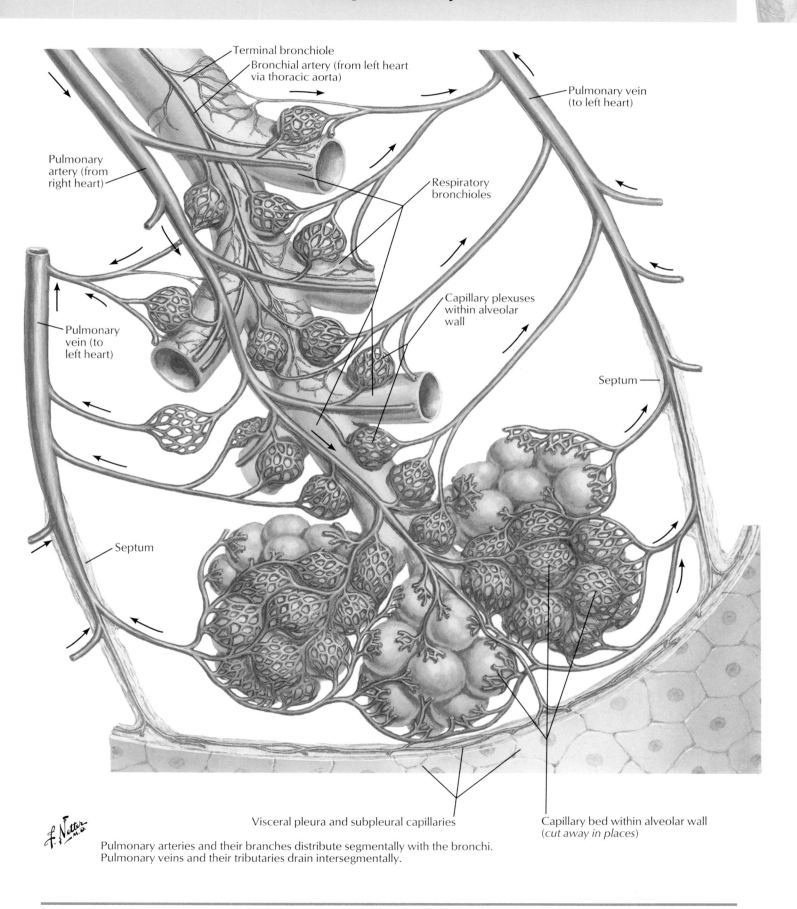

Terminal bronchiole
Bronchial artery (from left heart via thoracic aorta)
Pulmonary vein (to left heart)
Pulmonary artery (from right heart)
Respiratory bronchioles
Pulmonary vein (to left heart)
Capillary plexuses within alveolar wall
Septum
Septum
Visceral pleura and subpleural capillaries
Capillary bed within alveolar wall (*cut away in places*)

Pulmonary arteries and their branches distribute segmentally with the bronchi.
Pulmonary veins and their tributaries drain intersegmentally.

F. Netter
M.D.

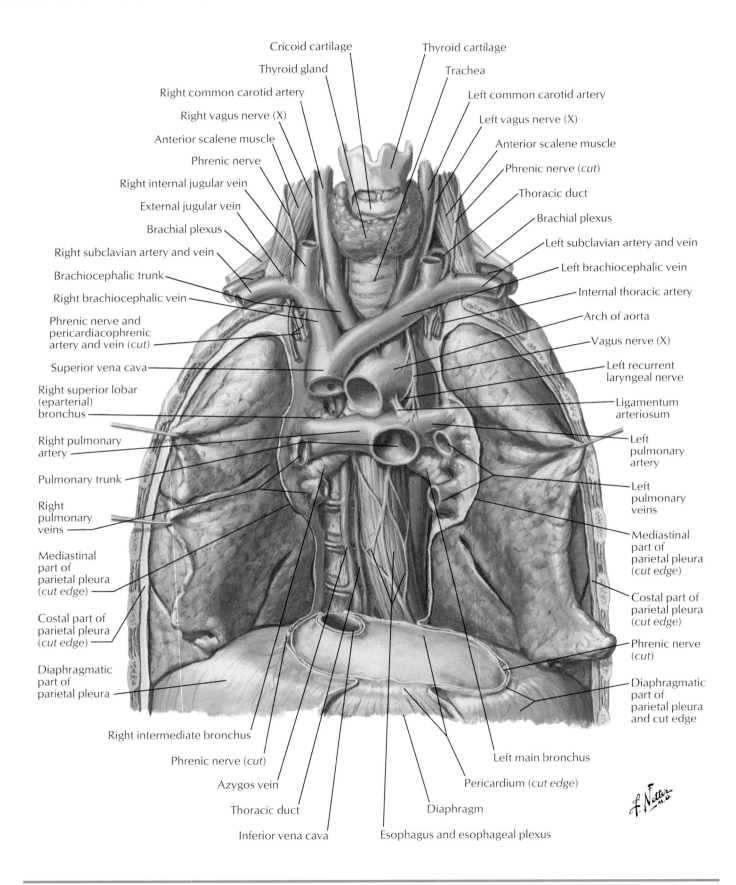

Cricoid cartilage

Thyroid cartilage

Thyroid gland

Trachea

Right common carotid artery

Left common carotid artery

Right vagus nerve (X)

Left vagus nerve (X)

Anterior scalene muscle

Anterior scalene muscle

Phrenic nerve

Phrenic nerve (*cut*)

Right internal jugular vein

Thoracic duct

External jugular vein

Brachial plexus

Brachial plexus

Left subclavian artery and vein

Right subclavian artery and vein

Left brachiocephalic vein

Brachiocephalic trunk

Internal thoracic artery

Right brachiocephalic vein

Arch of aorta

Phrenic nerve and
pericardiacophrenic
artery and vein (*cut*)

Vagus nerve (X)

Superior vena cava

Left recurrent
laryngeal nerve

Right superior lobar
(eparterial)
bronchus

Ligamentum
arteriosum

Right pulmonary
artery

Left
pulmonary
artery

Pulmonary trunk

Left
pulmonary
veins

Right
pulmonary
veins

Mediastinal
part of
parietal pleura
(*cut edge*)

Mediastinal
part of
parietal pleura
(*cut edge*)

Costal part of
parietal pleura
(*cut edge*)

Costal part of
parietal pleura
(*cut edge*)

Phrenic nerve
(*cut*)

Diaphragmatic
part of
parietal pleura

Diaphragmatic
part of
parietal pleura
and cut edge

Right intermediate bronchus

Left main bronchus

Phrenic nerve (*cut*)

Pericardium (*cut edge*)

Azygos vein

Diaphragm

Thoracic duct

Inferior vena cava

Esophagus and esophageal plexus

f. Netter.
m.d.

Plate 200

Lungs

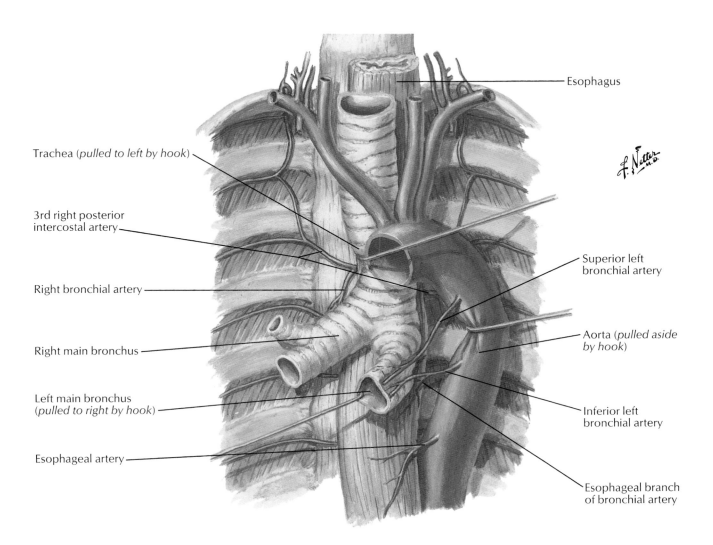

Esophagus

Trachea (*pulled to left by hook*)

3rd right posterior intercostal artery

Right bronchial artery

Right main bronchus

Left main bronchus (*pulled to right by hook*)

Esophageal artery

Superior left bronchial artery

Aorta (*pulled aside by hook*)

Inferior left bronchial artery

Esophageal branch of bronchial artery

Bronchial veins

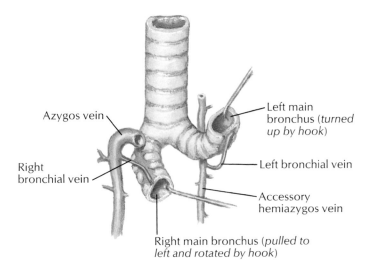

Azygos vein

Right bronchial vein

Left main bronchus (*turned up by hook*)

Left bronchial vein

Accessory hemiazygos vein

Right main bronchus (*pulled to left and rotated by hook*)

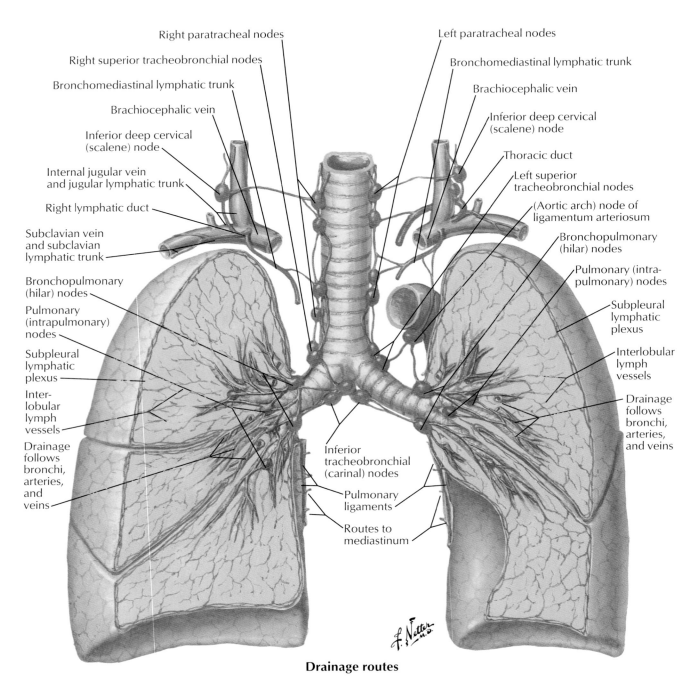

Right paratracheal nodes

Right superior tracheobronchial nodes

Bronchomediastinal lymphatic trunk

Brachiocephalic vein

Inferior deep cervical (scalene) node

Internal jugular vein and jugular lymphatic trunk

Right lymphatic duct

Subclavian vein and subclavian lymphatic trunk

Bronchopulmonary (hilar) nodes

Pulmonary (intrapulmonary) nodes

Subpleural lymphatic plexus

Interlobular lymph vessels

Drainage follows bronchi, arteries, and veins

Left paratracheal nodes

Bronchomediastinal lymphatic trunk

Brachiocephalic vein

Inferior deep cervical (scalene) node

Thoracic duct

Left superior tracheobronchial nodes

(Aortic arch) node of ligamentum arteriosum

Bronchopulmonary (hilar) nodes

Pulmonary (intra- pulmonary) nodes

Subpleural lymphatic plexus

Interlobular lymph vessels

Drainage follows bronchi, arteries, and veins

Inferior tracheobronchial (carinal) nodes

Pulmonary ligaments

Routes to mediastinum

Drainage routes

Right lung: All lobes drain to pulmonary and bronchopulmonary (hilar) nodes, then to inferior tracheobronchial (carinal) nodes, right superior tracheobronchial nodes, and right paratracheal nodes on the way to the brachiocephalic vein via the bronchomediastinal lymphatic trunk and/ or inferior deep cervical (scalene) node.

Left lung: The superior lobe drains to pulmonary and broncho- pulmonary (hilar) nodes, inferior tracheobronchial (carinal) nodes, left superior tracheobronchial nodes, left paratracheal nodes and/or (aortic arch) node of ligamentum arteriosum, then to the brachiocephalic vein via the left bronchomediastinal trunk and thoracic duct. The left inferior lobe also drains to the pulmonary and bronchopulmonary (hilar) nodes and to inferior tracheobronchial (carinal) nodes, but then mostly to right superior tracheobronchial nodes, where it follows the same route as lymph from the right lung.

Plate 202

Lungs

See also **Plates 129, 130, 297**

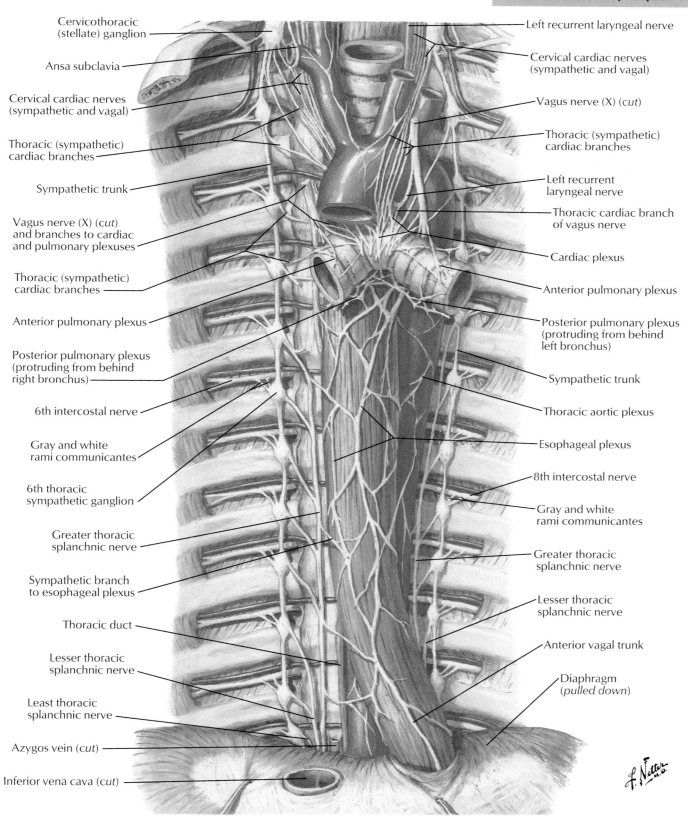

Cervicothoracic (stellate) ganglion

Ansa subclavia

Cervical cardiac nerves (sympathetic and vagal)

Thoracic (sympathetic) cardiac branches

Sympathetic trunk

Vagus nerve (X) (cut) and branches to cardiac and pulmonary plexuses

Thoracic (sympathetic) cardiac branches

Anterior pulmonary plexus

Posterior pulmonary plexus (protruding from behind right bronchus)

6th intercostal nerve

Gray and white rami communicantes

6th thoracic sympathetic ganglion

Greater thoracic splanchnic nerve

Sympathetic branch to esophageal plexus

Thoracic duct

Lesser thoracic splanchnic nerve

Least thoracic splanchnic nerve

Azygos vein (cut)

Inferior vena cava (cut)

Left recurrent laryngeal nerve

Cervical cardiac nerves (sympathetic and vagal)

Vagus nerve (X) (cut)

Thoracic (sympathetic) cardiac branches

Left recurrent laryngeal nerve

Thoracic cardiac branch of vagus nerve

Cardiac plexus

Anterior pulmonary plexus

Posterior pulmonary plexus (protruding from behind left bronchus)

Sympathetic trunk

Thoracic aortic plexus

Esophageal plexus

8th intercostal nerve

Gray and white rami communicantes

Greater thoracic splanchnic nerve

Lesser thoracic splanchnic nerve

Anterior vagal trunk

Diaphragm (pulled down)

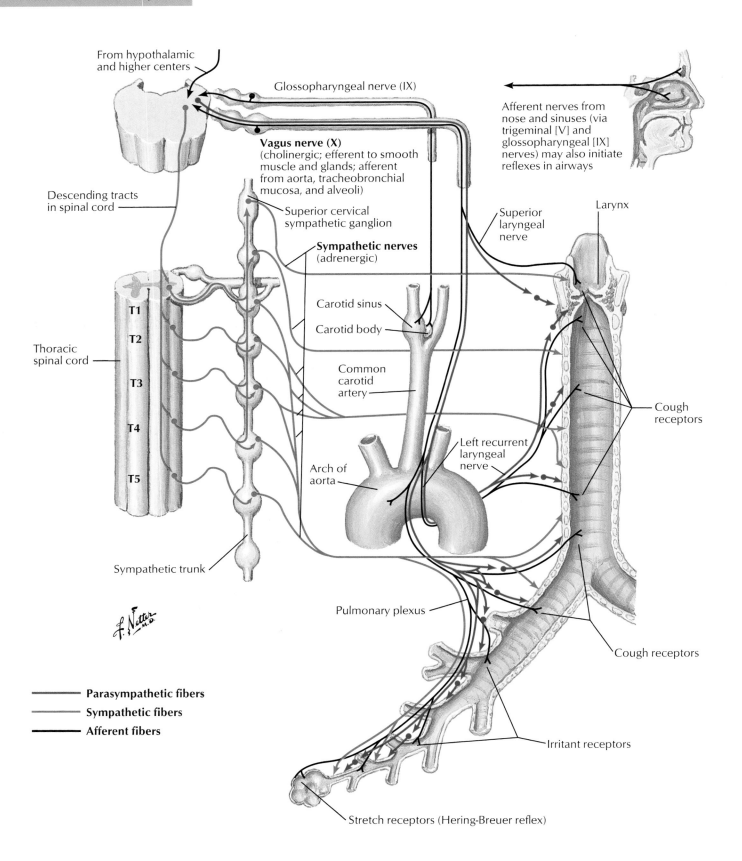

From hypothalamic and higher centers

Glossopharyngeal nerve (IX)

Afferent nerves from nose and sinuses (via trigeminal [V] and glossopharyngeal [IX] nerves) may also initiate reflexes in airways

Vagus nerve (X)
(cholinergic; efferent to smooth muscle and glands; afferent from aorta, tracheobronchial mucosa, and alveoli)

Descending tracts in spinal cord

Superior cervical sympathetic ganglion

Superior laryngeal nerve

Larynx

Sympathetic nerves
(adrenergic)

T1

Carotid sinus

Carotid body

T2

Thoracic spinal cord

Common carotid artery

T3

Cough receptors

T4

Left recurrent laryngeal nerve

T5

Arch of aorta

Sympathetic trunk

Pulmonary plexus

Cough receptors

Irritant receptors

— **Parasympathetic fibers**
— **Sympathetic fibers**
— **Afferent fibers**

Stretch receptors (Hering-Breuer reflex)

Plate 204

Lungs

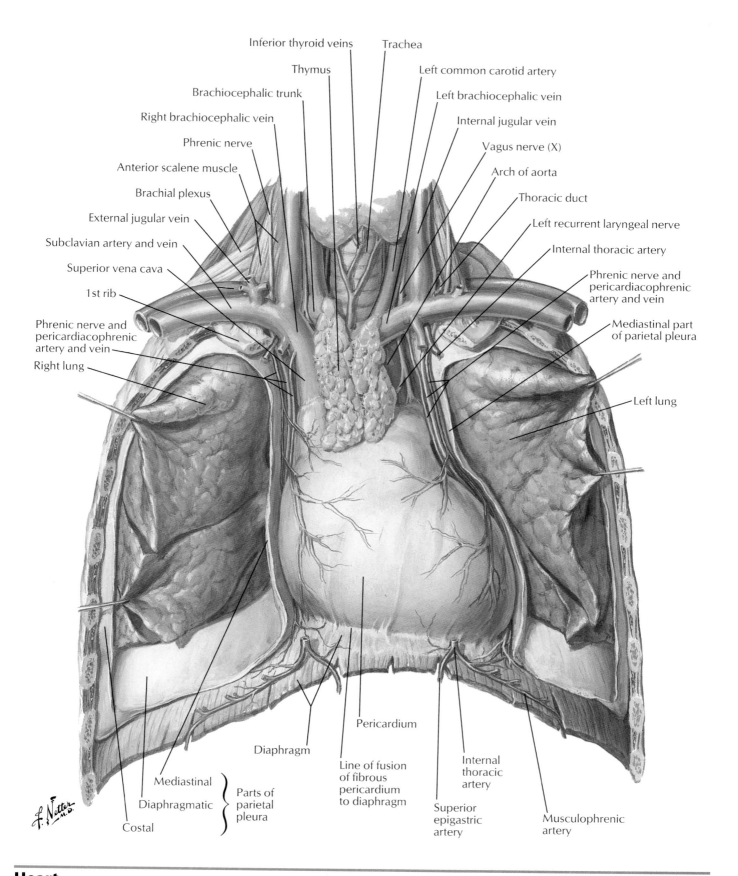

Inferior thyroid veins

Trachea

Thymus

Left common carotid artery

Brachiocephalic trunk

Left brachiocephalic vein

Right brachiocephalic vein

Internal jugular vein

Phrenic nerve

Vagus nerve (X)

Anterior scalene muscle

Arch of aorta

Brachial plexus

Thoracic duct

External jugular vein

Left recurrent laryngeal nerve

Subclavian artery and vein

Internal thoracic artery

Superior vena cava

Phrenic nerve and pericardiacophrenic artery and vein

1st rib

Phrenic nerve and pericardiacophrenic artery and vein

Mediastinal part of parietal pleura

Right lung

Left lung

Mediastinal

Diaphragmatic   } Parts of parietal pleura

Costal

Diaphragm

Pericardium

Line of fusion of fibrous pericardium to diaphragm

Internal thoracic artery

Superior epigastric artery

Musculophrenic artery

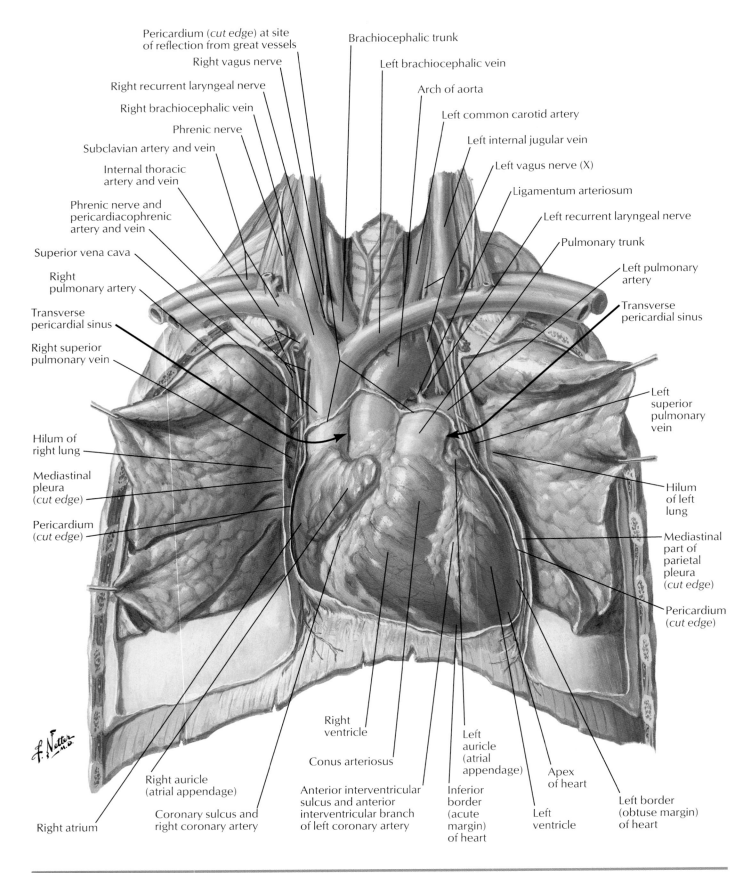

Pericardium (*cut edge*) at site of reflection from great vessels

Right vagus nerve

Right recurrent laryngeal nerve

Right brachiocephalic vein

Phrenic nerve

Subclavian artery and vein

Internal thoracic artery and vein

Phrenic nerve and pericardiacophrenic artery and vein

Superior vena cava

Right pulmonary artery

Transverse pericardial sinus

Right superior pulmonary vein

Hilum of right lung

Mediastinal pleura (*cut edge*)

Pericardium (*cut edge*)

Brachiocephalic trunk

Left brachiocephalic vein

Arch of aorta

Left common carotid artery

Left internal jugular vein

Left vagus nerve (X)

Ligamentum arteriosum

Left recurrent laryngeal nerve

Pulmonary trunk

Left pulmonary artery

Transverse pericardial sinus

Left superior pulmonary vein

Hilum of left lung

Mediastinal part of parietal pleura (*cut edge*)

Pericardium (*cut edge*)

Right ventricle

Conus arteriosus

Right auricle (atrial appendage)

Coronary sulcus and right coronary artery

Right atrium

Anterior interventricular sulcus and anterior interventricular branch of left coronary artery

Left auricle (atrial appendage)

Inferior border (acute margin) of heart

Left ventricle

Apex of heart

Left border (obtuse margin) of heart

Plate 206

Heart

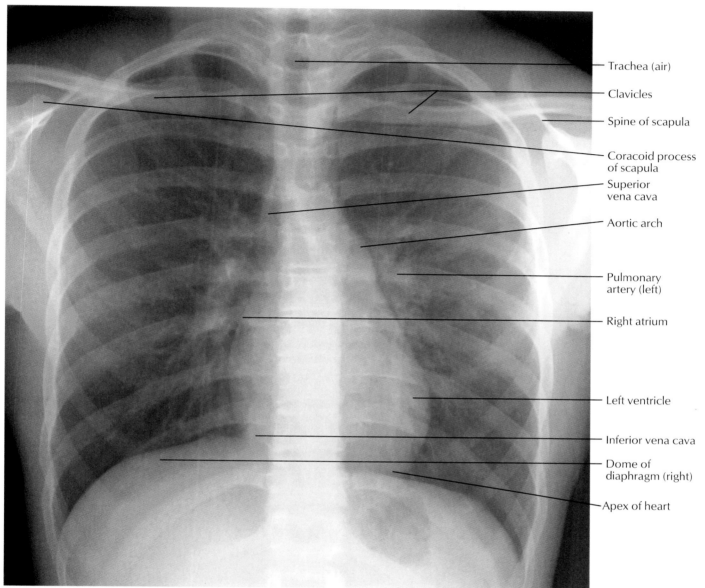

Trachea (air)

Clavicles

Spine of scapula

Coracoid process of scapula

Superior vena cava

Aortic arch

Pulmonary artery (left)

Right atrium

Left ventricle

Inferior vena cava

Dome of diaphragm (right)

Apex of heart

Precordial areas of auscultation

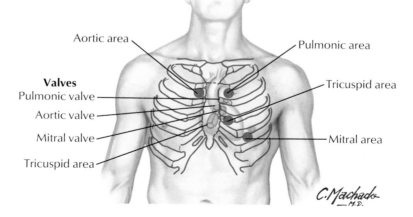

Aortic area

Pulmonic area

Valves

Pulmonic valve

Aortic valve

Mitral valve

Tricuspid area

Tricuspid area

Mitral area

C. Machado
M.D.

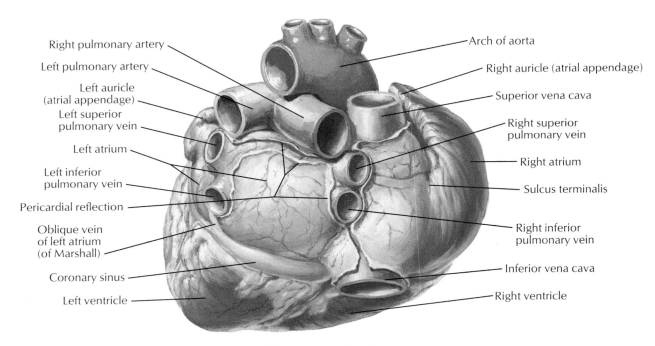

Right pulmonary artery

Left pulmonary artery

Left auricle (atrial appendage)

Left superior pulmonary vein

Left atrium

Left inferior pulmonary vein

Pericardial reflection

Oblique vein of left atrium (of Marshall)

Coronary sinus

Left ventricle

Arch of aorta

Right auricle (atrial appendage)

Superior vena cava

Right superior pulmonary vein

Right atrium

Sulcus terminalis

Right inferior pulmonary vein

Inferior vena cava

Right ventricle

Base of heart: posterior view

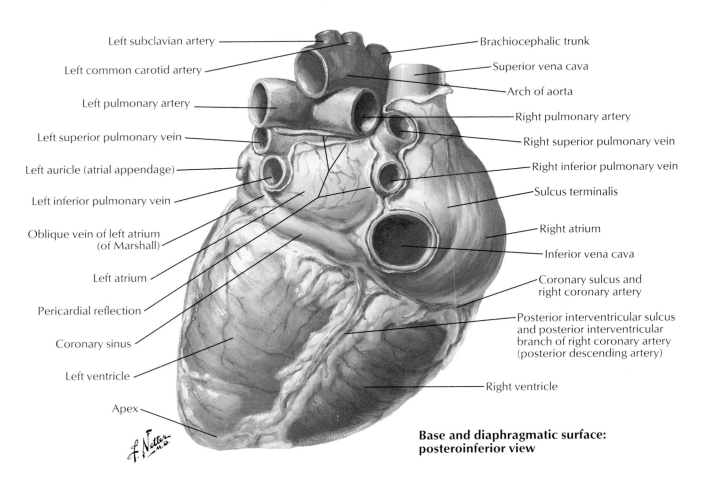

Left subclavian artery

Left common carotid artery

Left pulmonary artery

Left superior pulmonary vein

Left auricle (atrial appendage)

Left inferior pulmonary vein

Oblique vein of left atrium (of Marshall)

Left atrium

Pericardial reflection

Coronary sinus

Left ventricle

Apex

Brachiocephalic trunk

Superior vena cava

Arch of aorta

Right pulmonary artery

Right superior pulmonary vein

Right inferior pulmonary vein

Sulcus terminalis

Right atrium

Inferior vena cava

Coronary sulcus and right coronary artery

Posterior interventricular sulcus and posterior interventricular branch of right coronary artery (posterior descending artery)

Right ventricle

Base and diaphragmatic surface: posteroinferior view

Plate 208 **Heart**

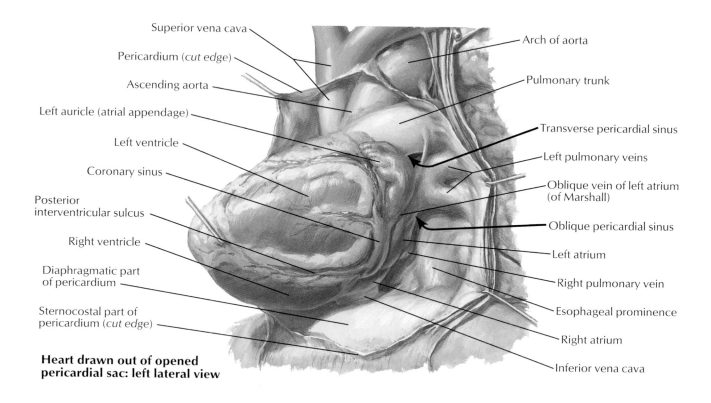

Superior vena cava

Pericardium (*cut edge*)

Ascending aorta

Left auricle (atrial appendage)

Left ventricle

Coronary sinus

Posterior interventricular sulcus

Right ventricle

Diaphragmatic part of pericardium

Sternocostal part of pericardium (*cut edge*)

Arch of aorta

Pulmonary trunk

Transverse pericardial sinus

Left pulmonary veins

Oblique vein of left atrium (of Marshall)

Oblique pericardial sinus

Left atrium

Right pulmonary vein

Esophageal prominence

Right atrium

Inferior vena cava

Heart drawn out of opened pericardial sac: left lateral view

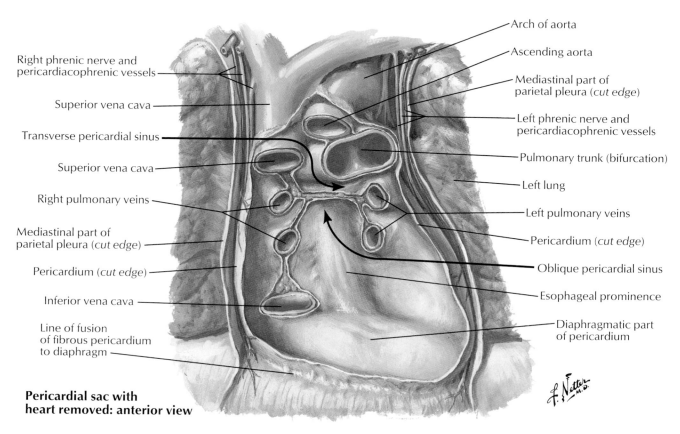

Right phrenic nerve and pericardiacophrenic vessels

Superior vena cava

Transverse pericardial sinus

Superior vena cava

Right pulmonary veins

Mediastinal part of parietal pleura (*cut edge*)

Pericardium (*cut edge*)

Inferior vena cava

Line of fusion of fibrous pericardium to diaphragm

Arch of aorta

Ascending aorta

Mediastinal part of parietal pleura (*cut edge*)

Left phrenic nerve and pericardiacophrenic vessels

Pulmonary trunk (bifurcation)

Left lung

Left pulmonary veins

Pericardium (*cut edge*)

Oblique pericardial sinus

Esophageal prominence

Diaphragmatic part of pericardium

Pericardial sac with heart removed: anterior view

f. Netter
M.D.

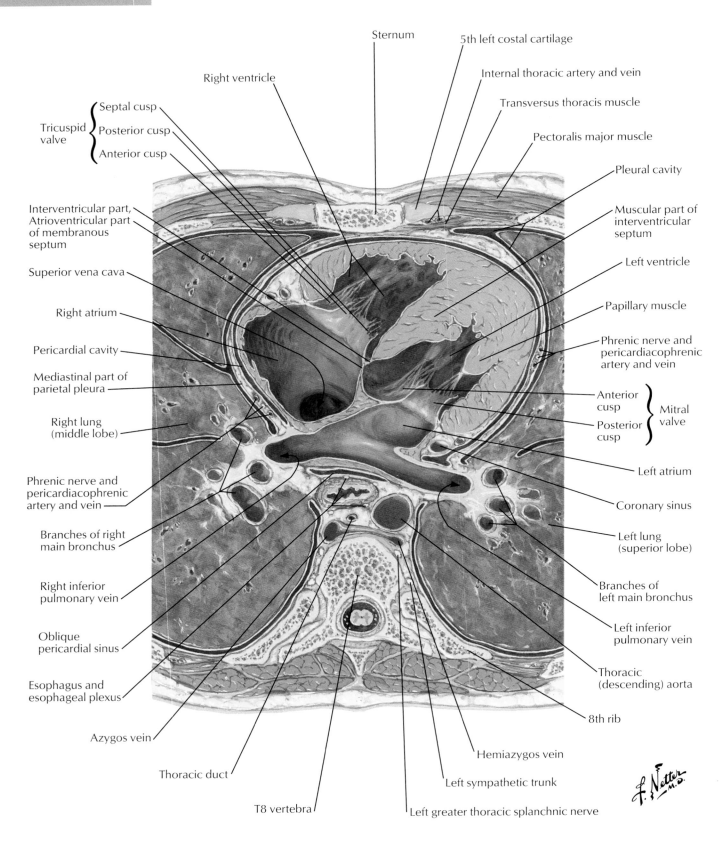

Sternum

5th left costal cartilage

Internal thoracic artery and vein

Right ventricle

Transversus thoracis muscle

Pectoralis major muscle

Tricuspid valve
{ Septal cusp
  Posterior cusp
  Anterior cusp

Pleural cavity

Muscular part of interventricular septum

Interventricular part, Atrioventricular part of membranous septum

Left ventricle

Superior vena cava

Papillary muscle

Right atrium

Phrenic nerve and pericardiacophrenic artery and vein

Pericardial cavity

Mediastinal part of parietal pleura

Anterior cusp
Posterior cusp
} Mitral valve

Right lung (middle lobe)

Left atrium

Phrenic nerve and pericardiacophrenic artery and vein

Coronary sinus

Branches of right main bronchus

Left lung (superior lobe)

Right inferior pulmonary vein

Branches of left main bronchus

Oblique pericardial sinus

Left inferior pulmonary vein

Esophagus and esophageal plexus

Thoracic (descending) aorta

8th rib

Azygos vein

Hemiazygos vein

Thoracic duct

Left sympathetic trunk

T8 vertebra

Left greater thoracic splanchnic nerve

f. Netter. m.d.

Plate 210

Heart

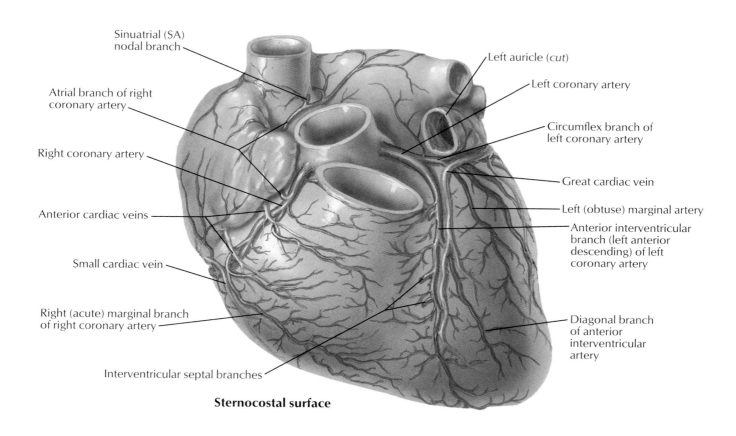

Sinuatrial (SA) nodal branch

Left auricle (*cut*)

Atrial branch of right coronary artery

Left coronary artery

Circumflex branch of left coronary artery

Right coronary artery

Great cardiac vein

Anterior cardiac veins

Left (obtuse) marginal artery

Small cardiac vein

Anterior interventricular branch (left anterior descending) of left coronary artery

Right (acute) marginal branch of right coronary artery

Diagonal branch of anterior interventricular artery

Interventricular septal branches

Sternocostal surface

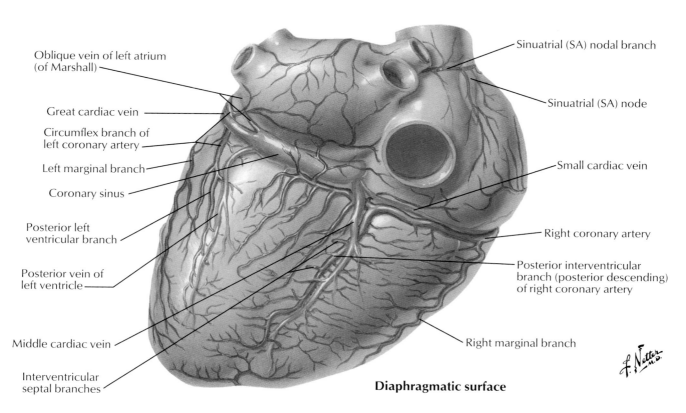

Oblique vein of left atrium (of Marshall)

Sinuatrial (SA) nodal branch

Great cardiac vein

Sinuatrial (SA) node

Circumflex branch of left coronary artery

Left marginal branch

Small cardiac vein

Coronary sinus

Posterior left ventricular branch

Right coronary artery

Posterior vein of left ventricle

Posterior interventricular branch (posterior descending) of right coronary artery

Middle cardiac vein

Interventricular septal branches

Right marginal branch

Diaphragmatic surface

f. Netter M.D.

Right coronary artery: left anterior oblique view

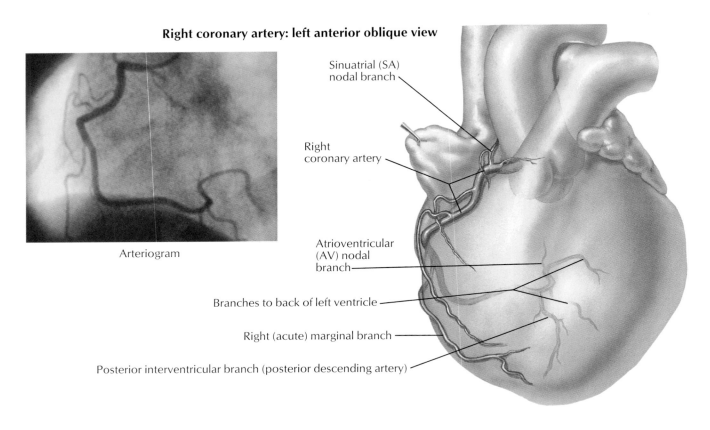

Arteriogram

Sinuatrial (SA) nodal branch

Right coronary artery

Atrioventricular (AV) nodal branch

Branches to back of left ventricle

Right (acute) marginal branch

Posterior interventricular branch (posterior descending artery)

Right coronary artery: right anterior oblique view

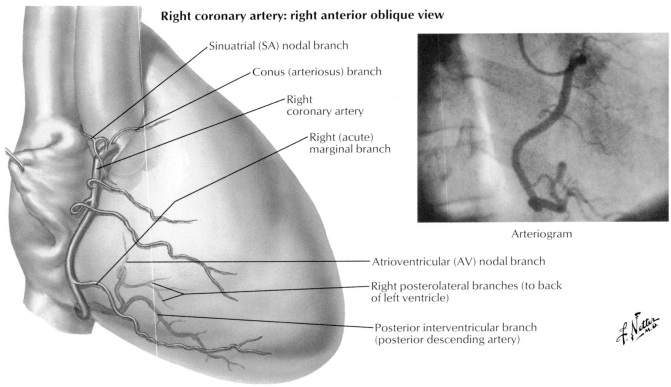

Sinuatrial (SA) nodal branch

Conus (arteriosus) branch

Right coronary artery

Right (acute) marginal branch

Arteriogram

Atrioventricular (AV) nodal branch

Right posterolateral branches (to back of left ventricle)

Posterior interventricular branch (posterior descending artery)

Plate 212   **Heart**

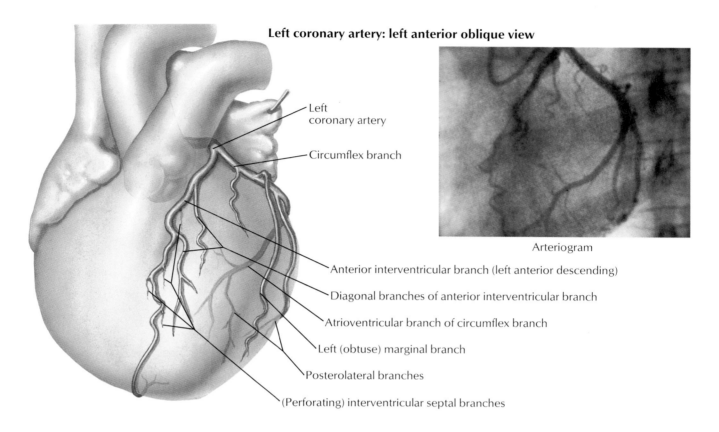

Left coronary artery: left anterior oblique view

Left coronary artery

Circumflex branch

Arteriogram

Anterior interventricular branch (left anterior descending)

Diagonal branches of anterior interventricular branch

Atrioventricular branch of circumflex branch

Left (obtuse) marginal branch

Posterolateral branches

(Perforating) interventricular septal branches

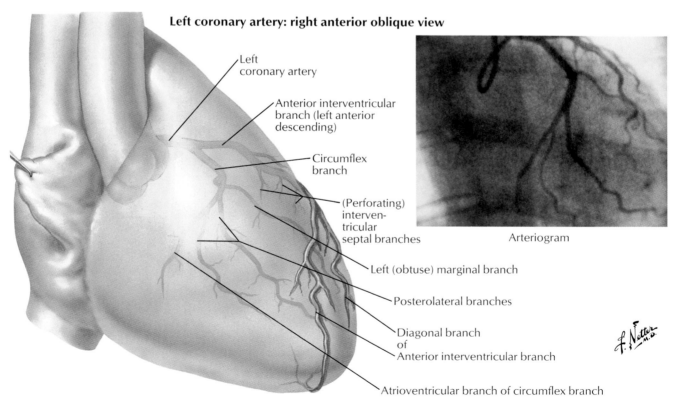

Left coronary artery: right anterior oblique view

Left coronary artery

Anterior interventricular branch (left anterior descending)

Circumflex branch

(Perforating) interventricular septal branches

Arteriogram

Left (obtuse) marginal branch

Posterolateral branches

Diagonal branch of Anterior interventricular branch

Atrioventricular branch of circumflex branch

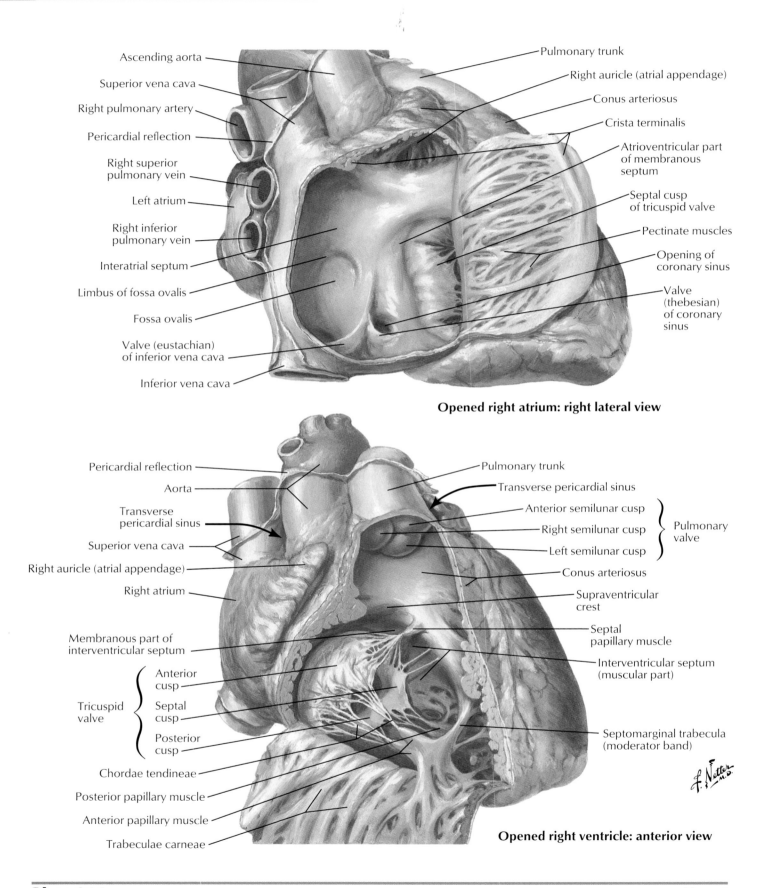

Ascending aorta

Superior vena cava

Right pulmonary artery

Pericardial reflection

Right superior pulmonary vein

Left atrium

Right inferior pulmonary vein

Interatrial septum

Limbus of fossa ovalis

Fossa ovalis

Valve (eustachian) of inferior vena cava

Inferior vena cava

Pulmonary trunk

Right auricle (atrial appendage)

Conus arteriosus

Crista terminalis

Atrioventricular part of membranous septum

Septal cusp of tricuspid valve

Pectinate muscles

Opening of coronary sinus

Valve (thebesian) of coronary sinus

Opened right atrium: right lateral view

Pericardial reflection

Aorta

Transverse pericardial sinus

Superior vena cava

Right auricle (atrial appendage)

Right atrium

Membranous part of interventricular septum

Anterior cusp

Tricuspid valve

Septal cusp

Posterior cusp

Chordae tendineae

Posterior papillary muscle

Anterior papillary muscle

Trabeculae carneae

Pulmonary trunk

Transverse pericardial sinus

Anterior semilunar cusp

Right semilunar cusp

Left semilunar cusp

Pulmonary valve

Conus arteriosus

Supraventricular crest

Septal papillary muscle

Interventricular septum (muscular part)

Septomarginal trabecula (moderator band)

Opened right ventricle: anterior view

Plate 214

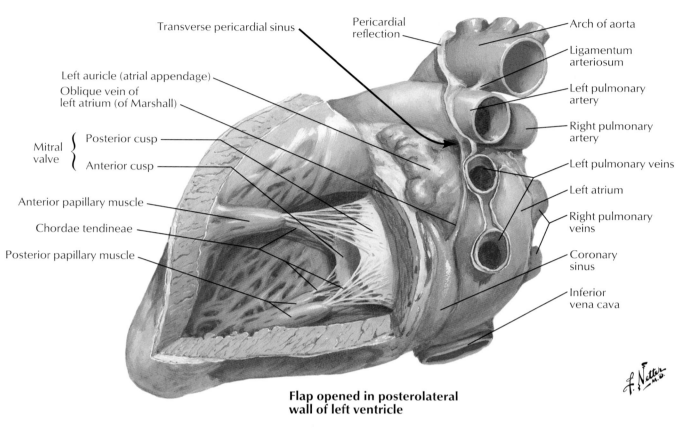

Transverse pericardial sinus

Pericardial reflection

Arch of aorta

Ligamentum arteriosum

Left auricle (atrial appendage)

Oblique vein of left atrium (of Marshall)

Left pulmonary artery

Right pulmonary artery

Mitral valve
{
Posterior cusp

Anterior cusp
}

Left pulmonary veins

Left atrium

Anterior papillary muscle

Right pulmonary veins

Chordae tendineae

Coronary sinus

Posterior papillary muscle

Inferior vena cava

Flap opened in posterolateral wall of left ventricle

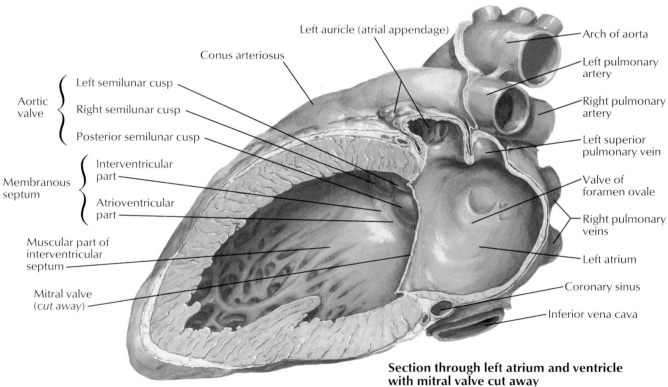

Left auricle (atrial appendage)

Conus arteriosus

Arch of aorta

Left pulmonary artery

Aortic valve
{
Left semilunar cusp

Right semilunar cusp

Posterior semilunar cusp
}

Right pulmonary artery

Membranous septum
{
Interventricular part

Atrioventricular part
}

Left superior pulmonary vein

Valve of foramen ovale

Muscular part of interventricular septum

Right pulmonary veins

Left atrium

Mitral valve (cut away)

Coronary sinus

Inferior vena cava

Section through left atrium and ventricle with mitral valve cut away

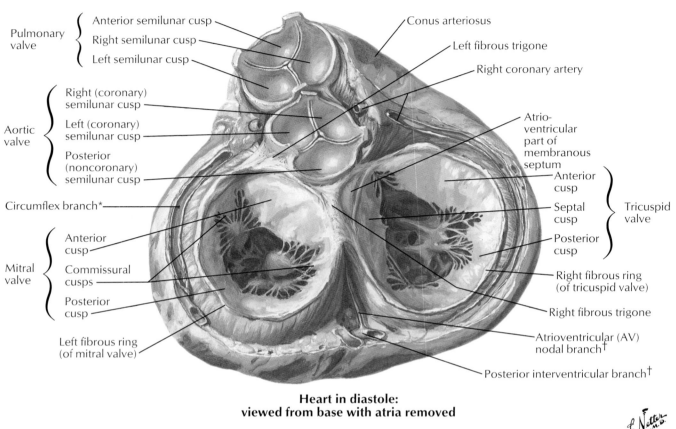

Pulmonary valve
- Anterior semilunar cusp
- Right semilunar cusp
- Left semilunar cusp

Aortic valve
- Right (coronary) semilunar cusp
- Left (coronary) semilunar cusp
- Posterior (noncoronary) semilunar cusp

Circumflex branch*

Mitral valve
- Anterior cusp
- Commissural cusps
- Posterior cusp

Left fibrous ring (of mitral valve)

Conus arteriosus

Left fibrous trigone

Right coronary artery

Atrio-ventricular part of membranous septum

Anterior cusp
Septal cusp
Posterior cusp
} Tricuspid valve

Right fibrous ring (of tricuspid valve)

Right fibrous trigone

Atrioventricular (AV) nodal branch†

Posterior interventricular branch†

Heart in diastole:
viewed from base with atria removed

f. Netter

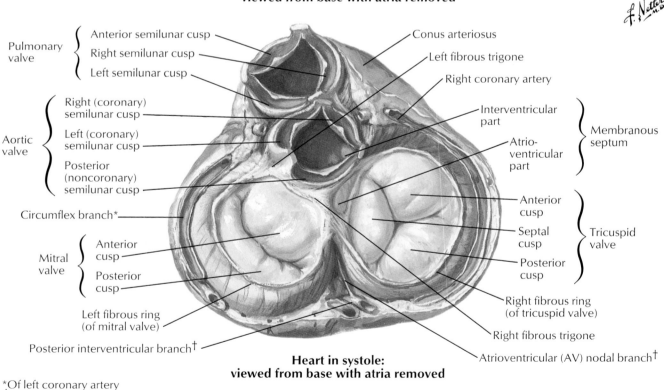

Pulmonary valve
- Anterior semilunar cusp
- Right semilunar cusp
- Left semilunar cusp

Aortic valve
- Right (coronary) semilunar cusp
- Left (coronary) semilunar cusp
- Posterior (noncoronary) semilunar cusp

Circumflex branch*

Mitral valve
- Anterior cusp
- Posterior cusp

Left fibrous ring (of mitral valve)

Posterior interventricular branch†

Conus arteriosus

Left fibrous trigone

Right coronary artery

Interventricular part
Atrio-ventricular part
} Membranous septum

Anterior cusp
Septal cusp
Posterior cusp
} Tricuspid valve

Right fibrous ring (of tricuspid valve)

Right fibrous trigone

Atrioventricular (AV) nodal branch†

Heart in systole:
viewed from base with atria removed

*Of left coronary artery
†Of right coronary artery

Plate 216   **Heart**

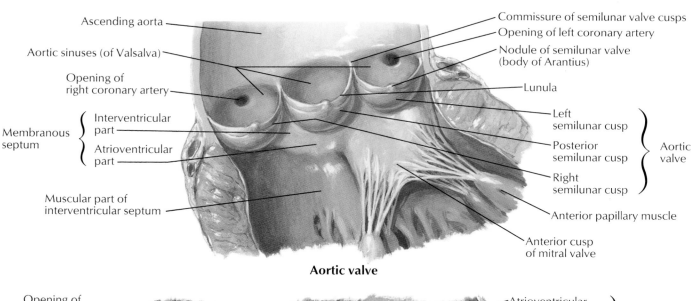

Ascending aorta

Aortic sinuses (of Valsalva)

Opening of right coronary artery

Membranous septum { Interventricular part / Atrioventricular part

Muscular part of interventricular septum

Commissure of semilunar valve cusps

Opening of left coronary artery

Nodule of semilunar valve (body of Arantius)

Lunula

Left semilunar cusp
Posterior semilunar cusp } Aortic valve
Right semilunar cusp

Anterior papillary muscle

Anterior cusp of mitral valve

Aortic valve

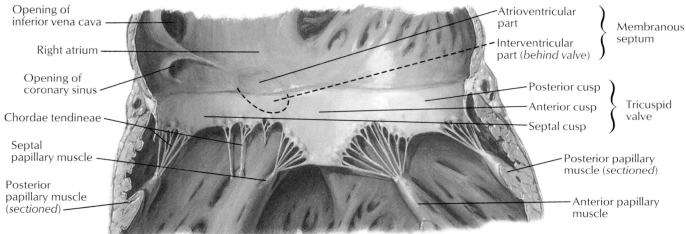

Opening of inferior vena cava

Right atrium

Opening of coronary sinus

Chordae tendineae

Septal papillary muscle

Posterior papillary muscle (*sectioned*)

Atrioventricular part } Membranous septum
Interventricular part (*behind valve*)

Posterior cusp
Anterior cusp } Tricuspid valve
Septal cusp

Posterior papillary muscle (*sectioned*)

Anterior papillary muscle

Tricuspid (right atrioventricular) valve

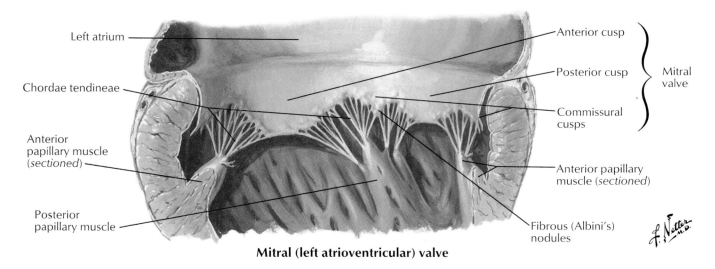

Left atrium

Chordae tendineae

Anterior papillary muscle (*sectioned*)

Posterior papillary muscle

Anterior cusp

Posterior cusp } Mitral valve

Commissural cusps

Anterior papillary muscle (*sectioned*)

Fibrous (Albini's) nodules

Mitral (left atrioventricular) valve

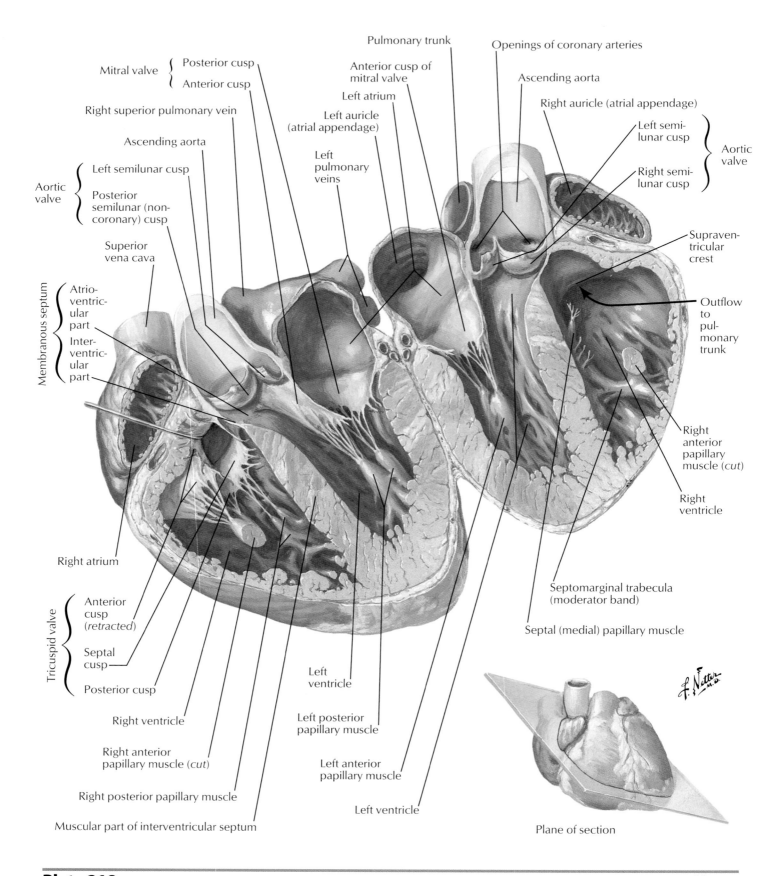

Mitral valve { Posterior cusp / Anterior cusp

Right superior pulmonary vein

Ascending aorta

Aortic valve { Left semilunar cusp / Posterior semilunar (non-coronary) cusp

Superior vena cava

Membranous septum { Atrio-ventric-ular part / Inter-ventric-ular part

Right atrium

Tricuspid valve { Anterior cusp (*retracted*) / Septal cusp / Posterior cusp

Right ventricle

Right anterior papillary muscle (*cut*)

Right posterior papillary muscle

Muscular part of interventricular septum

Pulmonary trunk

Anterior cusp of mitral valve

Left atrium

Left auricle (atrial appendage)

Left pulmonary veins

Openings of coronary arteries

Ascending aorta

Right auricle (atrial appendage)

Left semi-lunar cusp

Right semi-lunar cusp

} Aortic valve

Supraventricular crest

Outflow to pulmonary trunk

Right anterior papillary muscle (*cut*)

Right ventricle

Septomarginal trabecula (moderator band)

Septal (medial) papillary muscle

Left ventricle

Left posterior papillary muscle

Left anterior papillary muscle

Left ventricle

Plane of section

Plate 218   **Heart**

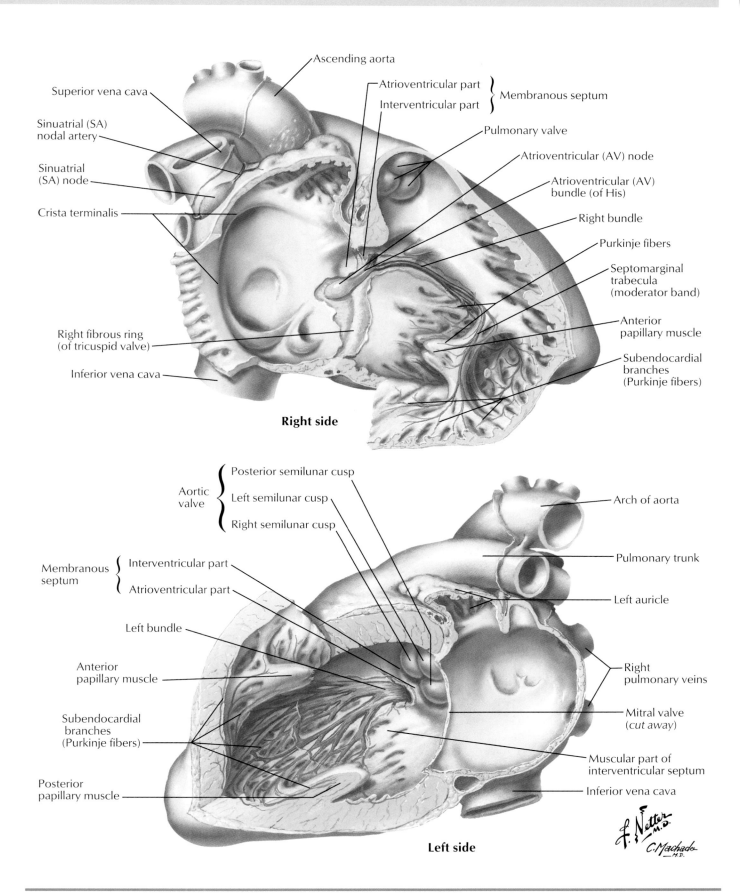

Ascending aorta

Superior vena cava

Sinuatrial (SA) nodal artery

Sinuatrial (SA) node

Crista terminalis

Atrioventricular part
Interventricular part } Membranous septum

Pulmonary valve

Atrioventricular (AV) node

Atrioventricular (AV) bundle (of His)

Right bundle

Purkinje fibers

Septomarginal trabecula (moderator band)

Right fibrous ring (of tricuspid valve)

Inferior vena cava

Anterior papillary muscle

Subendocardial branches (Purkinje fibers)

Right side

Posterior semilunar cusp

Aortic valve { Left semilunar cusp

Right semilunar cusp

Arch of aorta

Pulmonary trunk

Membranous septum { Interventricular part

Atrioventricular part

Left auricle

Left bundle

Anterior papillary muscle

Right pulmonary veins

Subendocardial branches (Purkinje fibers)

Mitral valve (cut away)

Muscular part of interventricular septum

Posterior papillary muscle

Inferior vena cava

Left side

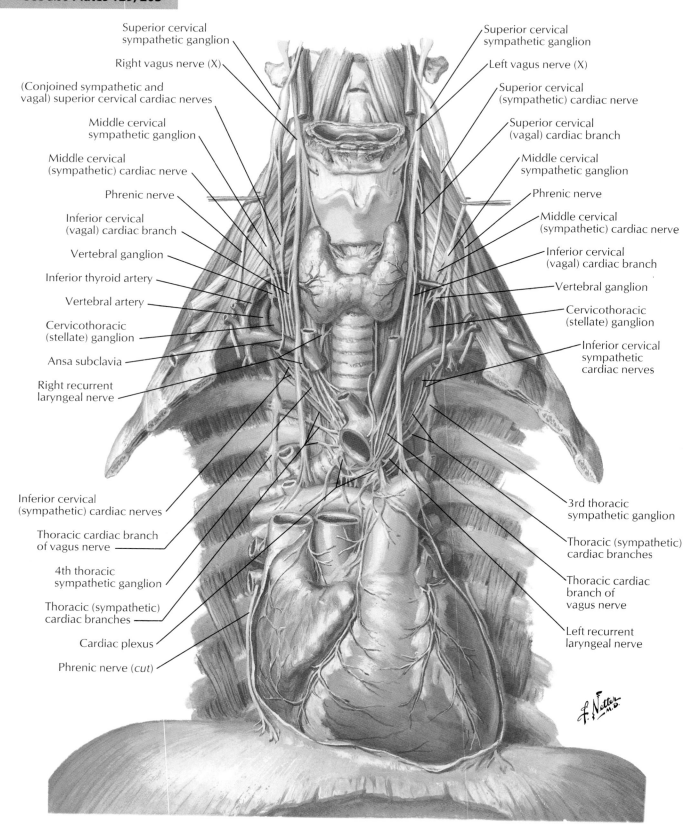

Superior cervical sympathetic ganglion

Right vagus nerve (X)

(Conjoined sympathetic and vagal) superior cervical cardiac nerves

Middle cervical sympathetic ganglion

Middle cervical (sympathetic) cardiac nerve

Phrenic nerve

Inferior cervical (vagal) cardiac branch

Vertebral ganglion

Inferior thyroid artery

Vertebral artery

Cervicothoracic (stellate) ganglion

Ansa subclavia

Right recurrent laryngeal nerve

Inferior cervical (sympathetic) cardiac nerves

Thoracic cardiac branch of vagus nerve

4th thoracic sympathetic ganglion

Thoracic (sympathetic) cardiac branches

Cardiac plexus

Phrenic nerve (cut)

Superior cervical sympathetic ganglion

Left vagus nerve (X)

Superior cervical (sympathetic) cardiac nerve

Superior cervical (vagal) cardiac branch

Middle cervical sympathetic ganglion

Phrenic nerve

Middle cervical (sympathetic) cardiac nerve

Inferior cervical (vagal) cardiac branch

Vertebral ganglion

Cervicothoracic (stellate) ganglion

Inferior cervical sympathetic cardiac nerves

3rd thoracic sympathetic ganglion

Thoracic (sympathetic) cardiac branches

Thoracic cardiac branch of vagus nerve

Left recurrent laryngeal nerve

Plate 220

Heart

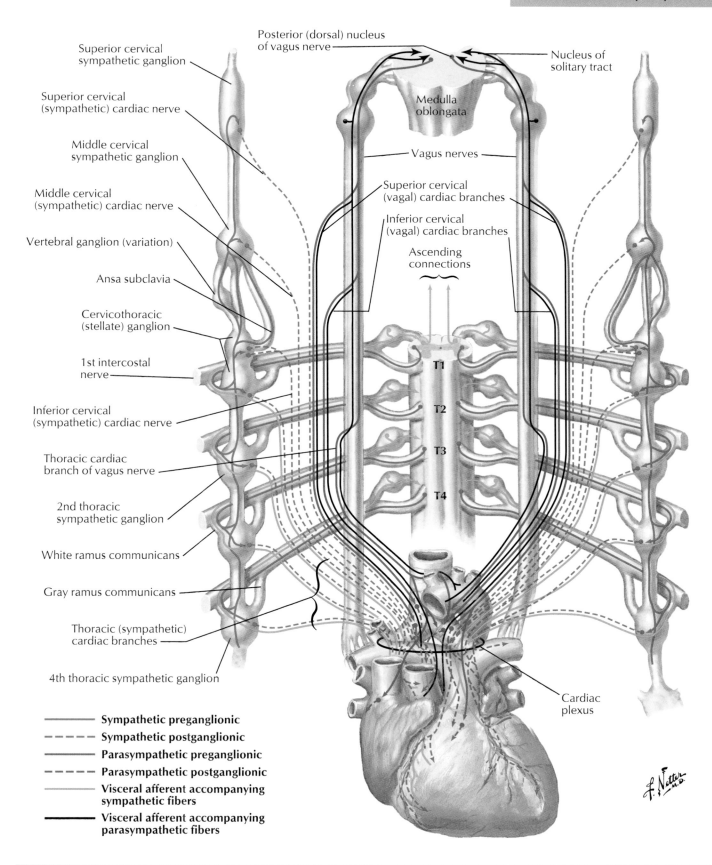

Superior cervical sympathetic ganglion

Superior cervical (sympathetic) cardiac nerve

Middle cervical sympathetic ganglion

Middle cervical (sympathetic) cardiac nerve

Vertebral ganglion (variation)

Ansa subclavia

Cervicothoracic (stellate) ganglion

1st intercostal nerve

Inferior cervical (sympathetic) cardiac nerve

Thoracic cardiac branch of vagus nerve

2nd thoracic sympathetic ganglion

White ramus communicans

Gray ramus communicans

Thoracic (sympathetic) cardiac branches

4th thoracic sympathetic ganglion

Posterior (dorsal) nucleus of vagus nerve

Nucleus of solitary tract

Medulla oblongata

Vagus nerves

Superior cervical (vagal) cardiac branches

Inferior cervical (vagal) cardiac branches

Ascending connections

T1
T2
T3
T4

Cardiac plexus

—————— **Sympathetic preganglionic**

- - - - - **Sympathetic postganglionic**

—————— **Parasympathetic preganglionic**

- - - - - **Parasympathetic postganglionic**

—————— **Visceral afferent accompanying sympathetic fibers**

—————— **Visceral afferent accompanying parasympathetic fibers**

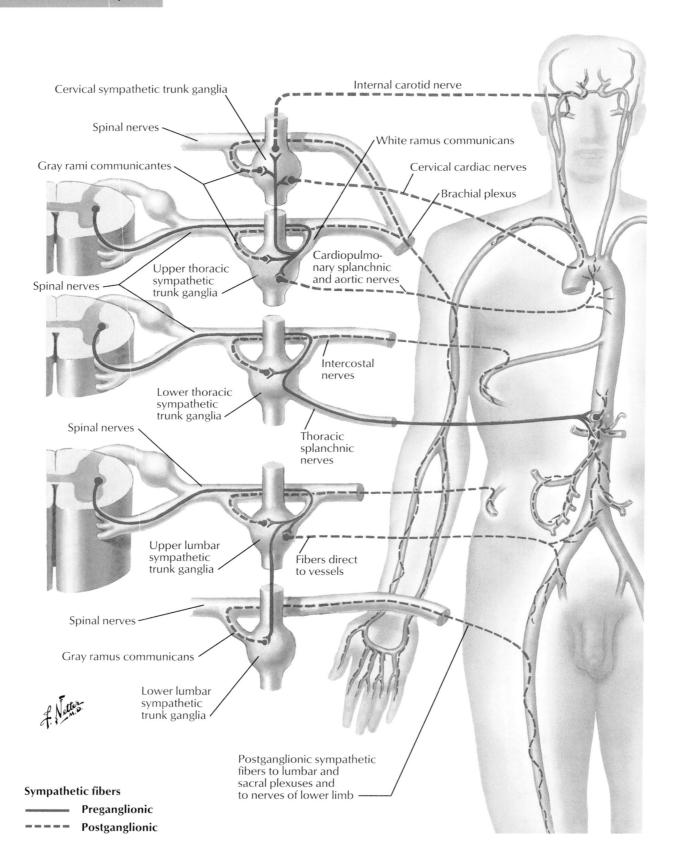

Cervical sympathetic trunk ganglia

Spinal nerves

Gray rami communicantes

Spinal nerves

Upper thoracic sympathetic trunk ganglia

Internal carotid nerve

White ramus communicans

Cervical cardiac nerves

Brachial plexus

Cardiopulmonary splanchnic and aortic nerves

Intercostal nerves

Lower thoracic sympathetic trunk ganglia

Thoracic splanchnic nerves

Spinal nerves

Upper lumbar sympathetic trunk ganglia

Fibers direct to vessels

Spinal nerves

Gray ramus communicans

Lower lumbar sympathetic trunk ganglia

Postganglionic sympathetic fibers to lumbar and sacral plexuses and to nerves of lower limb

Sympathetic fibers

———— Preganglionic

- - - - - Postganglionic

Plate 222

Heart

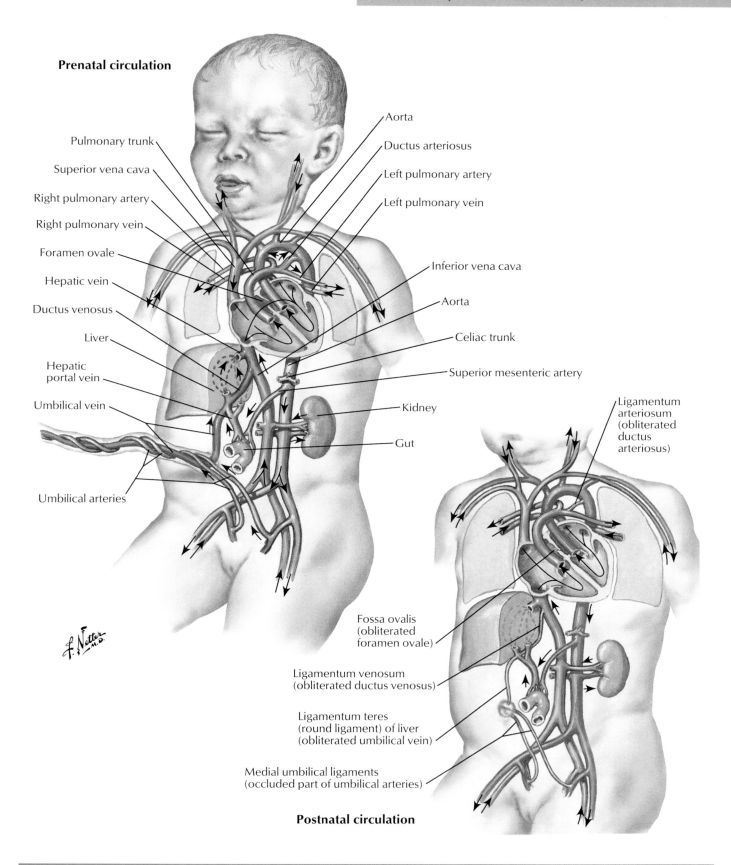

Prenatal circulation

Pulmonary trunk

Superior vena cava

Right pulmonary artery

Right pulmonary vein

Foramen ovale

Hepatic vein

Ductus venosus

Liver

Hepatic portal vein

Umbilical vein

Umbilical arteries

Aorta

Ductus arteriosus

Left pulmonary artery

Left pulmonary vein

Inferior vena cava

Aorta

Celiac trunk

Superior mesenteric artery

Kidney

Gut

Ligamentum arteriosum (obliterated ductus arteriosus)

Fossa ovalis (obliterated foramen ovale)

Ligamentum venosum (obliterated ductus venosus)

Ligamentum teres (round ligament) of liver (obliterated umbilical vein)

Medial umbilical ligaments (occluded part of umbilical arteries)

Postnatal circulation

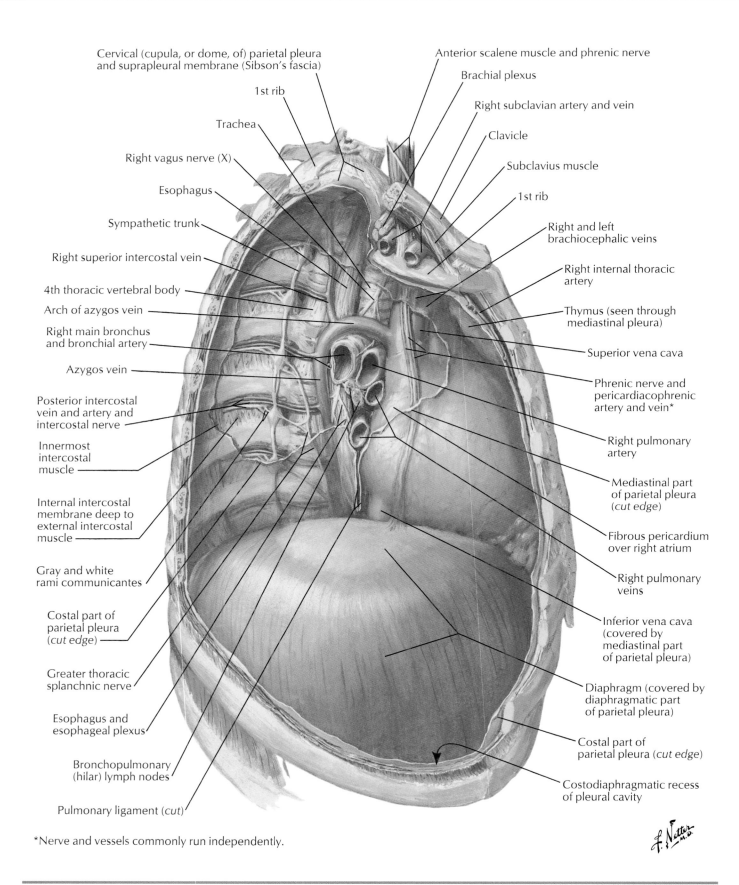

Cervical (cupula, or dome, of) parietal pleura and suprapleural membrane (Sibson's fascia)

1st rib

Trachea

Right vagus nerve (X)

Esophagus

Sympathetic trunk

Right superior intercostal vein

4th thoracic vertebral body

Arch of azygos vein

Right main bronchus and bronchial artery

Azygos vein

Posterior intercostal vein and artery and intercostal nerve

Innermost intercostal muscle

Internal intercostal membrane deep to external intercostal muscle

Gray and white rami communicantes

Costal part of parietal pleura (cut edge)

Greater thoracic splanchnic nerve

Esophagus and esophageal plexus

Bronchopulmonary (hilar) lymph nodes

Pulmonary ligament (cut)

Anterior scalene muscle and phrenic nerve

Brachial plexus

Right subclavian artery and vein

Clavicle

Subclavius muscle

1st rib

Right and left brachiocephalic veins

Right internal thoracic artery

Thymus (seen through mediastinal pleura)

Superior vena cava

Phrenic nerve and pericardiacophrenic artery and vein*

Right pulmonary artery

Mediastinal part of parietal pleura (cut edge)

Fibrous pericardium over right atrium

Right pulmonary veins

Inferior vena cava (covered by mediastinal part of parietal pleura)

Diaphragm (covered by diaphragmatic part of parietal pleura)

Costal part of parietal pleura (cut edge)

Costodiaphragmatic recess of pleural cavity

*Nerve and vessels commonly run independently.

Plate 224

Mediastinum

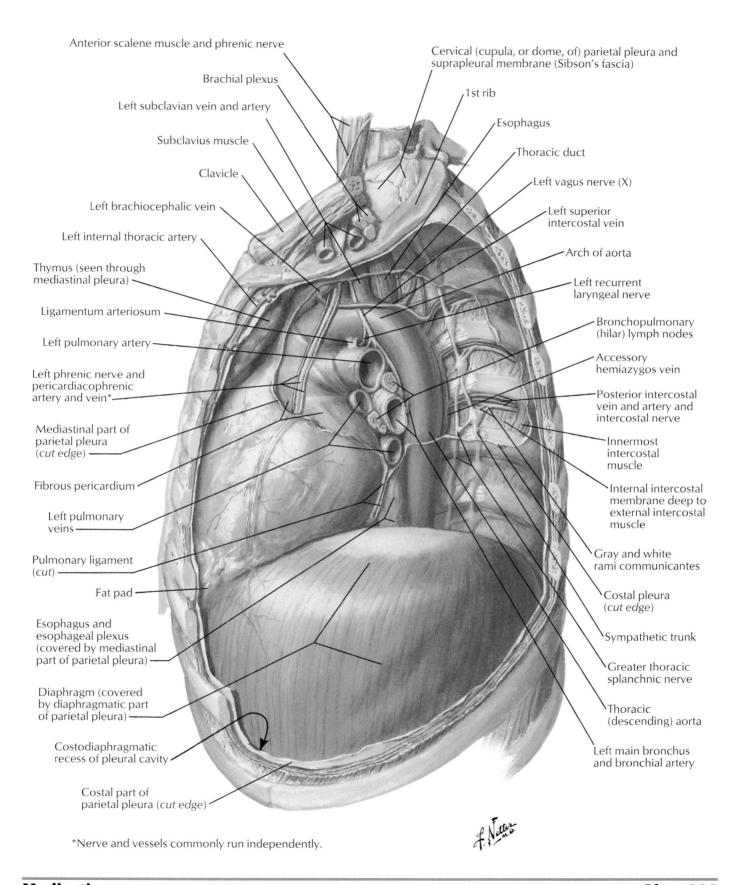

Anterior scalene muscle and phrenic nerve

Brachial plexus

Left subclavian vein and artery

Subclavius muscle

Clavicle

Left brachiocephalic vein

Left internal thoracic artery

Thymus (seen through mediastinal pleura)

Ligamentum arteriosum

Left pulmonary artery

Left phrenic nerve and pericardiacophrenic artery and vein*

Mediastinal part of parietal pleura (*cut edge*)

Fibrous pericardium

Left pulmonary veins

Pulmonary ligament (*cut*)

Fat pad

Esophagus and esophageal plexus (covered by mediastinal part of parietal pleura)

Diaphragm (covered by diaphragmatic part of parietal pleura)

Costodiaphragmatic recess of pleural cavity

Costal part of parietal pleura (*cut edge*)

Cervical (cupula, or dome, of) parietal pleura and suprapleural membrane (Sibson's fascia)

1st rib

Esophagus

Thoracic duct

Left vagus nerve (X)

Left superior intercostal vein

Arch of aorta

Left recurrent laryngeal nerve

Bronchopulmonary (hilar) lymph nodes

Accessory hemiazygos vein

Posterior intercostal vein and artery and intercostal nerve

Innermost intercostal muscle

Internal intercostal membrane deep to external intercostal muscle

Gray and white rami communicantes

Costal pleura (*cut edge*)

Sympathetic trunk

Greater thoracic splanchnic nerve

Thoracic (descending) aorta

Left main bronchus and bronchial artery

*Nerve and vessels commonly run independently.

Mediastinum

Plate 225

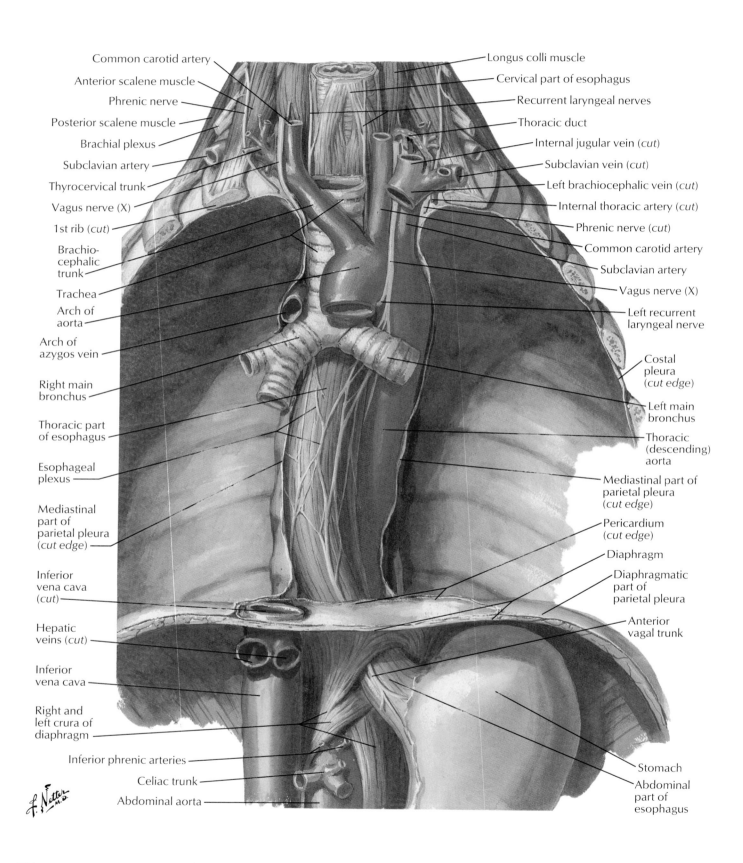

Common carotid artery

Anterior scalene muscle

Phrenic nerve

Posterior scalene muscle

Brachial plexus

Subclavian artery

Thyrocervical trunk

Vagus nerve (X)

1st rib (cut)

Brachio-cephalic trunk

Trachea

Arch of aorta

Arch of azygos vein

Right main bronchus

Thoracic part of esophagus

Esophageal plexus

Mediastinal part of parietal pleura (cut edge)

Inferior vena cava (cut)

Hepatic veins (cut)

Inferior vena cava

Right and left crura of diaphragm

Inferior phrenic arteries

Celiac trunk

Abdominal aorta

Longus colli muscle

Cervical part of esophagus

Recurrent laryngeal nerves

Thoracic duct

Internal jugular vein (cut)

Subclavian vein (cut)

Left brachiocephalic vein (cut)

Internal thoracic artery (cut)

Phrenic nerve (cut)

Common carotid artery

Subclavian artery

Vagus nerve (X)

Left recurrent laryngeal nerve

Costal pleura (cut edge)

Left main bronchus

Thoracic (descending) aorta

Mediastinal part of parietal pleura (cut edge)

Pericardium (cut edge)

Diaphragm

Diaphragmatic part of parietal pleura

Anterior vagal trunk

Stomach

Abdominal part of esophagus

Plate 226   **Mediastinum**

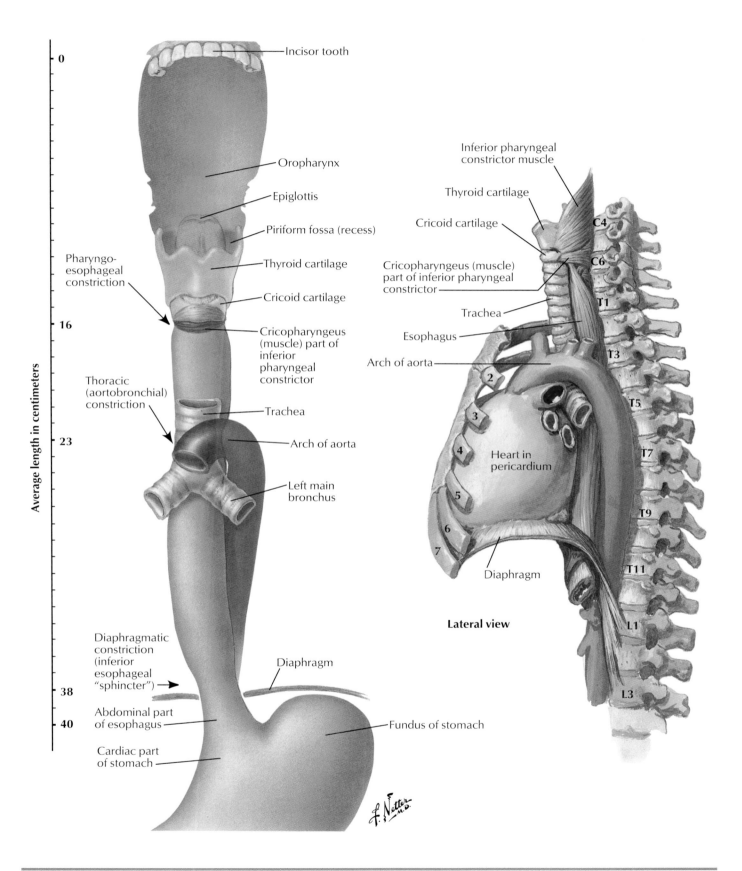

Incisor tooth

Oropharynx

Epiglottis

Piriform fossa (recess)

Pharyngo-esophageal constriction

Thyroid cartilage

Cricoid cartilage

Cricopharyngeus (muscle) part of inferior pharyngeal constrictor

Thoracic (aortobronchial) constriction

Trachea

Arch of aorta

Left main bronchus

0

Average length in centimeters

16

23

38

40

Diaphragmatic constriction (inferior esophageal "sphincter")

Diaphragm

Abdominal part of esophagus

Fundus of stomach

Cardiac part of stomach

Inferior pharyngeal constrictor muscle

Thyroid cartilage

Cricoid cartilage

Cricopharyngeus (muscle) part of inferior pharyngeal constrictor

Trachea

Esophagus

Arch of aorta

C4

C6

T1

T3

T5

T7

T9

T11

L1

L3

2

3

4

5

6

7

Heart in pericardium

Diaphragm

Lateral view

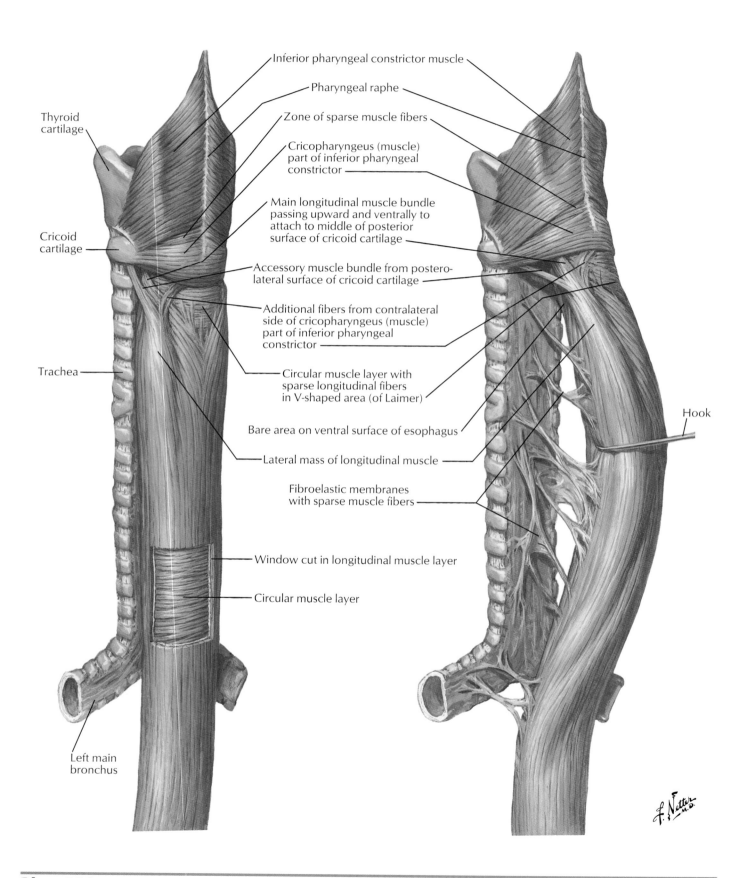

Inferior pharyngeal constrictor muscle

Pharyngeal raphe

Zone of sparse muscle fibers

Cricopharyngeus (muscle) part of inferior pharyngeal constrictor

Main longitudinal muscle bundle passing upward and ventrally to attach to middle of posterior surface of cricoid cartilage

Accessory muscle bundle from postero-lateral surface of cricoid cartilage

Additional fibers from contralateral side of cricopharyngeus (muscle) part of inferior pharyngeal constrictor

Circular muscle layer with sparse longitudinal fibers in V-shaped area (of Laimer)

Bare area on ventral surface of esophagus

Lateral mass of longitudinal muscle

Fibroelastic membranes with sparse muscle fibers

Window cut in longitudinal muscle layer

Circular muscle layer

Thyroid cartilage

Cricoid cartilage

Trachea

Left main bronchus

Hook

Plate 228

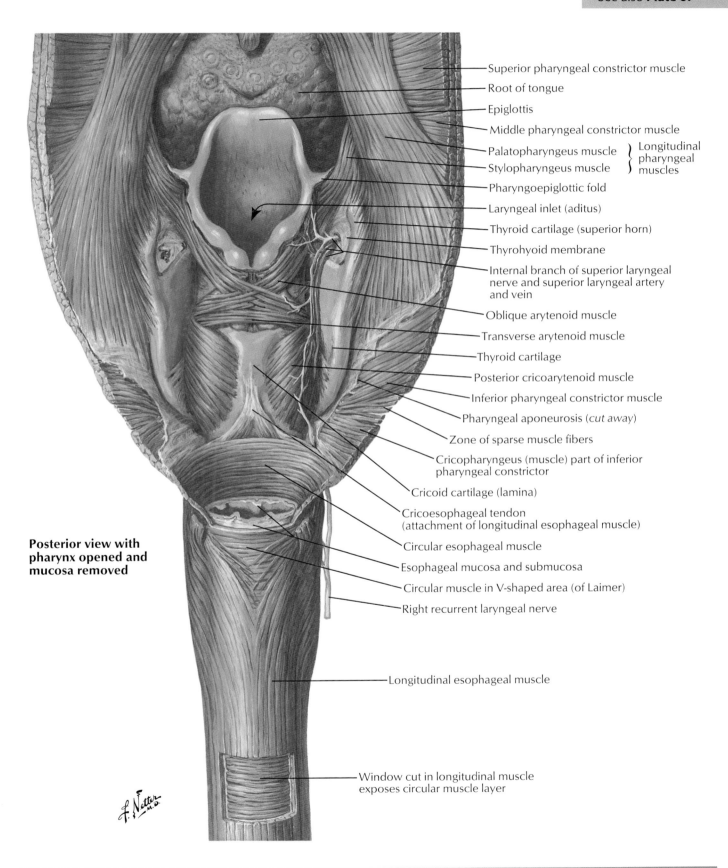

Superior pharyngeal constrictor muscle

Root of tongue

Epiglottis

Middle pharyngeal constrictor muscle

Palatopharyngeus muscle } Longitudinal pharyngeal muscles

Stylopharyngeus muscle

Pharyngoepiglottic fold

Laryngeal inlet (aditus)

Thyroid cartilage (superior horn)

Thyrohyoid membrane

Internal branch of superior laryngeal nerve and superior laryngeal artery and vein

Oblique arytenoid muscle

Transverse arytenoid muscle

Thyroid cartilage

Posterior cricoarytenoid muscle

Inferior pharyngeal constrictor muscle

Pharyngeal aponeurosis (*cut away*)

Zone of sparse muscle fibers

Cricopharyngeus (muscle) part of inferior pharyngeal constrictor

Cricoid cartilage (lamina)

Cricoesophageal tendon (attachment of longitudinal esophageal muscle)

Circular esophageal muscle

Esophageal mucosa and submucosa

Circular muscle in V-shaped area (of Laimer)

Right recurrent laryngeal nerve

Longitudinal esophageal muscle

Window cut in longitudinal muscle exposes circular muscle layer

Posterior view with pharynx opened and mucosa removed

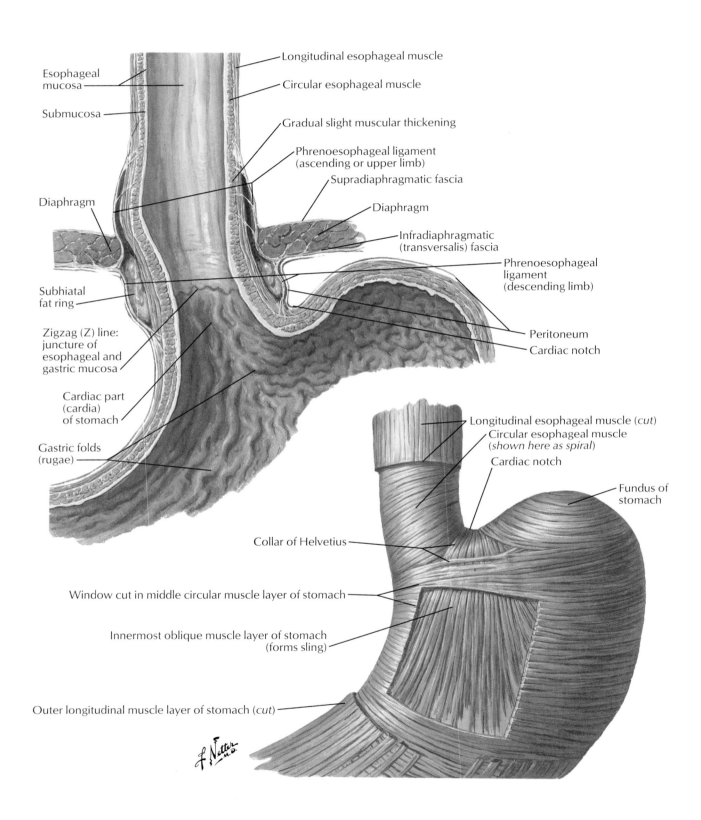

Longitudinal esophageal muscle

Circular esophageal muscle

Esophageal mucosa

Gradual slight muscular thickening

Submucosa

Phrenoesophageal ligament (ascending or upper limb)

Supradiaphragmatic fascia

Diaphragm

Diaphragm

Infradiaphragmatic (transversalis) fascia

Phrenoesophageal ligament (descending limb)

Subhiatal fat ring

Peritoneum

Cardiac notch

Zigzag (Z) line: juncture of esophageal and gastric mucosa

Cardiac part (cardia) of stomach

Gastric folds (rugae)

Longitudinal esophageal muscle (*cut*)

Circular esophageal muscle (*shown here as spiral*)

Cardiac notch

Fundus of stomach

Collar of Helvetius

Window cut in middle circular muscle layer of stomach

Innermost oblique muscle layer of stomach (forms sling)

Outer longitudinal muscle layer of stomach (*cut*)

Plate 230 **Mediastinum**

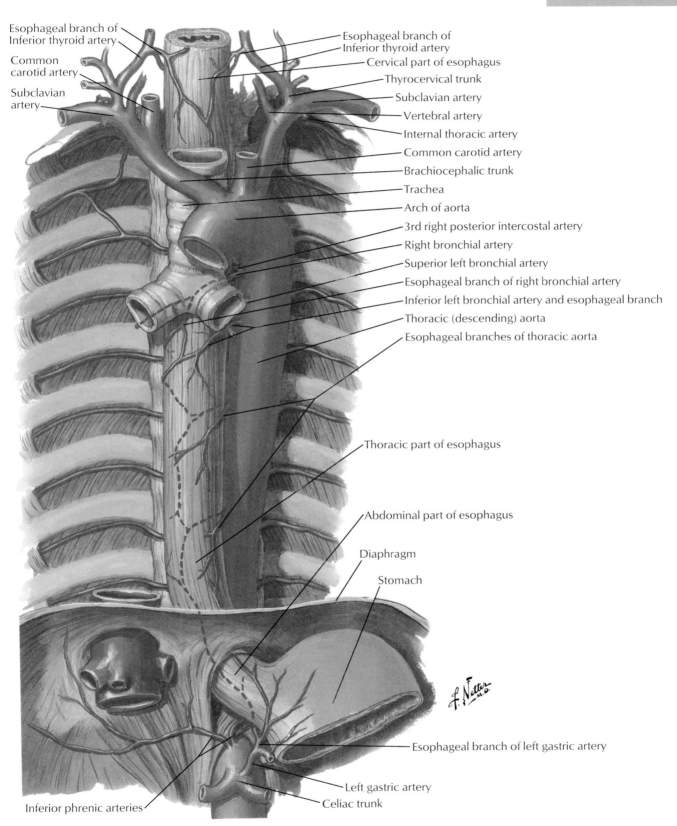

Esophageal branch of Inferior thyroid artery

Common carotid artery

Subclavian artery

Esophageal branch of Inferior thyroid artery

Cervical part of esophagus

Thyrocervical trunk

Subclavian artery

Vertebral artery

Internal thoracic artery

Common carotid artery

Brachiocephalic trunk

Trachea

Arch of aorta

3rd right posterior intercostal artery

Right bronchial artery

Superior left bronchial artery

Esophageal branch of right bronchial artery

Inferior left bronchial artery and esophageal branch

Thoracic (descending) aorta

Esophageal branches of thoracic aorta

Thoracic part of esophagus

Abdominal part of esophagus

Diaphragm

Stomach

Esophageal branch of left gastric artery

Left gastric artery

Celiac trunk

Inferior phrenic arteries

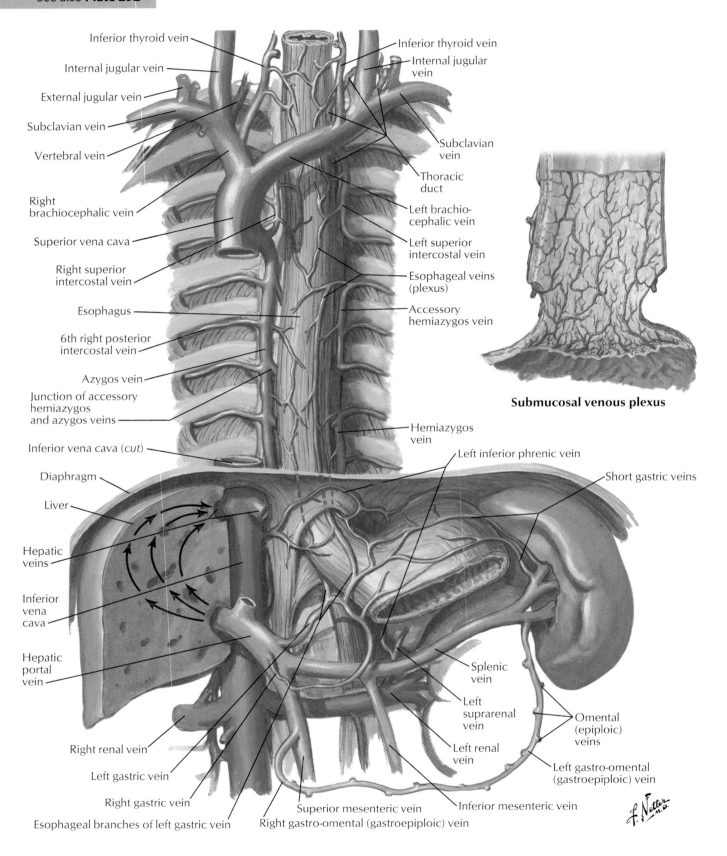

Inferior thyroid vein

Internal jugular vein

External jugular vein

Subclavian vein

Vertebral vein

Right brachiocephalic vein

Superior vena cava

Right superior intercostal vein

Esophagus

6th right posterior intercostal vein

Azygos vein

Junction of accessory hemiazygos and azygos veins

Inferior vena cava (*cut*)

Diaphragm

Liver

Hepatic veins

Inferior vena cava

Hepatic portal vein

Right renal vein

Left gastric vein

Right gastric vein

Esophageal branches of left gastric vein

Inferior thyroid vein

Internal jugular vein

Subclavian vein

Thoracic duct

Left brachio-cephalic vein

Left superior intercostal vein

Esophageal veins (plexus)

Accessory hemiazygos vein

Hemiazygos vein

Left inferior phrenic vein

Short gastric veins

Splenic vein

Left suprarenal vein

Left renal vein

Omental (epiploic) veins

Left gastro-omental (gastroepiploic) vein

Superior mesenteric vein

Right gastro-omental (gastroepiploic) vein

Inferior mesenteric vein

Submucosal venous plexus

Plate 232   **Mediastinum**

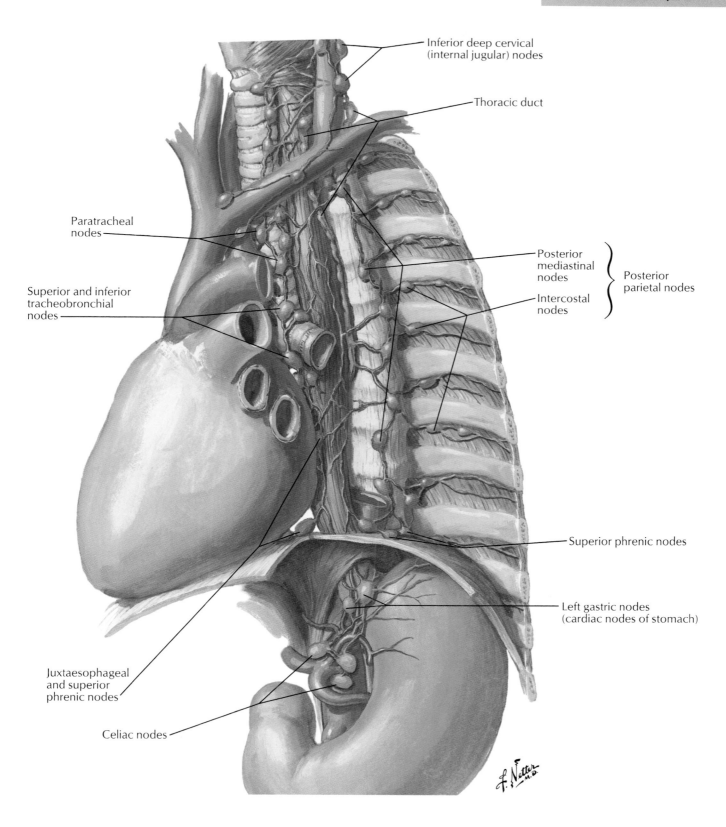

Inferior deep cervical (internal jugular) nodes

Thoracic duct

Paratracheal nodes

Superior and inferior tracheobronchial nodes

Posterior mediastinal nodes

Intercostal nodes

Posterior parietal nodes

Superior phrenic nodes

Left gastric nodes (cardiac nodes of stomach)

Juxtaesophageal and superior phrenic nodes

Celiac nodes

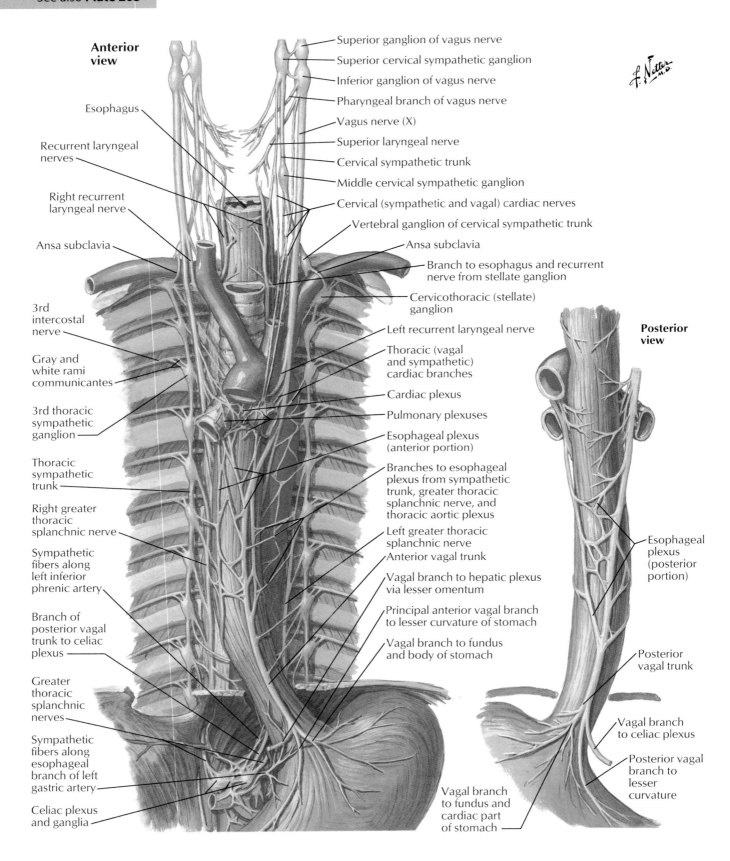

Anterior view

Superior ganglion of vagus nerve

Superior cervical sympathetic ganglion

Inferior ganglion of vagus nerve

Pharyngeal branch of vagus nerve

Esophagus

Vagus nerve (X)

Recurrent laryngeal nerves

Superior laryngeal nerve

Cervical sympathetic trunk

Middle cervical sympathetic ganglion

Right recurrent laryngeal nerve

Cervical (sympathetic and vagal) cardiac nerves

Vertebral ganglion of cervical sympathetic trunk

Ansa subclavia

Ansa subclavia

Branch to esophagus and recurrent nerve from stellate ganglion

Cervicothoracic (stellate) ganglion

3rd intercostal nerve

Left recurrent laryngeal nerve

Posterior view

Gray and white rami communicantes

Thoracic (vagal and sympathetic) cardiac branches

Cardiac plexus

3rd thoracic sympathetic ganglion

Pulmonary plexuses

Esophageal plexus (anterior portion)

Thoracic sympathetic trunk

Branches to esophageal plexus from sympathetic trunk, greater thoracic splanchnic nerve, and thoracic aortic plexus

Right greater thoracic splanchnic nerve

Left greater thoracic splanchnic nerve

Sympathetic fibers along left inferior phrenic artery

Anterior vagal trunk

Vagal branch to hepatic plexus via lesser omentum

Esophageal plexus (posterior portion)

Branch of posterior vagal trunk to celiac plexus

Principal anterior vagal branch to lesser curvature of stomach

Greater thoracic splanchnic nerves

Vagal branch to fundus and body of stomach

Posterior vagal trunk

Sympathetic fibers along esophageal branch of left gastric artery

Vagal branch to celiac plexus

Posterior vagal branch to lesser curvature

Celiac plexus and ganglia

Vagal branch to fundus and cardiac part of stomach

Plate 234

Mediastinum

Series of chest axial CT images from superior (A) to inferior (C)

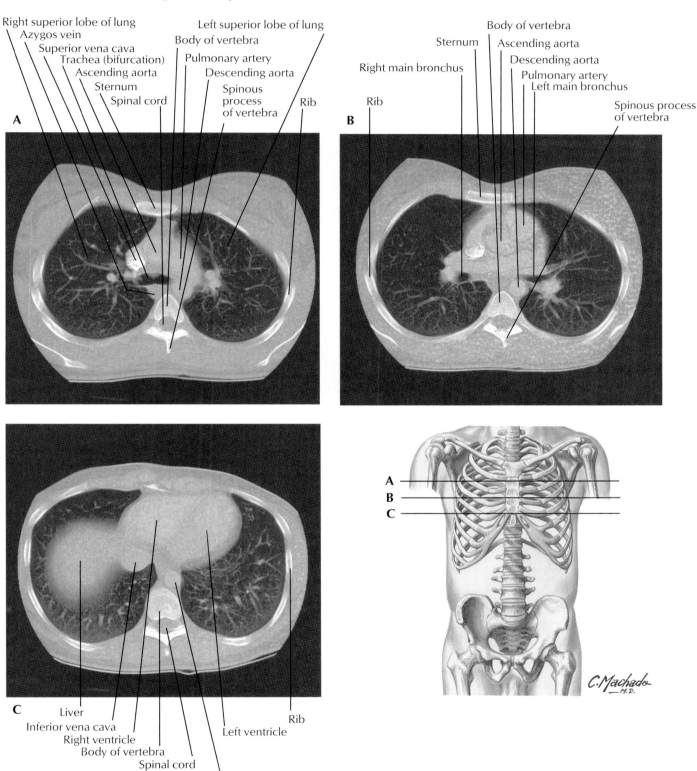

Right superior lobe of lung
Azygos vein
Superior vena cava
Trachea (bifurcation)
Ascending aorta
Sternum
Spinal cord

Left superior lobe of lung
Body of vertebra
Pulmonary artery
Descending aorta
Spinous process of vertebra
Rib

A

Body of vertebra
Sternum
Ascending aorta
Right main bronchus
Descending aorta
Pulmonary artery
Left main bronchus
Rib
Spinous process of vertebra

B

C
Liver
Inferior vena cava
Right ventricle
Body of vertebra
Spinal cord
Descending aorta
Left ventricle
Rib

A
B
C

C. Machado
M.D.

Transverse Section: Lower Level of T3, Sternoclavicular Joint

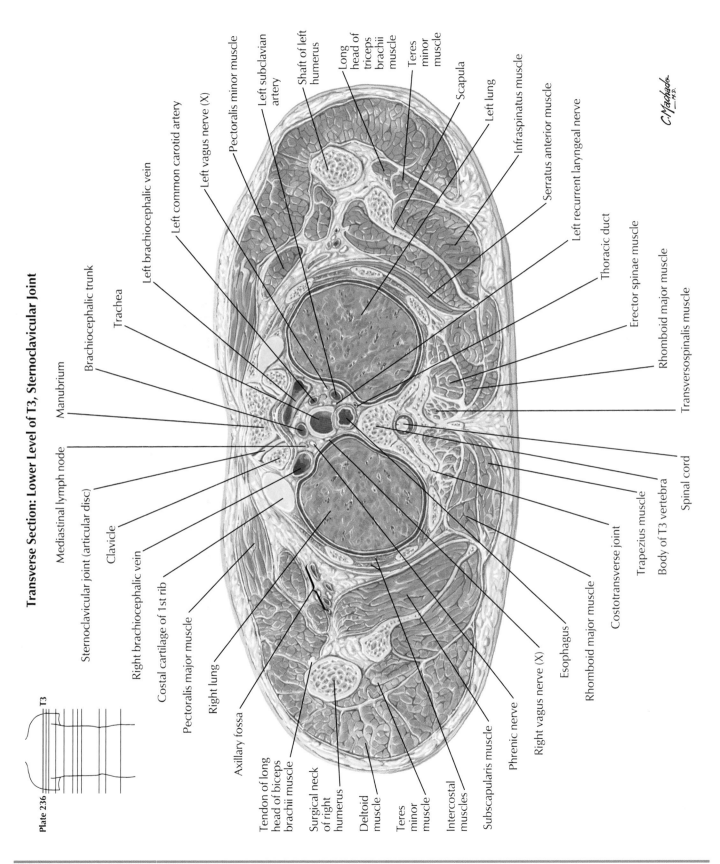

Mediastinal lymph node

Manubrium

Brachiocephalic trunk

Trachea

Left brachiocephalic vein

Left common carotid artery

Left vagus nerve (X)

Pectoralis minor muscle

Left subclavian artery

Shaft of left humerus

Long head of triceps brachii muscle

Teres minor muscle

Scapula

Left lung

Infraspinatus muscle

Serratus anterior muscle

Left recurrent laryngeal nerve

Thoracic duct

Erector spinae muscle

Rhomboid major muscle

Transversospinalis muscle

Sternoclavicular joint (articular disc)

Clavicle

Right brachiocephalic vein

Costal cartilage of 1st rib

Pectoralis major muscle

Right lung

Axillary fossa

Tendon of long head of biceps brachii muscle

Surgical neck of right humerus

Deltoid muscle

Teres minor muscle

Intercostal muscles

Subscapularis muscle

Phrenic nerve

Right vagus nerve (X)

Esophagus

Rhomboid major muscle

Costotransverse joint

Trapezius muscle

Body of T3 vertebra

Spinal cord

Plate 236

Plate 236

Cross-sectional Anatomy

Transverse Section: T3–4 Intervertebral Disc, Manubrium

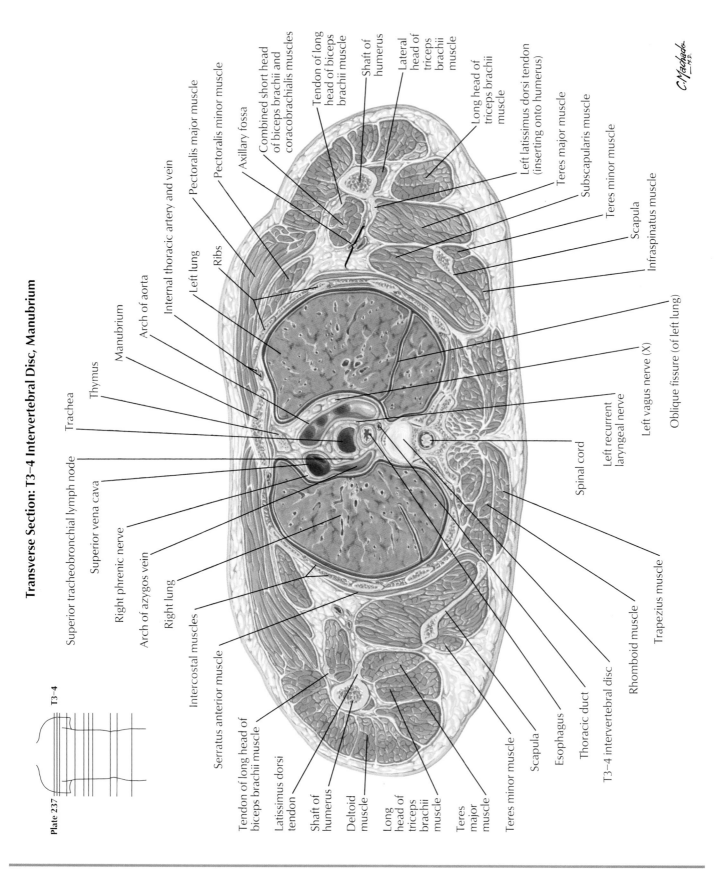

Pectoralis minor muscle

Pectoralis major muscle

Axillary fossa

Combined short head of biceps brachii and coracobrachialis muscles

Tendon of long head of biceps brachii muscle

Shaft of humerus

Lateral head of triceps brachii muscle

Long head of triceps brachii muscle

Left latissimus dorsi tendon (inserting onto humerus)

Teres major muscle

Subscapularis muscle

Teres minor muscle

Scapula

Infraspinatus muscle

Internal thoracic artery and vein

Left lung

Ribs

Arch of aorta

Manubrium

Thymus

Trachea

Superior tracheobronchial lymph node

Superior vena cava

Right phrenic nerve

Arch of azygos vein

Right lung

Intercostal muscles

Serratus anterior muscle

Tendon of long head of biceps brachii muscle

Latissimus dorsi tendon

Shaft of humerus

Deltoid muscle

Long head of triceps brachii muscle

Teres major muscle

Teres minor muscle

Scapula

Esophagus

Thoracic duct

T3–4 intervertebral disc

Rhomboid muscle

Trapezius muscle

Spinal cord

Left recurrent laryngeal nerve

Left vagus nerve (X)

Oblique fissure (of left lung)

C. Machado —MD.

T3–4

Plate 237

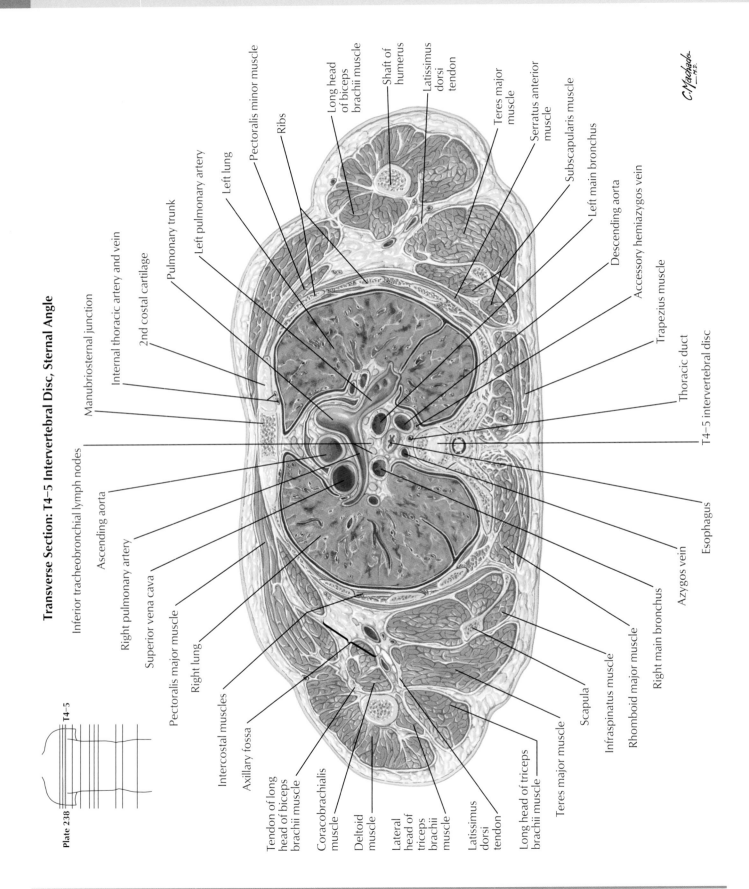

Transverse Section: T4–5 Intervertebral Disc, Sternal Angle

Inferior tracheobronchial lymph nodes

Ascending aorta

Right pulmonary artery

Superior vena cava

Pectoralis major muscle

Right lung

Intercostal muscles

Axillary fossa

Tendon of long head of biceps brachii muscle

Coracobrachialis muscle

Deltoid muscle

Lateral head of triceps brachii muscle

Latissimus dorsi tendon

Long head of triceps brachii muscle

Teres major muscle

Scapula

Infraspinatus muscle

Rhomboid major muscle

Right main bronchus

Azygos vein

Esophagus

T4–5 intervertebral disc

Thoracic duct

Trapezius muscle

Accessory hemiazygos vein

Descending aorta

Left main bronchus

Subscapularis muscle

Serratus anterior muscle

Teres major muscle

Latissimus dorsi tendon

Shaft of humerus

Long head of biceps brachii muscle

Pectoralis minor muscle

Ribs

Left lung

Left pulmonary artery

Pulmonary trunk

2nd costal cartilage

Internal thoracic artery and vein

Manubriosternal junction

Manubriosternal junction

Plate 238

T4–5

Plate 238

Cross-sectional Anatomy

Transverse Section: Level of T7, 3rd Interchondral Space

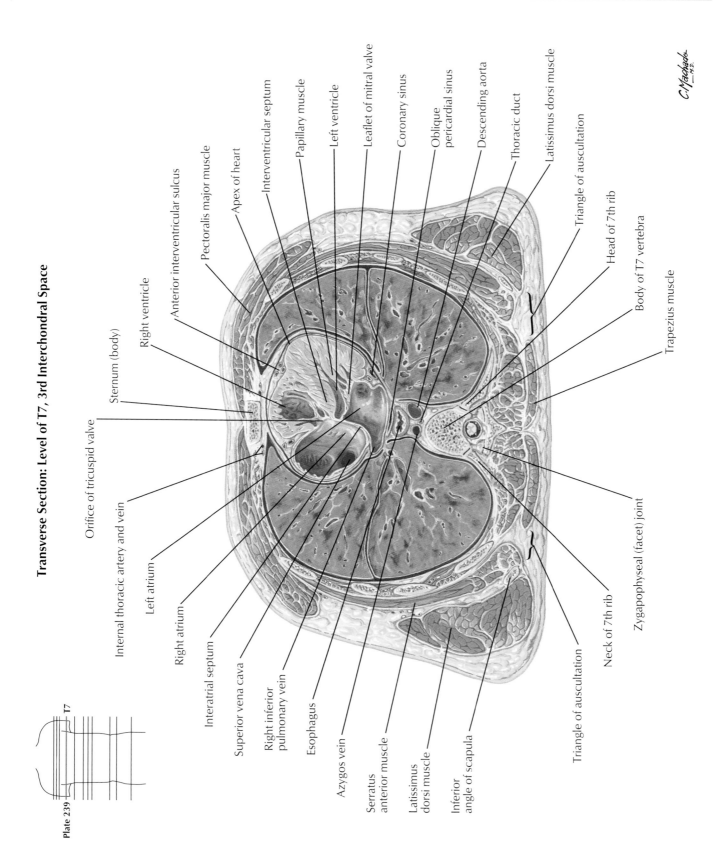

Pectoralis major muscle

Anterior interventricular sulcus

Apex of heart

Interventricular septum

Papillary muscle

Left ventricle

Leaflet of mitral valve

Coronary sinus

Oblique pericardial sinus

Descending aorta

Thoracic duct

Latissimus dorsi muscle

Triangle of auscultation

Head of 7th rib

Body of T7 vertebra

Trapezius muscle

Right ventricle

Sternum (body)

Orifice of tricuspid valve

Internal thoracic artery and vein

Left atrium

Right atrium

Interatrial septum

Superior vena cava

Right inferior pulmonary vein

Esophagus

Azygos vein

Serratus anterior muscle

Latissimus dorsi muscle

Inferior angle of scapula

Triangle of auscultation

Neck of 7th rib

Zygapophyseal (facet) joint

T7

Plate 239

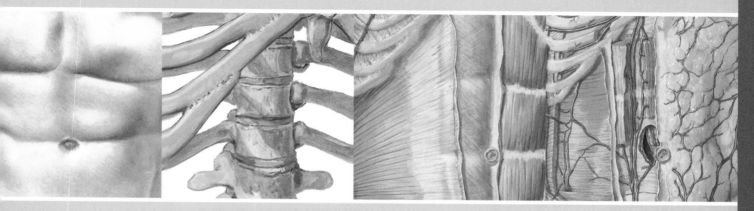

Section 4 ABDOMEN

Topographic Anatomy

Plate 240

240   Abdomen

Body Wall

Plates 241-260

241   Bony Framework of Abdomen

242   Regions and Planes of Abdomen

243   Anterior Abdominal Wall: Superficial Dissection

244   Anterior Abdominal Wall: Intermediate Dissection

245   Anterior Abdominal Wall: Deep Dissection

246   Rectus Sheath: Cross Section

247   Anterior Abdominal Wall: Internal View

248   Posterolateral Abdominal Wall

249   Arteries of Anterior Abdominal Wall

250   Veins of Anterior Abdominal Wall

251   Nerves of Anterior Abdominal Wall

252   Thoracoabdominal Nerves

253   Inguinal Region: Dissections

254   Inguinal Canal and Spermatic Cord

255   Femoral Sheath and Inguinal Canal

256   Posterior Abdominal Wall: Internal View

257   Arteries of Posterior Abdominal Wall

258   Veins of Posterior Abdominal Wall

259   Lymph Vessels and Nodes of Posterior
      Abdominal Wall

260   Nerves of Posterior Abdominal Wall

4 ABDOMEN

Peritoneal Cavity
Plates 261-266

261 Greater Omentum and Abdominal Viscera

262 Mesenteric Relations of Intestines

263 Mesenteric Relations of Intestines (continued)

264 Omental Bursa: Stomach Reflected

265 Omental Bursa: Cross Section

266 Peritoneum of Posterior Abdominal Wall

Viscera (Gut)
Plates 267-276

267 Stomach in Situ

268 Mucosa of Stomach

269 Musculature of Stomach

270 Duodenum in Situ

271 Mucosa and Musculature of Duodenum

272 Mucosa and Musculature of Small Intestine

273 Ileocecal Region

274 Ileocecal Region (continued)

275 (Vermiform) Appendix

276 Mucosa and Musculature of Large Intestine

Viscera (Accessory Organs)
Plates 277-282

277 Surfaces and Bed of Liver

278 Liver in Situ: Vascular and Duct Systems

279 Liver Structure: Schema

280 Gallbladder, Extrahepatic Bile Ducts, and Pancreatic Duct

281 Pancreas in Situ

282 Spleen

Visceral Vasculature
Plates 283-296

283 Arteries of Stomach, Liver, and Spleen

284 Arteries of Liver, Pancreas, Duodenum, and Spleen

285 Celiac Arteriogram

286 Arteries of Duodenum and Head of Pancreas

287 Arteries of Small Intestine

288 Arteries of Large Intestine

289 Veins of Stomach, Duodenum, Pancreas, and Spleen

290 Veins of Small Intestine

291 Veins of Large Intestine

292 Hepatic Portal Vein Tributaries: Portacaval Anastomoses

293 Lymph Vessels and Nodes of Stomach

294 Lymph Vessels and Nodes of Pancreas

295 Lymph Vessels and Nodes of Small Intestine

296 Lymph Vessels and Nodes of Large Intestine

Innervation
Plates 297-307

297 Autonomic Nerves and Ganglia of Abdomen

298 Autonomic Innervation of Stomach and Duodenum

299 Autonomic Innervation of Stomach and Duodenum (continued)

300 Autonomic Innervation of Stomach and Duodenum: Schema

301 Autonomic Innervation of Small Intestine

302 Autonomic Innervation of Large Intestine

303 Autonomic Innervation of Small and Large Intestines: Schema

304 Autonomic Reflex Pathways: Schema

305 Intrinsic Autonomic Plexuses of Intestine: Schema

306 Autonomic Innervation of Liver and Biliary Tract: Schema

307 Autonomic Innervation of Pancreas: Schema

Kidneys and Suprarenal Glands
Plates 308-322

308 Kidneys in Situ: Anterior Views

309 Kidneys in Situ: Posterior Views

310 Renal Artery and Vein in Situ

311 Gross Structure of Kidney

312 Intrarenal Arteries and Renal Segments

313 Nephron and Collecting Tubule: Schema

314 Blood Vessels in Parenchyma of Kidney: Schema

315 Ureters in the Abdomen and Pelvis

316 Arteries of Ureters and Urinary Bladder

317 Renal Fasciae

318 Lymph Vessels and Nodes of Kidneys and Urinary Bladder

319 Autonomic Nerves of Kidneys, Ureters, and Urinary Bladder

320 Autonomic Innervation of Kidneys and Upper Ureters: Schema

321 Autonomic Nerves of Suprarenal Glands: Dissection and Schema

322 Arteries and Veins of Suprarenal Glands in Situ

Cross-sectional Anatomy

Plates 323-330

323 Abdominal Wall and Viscera: Paramedian (Parasagittal) Section

324 Abdominal Scans: Axial CT Images

325 Schematic Cross Section of Abdomen at T10

326 Schematic Cross Section of Abdomen at Upper T12

327 Schematic Cross Section of Abdomen at Middle T12

328 Schematic Cross Section of Abdomen at T12-L1

329 Schematic Cross Section of Abdomen at L1-L2

330 Schematic Cross Section of Abdomen at L3, 4

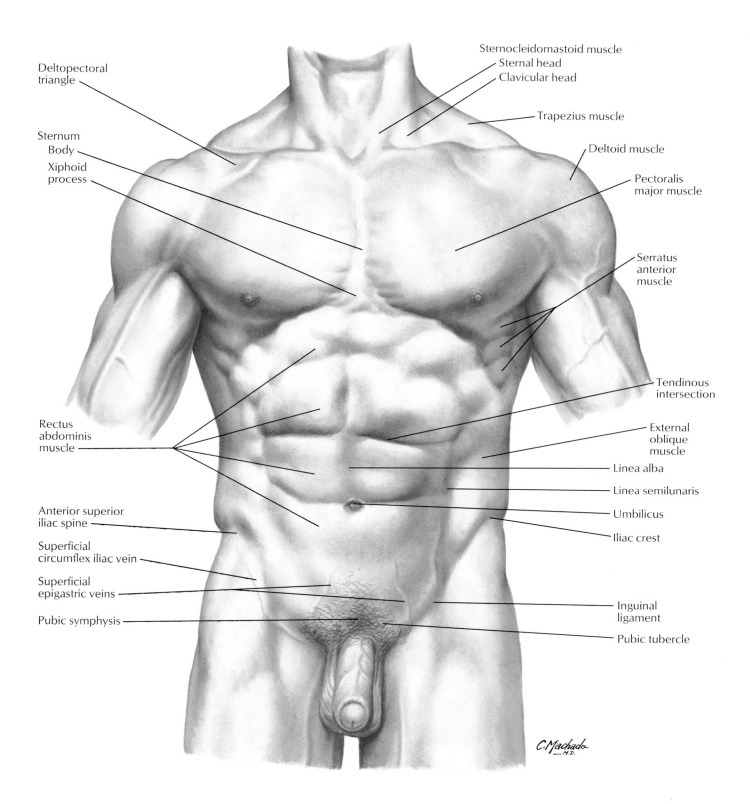

Deltopectoral triangle

Sternum
Body
Xiphoid process

Rectus abdominis muscle

Anterior superior iliac spine

Superficial circumflex iliac vein

Superficial epigastric veins

Pubic symphysis

Sternocleidomastoid muscle
Sternal head
Clavicular head

Trapezius muscle

Deltoid muscle

Pectoralis major muscle

Serratus anterior muscle

Tendinous intersection

External oblique muscle

Linea alba

Linea semilunaris

Umbilicus

Iliac crest

Inguinal ligament

Pubic tubercle

C. Machado
—M.D.—

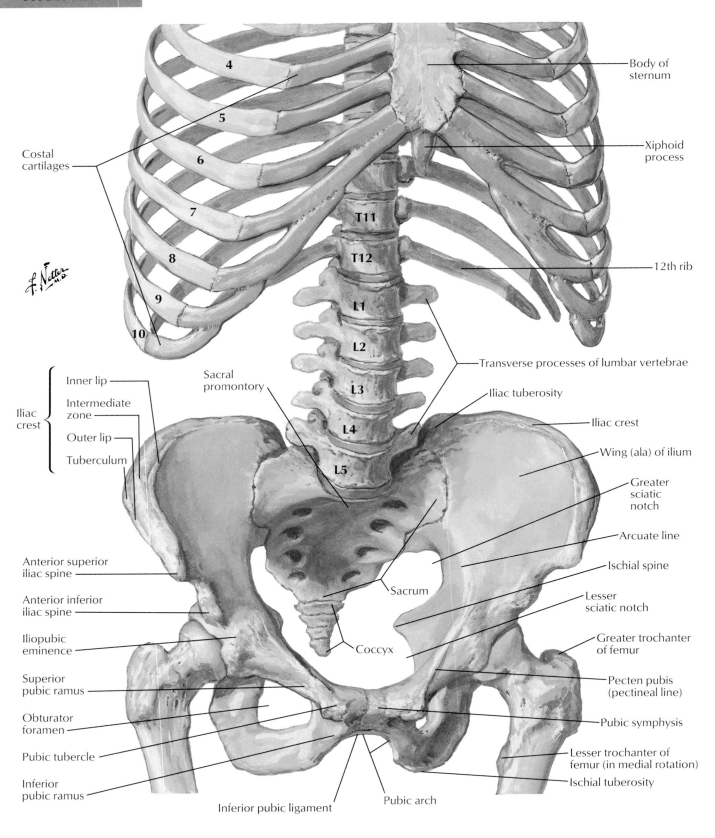

Body of sternum

Xiphoid process

Costal cartilages

12th rib

Transverse processes of lumbar vertebrae

Iliac tuberosity

Iliac crest

Sacral promontory

Wing (ala) of ilium

Greater sciatic notch

Iliac crest — Inner lip, Intermediate zone, Outer lip, Tuberculum

Arcuate line

Ischial spine

Anterior superior iliac spine

Lesser sciatic notch

Sacrum

Anterior inferior iliac spine

Greater trochanter of femur

Iliopubic eminence

Coccyx

Pecten pubis (pectineal line)

Superior pubic ramus

Pubic symphysis

Obturator foramen

Lesser trochanter of femur (in medial rotation)

Pubic tubercle

Ischial tuberosity

Inferior pubic ramus

Inferior pubic ligament

Pubic arch

Plate 241

Body Wall

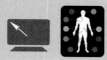

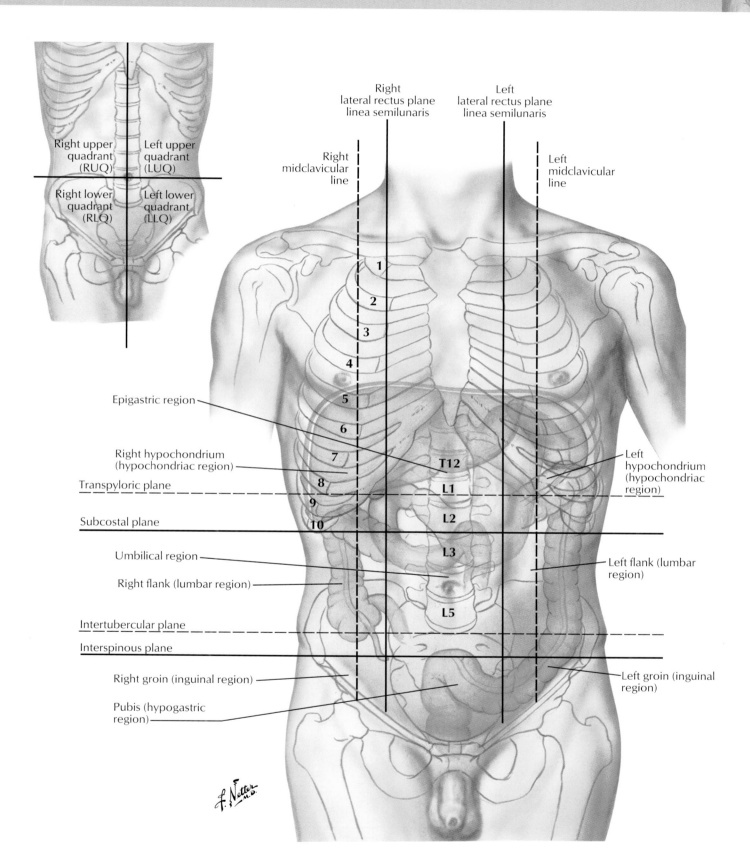

Right upper quadrant (RUQ)

Left upper quadrant (LUQ)

Right lower quadrant (RLQ)

Left lower quadrant (LLQ)

Right lateral rectus plane linea semilunaris

Left lateral rectus plane linea semilunaris

Right midclavicular line

Left midclavicular line

Epigastric region

Right hypochondrium (hypochondriac region)

Transpyloric plane

Subcostal plane

Umbilical region

Right flank (lumbar region)

Intertubercular plane

Interspinous plane

Right groin (inguinal region)

Pubis (hypogastric region)

Left hypochondrium (hypochondriac region)

Left flank (lumbar region)

Left groin (inguinal region)

T12
L1
L2
L3
L5

1
2
3
4
5
6
7
8
9
10

Anterior Abdominal Wall: Superficial Dissection

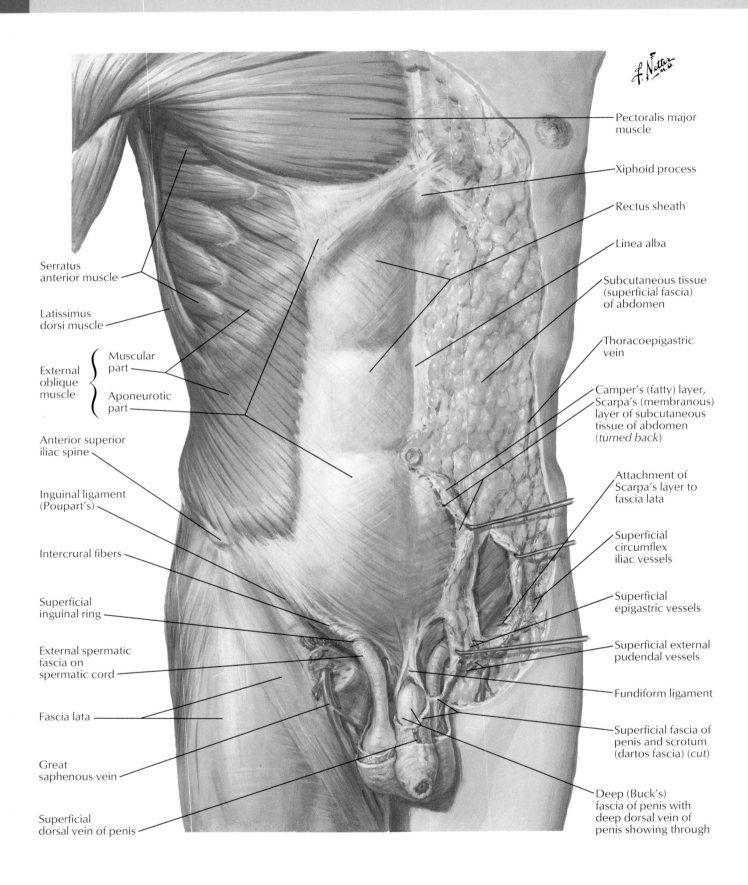

Pectoralis major muscle

Xiphoid process

Rectus sheath

Linea alba

Subcutaneous tissue (superficial fascia) of abdomen

Thoracoepigastric vein

Camper's (fatty) layer, Scarpa's (membranous) layer of subcutaneous tissue of abdomen (*turned back*)

Attachment of Scarpa's layer to fascia lata

Superficial circumflex iliac vessels

Superficial epigastric vessels

Superficial external pudendal vessels

Fundiform ligament

Superficial fascia of penis and scrotum (dartos fascia) (*cut*)

Deep (Buck's) fascia of penis with deep dorsal vein of penis showing through

Serratus anterior muscle

Latissimus dorsi muscle

External oblique muscle { Muscular part / Aponeurotic part }

Anterior superior iliac spine

Inguinal ligament (Poupart's)

Intercrural fibers

Superficial inguinal ring

External spermatic fascia on spermatic cord

Fascia lata

Great saphenous vein

Superficial dorsal vein of penis

Plate 243 **Body Wall**

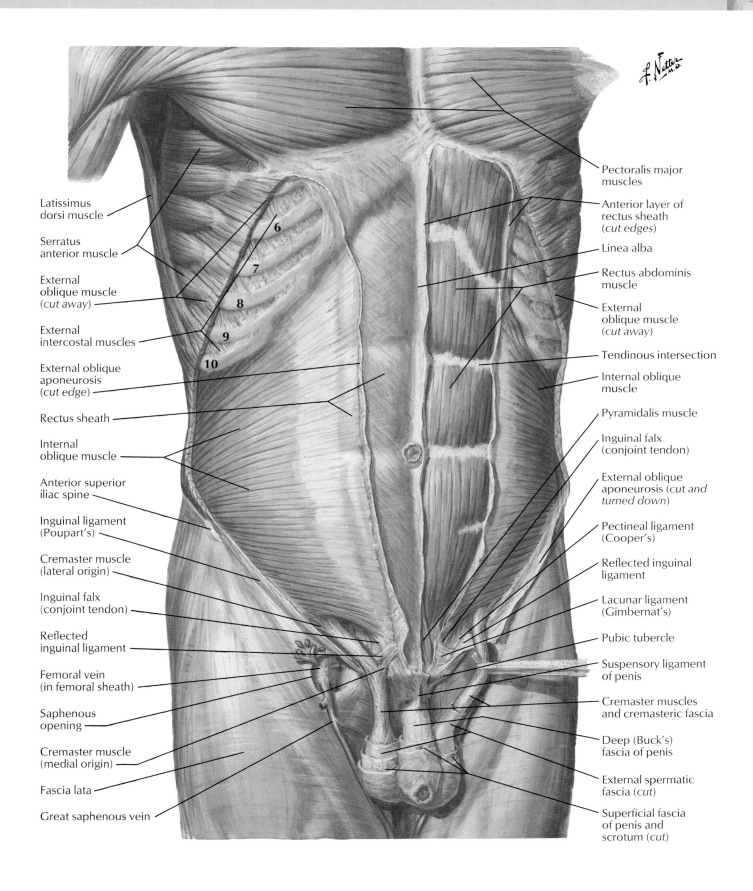

Latissimus
dorsi muscle

Serratus
anterior muscle

External
oblique muscle
(*cut away*)

External
intercostal muscles

External oblique
aponeurosis
(*cut edge*)

Rectus sheath

Internal
oblique muscle

Anterior superior
iliac spine

Inguinal ligament
(Poupart's)

Cremaster muscle
(lateral origin)

Inguinal falx
(conjoint tendon)

Reflected
inguinal ligament

Femoral vein
(in femoral sheath)

Saphenous
opening

Cremaster muscle
(medial origin)

Fascia lata

Great saphenous vein

6
7
8
9
10

f. Netter
M.D.

Pectoralis major
muscles

Anterior layer of
rectus sheath
(*cut edges*)

Linea alba

Rectus abdominis
muscle

External
oblique muscle
(*cut away*)

Tendinous intersection

Internal oblique
muscle

Pyramidalis muscle

Inguinal falx
(conjoint tendon)

External oblique
aponeurosis (*cut and
turned down*)

Pectineal ligament
(Cooper's)

Reflected inguinal
ligament

Lacunar ligament
(Gimbernat's)

Pubic tubercle

Suspensory ligament
of penis

Cremaster muscles
and cremasteric fascia

Deep (Buck's)
fascia of penis

External spermatic
fascia (*cut*)

Superficial fascia
of penis and
scrotum (*cut*)

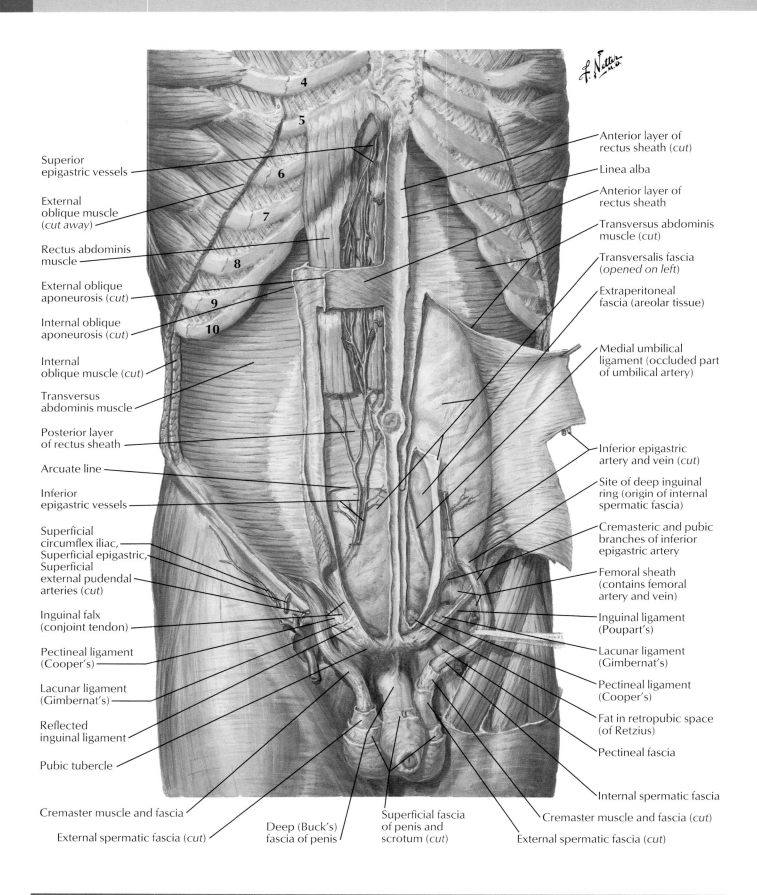

Superior epigastric vessels

External oblique muscle (cut away)

Rectus abdominis muscle

External oblique aponeurosis (cut)

Internal oblique aponeurosis (cut)

Internal oblique muscle (cut)

Transversus abdominis muscle

Posterior layer of rectus sheath

Arcuate line

Inferior epigastric vessels

Superficial circumflex iliac, Superficial epigastric, Superficial external pudendal arteries (cut)

Inguinal falx (conjoint tendon)

Pectineal ligament (Cooper's)

Lacunar ligament (Gimbernat's)

Reflected inguinal ligament

Pubic tubercle

Cremaster muscle and fascia

External spermatic fascia (cut)

Deep (Buck's) fascia of penis

Superficial fascia of penis and scrotum (cut)

Anterior layer of rectus sheath (cut)

Linea alba

Anterior layer of rectus sheath

Transversus abdominis muscle (cut)

Transversalis fascia (opened on left)

Extraperitoneal fascia (areolar tissue)

Medial umbilical ligament (occluded part of umbilical artery)

Inferior epigastric artery and vein (cut)

Site of deep inguinal ring (origin of internal spermatic fascia)

Cremasteric and pubic branches of inferior epigastric artery

Femoral sheath (contains femoral artery and vein)

Inguinal ligament (Poupart's)

Lacunar ligament (Gimbernat's)

Pectineal ligament (Cooper's)

Fat in retropubic space (of Retzius)

Pectineal fascia

Internal spermatic fascia

Cremaster muscle and fascia (cut)

External spermatic fascia (cut)

Plate 245 **Body Wall**

Section above arcuate line

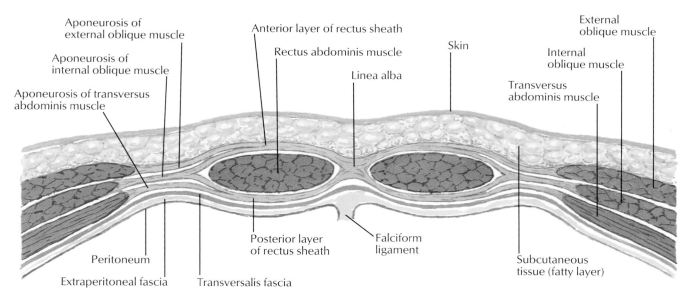

Aponeurosis of external oblique muscle

Aponeurosis of internal oblique muscle

Aponeurosis of transversus abdominis muscle

Anterior layer of rectus sheath

Rectus abdominis muscle

Linea alba

Skin

External oblique muscle

Internal oblique muscle

Transversus abdominis muscle

Peritoneum

Extraperitoneal fascia

Transversalis fascia

Posterior layer of rectus sheath

Falciform ligament

Subcutaneous tissue (fatty layer)

Aponeurosis of internal oblique muscle splits to form anterior and posterior layers of rectus sheath. Aponeurosis of external oblique muscle joins anterior layer of sheath; aponeurosis of transversus abdominis muscle joins posterior layer. Anterior and posterior layers of rectus sheath unite medially to form linea alba.

Section below arcuate line

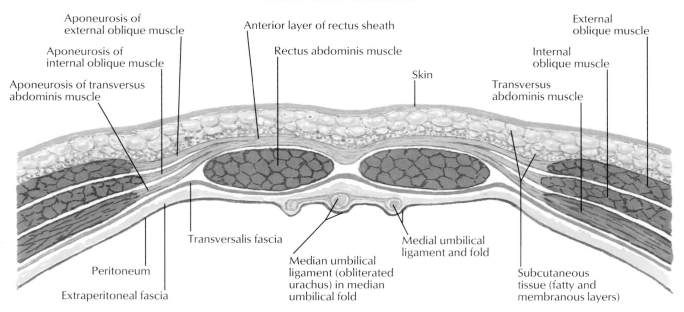

Aponeurosis of external oblique muscle

Aponeurosis of internal oblique muscle

Aponeurosis of transversus abdominis muscle

Anterior layer of rectus sheath

Rectus abdominis muscle

Skin

External oblique muscle

Internal oblique muscle

Transversus abdominis muscle

Transversalis fascia

Median umbilical ligament (obliterated urachus) in median umbilical fold

Medial umbilical ligament and fold

Peritoneum

Extraperitoneal fascia

Subcutaneous tissue (fatty and membranous layers)

Aponeurosis of internal oblique muscle does not split at this level but passes completely anterior to rectus abdominis muscle and is fused there with both aponeurosis of external oblique muscle and that of transversus abdominis muscle. Thus, posterior wall of rectus sheath is absent below arcuate line and is composed of only transversalis fascia.

F. Netter m.d.

For umbilical vessels see **Plate 223**

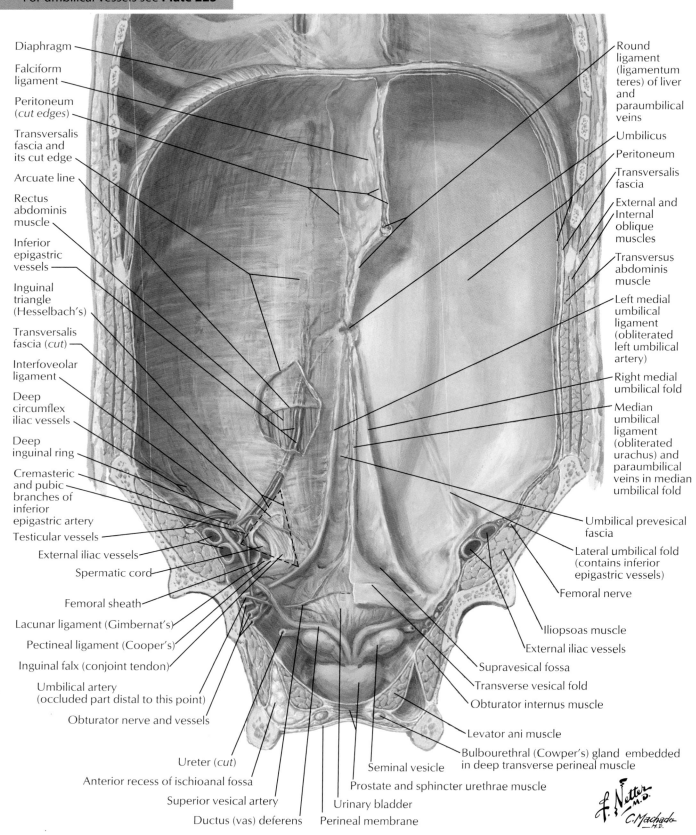

Diaphragm

Falciform ligament

Peritoneum (*cut edges*)

Transversalis fascia and its cut edge

Arcuate line

Rectus abdominis muscle

Inferior epigastric vessels

Inguinal triangle (Hesselbach's)

Transversalis fascia (*cut*)

Interfoveolar ligament

Deep circumflex iliac vessels

Deep inguinal ring

Cremasteric and pubic branches of inferior epigastric artery

Testicular vessels

External iliac vessels

Spermatic cord

Femoral sheath

Lacunar ligament (Gimbernat's)

Pectineal ligament (Cooper's)

Inguinal falx (conjoint tendon)

Umbilical artery (occluded part distal to this point)

Obturator nerve and vessels

Ureter (*cut*)

Anterior recess of ischioanal fossa

Superior vesical artery

Ductus (vas) deferens

Round ligament (ligamentum teres) of liver and paraumbilical veins

Umbilicus

Peritoneum

Transversalis fascia

External and Internal oblique muscles

Transversus abdominis muscle

Left medial umbilical ligament (obliterated left umbilical artery)

Right medial umbilical fold

Median umbilical ligament (obliterated urachus) and paraumbilical veins in median umbilical fold

Umbilical prevesical fascia

Lateral umbilical fold (contains inferior epigastric vessels)

Femoral nerve

Iliopsoas muscle

External iliac vessels

Supravesical fossa

Transverse vesical fold

Obturator internus muscle

Levator ani muscle

Bulbourethral (Cowper's) gland embedded in deep transverse perineal muscle

Prostate and sphincter urethrae muscle

Seminal vesicle

Urinary bladder

Perineal membrane

Plate 247   **Body Wall**

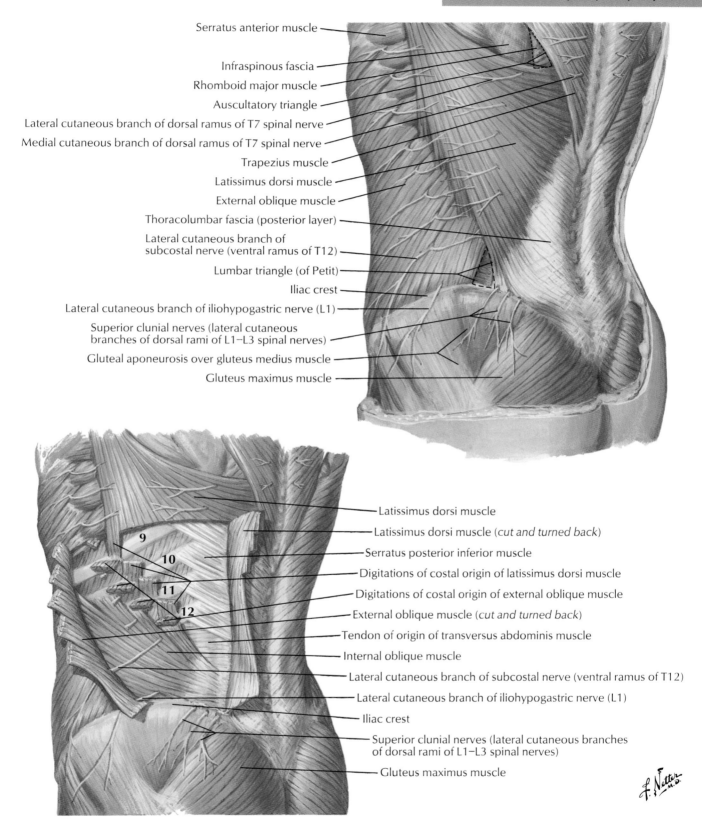

Serratus anterior muscle

Infraspinous fascia

Rhomboid major muscle

Auscultatory triangle

Lateral cutaneous branch of dorsal ramus of T7 spinal nerve

Medial cutaneous branch of dorsal ramus of T7 spinal nerve

Trapezius muscle

Latissimus dorsi muscle

External oblique muscle

Thoracolumbar fascia (posterior layer)

Lateral cutaneous branch of subcostal nerve (ventral ramus of T12)

Lumbar triangle (of Petit)

Iliac crest

Lateral cutaneous branch of iliohypogastric nerve (L1)

Superior clunial nerves (lateral cutaneous branches of dorsal rami of L1–L3 spinal nerves)

Gluteal aponeurosis over gluteus medius muscle

Gluteus maximus muscle

9
10
11
12

Latissimus dorsi muscle

Latissimus dorsi muscle (*cut and turned back*)

Serratus posterior inferior muscle

Digitations of costal origin of latissimus dorsi muscle

Digitations of costal origin of external oblique muscle

External oblique muscle (*cut and turned back*)

Tendon of origin of transversus abdominis muscle

Internal oblique muscle

Lateral cutaneous branch of subcostal nerve (ventral ramus of T12)

Lateral cutaneous branch of iliohypogastric nerve (L1)

Iliac crest

Superior clunial nerves (lateral cutaneous branches of dorsal rami of L1–L3 spinal nerves)

Gluteus maximus muscle

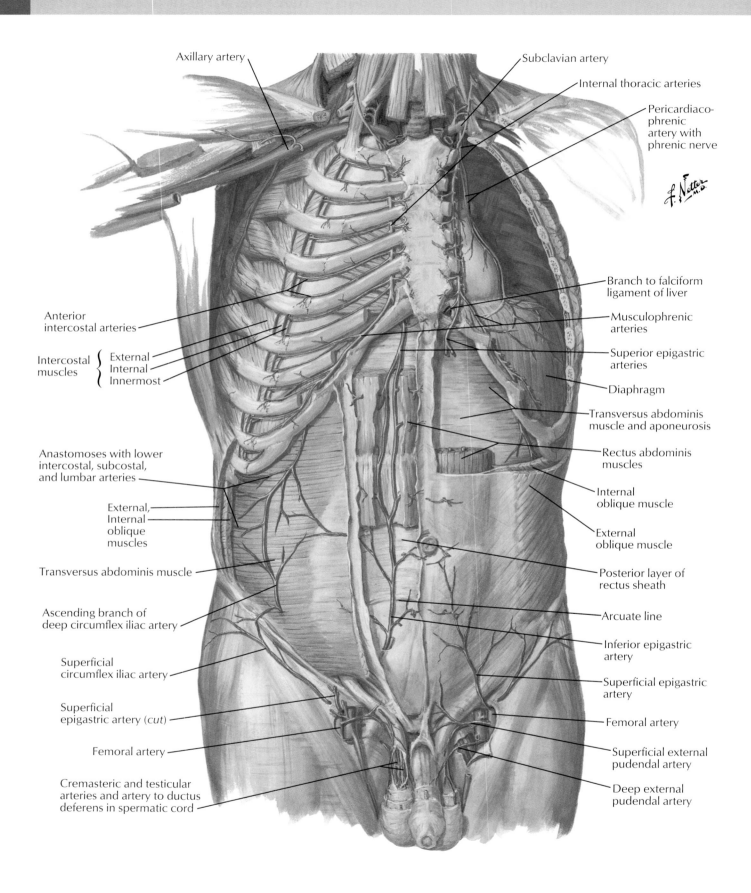

Axillary artery

Subclavian artery

Internal thoracic arteries

Pericardiaco-phrenic artery with phrenic nerve

Branch to falciform ligament of liver

Musculophrenic arteries

Superior epigastric arteries

Diaphragm

Transversus abdominis muscle and aponeurosis

Rectus abdominis muscles

Internal oblique muscle

External oblique muscle

Posterior layer of rectus sheath

Arcuate line

Inferior epigastric artery

Superficial epigastric artery

Femoral artery

Superficial external pudendal artery

Deep external pudendal artery

Anterior intercostal arteries

Intercostal muscles { External Internal Innermost

Anastomoses with lower intercostal, subcostal, and lumbar arteries

External, Internal oblique muscles

Transversus abdominis muscle

Ascending branch of deep circumflex iliac artery

Superficial circumflex iliac artery

Superficial epigastric artery (cut)

Femoral artery

Cremasteric and testicular arteries and artery to ductus deferens in spermatic cord

Plate 249　　　　　　　　　　　　　　　　　　　　　　　　**Body Wall**

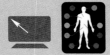

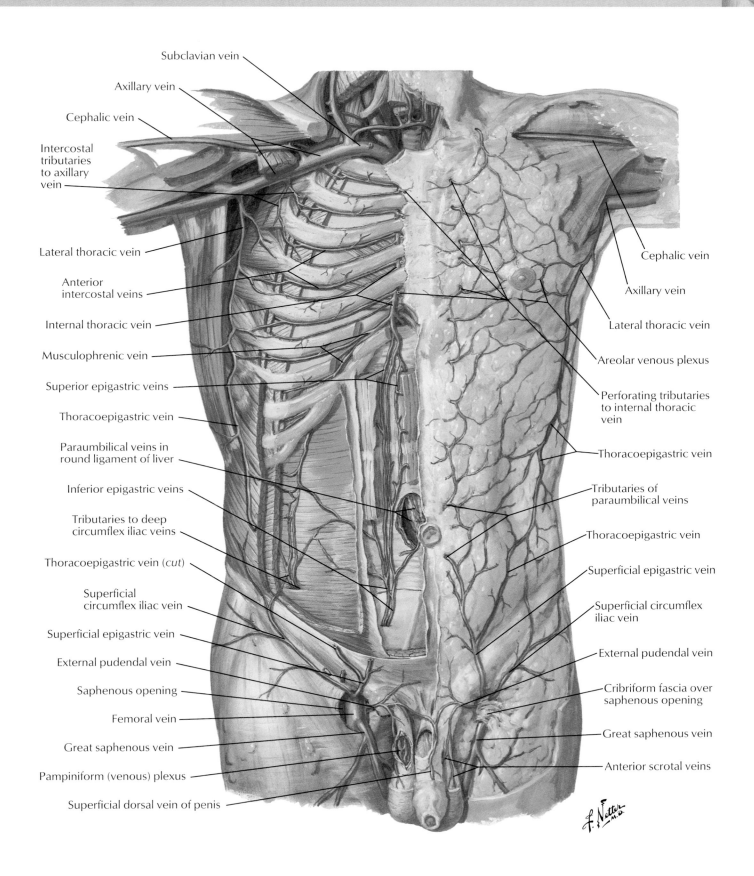

Subclavian vein

Axillary vein

Cephalic vein

Intercostal tributaries to axillary vein

Lateral thoracic vein

Anterior intercostal veins

Internal thoracic vein

Musculophrenic vein

Superior epigastric veins

Thoracoepigastric vein

Paraumbilical veins in round ligament of liver

Inferior epigastric veins

Tributaries to deep circumflex iliac veins

Thoracoepigastric vein (cut)

Superficial circumflex iliac vein

Superficial epigastric vein

External pudendal vein

Saphenous opening

Femoral vein

Great saphenous vein

Pampiniform (venous) plexus

Superficial dorsal vein of penis

Cephalic vein

Axillary vein

Lateral thoracic vein

Areolar venous plexus

Perforating tributaries to internal thoracic vein

Thoracoepigastric vein

Tributaries of paraumbilical veins

Thoracoepigastric vein

Superficial epigastric vein

Superficial circumflex iliac vein

External pudendal vein

Cribriform fascia over saphenous opening

Great saphenous vein

Anterior scrotal veins

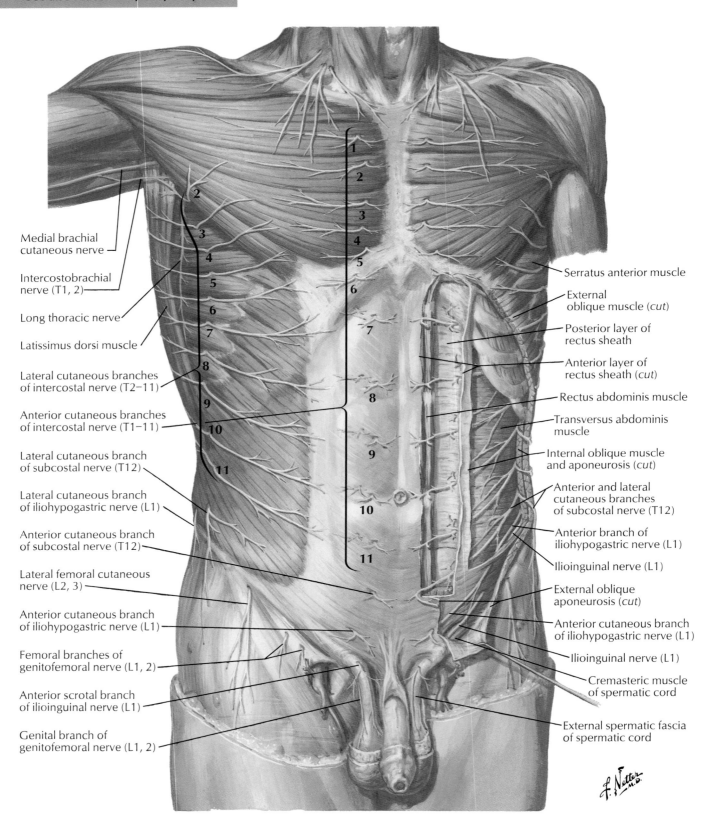

Medial brachial
cutaneous nerve

Intercostobrachial
nerve (T1, 2)

Long thoracic nerve

Latissimus dorsi muscle

Lateral cutaneous branches
of intercostal nerve (T2–11)

Anterior cutaneous branches
of intercostal nerve (T1–11)

Lateral cutaneous branch
of subcostal nerve (T12)

Lateral cutaneous branch
of iliohypogastric nerve (L1)

Anterior cutaneous branch
of subcostal nerve (T12)

Lateral femoral cutaneous
nerve (L2, 3)

Anterior cutaneous branch
of iliohypogastric nerve (L1)

Femoral branches of
genitofemoral nerve (L1, 2)

Anterior scrotal branch
of ilioinguinal nerve (L1)

Genital branch of
genitofemoral nerve (L1, 2)

Serratus anterior muscle

External
oblique muscle (*cut*)

Posterior layer of
rectus sheath

Anterior layer of
rectus sheath (*cut*)

Rectus abdominis muscle

Transversus abdominis
muscle

Internal oblique muscle
and aponeurosis (*cut*)

Anterior and lateral
cutaneous branches
of subcostal nerve (T12)

Anterior branch of
iliohypogastric nerve (L1)

Ilioinguinal nerve (L1)

External oblique
aponeurosis (*cut*)

Anterior cutaneous branch
of iliohypogastric nerve (L1)

Ilioinguinal nerve (L1)

Cremasteric muscle
of spermatic cord

External spermatic fascia
of spermatic cord

Plate 251

Body Wall

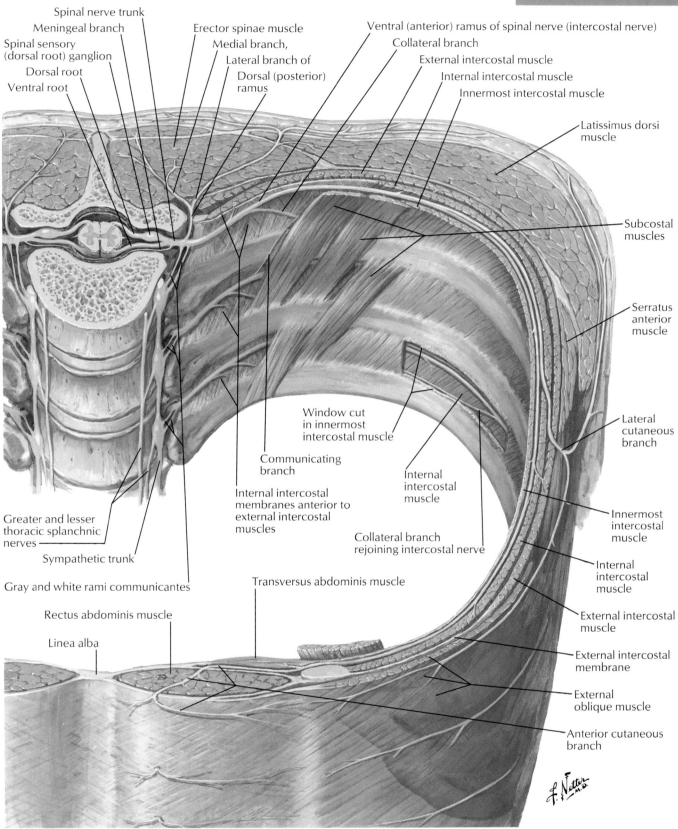

Spinal nerve trunk

Meningeal branch

Spinal sensory (dorsal root) ganglion

Dorsal root

Ventral root

Erector spinae muscle

Medial branch,

Lateral branch of

Dorsal (posterior) ramus

Ventral (anterior) ramus of spinal nerve (intercostal nerve)

Collateral branch

External intercostal muscle

Internal intercostal muscle

Innermost intercostal muscle

Latissimus dorsi muscle

Subcostal muscles

Serratus anterior muscle

Window cut in innermost intercostal muscle

Communicating branch

Internal intercostal membranes anterior to external intercostal muscles

Internal intercostal muscle

Collateral branch rejoining intercostal nerve

Lateral cutaneous branch

Innermost intercostal muscle

Internal intercostal muscle

Greater and lesser thoracic splanchnic nerves

Sympathetic trunk

Gray and white rami communicantes

Transversus abdominis muscle

External intercostal muscle

Rectus abdominis muscle

Linea alba

External intercostal membrane

External oblique muscle

Anterior cutaneous branch

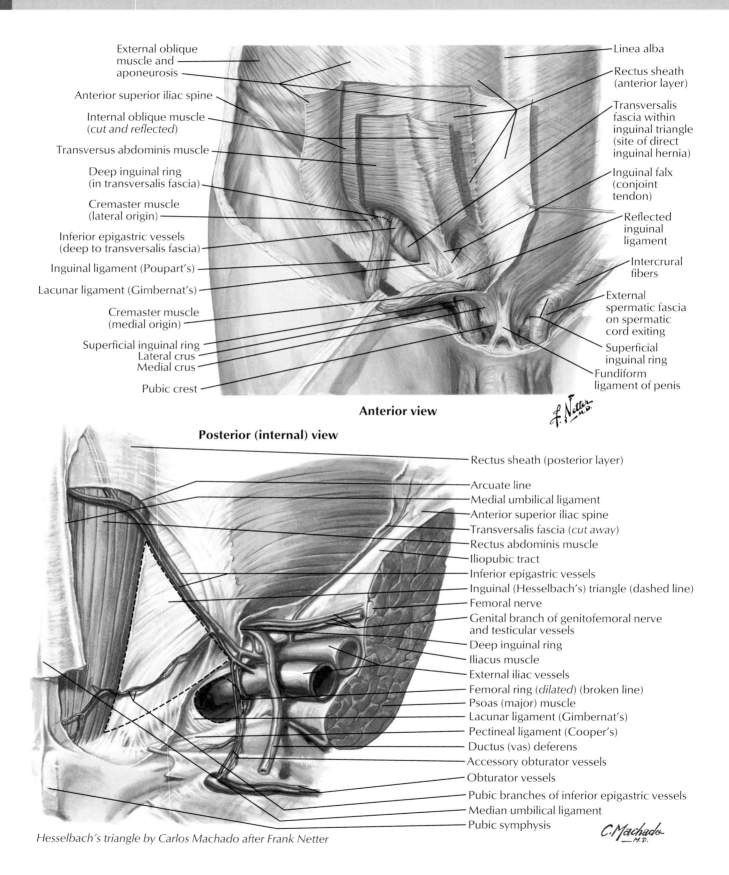

External oblique muscle and aponeurosis

Anterior superior iliac spine

Internal oblique muscle (*cut and reflected*)

Transversus abdominis muscle

Deep inguinal ring (in transversalis fascia)

Cremaster muscle (lateral origin)

Inferior epigastric vessels (deep to transversalis fascia)

Inguinal ligament (Poupart's)

Lacunar ligament (Gimbernat's)

Cremaster muscle (medial origin)

Superficial inguinal ring
Lateral crus
Medial crus

Pubic crest

Linea alba

Rectus sheath (anterior layer)

Transversalis fascia within inguinal triangle (site of direct inguinal hernia)

Inguinal falx (conjoint tendon)

Reflected inguinal ligament

Intercrural fibers

External spermatic fascia on spermatic cord exiting

Superficial inguinal ring

Fundiform ligament of penis

Anterior view

Posterior (internal) view

Rectus sheath (posterior layer)

Arcuate line
Medial umbilical ligament
Anterior superior iliac spine
Transversalis fascia (*cut away*)
Rectus abdominis muscle
Iliopubic tract
Inferior epigastric vessels
Inguinal (Hesselbach's) triangle (dashed line)
Femoral nerve
Genital branch of genitofemoral nerve and testicular vessels
Deep inguinal ring
Iliacus muscle
External iliac vessels
Femoral ring (*dilated*) (broken line)
Psoas (major) muscle
Lacunar ligament (Gimbernat's)
Pectineal ligament (Cooper's)
Ductus (vas) deferens
Accessory obturator vessels
Obturator vessels
Pubic branches of inferior epigastric vessels
Median umbilical ligament
Pubic symphysis

Hesselbach's triangle by Carlos Machado after Frank Netter

Plate 253 **Body Wall**

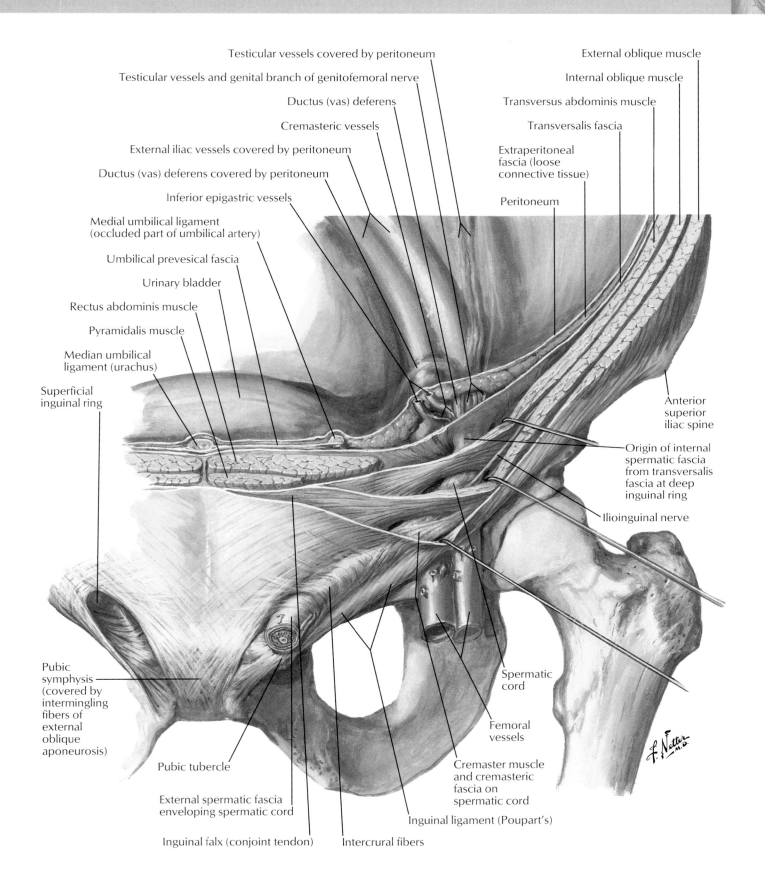

Testicular vessels covered by peritoneum

Testicular vessels and genital branch of genitofemoral nerve

Ductus (vas) deferens

Cremasteric vessels

External iliac vessels covered by peritoneum

Ductus (vas) deferens covered by peritoneum

Inferior epigastric vessels

Medial umbilical ligament (occluded part of umbilical artery)

Umbilical prevesical fascia

Urinary bladder

Rectus abdominis muscle

Pyramidalis muscle

Median umbilical ligament (urachus)

Superficial inguinal ring

Pubic symphysis (covered by intermingling fibers of external oblique aponeurosis)

Pubic tubercle

External spermatic fascia enveloping spermatic cord

Inguinal falx (conjoint tendon)

Intercrural fibers

External oblique muscle

Internal oblique muscle

Transversus abdominis muscle

Transversalis fascia

Extraperitoneal fascia (loose connective tissue)

Peritoneum

Anterior superior iliac spine

Origin of internal spermatic fascia from transversalis fascia at deep inguinal ring

Ilioinguinal nerve

Spermatic cord

Femoral vessels

Cremaster muscle and cremasteric fascia on spermatic cord

Inguinal ligament (Poupart's)

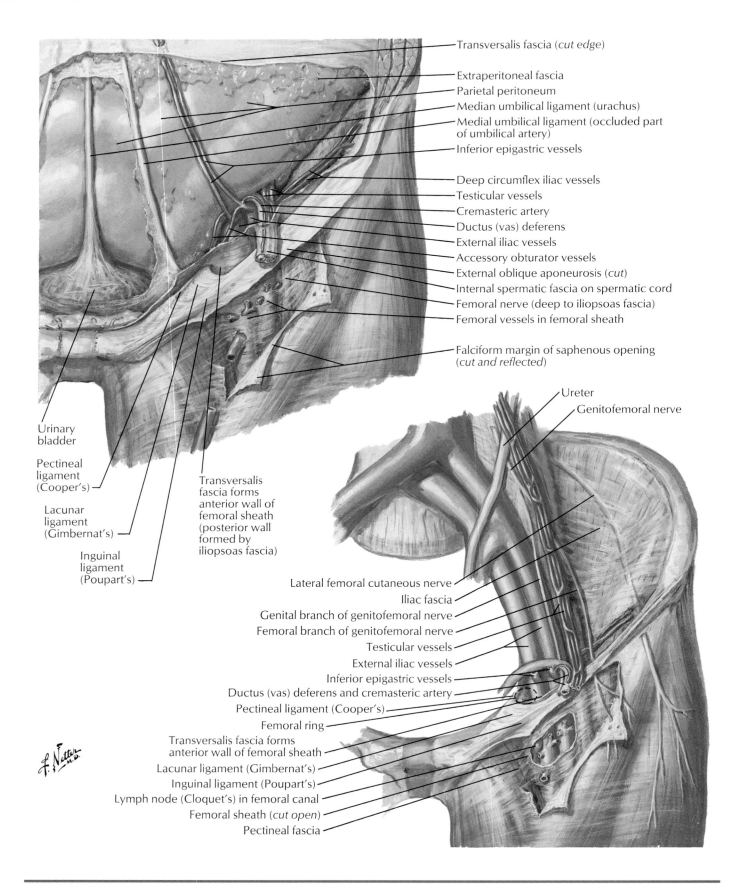

Transversalis fascia (*cut edge*)

Extraperitoneal fascia

Parietal peritoneum

Median umbilical ligament (urachus)

Medial umbilical ligament (occluded part of umbilical artery)

Inferior epigastric vessels

Deep circumflex iliac vessels

Testicular vessels

Cremasteric artery

Ductus (vas) deferens

External iliac vessels

Accessory obturator vessels

External oblique aponeurosis (*cut*)

Internal spermatic fascia on spermatic cord

Femoral nerve (deep to iliopsoas fascia)

Femoral vessels in femoral sheath

Falciform margin of saphenous opening (*cut and reflected*)

Ureter

Genitofemoral nerve

Urinary bladder

Pectineal ligament (Cooper's)

Lacunar ligament (Gimbernat's)

Inguinal ligament (Poupart's)

Transversalis fascia forms anterior wall of femoral sheath (posterior wall formed by iliopsoas fascia)

Lateral femoral cutaneous nerve

Iliac fascia

Genital branch of genitofemoral nerve

Femoral branch of genitofemoral nerve

Testicular vessels

External iliac vessels

Inferior epigastric vessels

Ductus (vas) deferens and cremasteric artery

Pectineal ligament (Cooper's)

Femoral ring

Transversalis fascia forms anterior wall of femoral sheath

Lacunar ligament (Gimbernat's)

Inguinal ligament (Poupart's)

Lymph node (Cloquet's) in femoral canal

Femoral sheath (*cut open*)

Pectineal fascia

Plate 255 **Body Wall**

For diaphragm see also **Plate 189**

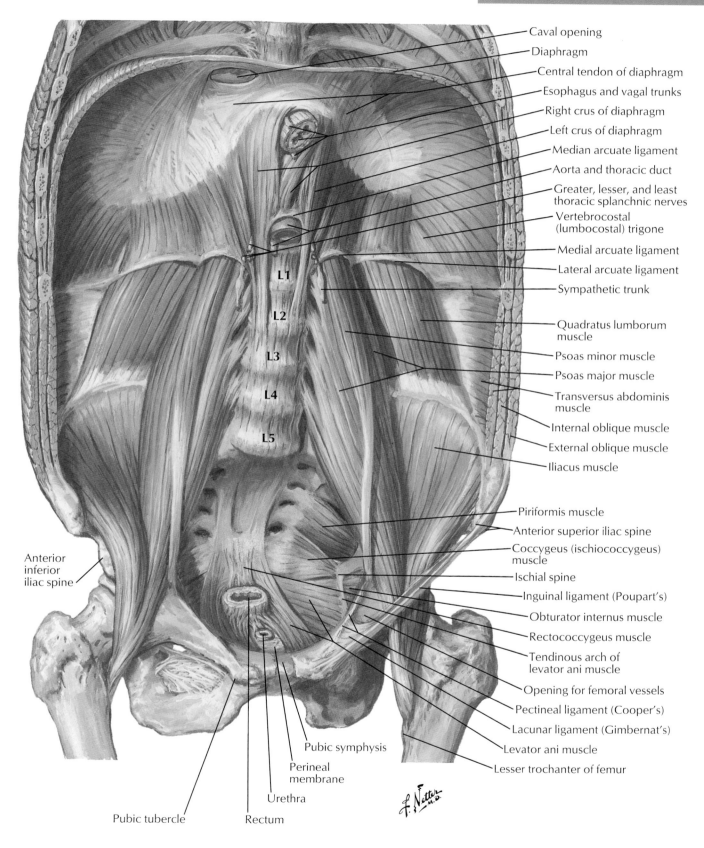

Caval opening

Diaphragm

Central tendon of diaphragm

Esophagus and vagal trunks

Right crus of diaphragm

Left crus of diaphragm

Median arcuate ligament

Aorta and thoracic duct

Greater, lesser, and least thoracic splanchnic nerves

Vertebrocostal (lumbocostal) trigone

Medial arcuate ligament

Lateral arcuate ligament

Sympathetic trunk

Quadratus lumborum muscle

Psoas minor muscle

Psoas major muscle

Transversus abdominis muscle

Internal oblique muscle

External oblique muscle

Iliacus muscle

Piriformis muscle

Anterior superior iliac spine

Coccygeus (ischiococcygeus) muscle

Ischial spine

Inguinal ligament (Poupart's)

Obturator internus muscle

Rectococcygeus muscle

Tendinous arch of levator ani muscle

Opening for femoral vessels

Pectineal ligament (Cooper's)

Lacunar ligament (Gimbernat's)

Levator ani muscle

Lesser trochanter of femur

L1

L2

L3

L4

L5

Anterior inferior iliac spine

Pubic tubercle

Rectum

Urethra

Perineal membrane

Pubic symphysis

Body Wall

Plate 256

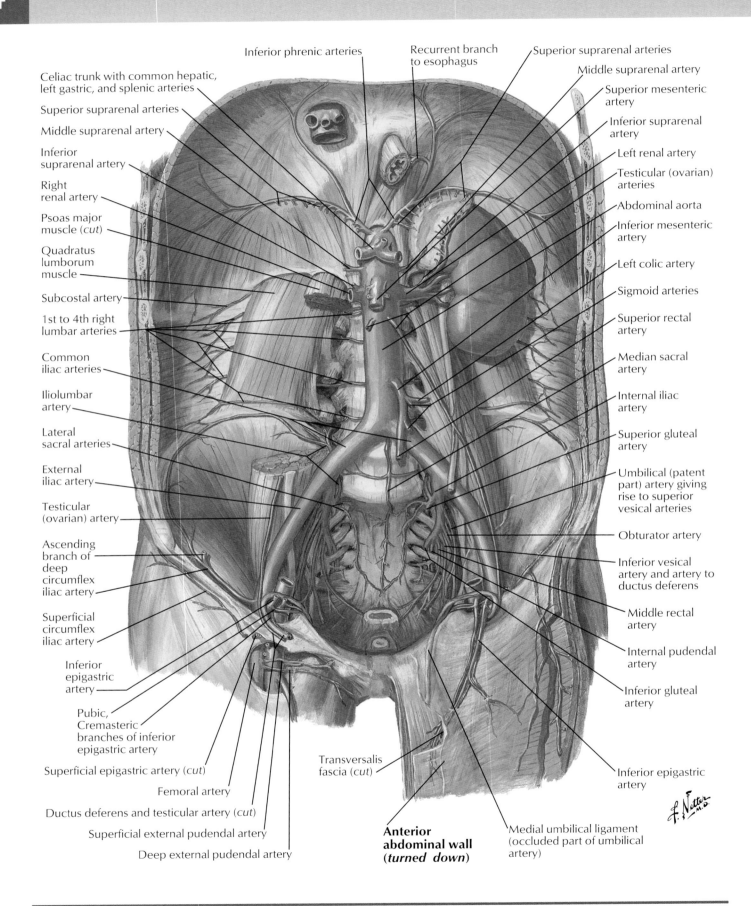

Inferior phrenic arteries

Recurrent branch to esophagus

Superior suprarenal arteries

Celiac trunk with common hepatic, left gastric, and splenic arteries

Superior suprarenal arteries

Middle suprarenal artery

Inferior suprarenal artery

Right renal artery

Psoas major muscle (cut)

Quadratus lumborum muscle

Subcostal artery

1st to 4th right lumbar arteries

Common iliac arteries

Iliolumbar artery

Lateral sacral arteries

External iliac artery

Testicular (ovarian) artery

Ascending branch of deep circumflex iliac artery

Superficial circumflex iliac artery

Inferior epigastric artery

Pubic, Cremasteric branches of inferior epigastric artery

Superficial epigastric artery (cut)

Femoral artery

Ductus deferens and testicular artery (cut)

Superficial external pudendal artery

Deep external pudendal artery

Middle suprarenal artery

Superior mesenteric artery

Inferior suprarenal artery

Left renal artery

Testicular (ovarian) arteries

Abdominal aorta

Inferior mesenteric artery

Left colic artery

Sigmoid arteries

Superior rectal artery

Median sacral artery

Internal iliac artery

Superior gluteal artery

Umbilical (patent part) artery giving rise to superior vesical arteries

Obturator artery

Inferior vesical artery and artery to ductus deferens

Middle rectal artery

Internal pudendal artery

Inferior gluteal artery

Inferior epigastric artery

Transversalis fascia (cut)

Anterior abdominal wall (turned down)

Medial umbilical ligament (occluded part of umbilical artery)

f. Netter M.D.

Plate 257

Body Wall

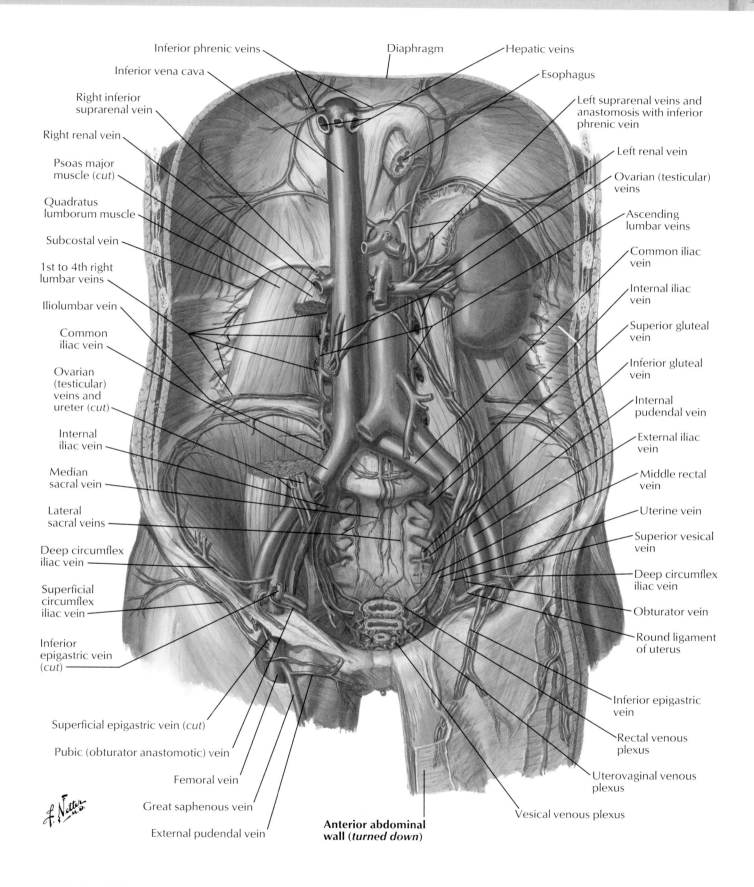

Inferior phrenic veins

Diaphragm

Hepatic veins

Inferior vena cava

Esophagus

Right inferior suprarenal vein

Left suprarenal veins and anastomosis with inferior phrenic vein

Right renal vein

Left renal vein

Psoas major muscle (cut)

Ovarian (testicular) veins

Quadratus lumborum muscle

Ascending lumbar veins

Subcostal vein

Common iliac vein

1st to 4th right lumbar veins

Internal iliac vein

Iliolumbar vein

Superior gluteal vein

Common iliac vein

Inferior gluteal vein

Ovarian (testicular) veins and ureter (cut)

Internal pudendal vein

Internal iliac vein

External iliac vein

Median sacral vein

Middle rectal vein

Lateral sacral veins

Uterine vein

Deep circumflex iliac vein

Superior vesical vein

Superficial circumflex iliac vein

Deep circumflex iliac vein

Obturator vein

Inferior epigastric vein (cut)

Round ligament of uterus

Inferior epigastric vein

Superficial epigastric vein (cut)

Rectal venous plexus

Pubic (obturator anastomotic) vein

Femoral vein

Uterovaginal venous plexus

Great saphenous vein

Vesical venous plexus

External pudendal vein

Anterior abdominal wall (turned down)

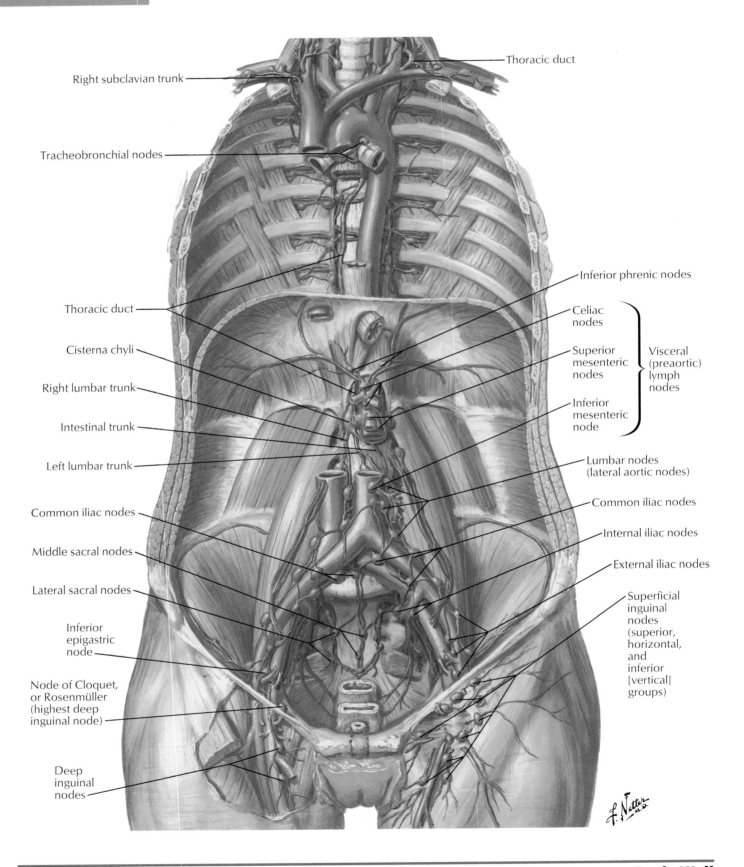

Right subclavian trunk

Tracheobronchial nodes

Thoracic duct

Cisterna chyli

Right lumbar trunk

Intestinal trunk

Left lumbar trunk

Common iliac nodes

Middle sacral nodes

Lateral sacral nodes

Inferior epigastric node

Node of Cloquet, or Rosenmüller (highest deep inguinal node)

Deep inguinal nodes

Thoracic duct

Inferior phrenic nodes

Celiac nodes

Superior mesenteric nodes

Inferior mesenteric node

Visceral (preaortic) lymph nodes

Lumbar nodes (lateral aortic nodes)

Common iliac nodes

Internal iliac nodes

External iliac nodes

Superficial inguinal nodes (superior, horizontal, and inferior [vertical] groups)

Plate 259

Body Wall

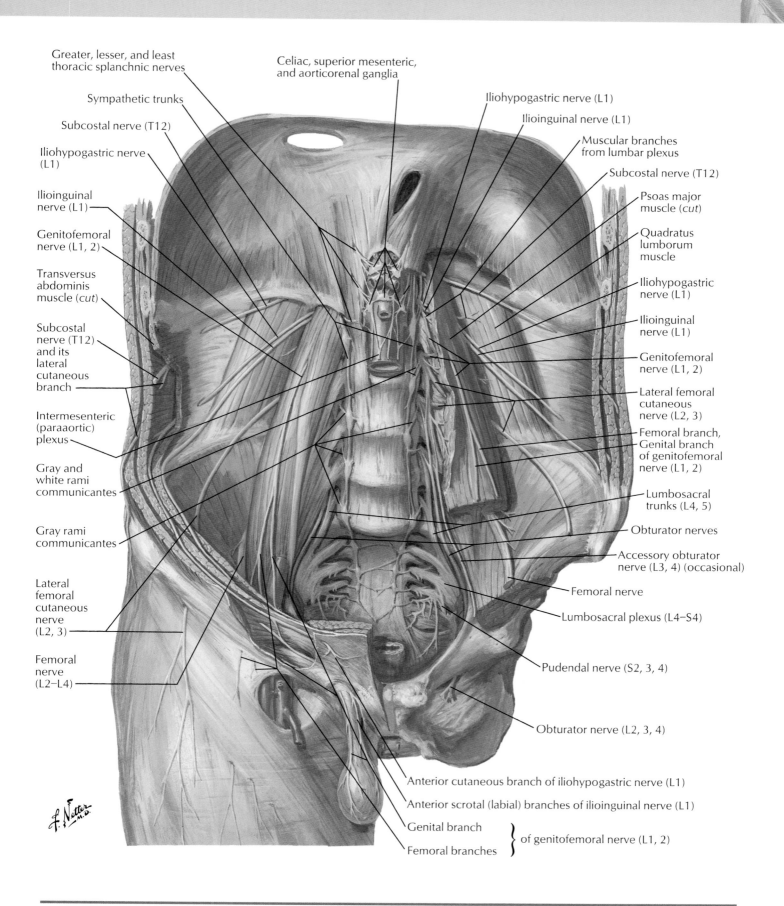

Greater, lesser, and least thoracic splanchnic nerves

Sympathetic trunks

Subcostal nerve (T12)

Iliohypogastric nerve (L1)

Ilioinguinal nerve (L1)

Genitofemoral nerve (L1, 2)

Transversus abdominis muscle (cut)

Subcostal nerve (T12) and its lateral cutaneous branch

Intermesenteric (paraaortic) plexus

Gray and white rami communicantes

Gray rami communicantes

Lateral femoral cutaneous nerve (L2, 3)

Femoral nerve (L2–L4)

Celiac, superior mesenteric, and aorticorenal ganglia

Iliohypogastric nerve (L1)

Ilioinguinal nerve (L1)

Muscular branches from lumbar plexus

Subcostal nerve (T12)

Psoas major muscle (cut)

Quadratus lumborum muscle

Iliohypogastric nerve (L1)

Ilioinguinal nerve (L1)

Genitofemoral nerve (L1, 2)

Lateral femoral cutaneous nerve (L2, 3)

Femoral branch, Genital branch of genitofemoral nerve (L1, 2)

Lumbosacral trunks (L4, 5)

Obturator nerves

Accessory obturator nerve (L3, 4) (occasional)

Femoral nerve

Lumbosacral plexus (L4–S4)

Pudendal nerve (S2, 3, 4)

Obturator nerve (L2, 3, 4)

Anterior cutaneous branch of iliohypogastric nerve (L1)

Anterior scrotal (labial) branches of ilioinguinal nerve (L1)

Genital branch
Femoral branches } of genitofemoral nerve (L1, 2)

J. Netter M.D.

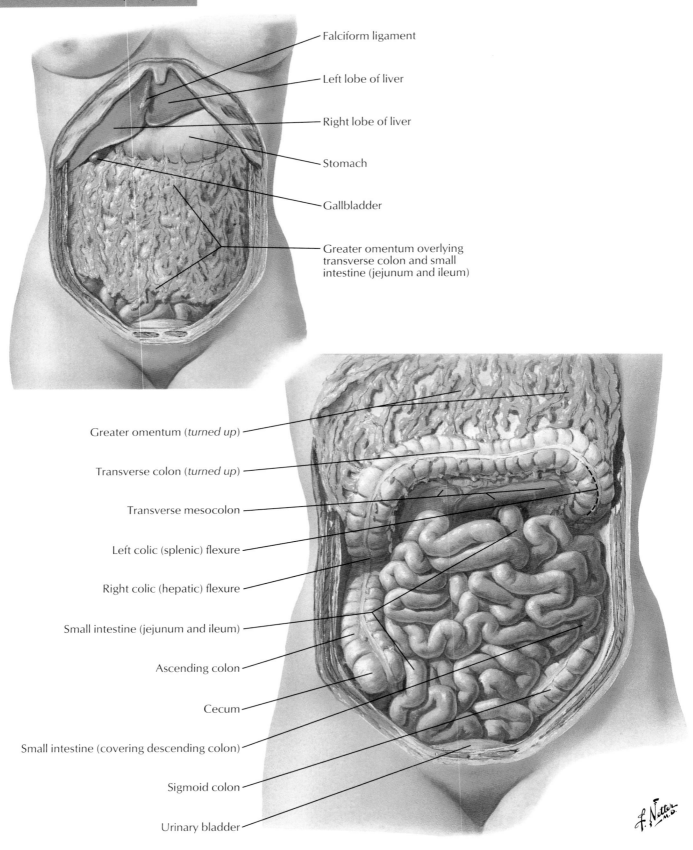

Falciform ligament

Left lobe of liver

Right lobe of liver

Stomach

Gallbladder

Greater omentum overlying transverse colon and small intestine (jejunum and ileum)

Greater omentum (*turned up*)

Transverse colon (*turned up*)

Transverse mesocolon

Left colic (splenic) flexure

Right colic (hepatic) flexure

Small intestine (jejunum and ileum)

Ascending colon

Cecum

Small intestine (covering descending colon)

Sigmoid colon

Urinary bladder

Plate 261   **Peritoneal Cavity**

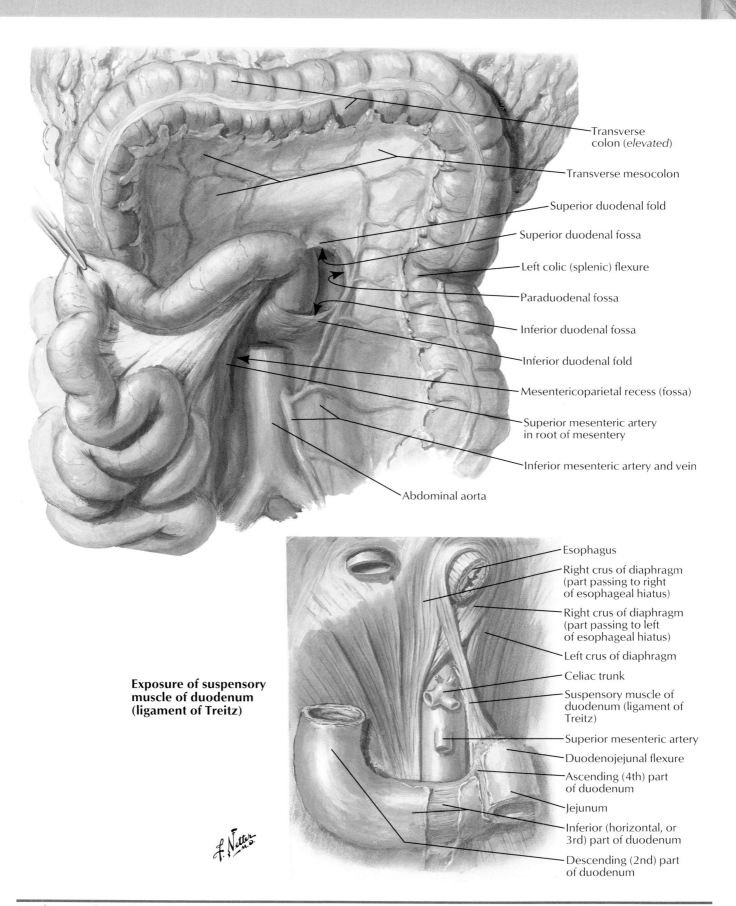

Transverse colon (*elevated*)

Transverse mesocolon

Superior duodenal fold

Superior duodenal fossa

Left colic (splenic) flexure

Paraduodenal fossa

Inferior duodenal fossa

Inferior duodenal fold

Mesentericoparietal recess (fossa)

Superior mesenteric artery in root of mesentery

Inferior mesenteric artery and vein

Abdominal aorta

Exposure of suspensory muscle of duodenum (ligament of Treitz)

Esophagus

Right crus of diaphragm (part passing to right of esophageal hiatus)

Right crus of diaphragm (part passing to left of esophageal hiatus)

Left crus of diaphragm

Celiac trunk

Suspensory muscle of duodenum (ligament of Treitz)

Superior mesenteric artery

Duodenojejunal flexure

Ascending (4th) part of duodenum

Jejunum

Inferior (horizontal, or 3rd) part of duodenum

Descending (2nd) part of duodenum

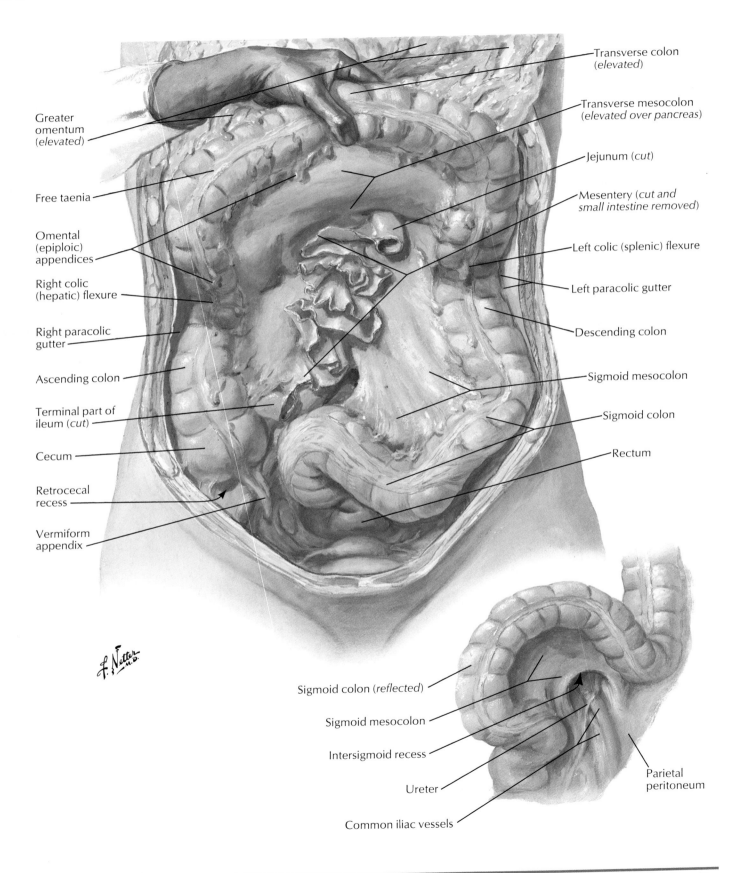

Transverse colon (*elevated*)

Transverse mesocolon (*elevated over pancreas*)

Jejunum (*cut*)

Mesentery (*cut and small intestine removed*)

Left colic (splenic) flexure

Left paracolic gutter

Descending colon

Sigmoid mesocolon

Sigmoid colon

Rectum

Greater omentum (*elevated*)

Free taenia

Omental (epiploic) appendices

Right colic (hepatic) flexure

Right paracolic gutter

Ascending colon

Terminal part of ileum (*cut*)

Cecum

Retrocecal recess

Vermiform appendix

Sigmoid colon (*reflected*)

Sigmoid mesocolon

Intersigmoid recess

Ureter

Common iliac vessels

Parietal peritoneum

Plate 263 **Peritoneal Cavity**

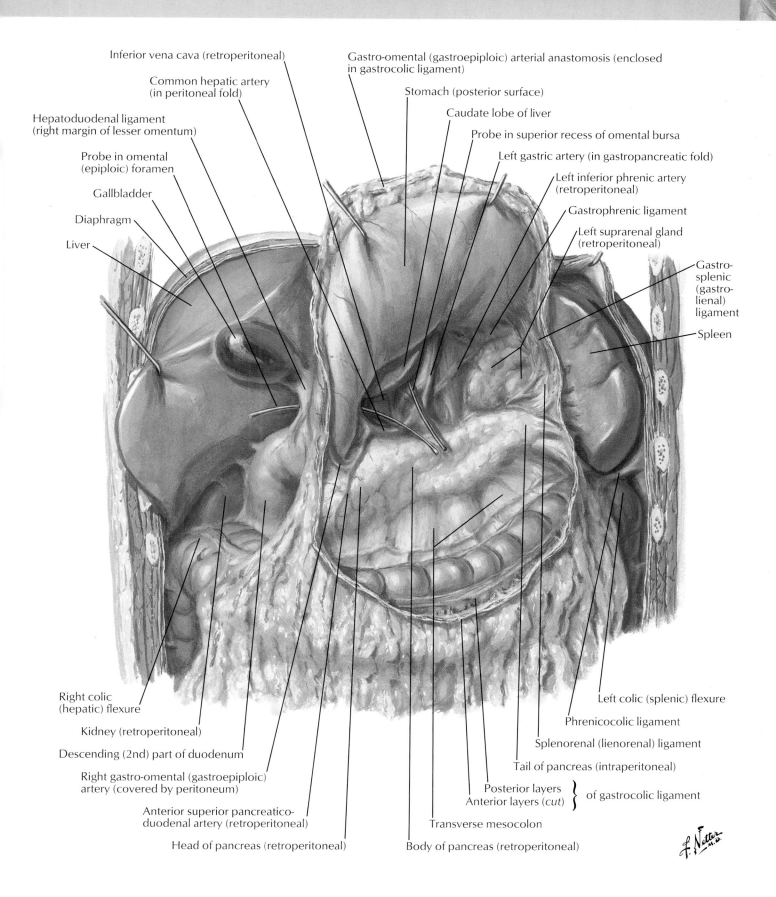

Inferior vena cava (retroperitoneal)

Common hepatic artery (in peritoneal fold)

Hepatoduodenal ligament (right margin of lesser omentum)

Probe in omental (epiploic) foramen

Gallbladder

Diaphragm

Liver

Gastro-omental (gastroepiploic) arterial anastomosis (enclosed in gastrocolic ligament)

Stomach (posterior surface)

Caudate lobe of liver

Probe in superior recess of omental bursa

Left gastric artery (in gastropancreatic fold)

Left inferior phrenic artery (retroperitoneal)

Gastrophrenic ligament

Left suprarenal gland (retroperitoneal)

Gastro-splenic (gastro-lienal) ligament

Spleen

Right colic (hepatic) flexure

Kidney (retroperitoneal)

Descending (2nd) part of duodenum

Right gastro-omental (gastroepiploic) artery (covered by peritoneum)

Anterior superior pancreatico-duodenal artery (retroperitoneal)

Head of pancreas (retroperitoneal)

Transverse mesocolon

Body of pancreas (retroperitoneal)

Posterior layers
Anterior layers (cut) } of gastrocolic ligament

Tail of pancreas (intraperitoneal)

Splenorenal (lienorenal) ligament

Phrenicocolic ligament

Left colic (splenic) flexure

f. Netter m.d.

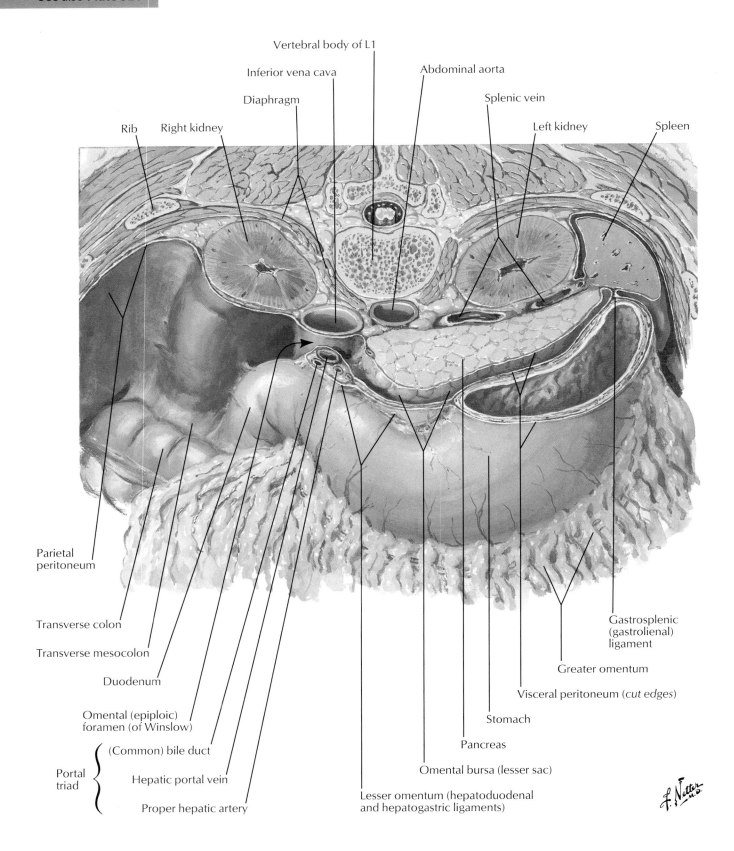

Vertebral body of L1

Inferior vena cava

Diaphragm

Abdominal aorta

Splenic vein

Rib   Right kidney

Left kidney

Spleen

Parietal
peritoneum

Transverse colon

Transverse mesocolon

Duodenum

Omental (epiploic)
foramen (of Winslow)

(Common) bile duct

Portal
triad

Hepatic portal vein

Proper hepatic artery

Lesser omentum (hepatoduodenal
and hepatogastric ligaments)

Omental bursa (lesser sac)

Pancreas

Stomach

Visceral peritoneum (*cut edges*)

Greater omentum

Gastrosplenic
(gastrolienal)
ligament

f. Netter
m.d.

Plate 265

Peritoneal Cavity

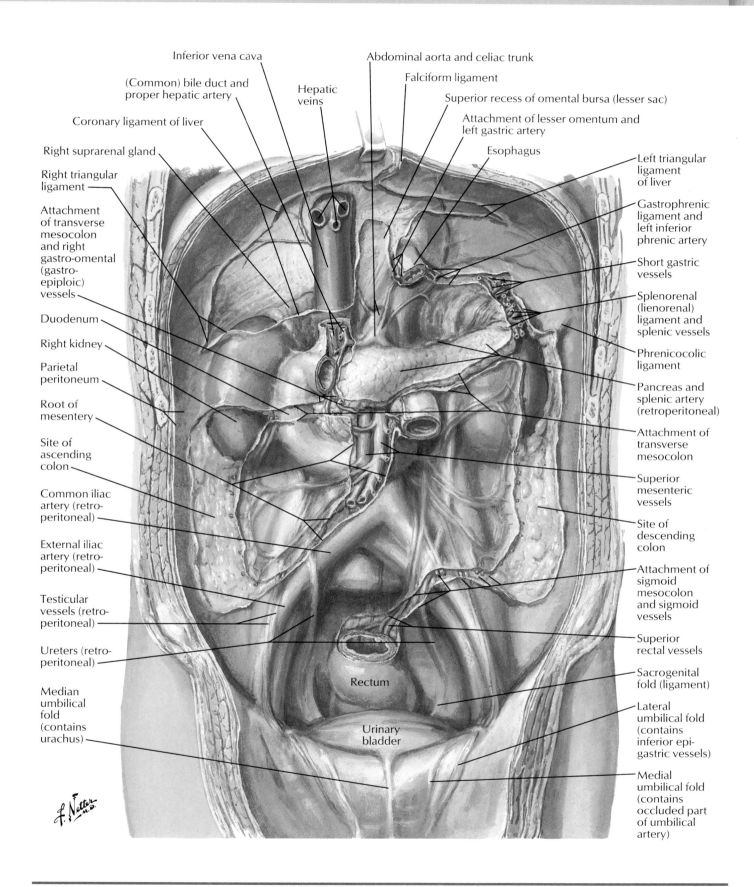

Inferior vena cava

(Common) bile duct and proper hepatic artery

Hepatic veins

Abdominal aorta and celiac trunk

Falciform ligament

Superior recess of omental bursa (lesser sac)

Attachment of lesser omentum and left gastric artery

Coronary ligament of liver

Esophagus

Right suprarenal gland

Left triangular ligament of liver

Right triangular ligament

Gastrophrenic ligament and left inferior phrenic artery

Attachment of transverse mesocolon and right gastro-omental (gastro-epiploic) vessels

Short gastric vessels

Splenorenal (lienorenal) ligament and splenic vessels

Duodenum

Right kidney

Phrenicocolic ligament

Parietal peritoneum

Pancreas and splenic artery (retroperitoneal)

Root of mesentery

Attachment of transverse mesocolon

Site of ascending colon

Superior mesenteric vessels

Common iliac artery (retro-peritoneal)

Site of descending colon

External iliac artery (retro-peritoneal)

Attachment of sigmoid mesocolon and sigmoid vessels

Testicular vessels (retro-peritoneal)

Superior rectal vessels

Ureters (retro-peritoneal)

Sacrogenital fold (ligament)

Median umbilical fold (contains urachus)

Rectum

Lateral umbilical fold (contains inferior epi-gastric vessels)

Urinary bladder

Medial umbilical fold (contains occluded part of umbilical artery)

f. Netter M.D.

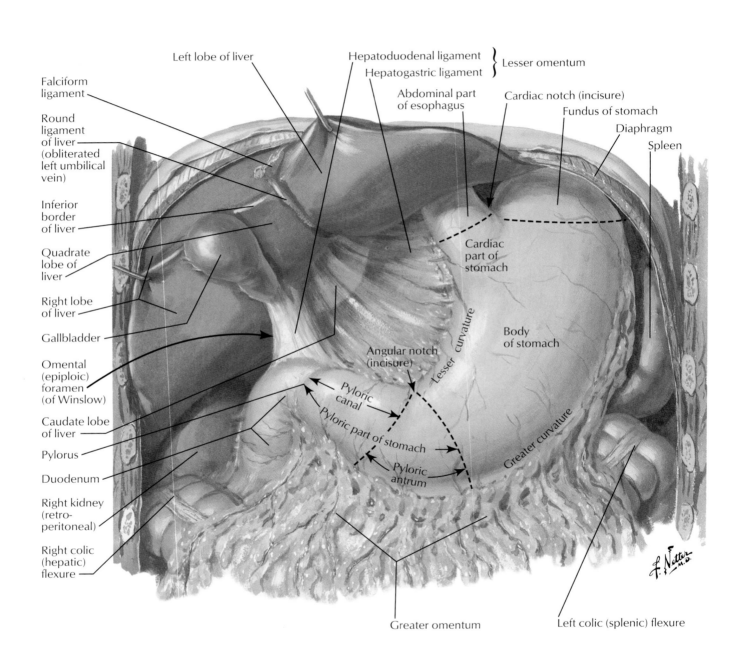

Falciform ligament

Round ligament of liver (obliterated left umbilical vein)

Inferior border of liver

Quadrate lobe of liver

Right lobe of liver

Gallbladder

Omental (epiploic) foramen (of Winslow)

Caudate lobe of liver

Pylorus

Duodenum

Right kidney (retroperitoneal)

Right colic (hepatic) flexure

Left lobe of liver

Hepatoduodenal ligament
Hepatogastric ligament ⎫ Lesser omentum

Abdominal part of esophagus

Cardiac notch (incisure)

Fundus of stomach

Diaphragm

Spleen

Cardiac part of stomach

Body of stomach

Lesser curvature

Angular notch (incisure)

Pyloric canal

Pyloric part of stomach

Pyloric antrum

Greater curvature

Greater omentum

Left colic (splenic) flexure

Plate 267

Viscera (Gut)

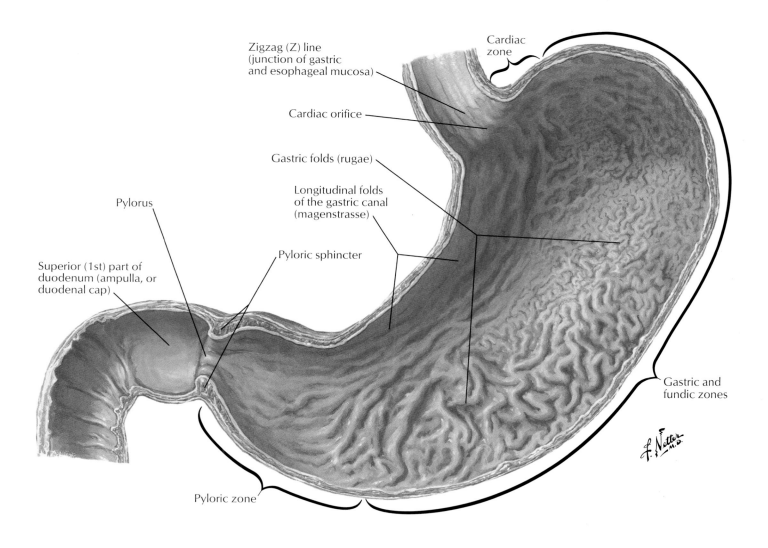

Zigzag (Z) line
(junction of gastric
and esophageal mucosa)

Cardiac
zone

Cardiac orifice

Gastric folds (rugae)

Longitudinal folds
of the gastric canal
(magenstrasse)

Pylorus

Pyloric sphincter

Superior (1st) part of
duodenum (ampulla, or
duodenal cap)

Gastric and
fundic zones

Pyloric zone

F. Netter M.D.

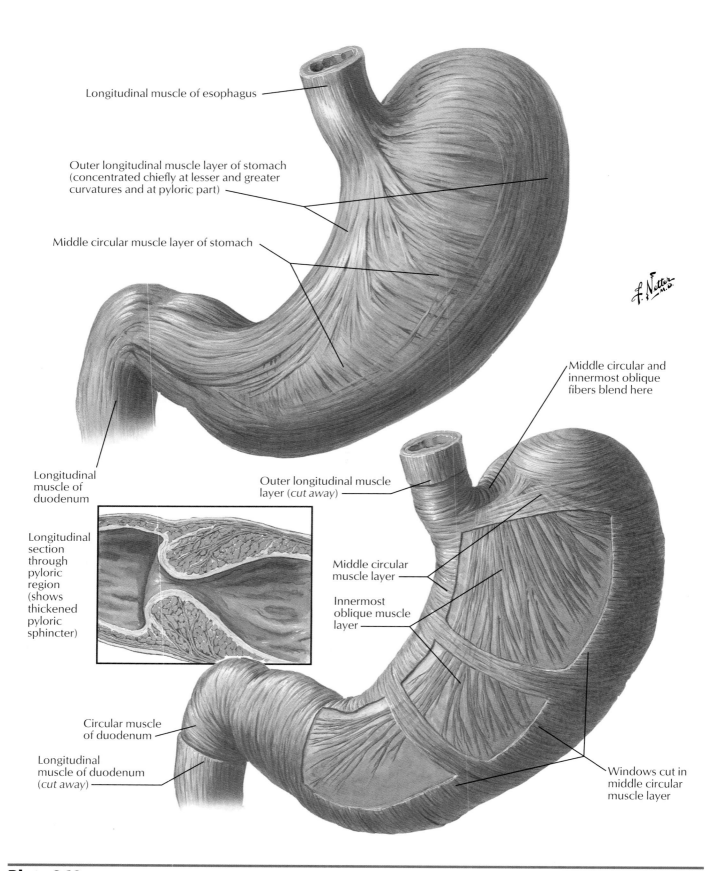

Longitudinal muscle of esophagus

Outer longitudinal muscle layer of stomach (concentrated chiefly at lesser and greater curvatures and at pyloric part)

Middle circular muscle layer of stomach

Middle circular and innermost oblique fibers blend here

Longitudinal muscle of duodenum

Outer longitudinal muscle layer (*cut away*)

Middle circular muscle layer

Longitudinal section through pyloric region (shows thickened pyloric sphincter)

Innermost oblique muscle layer

Circular muscle of duodenum

Longitudinal muscle of duodenum (*cut away*)

Windows cut in middle circular muscle layer

Plate 269   **Viscera (Gut)**

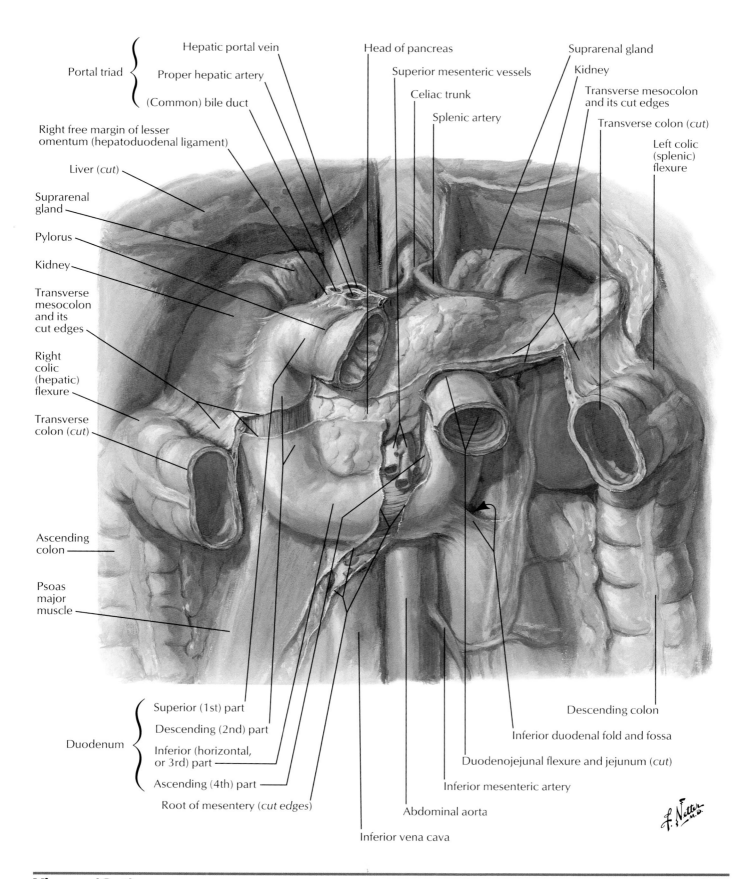

Portal triad
- Hepatic portal vein
- Proper hepatic artery
- (Common) bile duct

Head of pancreas

Superior mesenteric vessels

Celiac trunk

Splenic artery

Suprarenal gland

Kidney

Transverse mesocolon and its cut edges

Transverse colon (cut)

Left colic (splenic) flexure

Right free margin of lesser omentum (hepatoduodenal ligament)

Liver (cut)

Suprarenal gland

Pylorus

Kidney

Transverse mesocolon and its cut edges

Right colic (hepatic) flexure

Transverse colon (cut)

Ascending colon

Psoas major muscle

Suprarenal gland

Kidney

Transverse mesocolon and its cut edges

Descending colon

Inferior duodenal fold and fossa

Duodenum
- Superior (1st) part
- Descending (2nd) part
- Inferior (horizontal, or 3rd) part
- Ascending (4th) part

Root of mesentery (cut edges)

Duodenojejunal flexure and jejunum (cut)

Inferior mesenteric artery

Abdominal aorta

Inferior vena cava

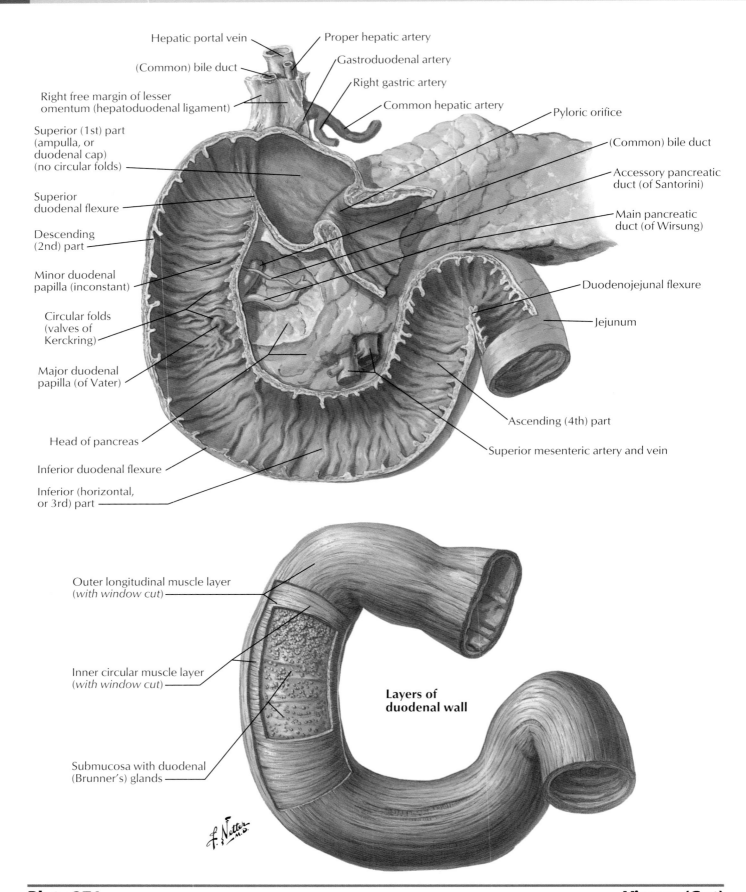

Hepatic portal vein

Proper hepatic artery

(Common) bile duct

Gastroduodenal artery

Right gastric artery

Right free margin of lesser omentum (hepatoduodenal ligament)

Common hepatic artery

Pyloric orifice

Superior (1st) part (ampulla, or duodenal cap) (no circular folds)

(Common) bile duct

Accessory pancreatic duct (of Santorini)

Superior duodenal flexure

Main pancreatic duct (of Wirsung)

Descending (2nd) part

Minor duodenal papilla (inconstant)

Duodenojejunal flexure

Circular folds (valves of Kerckring)

Jejunum

Major duodenal papilla (of Vater)

Head of pancreas

Ascending (4th) part

Inferior duodenal flexure

Superior mesenteric artery and vein

Inferior (horizontal, or 3rd) part

Outer longitudinal muscle layer (*with window cut*)

Inner circular muscle layer (*with window cut*)

Layers of duodenal wall

Submucosa with duodenal (Brunner's) glands

Plate 271

Viscera (Gut)

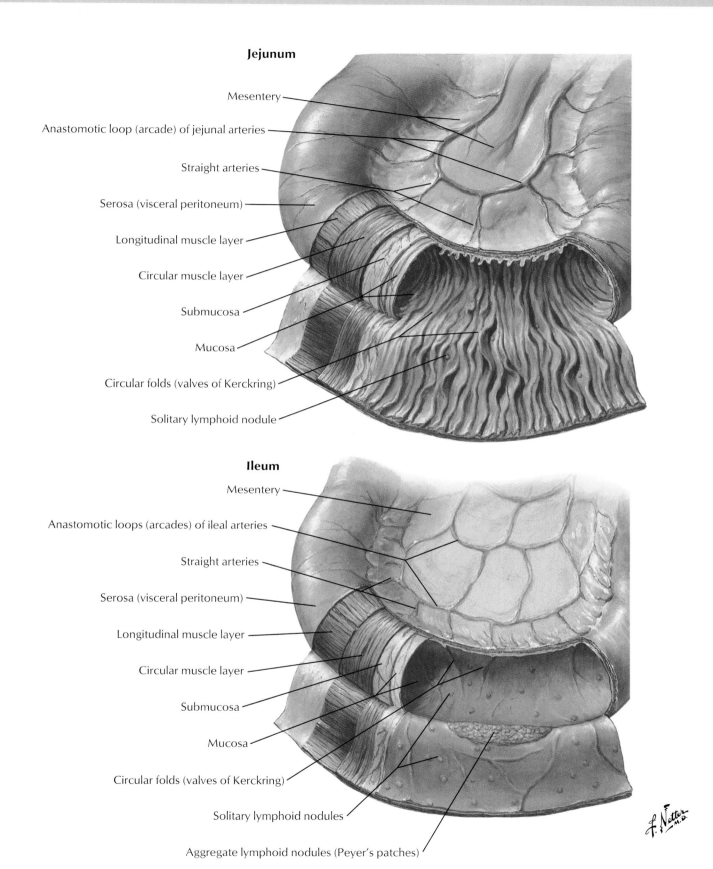

Jejunum

Mesentery

Anastomotic loop (arcade) of jejunal arteries

Straight arteries

Serosa (visceral peritoneum)

Longitudinal muscle layer

Circular muscle layer

Submucosa

Mucosa

Circular folds (valves of Kerckring)

Solitary lymphoid nodule

Ileum

Mesentery

Anastomotic loops (arcades) of ileal arteries

Straight arteries

Serosa (visceral peritoneum)

Longitudinal muscle layer

Circular muscle layer

Submucosa

Mucosa

Circular folds (valves of Kerckring)

Solitary lymphoid nodules

Aggregate lymphoid nodules (Peyer's patches)

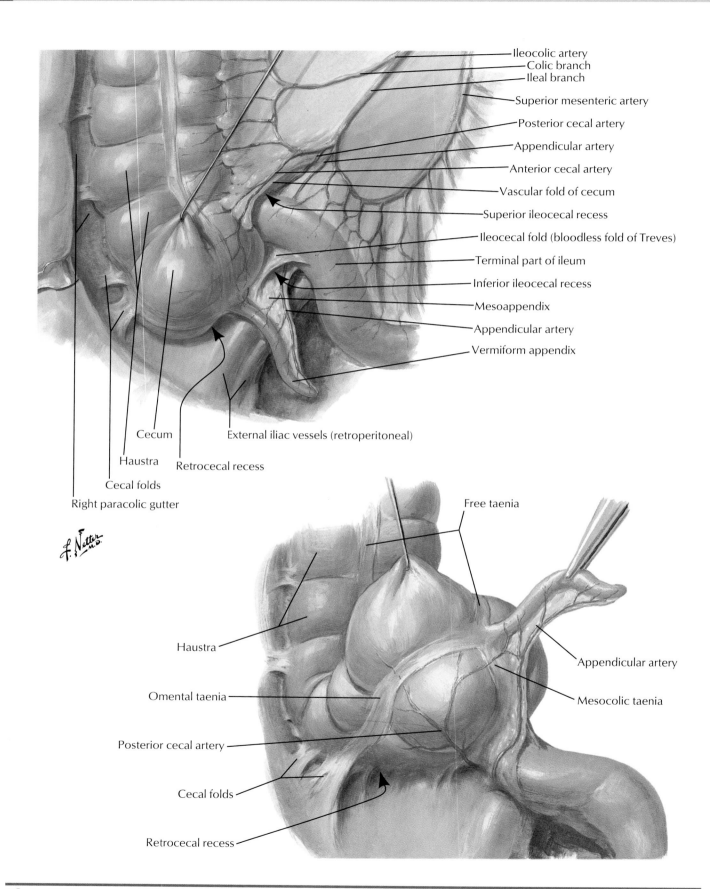

Ileocolic artery
Colic branch
Ileal branch
Superior mesenteric artery
Posterior cecal artery
Appendicular artery
Anterior cecal artery
Vascular fold of cecum
Superior ileocecal recess
Ileocecal fold (bloodless fold of Treves)
Terminal part of ileum
Inferior ileocecal recess
Mesoappendix
Appendicular artery
Vermiform appendix

External iliac vessels (retroperitoneal)
Cecum
Haustra
Retrocecal recess
Cecal folds
Right paracolic gutter

Free taenia

Haustra

Appendicular artery

Omental taenia

Mesocolic taenia

Posterior cecal artery

Cecal folds

Retrocecal recess

Plate 273

Viscera (Gut)

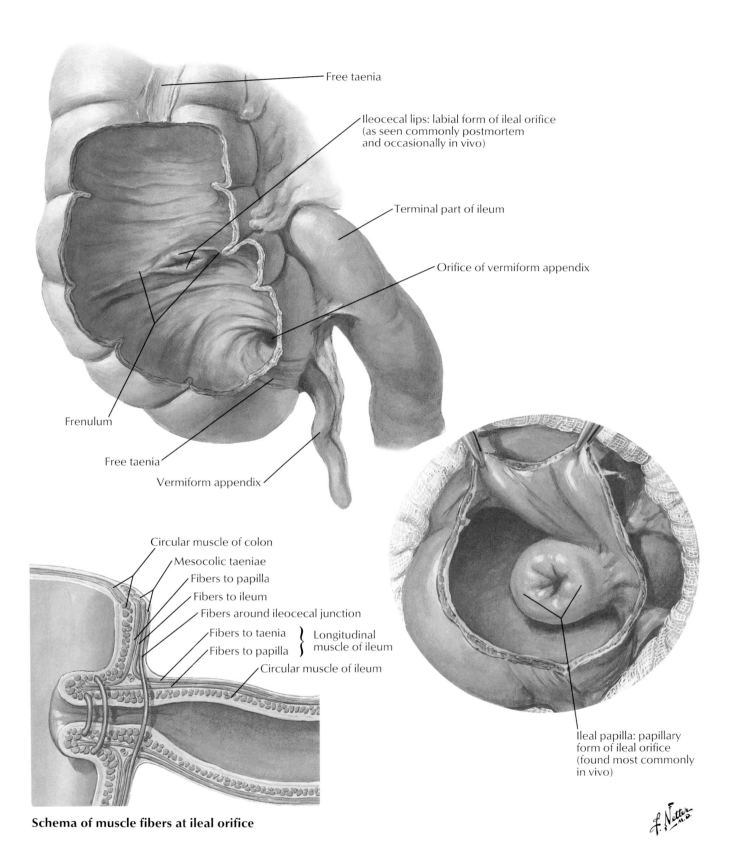

Free taenia

Ileocecal lips: labial form of ileal orifice (as seen commonly postmortem and occasionally in vivo)

Terminal part of ileum

Orifice of vermiform appendix

Frenulum

Free taenia

Vermiform appendix

Circular muscle of colon

Mesocolic taeniae

Fibers to papilla

Fibers to ileum

Fibers around ileocecal junction

Fibers to taenia } Longitudinal muscle of ileum

Fibers to papilla

Circular muscle of ileum

Schema of muscle fibers at ileal orifice

Ileal papilla: papillary form of ileal orifice (found most commonly in vivo)

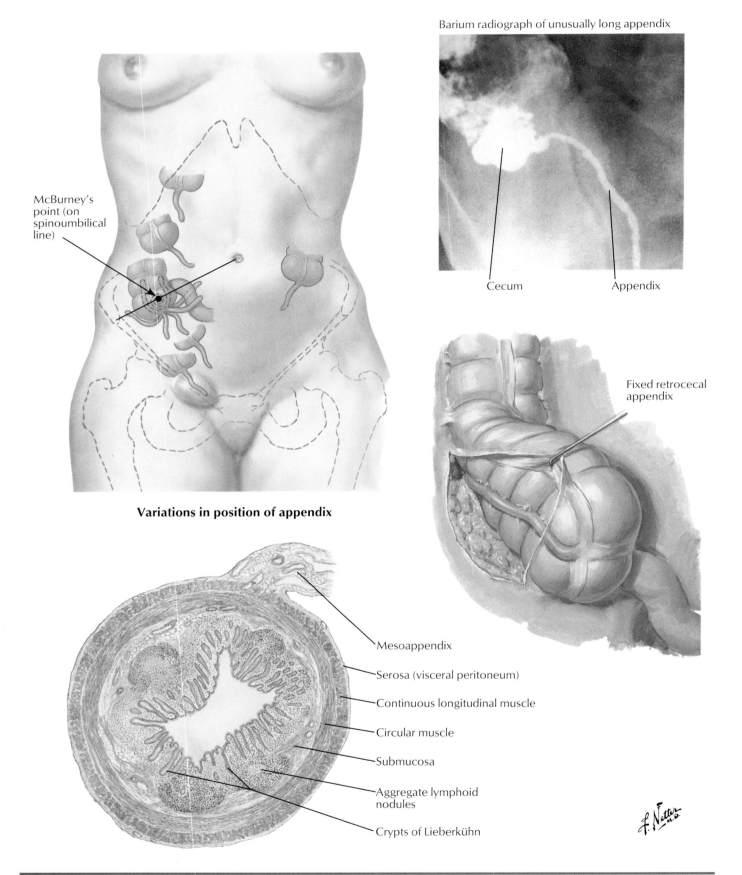

Barium radiograph of unusually long appendix

McBurney's point (on spinoumbilical line)

Cecum

Appendix

Variations in position of appendix

Fixed retrocecal appendix

Mesoappendix

Serosa (visceral peritoneum)

Continuous longitudinal muscle

Circular muscle

Submucosa

Aggregate lymphoid nodules

Crypts of Lieberkühn

Plate 275   **Viscera (Gut)**

For rectum and anal canal see **Plates 371-376**

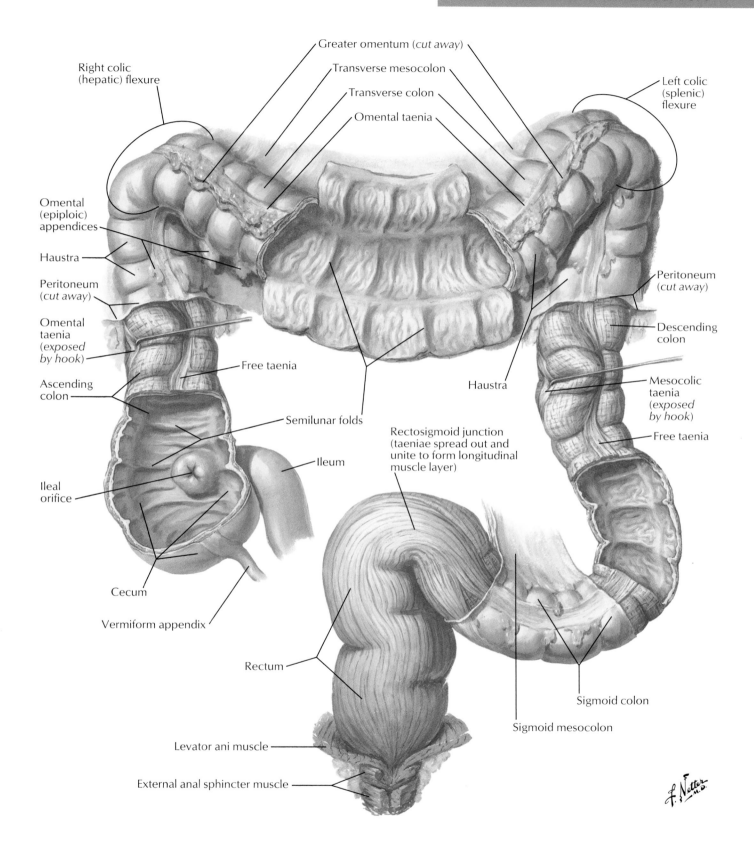

Greater omentum (*cut away*)

Transverse mesocolon

Transverse colon

Omental taenia

Right colic (hepatic) flexure

Left colic (splenic) flexure

Omental (epiploic) appendices

Haustra

Peritoneum (*cut away*)

Omental taenia (*exposed by hook*)

Ascending colon

Ileal orifice

Cecum

Vermiform appendix

Free taenia

Semilunar folds

Ileum

Rectum

Levator ani muscle

External anal sphincter muscle

Peritoneum (*cut away*)

Descending colon

Haustra

Mesocolic taenia (*exposed by hook*)

Free taenia

Rectosigmoid junction (taeniae spread out and unite to form longitudinal muscle layer)

Sigmoid colon

Sigmoid mesocolon

F. Netter M.D.

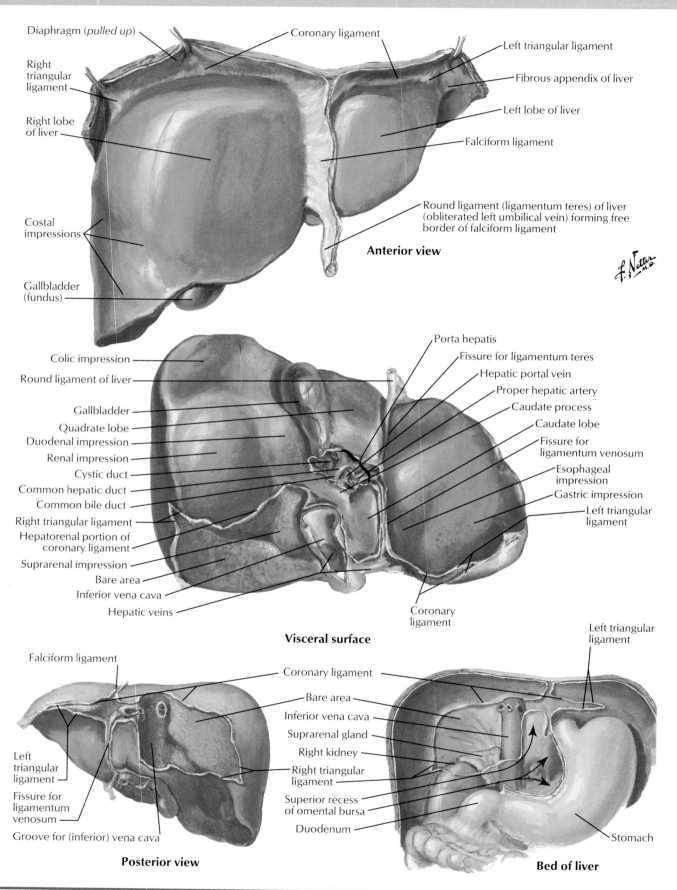

Diaphragm (*pulled up*)

Coronary ligament

Left triangular ligament

Right triangular ligament

Fibrous appendix of liver

Right lobe of liver

Left lobe of liver

Falciform ligament

Costal impressions

Round ligament (ligamentum teres) of liver (obliterated left umbilical vein) forming free border of falciform ligament

Gallbladder (fundus)

Anterior view

Colic impression

Porta hepatis

Round ligament of liver

Fissure for ligamentum teres

Hepatic portal vein

Gallbladder

Proper hepatic artery

Quadrate lobe

Caudate process

Duodenal impression

Caudate lobe

Renal impression

Fissure for ligamentum venosum

Cystic duct

Esophageal impression

Common hepatic duct

Gastric impression

Common bile duct

Left triangular ligament

Right triangular ligament

Hepatorenal portion of coronary ligament

Suprarenal impression

Bare area

Inferior vena cava

Hepatic veins

Coronary ligament

Visceral surface

Falciform ligament

Left triangular ligament

Coronary ligament

Bare area

Inferior vena cava

Suprarenal gland

Right kidney

Left triangular ligament

Right triangular ligament

Fissure for ligamentum venosum

Superior recess of omental bursa

Groove for (inferior) vena cava

Duodenum

Stomach

Posterior view

Bed of liver

Plate 277

Viscera (Accessory Organs)

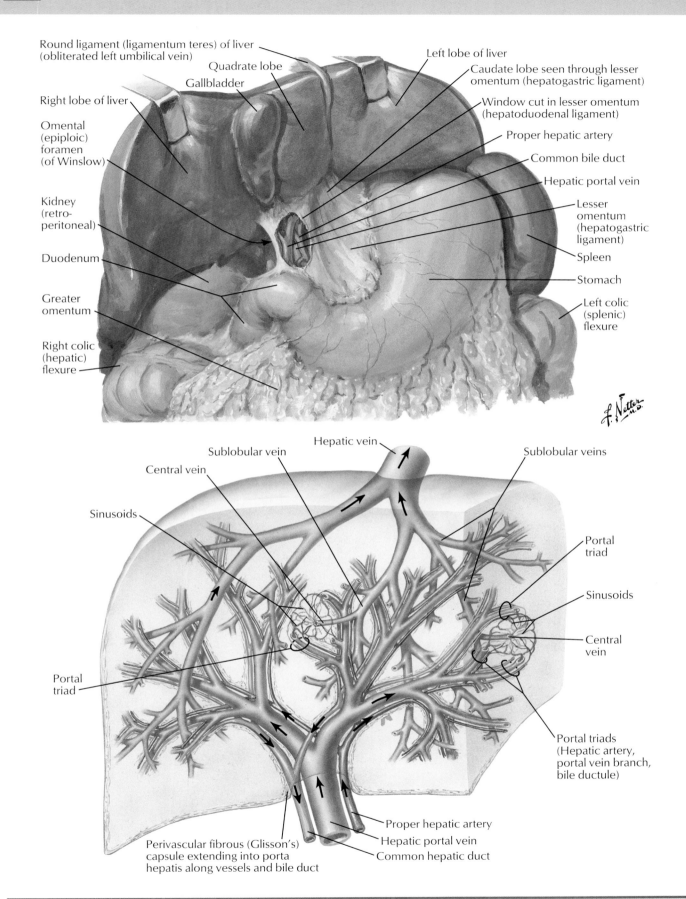

Round ligament (ligamentum teres) of liver (obliterated left umbilical vein)

Quadrate lobe

Gallbladder

Right lobe of liver

Omental (epiploic) foramen (of Winslow)

Kidney (retro-peritoneal)

Duodenum

Greater omentum

Right colic (hepatic) flexure

Left lobe of liver

Caudate lobe seen through lesser omentum (hepatogastric ligament)

Window cut in lesser omentum (hepatoduodenal ligament)

Proper hepatic artery

Common bile duct

Hepatic portal vein

Lesser omentum (hepatogastric ligament)

Spleen

Stomach

Left colic (splenic) flexure

Hepatic vein

Sublobular vein

Central vein

Sinusoids

Portal triad

Sublobular veins

Portal triad

Sinusoids

Central vein

Portal triads (Hepatic artery, portal vein branch, bile ductule)

Proper hepatic artery

Hepatic portal vein

Common hepatic duct

Perivascular fibrous (Glisson's) capsule extending into porta hepatis along vessels and bile duct

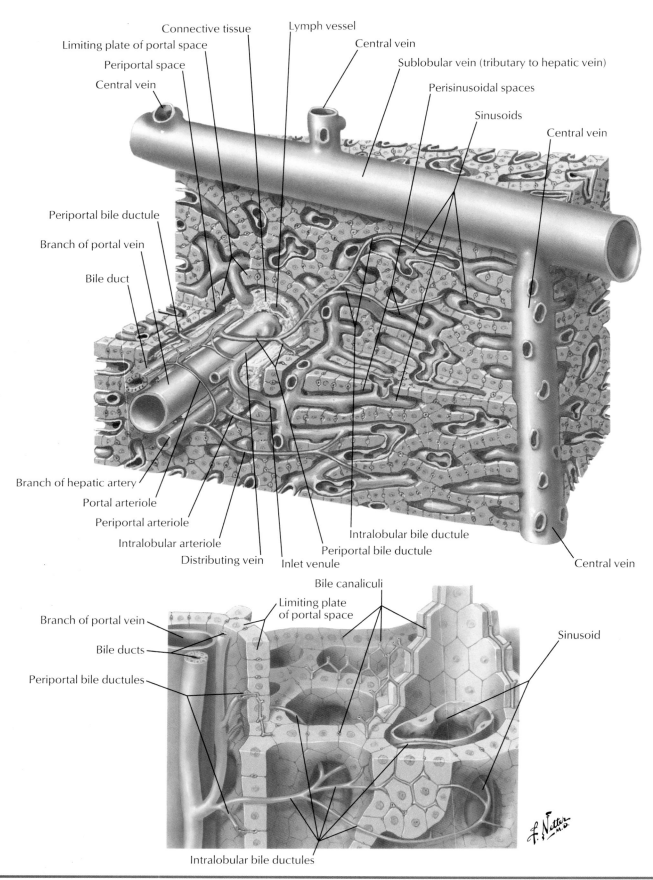

Connective tissue

Limiting plate of portal space

Periportal space

Central vein

Lymph vessel

Central vein

Sublobular vein (tributary to hepatic vein)

Perisinusoidal spaces

Sinusoids

Central vein

Periportal bile ductule

Branch of portal vein

Bile duct

Branch of hepatic artery

Portal arteriole

Periportal arteriole

Intralobular arteriole

Distributing vein

Inlet venule

Periportal bile ductule

Intralobular bile ductule

Central vein

Bile canaliculi

Limiting plate of portal space

Branch of portal vein

Bile ducts

Periportal bile ductules

Sinusoid

Intralobular bile ductules

Plate 279

Viscera (Accessory Organs)

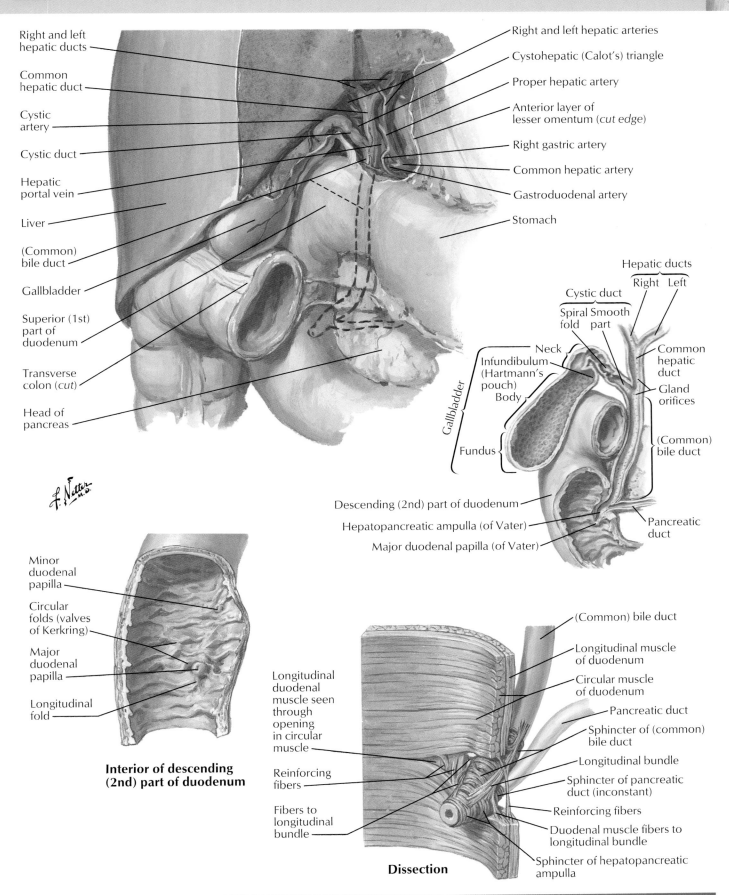

Right and left hepatic ducts

Common hepatic duct

Cystic artery

Cystic duct

Hepatic portal vein

Liver

(Common) bile duct

Gallbladder

Superior (1st) part of duodenum

Transverse colon (cut)

Head of pancreas

Right and left hepatic arteries

Cystohepatic (Calot's) triangle

Proper hepatic artery

Anterior layer of lesser omentum (cut edge)

Right gastric artery

Common hepatic artery

Gastroduodenal artery

Stomach

Hepatic ducts
Right   Left

Cystic duct

Spiral   Smooth
fold   part

Neck

Infundibulum (Hartmann's pouch)

Body

Gallbladder

Fundus

Common hepatic duct

Gland orifices

(Common) bile duct

Descending (2nd) part of duodenum

Hepatopancreatic ampulla (of Vater)

Major duodenal papilla (of Vater)

Pancreatic duct

Minor duodenal papilla

Circular folds (valves of Kerkring)

Major duodenal papilla

Longitudinal fold

Interior of descending (2nd) part of duodenum

Longitudinal duodenal muscle seen through opening in circular muscle

Reinforcing fibers

Fibers to longitudinal bundle

(Common) bile duct

Longitudinal muscle of duodenum

Circular muscle of duodenum

Pancreatic duct

Sphincter of (common) bile duct

Longitudinal bundle

Sphincter of pancreatic duct (inconstant)

Reinforcing fibers

Duodenal muscle fibers to longitudinal bundle

Sphincter of hepatopancreatic ampulla

Dissection

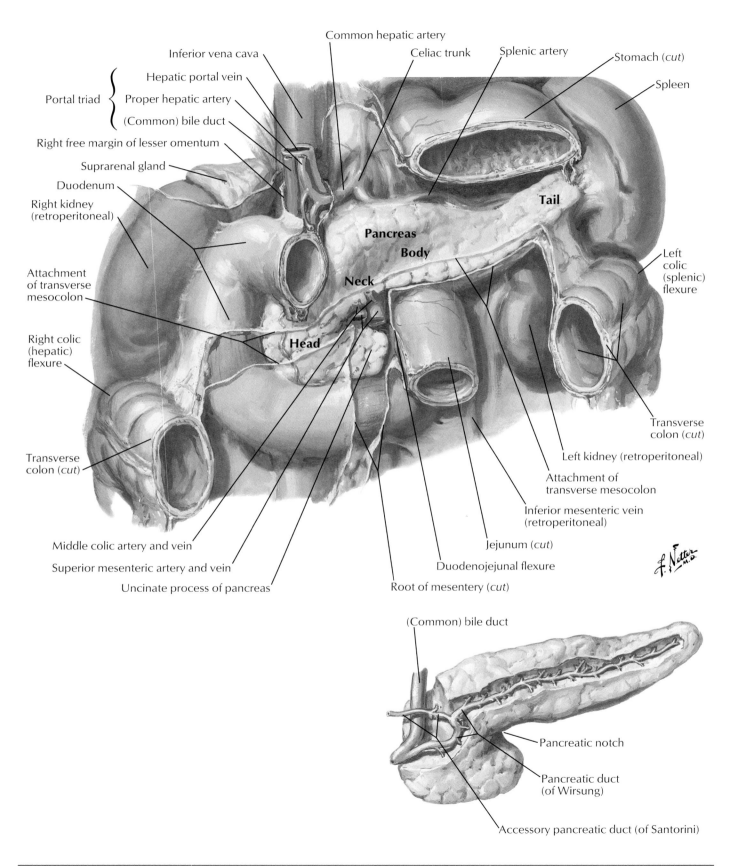

Common hepatic artery

Inferior vena cava

Celiac trunk

Splenic artery

Stomach (*cut*)

Hepatic portal vein

Spleen

Portal triad { Proper hepatic artery

(Common) bile duct

Right free margin of lesser omentum

Suprarenal gland

Tail

Duodenum

Pancreas

Right kidney
(retroperitoneal)

Body

Left
colic
(splenic)
flexure

Neck

Attachment
of transverse
mesocolon

Right colic
(hepatic)
flexure

Head

Transverse
colon (*cut*)

Transverse
colon (*cut*)

Left kidney (retroperitoneal)

Attachment of
transverse mesocolon

Inferior mesenteric vein
(retroperitoneal)

Middle colic artery and vein

Jejunum (*cut*)

Superior mesenteric artery and vein

Duodenojejunal flexure

Uncinate process of pancreas

Root of mesentery (*cut*)

(Common) bile duct

Pancreatic notch

Pancreatic duct
(of Wirsung)

Accessory pancreatic duct (of Santorini)

Plate 281   **Viscera (Accessory Organs)**

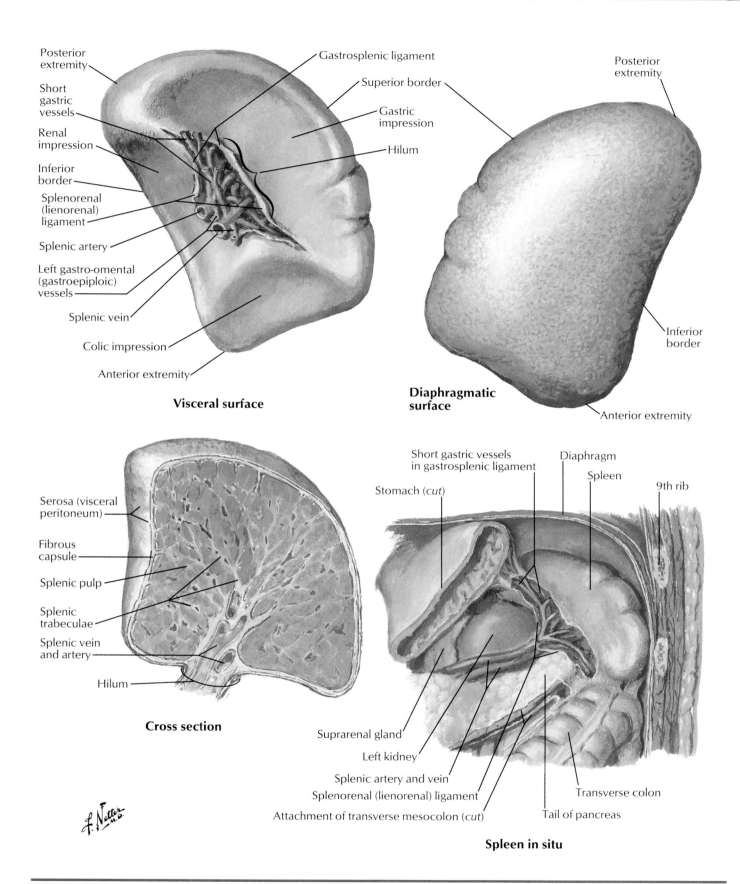

Posterior extremity

Short gastric vessels

Renal impression

Inferior border

Splenorenal (lienorenal) ligament

Splenic artery

Left gastro-omental (gastroepiploic) vessels

Splenic vein

Colic impression

Anterior extremity

Gastrosplenic ligament

Superior border

Gastric impression

Hilum

Visceral surface

Posterior extremity

Inferior border

Anterior extremity

Diaphragmatic surface

Serosa (visceral peritoneum)

Fibrous capsule

Splenic pulp

Splenic trabeculae

Splenic vein and artery

Hilum

Cross section

Short gastric vessels in gastrosplenic ligament

Stomach (cut)

Diaphragm

Spleen

9th rib

Suprarenal gland

Left kidney

Splenic artery and vein

Splenorenal (lienorenal) ligament

Attachment of transverse mesocolon (cut)

Tail of pancreas

Transverse colon

Spleen in situ

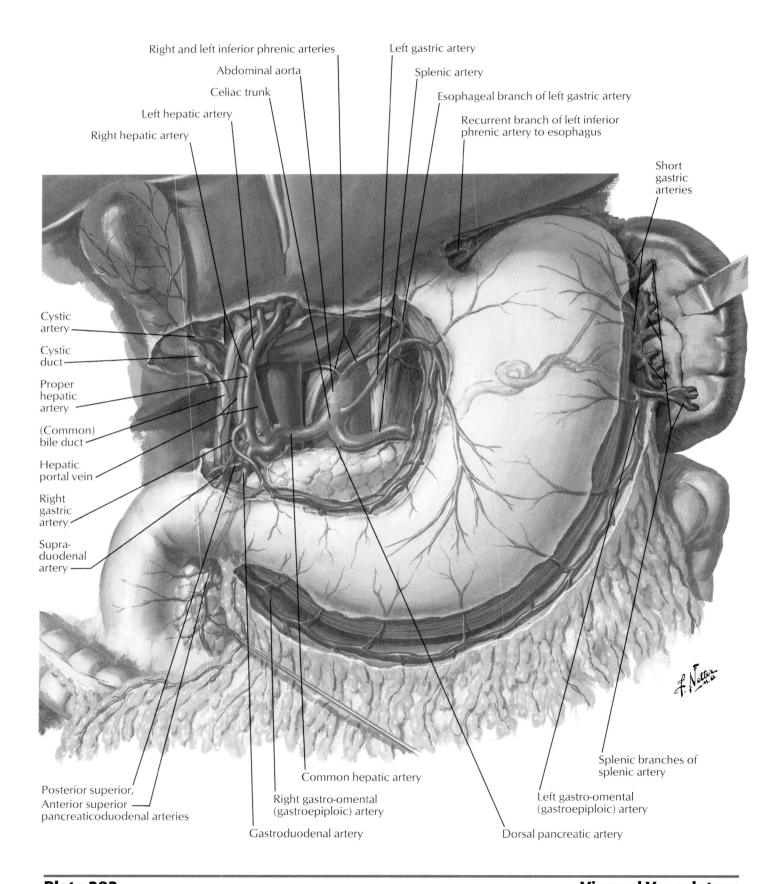

Right and left inferior phrenic arteries

Abdominal aorta

Celiac trunk

Left hepatic artery

Right hepatic artery

Left gastric artery

Splenic artery

Esophageal branch of left gastric artery

Recurrent branch of left inferior phrenic artery to esophagus

Short gastric arteries

Cystic artery

Cystic duct

Proper hepatic artery

(Common) bile duct

Hepatic portal vein

Right gastric artery

Supra-duodenal artery

Posterior superior, Anterior superior pancreaticoduodenal arteries

Right gastro-omental (gastroepiploic) artery

Gastroduodenal artery

Common hepatic artery

Dorsal pancreatic artery

Left gastro-omental (gastroepiploic) artery

Splenic branches of splenic artery

F. Netter M.D.

Plate 283   **Visceral Vasculature**

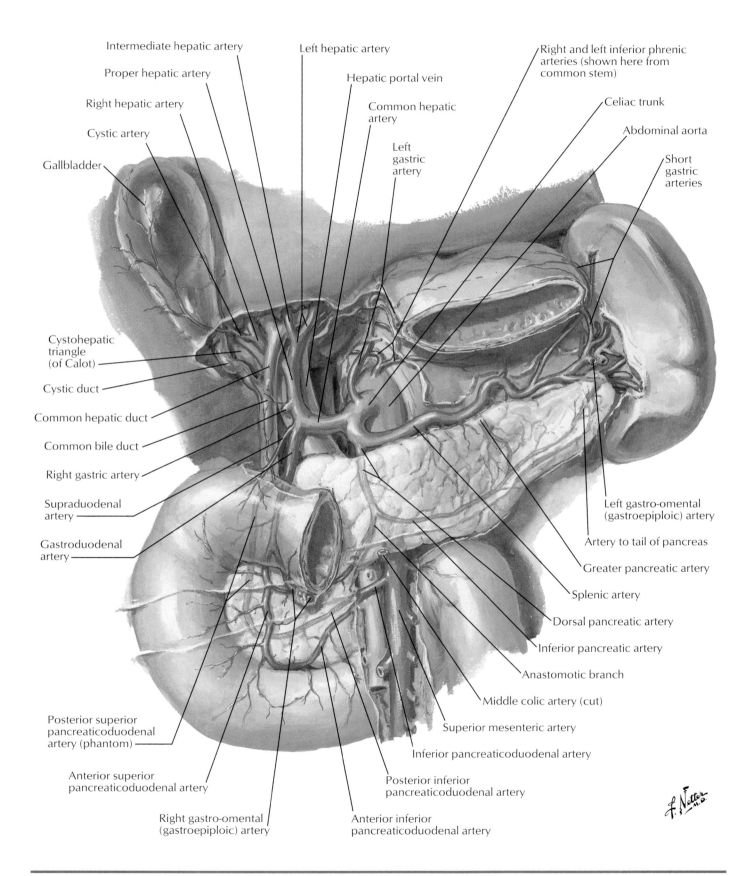

Intermediate hepatic artery

Proper hepatic artery

Right hepatic artery

Cystic artery

Gallbladder

Left hepatic artery

Hepatic portal vein

Common hepatic artery

Left gastric artery

Right and left inferior phrenic arteries (shown here from common stem)

Celiac trunk

Abdominal aorta

Short gastric arteries

Cystohepatic triangle (of Calot)

Cystic duct

Common hepatic duct

Common bile duct

Right gastric artery

Supraduodenal artery

Gastroduodenal artery

Posterior superior pancreaticoduodenal artery (phantom)

Anterior superior pancreaticoduodenal artery

Right gastro-omental (gastroepiploic) artery

Anterior inferior pancreaticoduodenal artery

Posterior inferior pancreaticoduodenal artery

Inferior pancreaticoduodenal artery

Superior mesenteric artery

Middle colic artery (cut)

Anastomotic branch

Inferior pancreatic artery

Dorsal pancreatic artery

Splenic artery

Greater pancreatic artery

Artery to tail of pancreas

Left gastro-omental (gastroepiploic) artery

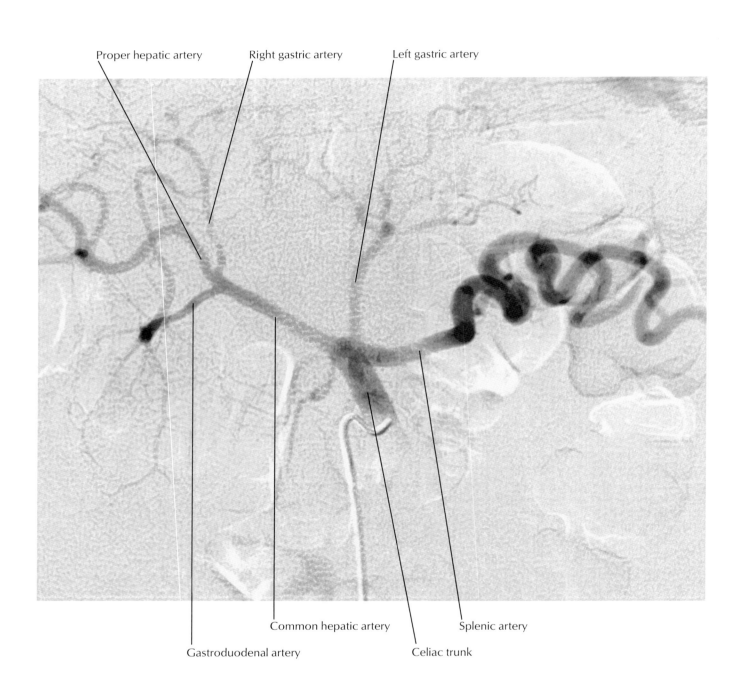

Proper hepatic artery   Right gastric artery   Left gastric artery

Gastroduodenal artery   Common hepatic artery   Celiac trunk   Splenic artery

Plate 285

Visceral Vasculature

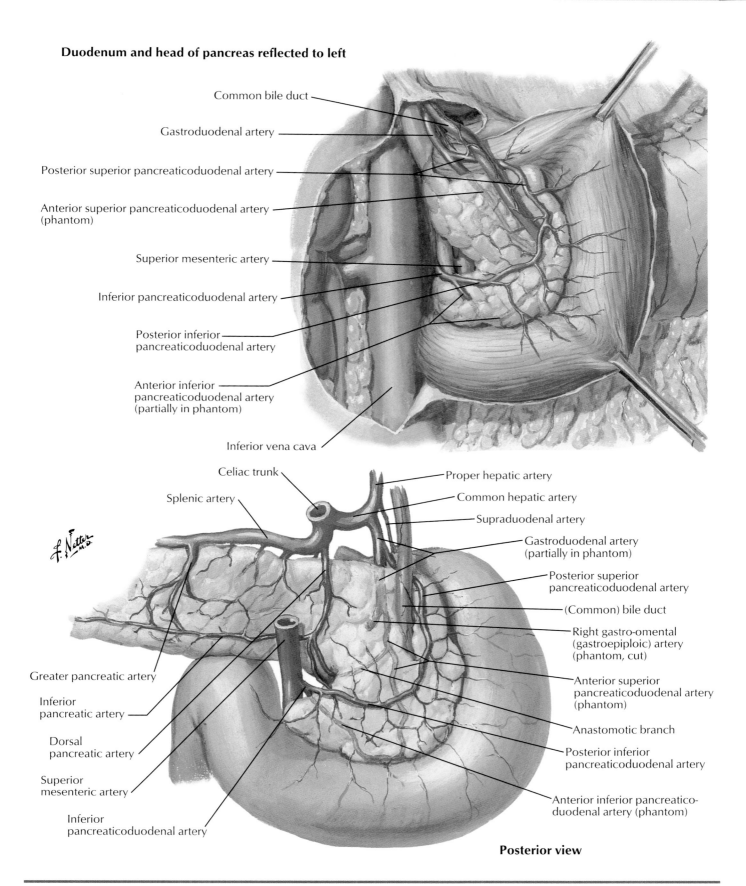

Duodenum and head of pancreas reflected to left

Common bile duct

Gastroduodenal artery

Posterior superior pancreaticoduodenal artery

Anterior superior pancreaticoduodenal artery (phantom)

Superior mesenteric artery

Inferior pancreaticoduodenal artery

Posterior inferior pancreaticoduodenal artery

Anterior inferior pancreaticoduodenal artery (partially in phantom)

Inferior vena cava

Celiac trunk

Splenic artery

Proper hepatic artery

Common hepatic artery

Supraduodenal artery

Gastroduodenal artery (partially in phantom)

Posterior superior pancreaticoduodenal artery

(Common) bile duct

Right gastro-omental (gastroepiploic) artery (phantom, cut)

Anterior superior pancreaticoduodenal artery (phantom)

Anastomotic branch

Posterior inferior pancreaticoduodenal artery

Greater pancreatic artery

Inferior pancreatic artery

Dorsal pancreatic artery

Superior mesenteric artery

Inferior pancreaticoduodenal artery

Anterior inferior pancreatico-duodenal artery (phantom)

Posterior view

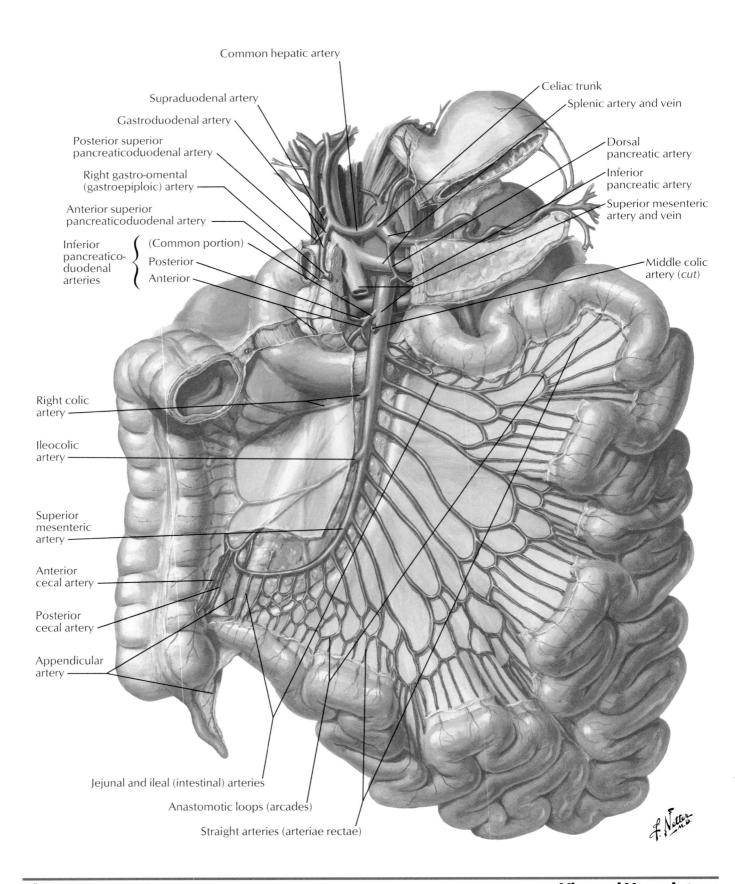

Common hepatic artery

Celiac trunk

Splenic artery and vein

Supraduodenal artery

Gastroduodenal artery

Posterior superior
pancreaticoduodenal artery

Dorsal
pancreatic artery

Inferior
pancreatic artery

Right gastro-omental
(gastroepiploic) artery

Superior mesenteric
artery and vein

Anterior superior
pancreaticoduodenal artery

Inferior
pancreatico-
duodenal
arteries

(Common portion)

Posterior

Anterior

Middle colic
artery (cut)

Right colic
artery

Ileocolic
artery

Superior
mesenteric
artery

Anterior
cecal artery

Posterior
cecal artery

Appendicular
artery

Jejunal and ileal (intestinal) arteries

Anastomotic loops (arcades)

Straight arteries (arteriae rectae)

Plate 287

Visceral Vasculature

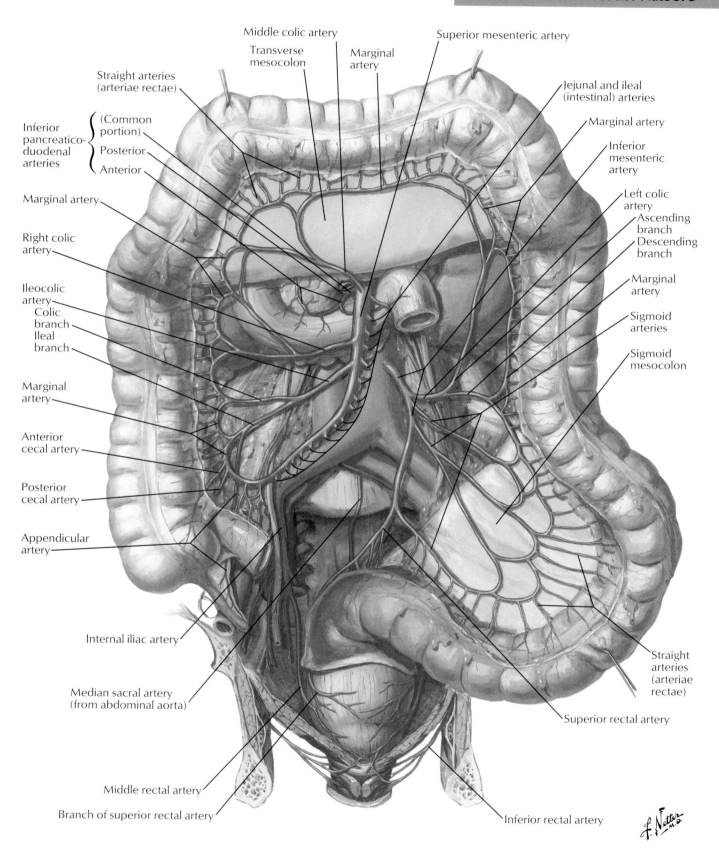

Middle colic artery

Transverse mesocolon

Marginal artery

Superior mesenteric artery

Jejunal and ileal (intestinal) arteries

Marginal artery

Inferior mesenteric artery

Left colic artery

Ascending branch

Descending branch

Marginal artery

Sigmoid arteries

Sigmoid mesocolon

Straight arteries (arteriae rectae)

Inferior pancreatico-duodenal arteries

(Common portion)

Posterior

Anterior

Marginal artery

Right colic artery

Ileocolic artery

Colic branch

Ileal branch

Marginal artery

Anterior cecal artery

Posterior cecal artery

Appendicular artery

Internal iliac artery

Median sacral artery (from abdominal aorta)

Straight arteries (arteriae rectae)

Superior rectal artery

Middle rectal artery

Branch of superior rectal artery

Inferior rectal artery

Veins of Stomach, Duodenum, Pancreas, and Spleen

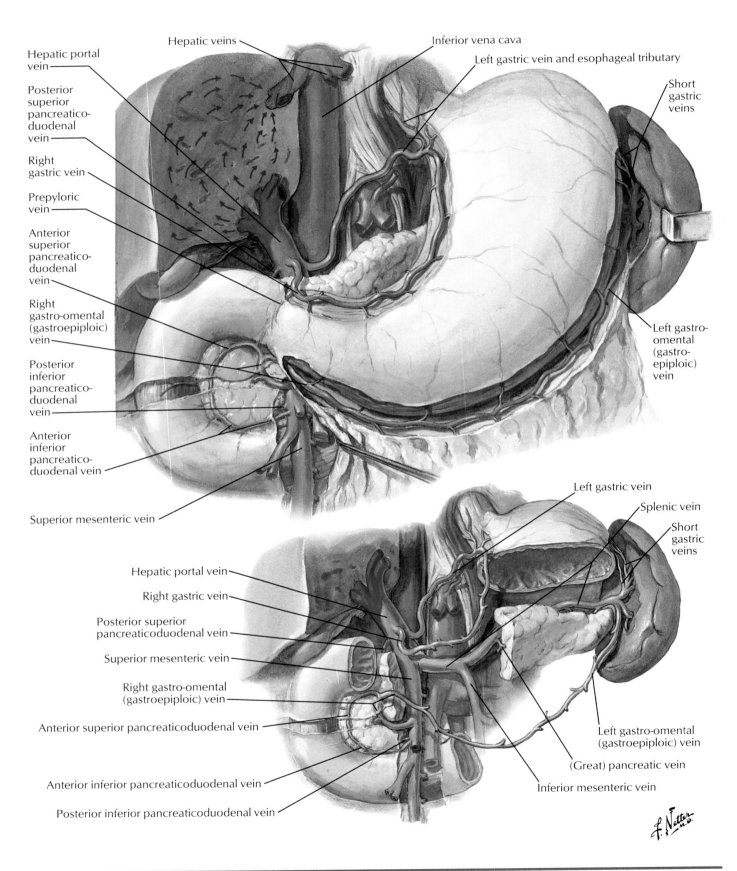

Hepatic veins

Inferior vena cava

Hepatic portal vein

Posterior superior pancreatico-duodenal vein

Right gastric vein

Prepyloric vein

Anterior superior pancreatico-duodenal vein

Right gastro-omental (gastroepiploic) vein

Posterior inferior pancreatico-duodenal vein

Anterior inferior pancreatico-duodenal vein

Superior mesenteric vein

Left gastric vein and esophageal tributary

Short gastric veins

Left gastro-omental (gastro-epiploic) vein

Hepatic portal vein

Right gastric vein

Posterior superior pancreaticoduodenal vein

Superior mesenteric vein

Right gastro-omental (gastroepiploic) vein

Anterior superior pancreaticoduodenal vein

Anterior inferior pancreaticoduodenal vein

Posterior inferior pancreaticoduodenal vein

Left gastric vein

Splenic vein

Short gastric veins

Left gastro-omental (gastroepiploic) vein

(Great) pancreatic vein

Inferior mesenteric vein

Plate 289

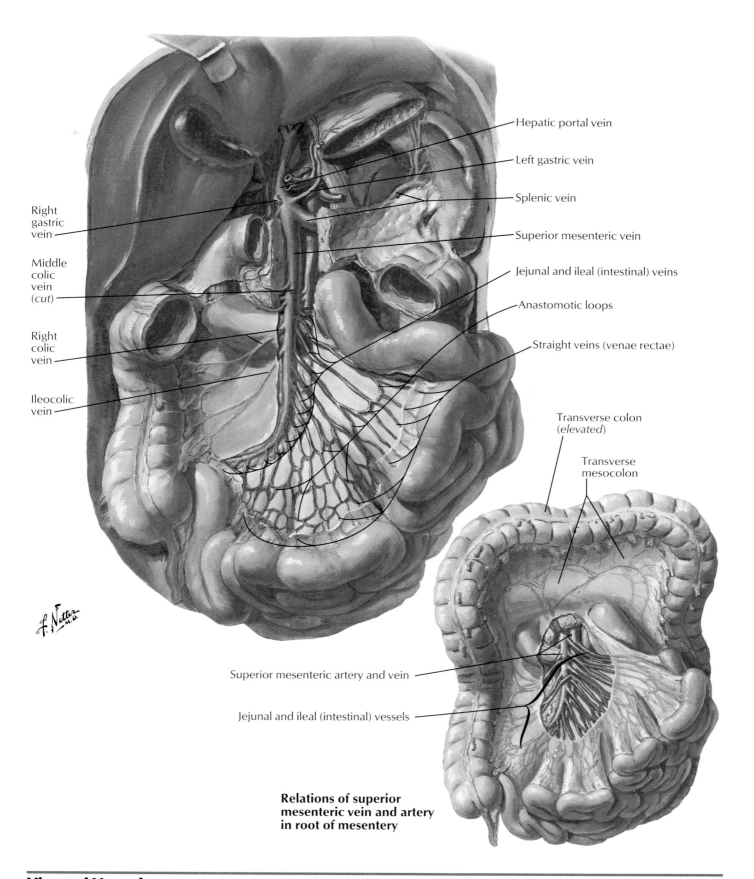

Right gastric vein

Middle colic vein (*cut*)

Right colic vein

Ileocolic vein

Hepatic portal vein

Left gastric vein

Splenic vein

Superior mesenteric vein

Jejunal and ileal (intestinal) veins

Anastomotic loops

Straight veins (venae rectae)

Transverse colon (*elevated*)

Transverse mesocolon

Superior mesenteric artery and vein

Jejunal and ileal (intestinal) vessels

Relations of superior mesenteric vein and artery in root of mesentery

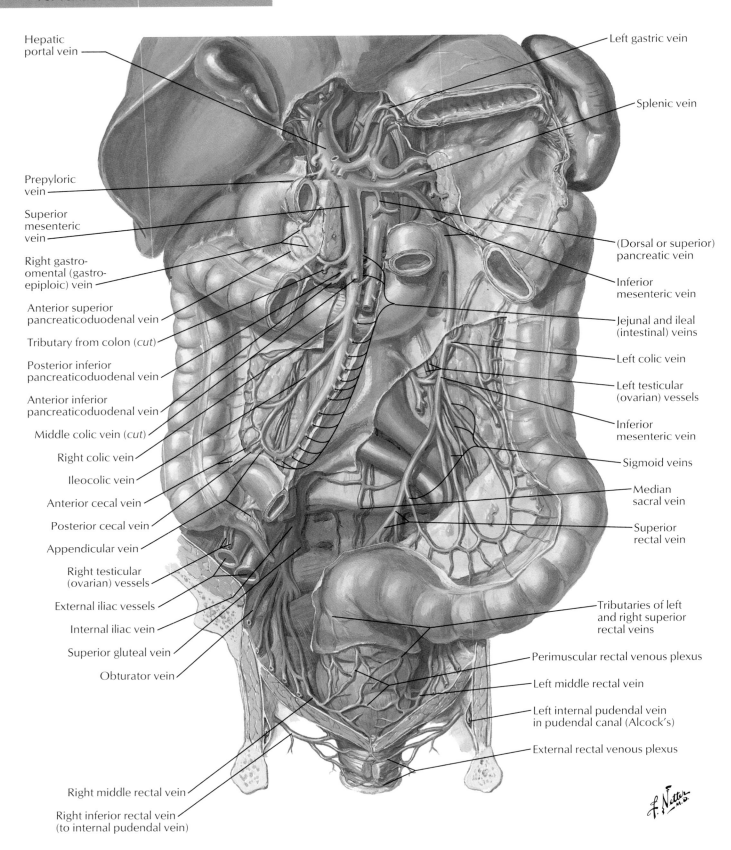

Hepatic portal vein

Left gastric vein

Splenic vein

Prepyloric vein

Superior mesenteric vein

Right gastro-omental (gastro-epiploic) vein

(Dorsal or superior) pancreatic vein

Inferior mesenteric vein

Anterior superior pancreaticoduodenal vein

Jejunal and ileal (intestinal) veins

Tributary from colon (cut)

Left colic vein

Posterior inferior pancreaticoduodenal vein

Left testicular (ovarian) vessels

Anterior inferior pancreaticoduodenal vein

Inferior mesenteric vein

Middle colic vein (cut)

Right colic vein

Sigmoid veins

Ileocolic vein

Median sacral vein

Anterior cecal vein

Superior rectal vein

Posterior cecal vein

Appendicular vein

Right testicular (ovarian) vessels

External iliac vessels

Tributaries of left and right superior rectal veins

Internal iliac vein

Perimuscular rectal venous plexus

Superior gluteal vein

Left middle rectal vein

Obturator vein

Left internal pudendal vein in pudendal canal (Alcock's)

External rectal venous plexus

Right middle rectal vein

Right inferior rectal vein (to internal pudendal vein)

Plate 291

Visceral Vasculature

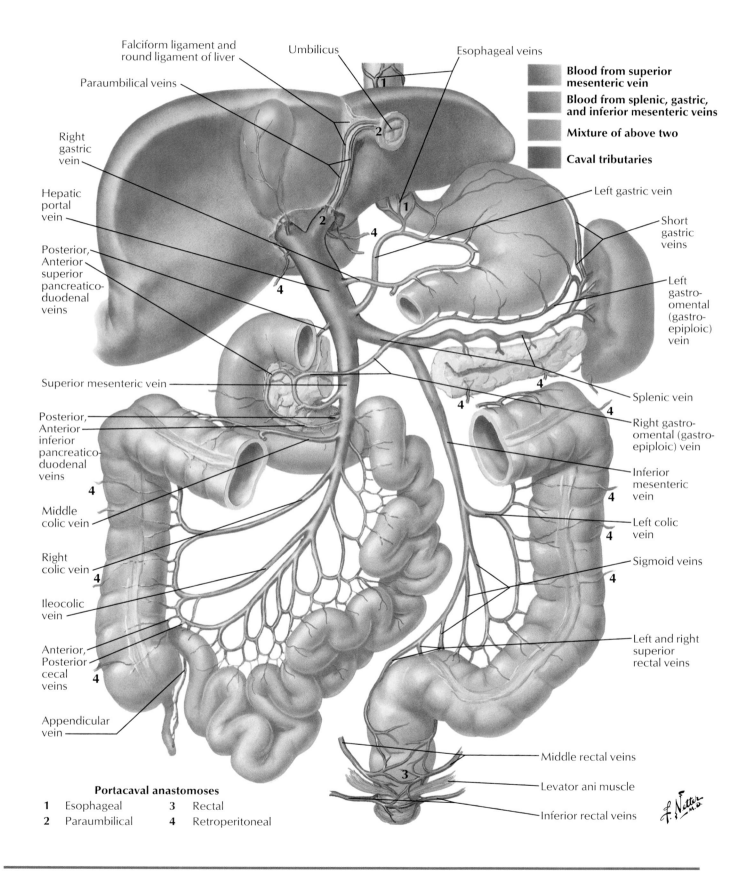

Falciform ligament and round ligament of liver

Umbilicus

Esophageal veins

Blood from superior mesenteric vein

Blood from splenic, gastric, and inferior mesenteric veins

Mixture of above two

Caval tributaries

Paraumbilical veins

Right gastric vein

Hepatic portal vein

Posterior, Anterior superior pancreatico-duodenal veins

Superior mesenteric vein

Posterior, Anterior inferior pancreatico-duodenal veins

Middle colic vein

Right colic vein

Ileocolic vein

Anterior, Posterior cecal veins

Appendicular vein

Left gastric vein

Short gastric veins

Left gastro-omental (gastro-epiploic) vein

Splenic vein

Right gastro-omental (gastro-epiploic) vein

Inferior mesenteric vein

Left colic vein

Sigmoid veins

Left and right superior rectal veins

Middle rectal veins

Levator ani muscle

Inferior rectal veins

Portacaval anastomoses

| 1 | Esophageal | 3 | Rectal |
| 2 | Paraumbilical | 4 | Retroperitoneal |

Visceral Vasculature

Plate 292

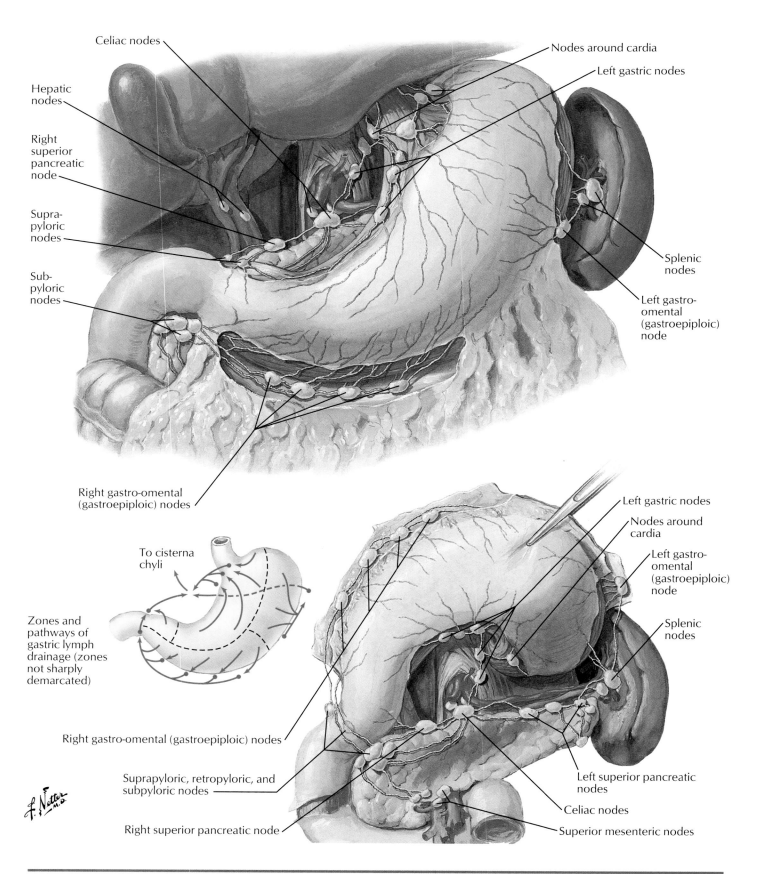

Celiac nodes

Hepatic nodes

Right superior pancreatic node

Supra-pyloric nodes

Sub-pyloric nodes

Right gastro-omental (gastroepiploic) nodes

Nodes around cardia

Left gastric nodes

Splenic nodes

Left gastro-omental (gastroepiploic) node

To cisterna chyli

Zones and pathways of gastric lymph drainage (zones not sharply demarcated)

Right gastro-omental (gastroepiploic) nodes

Suprapyloric, retropyloric, and subpyloric nodes

Right superior pancreatic node

Left gastric nodes

Nodes around cardia

Left gastro-omental (gastroepiploic) node

Splenic nodes

Left superior pancreatic nodes

Celiac nodes

Superior mesenteric nodes

F. Netter
M.D.

Plate 293 **Visceral Vasculature**

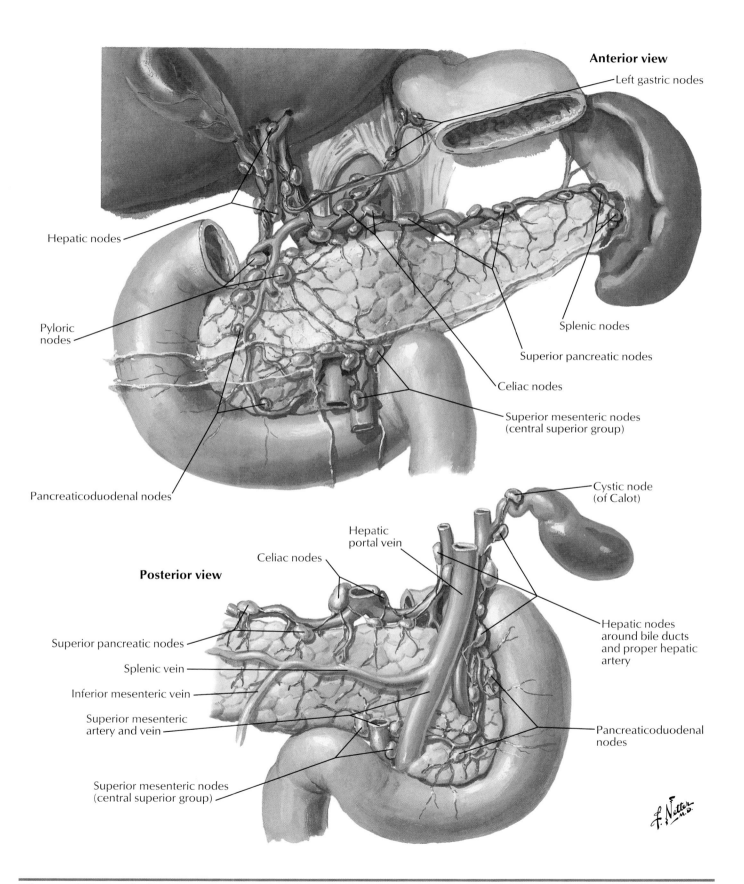

Anterior view

Left gastric nodes

Hepatic nodes

Pyloric nodes

Splenic nodes

Superior pancreatic nodes

Celiac nodes

Superior mesenteric nodes (central superior group)

Pancreaticoduodenal nodes

Cystic node (of Calot)

Hepatic portal vein

Celiac nodes

Posterior view

Hepatic nodes around bile ducts and proper hepatic artery

Superior pancreatic nodes

Splenic vein

Inferior mesenteric vein

Superior mesenteric artery and vein

Pancreaticoduodenal nodes

Superior mesenteric nodes (central superior group)

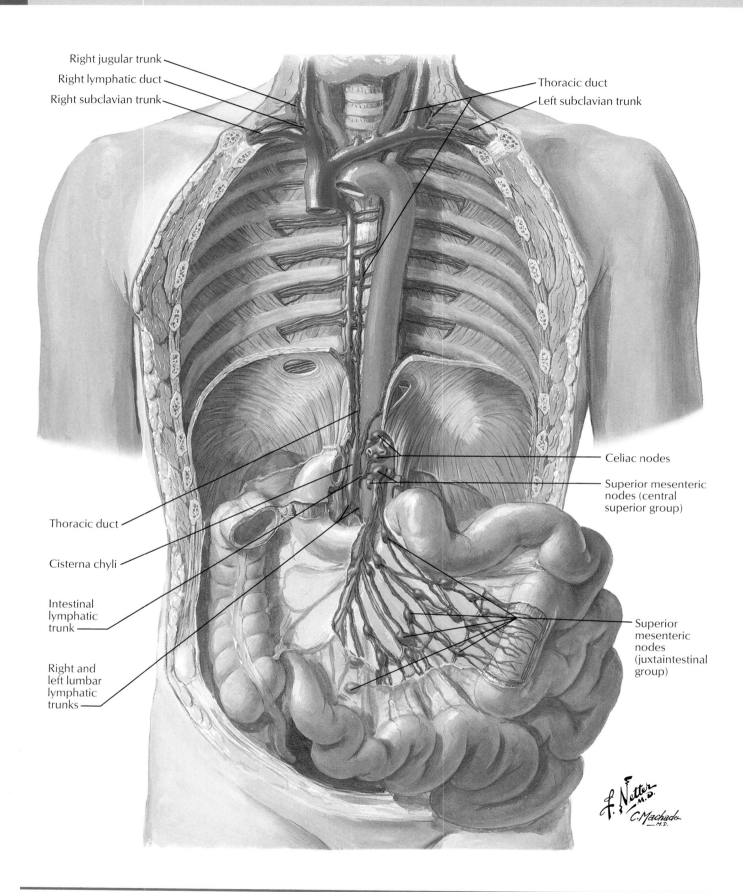

Right jugular trunk

Right lymphatic duct

Right subclavian trunk

Thoracic duct

Left subclavian trunk

Celiac nodes

Superior mesenteric nodes (central superior group)

Thoracic duct

Cisterna chyli

Intestinal lymphatic trunk

Right and left lumbar lymphatic trunks

Superior mesenteric nodes (juxtaintestinal group)

Plate 295 **Visceral Vasculature**

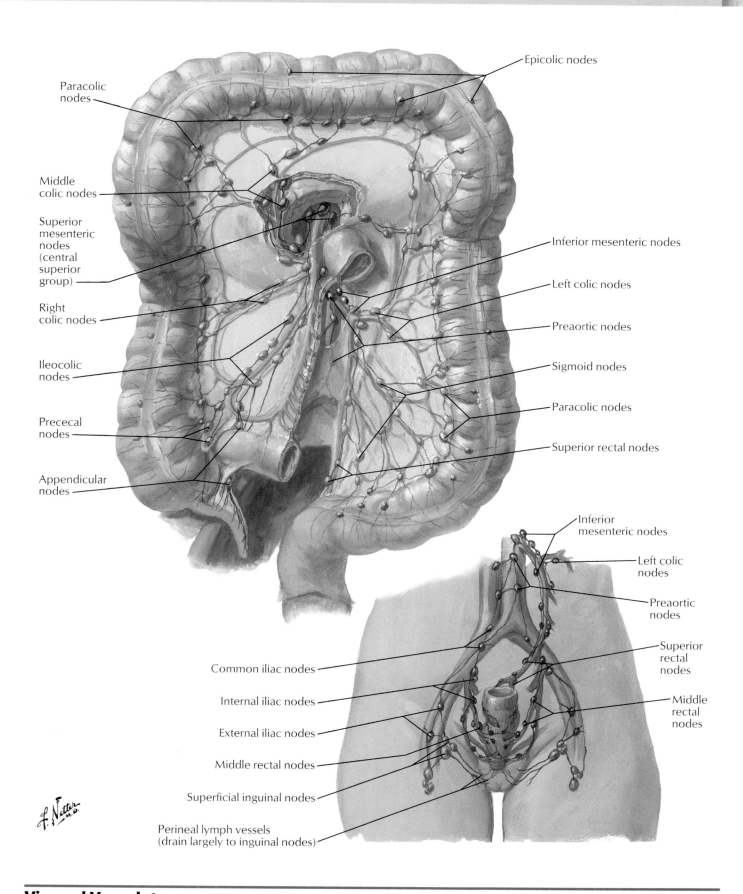

Epicolic nodes

Paracolic nodes

Middle colic nodes

Superior mesenteric nodes (central superior group)

Right colic nodes

Ileocolic nodes

Prececal nodes

Appendicular nodes

Inferior mesenteric nodes

Left colic nodes

Preaortic nodes

Sigmoid nodes

Paracolic nodes

Superior rectal nodes

Inferior mesenteric nodes

Left colic nodes

Preaortic nodes

Superior rectal nodes

Middle rectal nodes

Common iliac nodes

Internal iliac nodes

External iliac nodes

Middle rectal nodes

Superficial inguinal nodes

Perineal lymph vessels (drain largely to inguinal nodes)

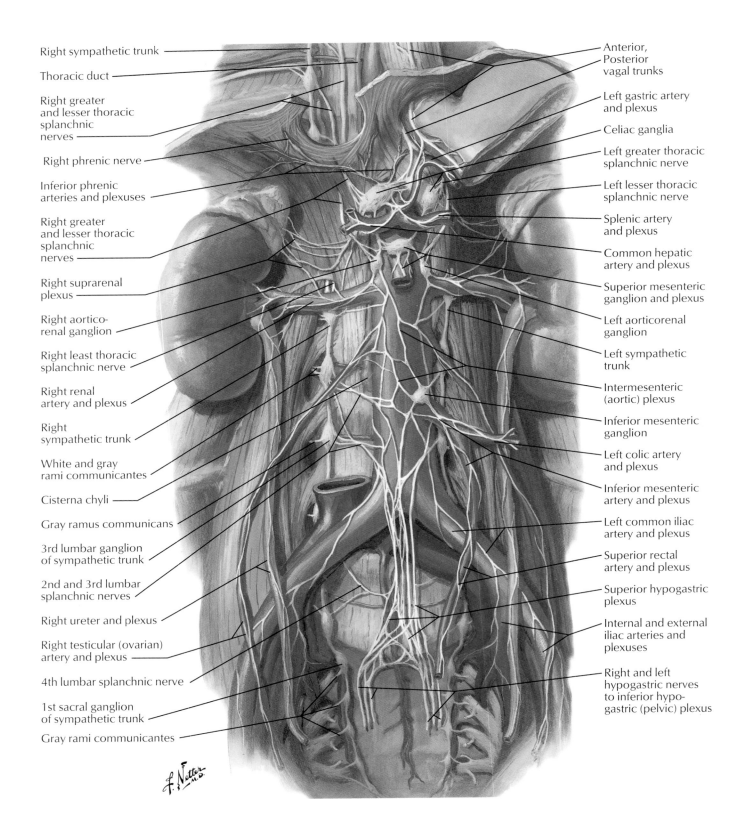

Right sympathetic trunk

Thoracic duct

Right greater and lesser thoracic splanchnic nerves

Right phrenic nerve

Inferior phrenic arteries and plexuses

Right greater and lesser thoracic splanchnic nerves

Right suprarenal plexus

Right aortico-renal ganglion

Right least thoracic splanchnic nerve

Right renal artery and plexus

Right sympathetic trunk

White and gray rami communicantes

Cisterna chyli

Gray ramus communicans

3rd lumbar ganglion of sympathetic trunk

2nd and 3rd lumbar splanchnic nerves

Right ureter and plexus

Right testicular (ovarian) artery and plexus

4th lumbar splanchnic nerve

1st sacral ganglion of sympathetic trunk

Gray rami communicantes

Anterior, Posterior vagal trunks

Left gastric artery and plexus

Celiac ganglia

Left greater thoracic splanchnic nerve

Left lesser thoracic splanchnic nerve

Splenic artery and plexus

Common hepatic artery and plexus

Superior mesenteric ganglion and plexus

Left aorticorenal ganglion

Left sympathetic trunk

Intermesenteric (aortic) plexus

Inferior mesenteric ganglion

Left colic artery and plexus

Inferior mesenteric artery and plexus

Left common iliac artery and plexus

Superior rectal artery and plexus

Superior hypogastric plexus

Internal and external iliac arteries and plexuses

Right and left hypogastric nerves to inferior hypo-gastric (pelvic) plexus

Plate 297   **Innervation**

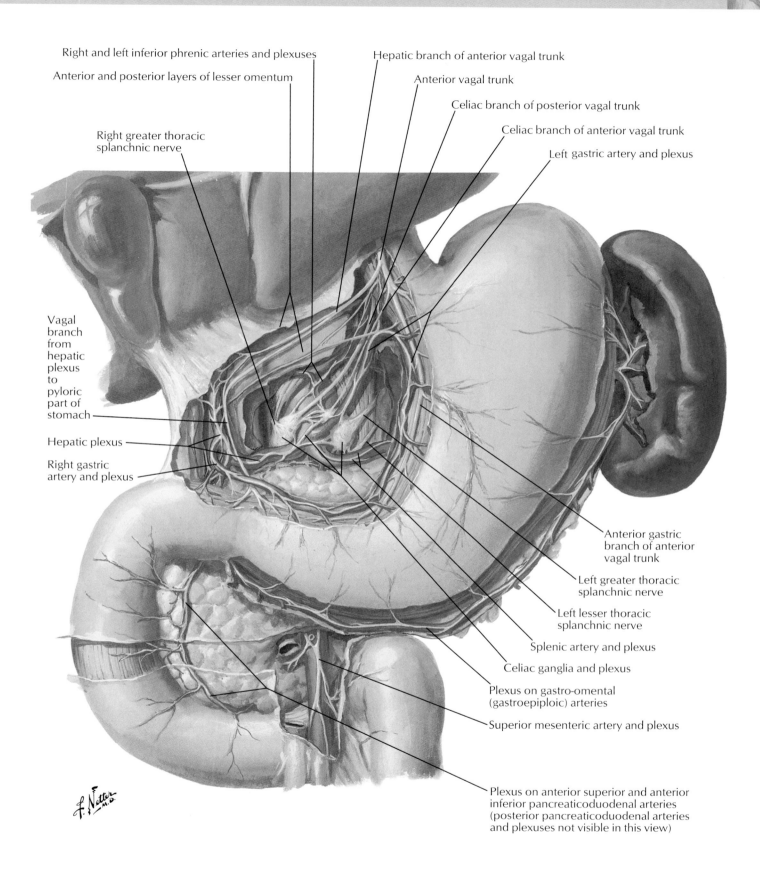

Right and left inferior phrenic arteries and plexuses

Anterior and posterior layers of lesser omentum

Right greater thoracic splanchnic nerve

Hepatic branch of anterior vagal trunk

Anterior vagal trunk

Celiac branch of posterior vagal trunk

Celiac branch of anterior vagal trunk

Left gastric artery and plexus

Vagal branch from hepatic plexus to pyloric part of stomach

Hepatic plexus

Right gastric artery and plexus

Anterior gastric branch of anterior vagal trunk

Left greater thoracic splanchnic nerve

Left lesser thoracic splanchnic nerve

Splenic artery and plexus

Celiac ganglia and plexus

Plexus on gastro-omental (gastroepiploic) arteries

Superior mesenteric artery and plexus

Plexus on anterior superior and anterior inferior pancreaticoduodenal arteries (posterior pancreaticoduodenal arteries and plexuses not visible in this view)

f. Netter. M.D.

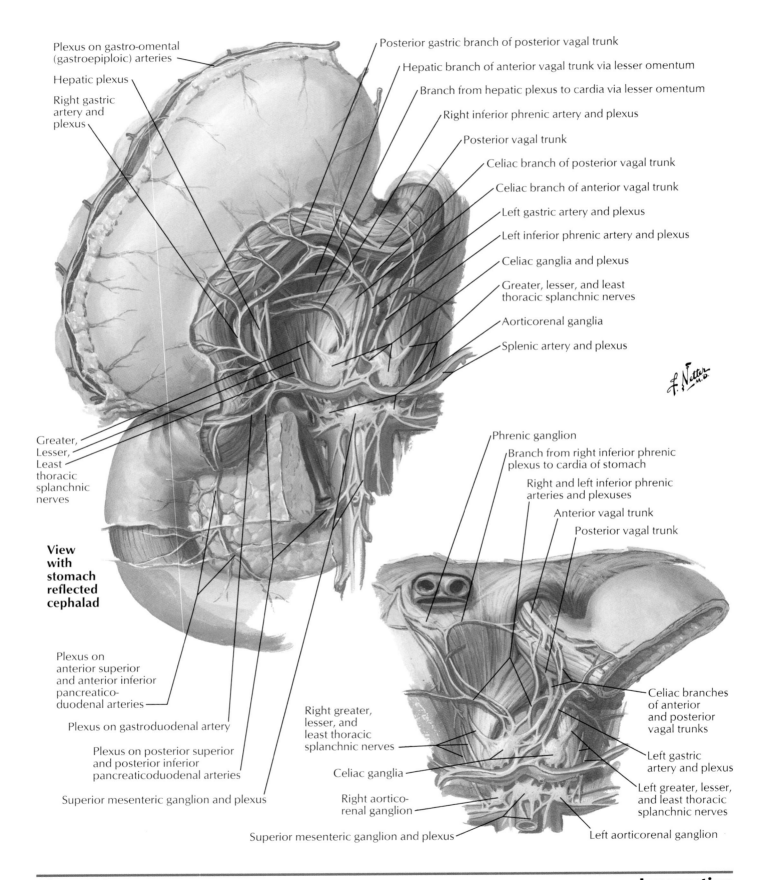

Plexus on gastro-omental (gastroepiploic) arteries

Hepatic plexus

Right gastric artery and plexus

Posterior gastric branch of posterior vagal trunk

Hepatic branch of anterior vagal trunk via lesser omentum

Branch from hepatic plexus to cardia via lesser omentum

Right inferior phrenic artery and plexus

Posterior vagal trunk

Celiac branch of posterior vagal trunk

Celiac branch of anterior vagal trunk

Left gastric artery and plexus

Left inferior phrenic artery and plexus

Celiac ganglia and plexus

Greater, lesser, and least thoracic splanchnic nerves

Aorticorenal ganglia

Splenic artery and plexus

Greater, Lesser, Least thoracic splanchnic nerves

View with stomach reflected cephalad

Phrenic ganglion

Branch from right inferior phrenic plexus to cardia of stomach

Right and left inferior phrenic arteries and plexuses

Anterior vagal trunk

Posterior vagal trunk

Plexus on anterior superior and anterior inferior pancreatico-duodenal arteries

Plexus on gastroduodenal artery

Plexus on posterior superior and posterior inferior pancreaticoduodenal arteries

Superior mesenteric ganglion and plexus

Right greater, lesser, and least thoracic splanchnic nerves

Celiac ganglia

Right aortico-renal ganglion

Superior mesenteric ganglion and plexus

Celiac branches of anterior and posterior vagal trunks

Left gastric artery and plexus

Left greater, lesser, and least thoracic splanchnic nerves

Left aorticorenal ganglion

Plate 299   **Innervation**

Right 6th thoracic ganglion of sympathetic trunk

Gray, White rami communicantes

Spinal sensory (dorsal root) ganglion

Anterior (ventral) root of spinal nerve

Right greater thoracic splanchnic nerve

Right lesser thoracic splanchnic nerve

Celiac ganglia

Least thoracic splanchnic nerve

Common hepatic artery

Proper hepatic artery

Superior mesenteric ganglion

Aorticorenal ganglia

Right gastric artery

Right renal artery

Gastroduodenal artery

Posterior and anterior superior pancreatico-duodenal arteries

Superior mesenteric artery

Posterior and anterior inferior pancreatico-duodenal arteries

Esophageal plexus

Left greater thoracic splanchnic nerve

Aortic plexus

Left 9th thoracic ganglion of sympathetic trunk

Posterior vagal trunk and celiac branch

Anterior vagal trunk and celiac branch of vagus nerve (X)

Left gastric artery

Celiac trunk

Splenic artery

Short gastric arteries

Left, Right gastro-omental (gastroepiploic) arteries

Sympathetic fibers

Preganglionic ————

Postganglionic - - - - - -

Parasympathetic fibers

Preganglionic ————

Postganglionic - - - - - -

Afferent fibers ————

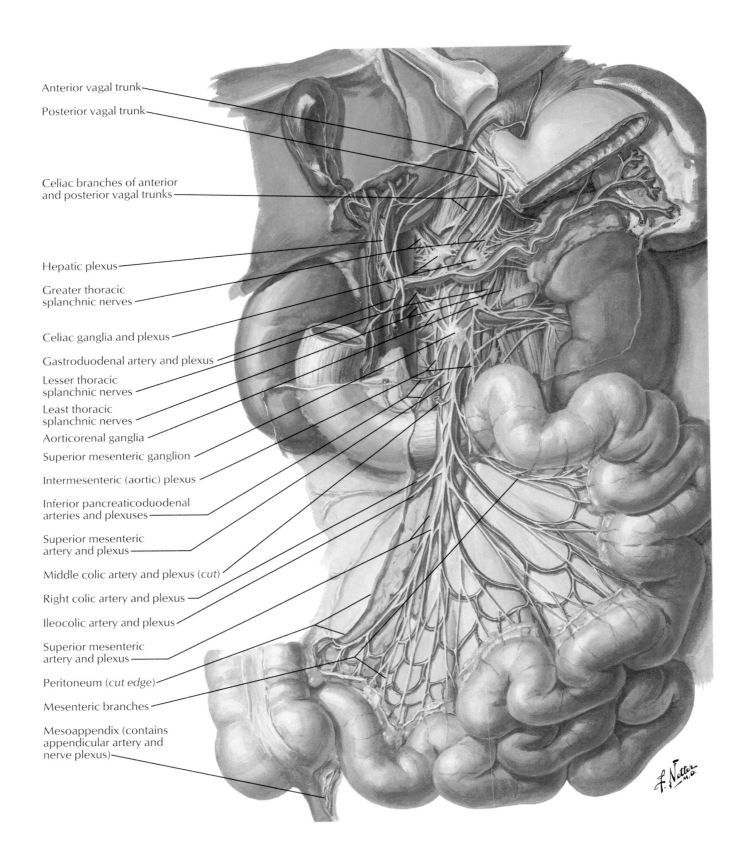

Anterior vagal trunk

Posterior vagal trunk

Celiac branches of anterior and posterior vagal trunks

Hepatic plexus

Greater thoracic splanchnic nerves

Celiac ganglia and plexus

Gastroduodenal artery and plexus

Lesser thoracic splanchnic nerves

Least thoracic splanchnic nerves

Aorticorenal ganglia

Superior mesenteric ganglion

Intermesenteric (aortic) plexus

Inferior pancreaticoduodenal arteries and plexuses

Superior mesenteric artery and plexus

Middle colic artery and plexus (cut)

Right colic artery and plexus

Ileocolic artery and plexus

Superior mesenteric artery and plexus

Peritoneum (cut edge)

Mesenteric branches

Mesoappendix (contains appendicular artery and nerve plexus)

Plate 301

Innervation

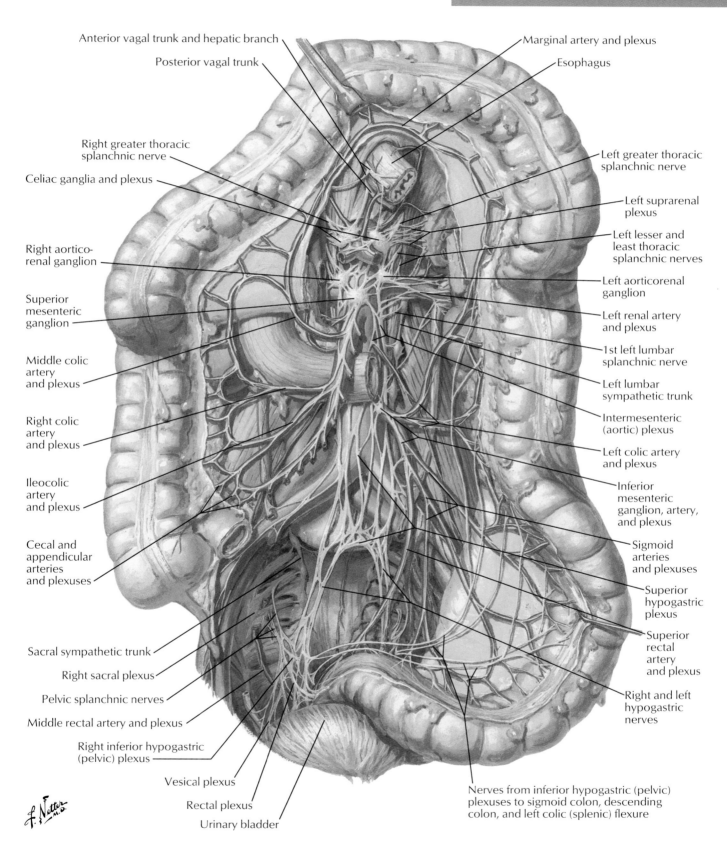

Anterior vagal trunk and hepatic branch

Posterior vagal trunk

Right greater thoracic splanchnic nerve

Celiac ganglia and plexus

Right aortico-renal ganglion

Superior mesenteric ganglion

Middle colic artery and plexus

Right colic artery and plexus

Ileocolic artery and plexus

Cecal and appendicular arteries and plexuses

Sacral sympathetic trunk

Right sacral plexus

Pelvic splanchnic nerves

Middle rectal artery and plexus

Right inferior hypogastric (pelvic) plexus

Vesical plexus

Rectal plexus

Urinary bladder

Marginal artery and plexus

Esophagus

Left greater thoracic splanchnic nerve

Left suprarenal plexus

Left lesser and least thoracic splanchnic nerves

Left aorticorenal ganglion

Left renal artery and plexus

1st left lumbar splanchnic nerve

Left lumbar sympathetic trunk

Intermesenteric (aortic) plexus

Left colic artery and plexus

Inferior mesenteric ganglion, artery, and plexus

Sigmoid arteries and plexuses

Superior hypogastric plexus

Superior rectal artery and plexus

Right and left hypogastric nerves

Nerves from inferior hypogastric (pelvic) plexuses to sigmoid colon, descending colon, and left colic (splenic) flexure

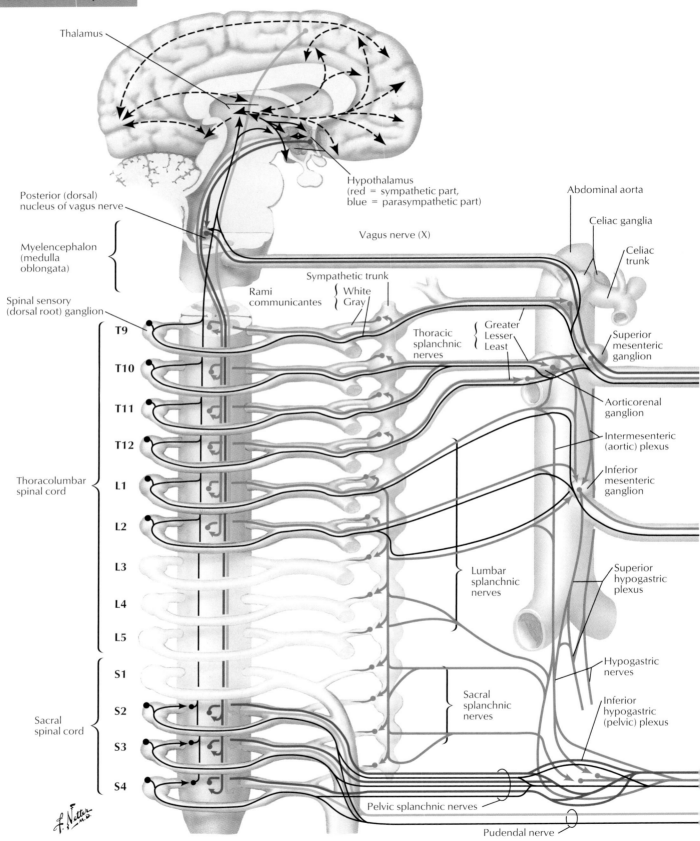

Thalamus

Hypothalamus
(red = sympathetic part,
blue = parasympathetic part)

Abdominal aorta

Celiac ganglia

Celiac trunk

Vagus nerve (X)

Posterior (dorsal)
nucleus of vagus nerve

Myelencephalon
(medulla
oblongata)

Spinal sensory
(dorsal root) ganglion

Sympathetic trunk

Rami
communicantes { White
Gray

Thoracic
splanchnic
nerves { Greater
Lesser
Least

Superior
mesenteric
ganglion

T9

T10

Aorticorenal
ganglion

T11

Intermesenteric
(aortic) plexus

T12

Inferior
mesenteric
ganglion

Thoracolumbar
spinal cord

L1

L2

L3

Lumbar
splanchnic
nerves

Superior
hypogastric
plexus

L4

L5

S1

Hypogastric
nerves

Sacral
splanchnic
nerves

S2

Inferior
hypogastric
(pelvic) plexus

Sacral
spinal cord

S3

S4

Pelvic splanchnic nerves

Pudendal nerve

Plate 303

Innervation

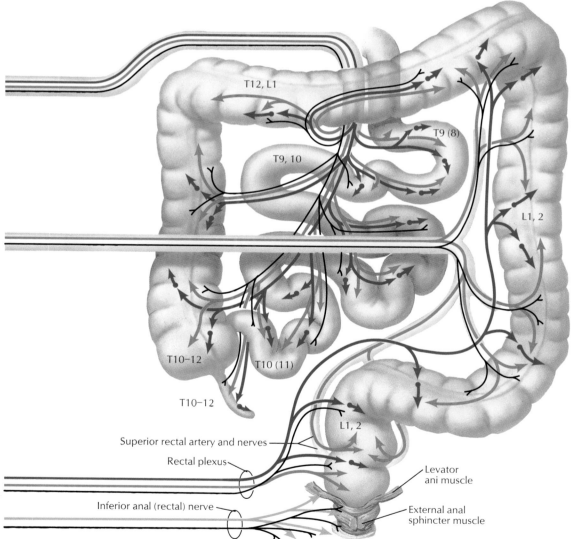

Sympathetic efferents
Parasympathetic efferents
Somatic efferents
Afferents and CNS connections
Indefinite paths

T12, L1

T9 (8)

T9, 10

L1, 2

T10–12

T10 (11)

T10–12

L1, 2

Superior rectal artery and nerves

Rectal plexus

Levator ani muscle

Inferior anal (rectal) nerve

External anal sphincter muscle

Chief segmental sources of sympathetic fibers innervating different regions of intestinal tract are indicated. Numerous afferent fibers are carried centripetally through approximately the same sympathetic splanchnic nerves that transmit preganglionic fibers.

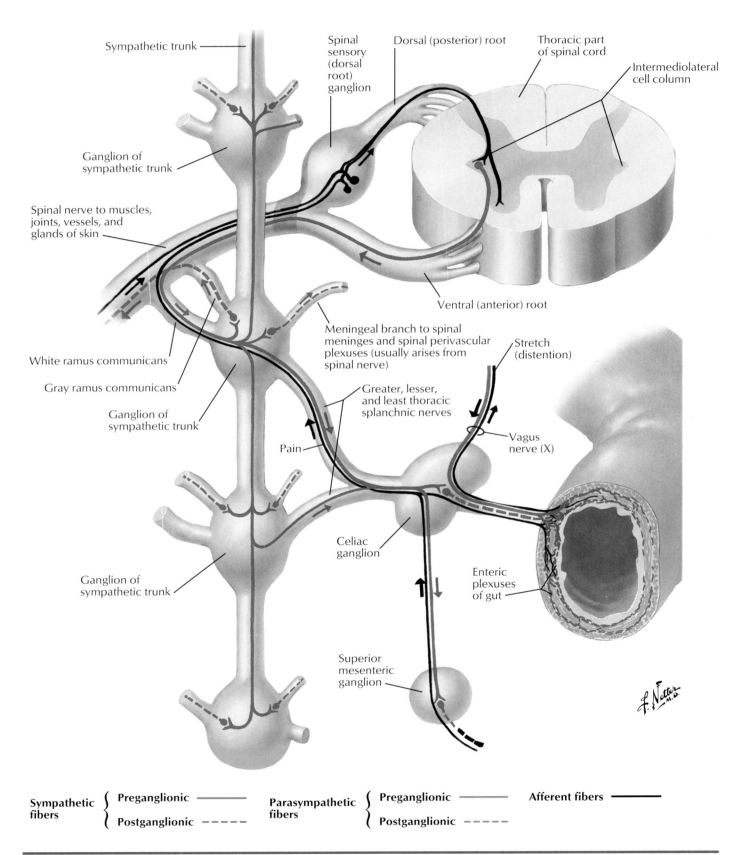

Sympathetic trunk

Spinal sensory (dorsal root) ganglion

Dorsal (posterior) root

Thoracic part of spinal cord

Intermediolateral cell column

Ganglion of sympathetic trunk

Spinal nerve to muscles, joints, vessels, and glands of skin

Ventral (anterior) root

White ramus communicans

Gray ramus communicans

Ganglion of sympathetic trunk

Meningeal branch to spinal meninges and spinal perivascular plexuses (usually arises from spinal nerve)

Greater, lesser, and least thoracic splanchnic nerves

Pain

Stretch (distention)

Vagus nerve (X)

Celiac ganglion

Enteric plexuses of gut

Ganglion of sympathetic trunk

Superior mesenteric ganglion

Sympathetic fibers { Preganglionic ——— Postganglionic - - - -

Parasympathetic fibers { Preganglionic ——— Postganglionic - - - -

Afferent fibers ———

Plate 304 **Innervation**

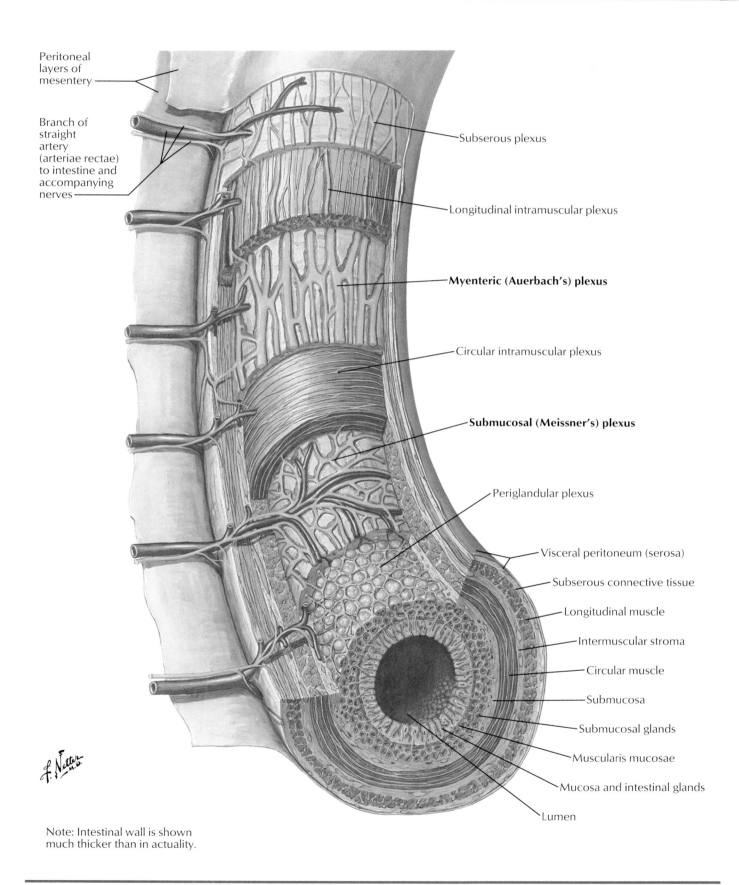

Peritoneal layers of mesentery

Branch of straight artery (arteriae rectae) to intestine and accompanying nerves

Subserous plexus

Longitudinal intramuscular plexus

Myenteric (Auerbach's) plexus

Circular intramuscular plexus

Submucosal (Meissner's) plexus

Periglandular plexus

Visceral peritoneum (serosa)

Subserous connective tissue

Longitudinal muscle

Intermuscular stroma

Circular muscle

Submucosa

Submucosal glands

Muscularis mucosae

Mucosa and intestinal glands

Lumen

Note: Intestinal wall is shown much thicker than in actuality.

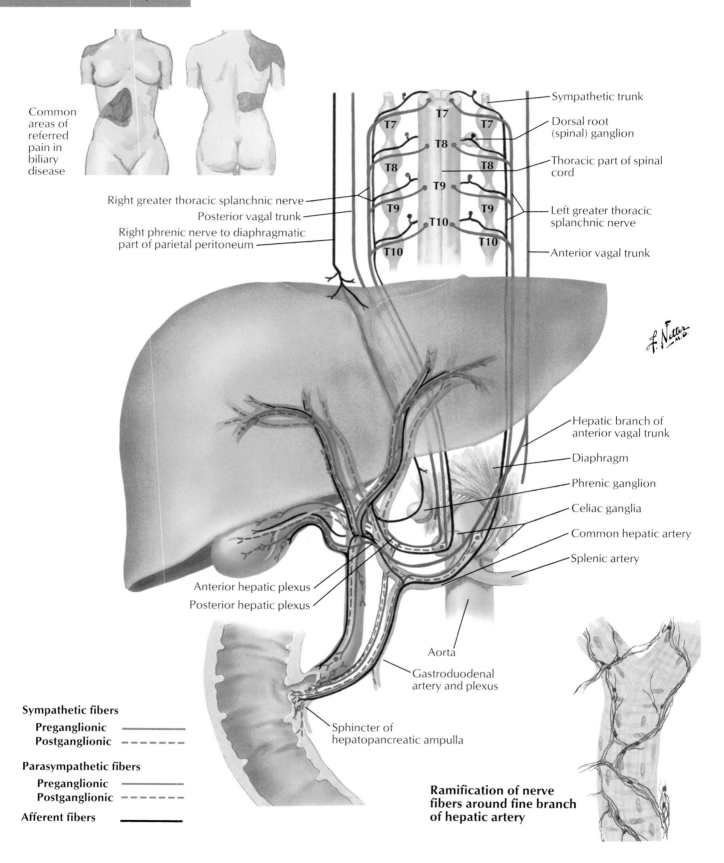

Common areas of referred pain in biliary disease

Right greater thoracic splanchnic nerve
Posterior vagal trunk
Right phrenic nerve to diaphragmatic part of parietal peritoneum

Sympathetic trunk
Dorsal root (spinal) ganglion
Thoracic part of spinal cord
Left greater thoracic splanchnic nerve
Anterior vagal trunk

Hepatic branch of anterior vagal trunk
Diaphragm
Phrenic ganglion
Celiac ganglia
Common hepatic artery
Splenic artery

Anterior hepatic plexus
Posterior hepatic plexus

Aorta
Gastroduodenal artery and plexus

Sphincter of hepatopancreatic ampulla

Sympathetic fibers
  Preganglionic ————
  Postganglionic ——————

Parasympathetic fibers
  Preganglionic ————
  Postganglionic ——————

Afferent fibers ————

Ramification of nerve fibers around fine branch of hepatic artery

Plate 306

Innervation

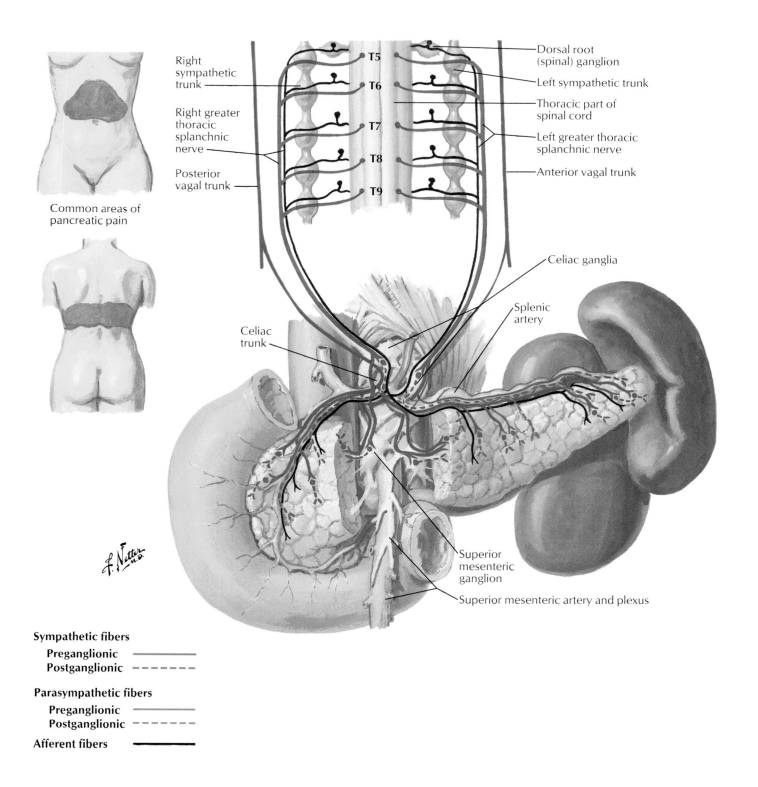

Common areas of
pancreatic pain

Right
sympathetic
trunk

Right greater
thoracic
splanchnic
nerve

Posterior
vagal trunk

T5
T6
T7
T8
T9

Dorsal root
(spinal) ganglion

Left sympathetic trunk

Thoracic part of
spinal cord

Left greater thoracic
splanchnic nerve

Anterior vagal trunk

Celiac ganglia

Splenic
artery

Celiac
trunk

Superior
mesenteric
ganglion

Superior mesenteric artery and plexus

Sympathetic fibers
   Preganglionic
   Postganglionic

Parasympathetic fibers
   Preganglionic
   Postganglionic

Afferent fibers

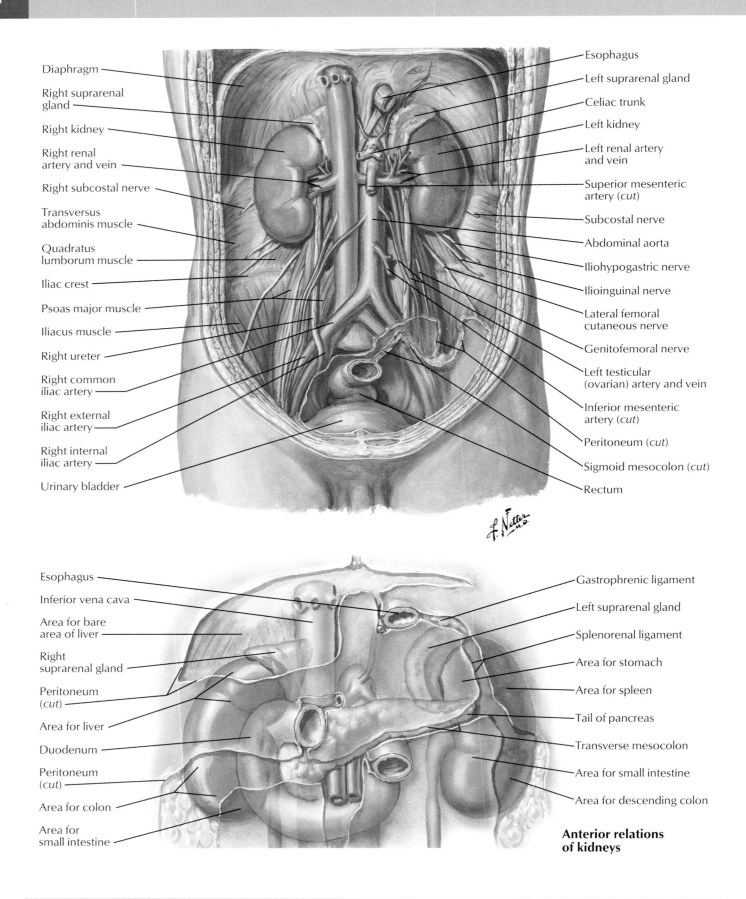

Diaphragm

Right suprarenal gland

Right kidney

Right renal artery and vein

Right subcostal nerve

Transversus abdominis muscle

Quadratus lumborum muscle

Iliac crest

Psoas major muscle

Iliacus muscle

Right ureter

Right common iliac artery

Right external iliac artery

Right internal iliac artery

Urinary bladder

Esophagus

Left suprarenal gland

Celiac trunk

Left kidney

Left renal artery and vein

Superior mesenteric artery (cut)

Subcostal nerve

Abdominal aorta

Iliohypogastric nerve

Ilioinguinal nerve

Lateral femoral cutaneous nerve

Genitofemoral nerve

Left testicular (ovarian) artery and vein

Inferior mesenteric artery (cut)

Peritoneum (cut)

Sigmoid mesocolon (cut)

Rectum

Esophagus

Inferior vena cava

Area for bare area of liver

Right suprarenal gland

Peritoneum (cut)

Area for liver

Duodenum

Peritoneum (cut)

Area for colon

Area for small intestine

Gastrophrenic ligament

Left suprarenal gland

Splenorenal ligament

Area for stomach

Area for spleen

Tail of pancreas

Transverse mesocolon

Area for small intestine

Area for descending colon

Anterior relations of kidneys

Plate 308   **Kidneys and Suprarenal Glands**

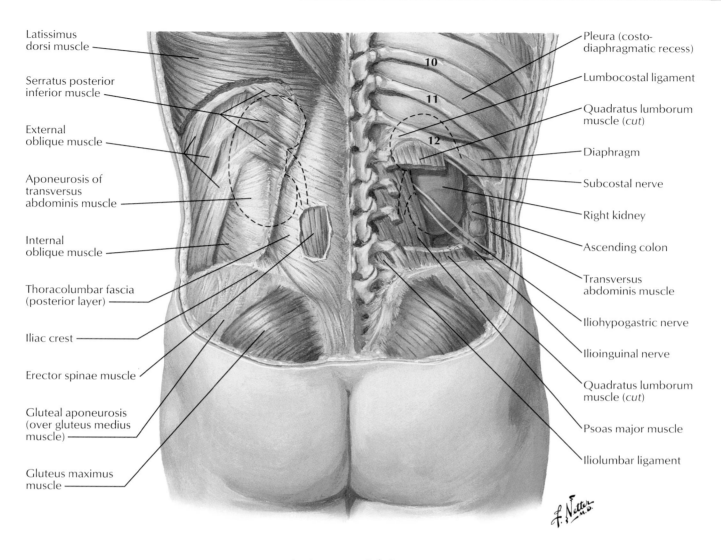

Latissimus dorsi muscle

Serratus posterior inferior muscle

External oblique muscle

Aponeurosis of transversus abdominis muscle

Internal oblique muscle

Thoracolumbar fascia (posterior layer)

Iliac crest

Erector spinae muscle

Gluteal aponeurosis (over gluteus medius muscle)

Gluteus maximus muscle

10

11

12

Pleura (costo-diaphragmatic recess)

Lumbocostal ligament

Quadratus lumborum muscle (cut)

Diaphragm

Subcostal nerve

Right kidney

Ascending colon

Transversus abdominis muscle

Iliohypogastric nerve

Ilioinguinal nerve

Quadratus lumborum muscle (cut)

Psoas major muscle

Iliolumbar ligament

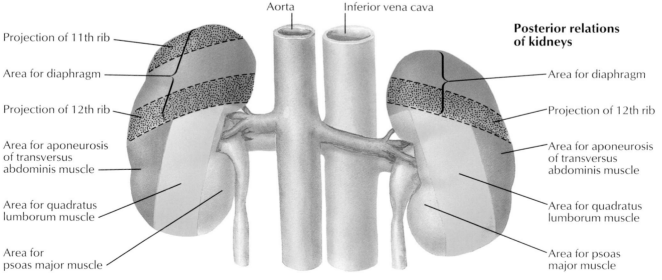

Aorta

Inferior vena cava

Posterior relations of kidneys

Projection of 11th rib

Area for diaphragm

Projection of 12th rib

Area for aponeurosis of transversus abdominis muscle

Area for quadratus lumborum muscle

Area for psoas major muscle

Area for diaphragm

Projection of 12th rib

Area for aponeurosis of transversus abdominis muscle

Area for quadratus lumborum muscle

Area for psoas major muscle

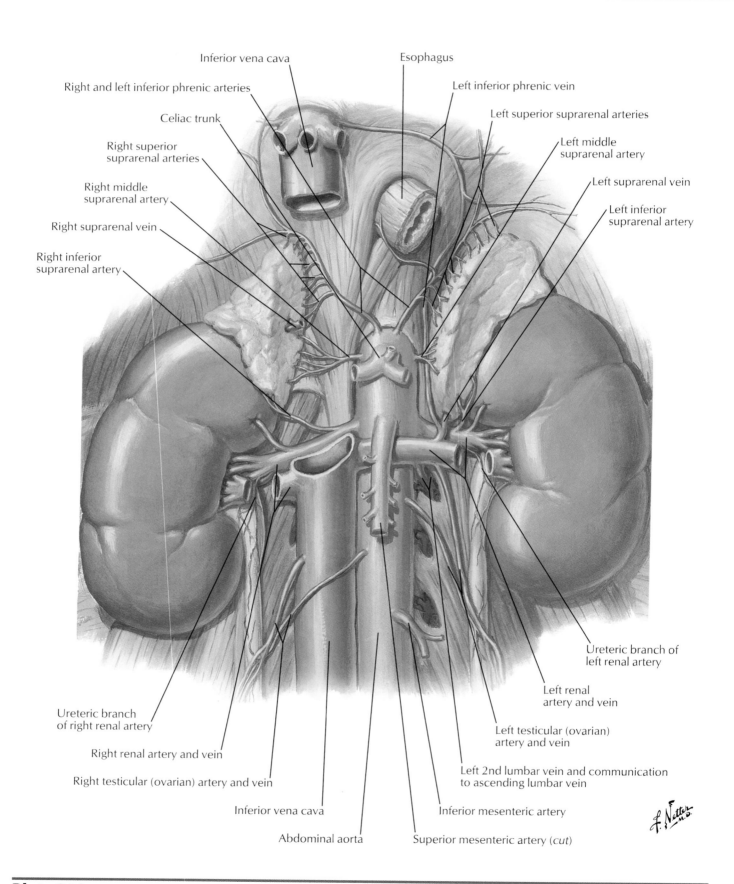

Inferior vena cava

Right and left inferior phrenic arteries

Celiac trunk

Right superior suprarenal arteries

Right middle suprarenal artery

Right suprarenal vein

Right inferior suprarenal artery

Esophagus

Left inferior phrenic vein

Left superior suprarenal arteries

Left middle suprarenal artery

Left suprarenal vein

Left inferior suprarenal artery

Ureteric branch of left renal artery

Left renal artery and vein

Left testicular (ovarian) artery and vein

Left 2nd lumbar vein and communication to ascending lumbar vein

Inferior mesenteric artery

Superior mesenteric artery (cut)

Ureteric branch of right renal artery

Right renal artery and vein

Right testicular (ovarian) artery and vein

Inferior vena cava

Abdominal aorta

Plate 310   **Kidneys and Suprarenal Glands**

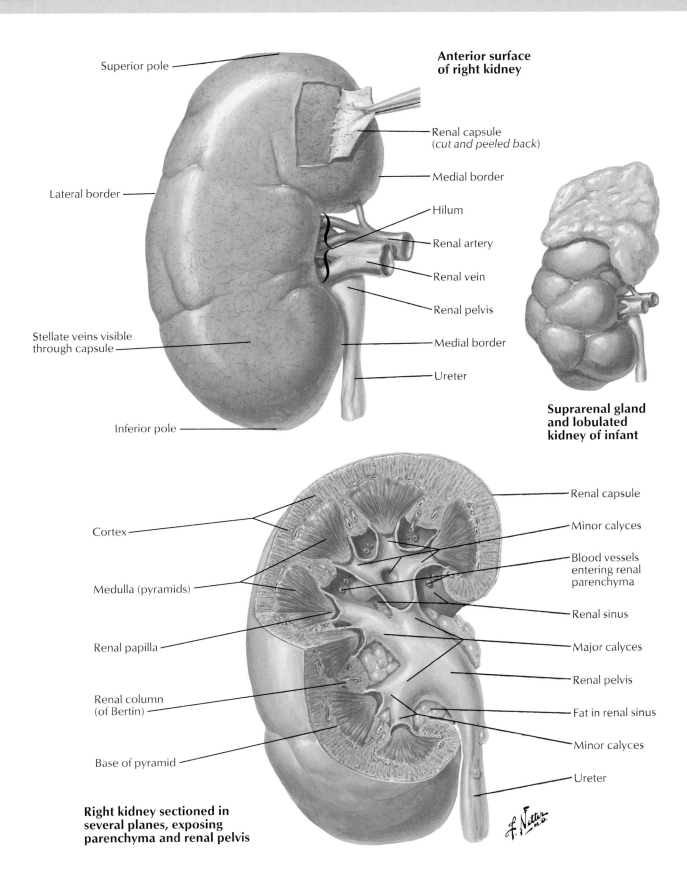

Superior pole

**Anterior surface
of right kidney**

Renal capsule
(*cut and peeled back*)

Medial border

Lateral border

Hilum

Renal artery

Renal vein

Renal pelvis

Stellate veins visible
through capsule

Medial border

Ureter

Inferior pole

**Suprarenal gland
and lobulated
kidney of infant**

Cortex

Renal capsule

Minor calyces

Blood vessels
entering renal
parenchyma

Medulla (pyramids)

Renal sinus

Renal papilla

Major calyces

Renal pelvis

Renal column
(of Bertin)

Fat in renal sinus

Minor calyces

Base of pyramid

Ureter

**Right kidney sectioned in
several planes, exposing
parenchyma and renal pelvis**

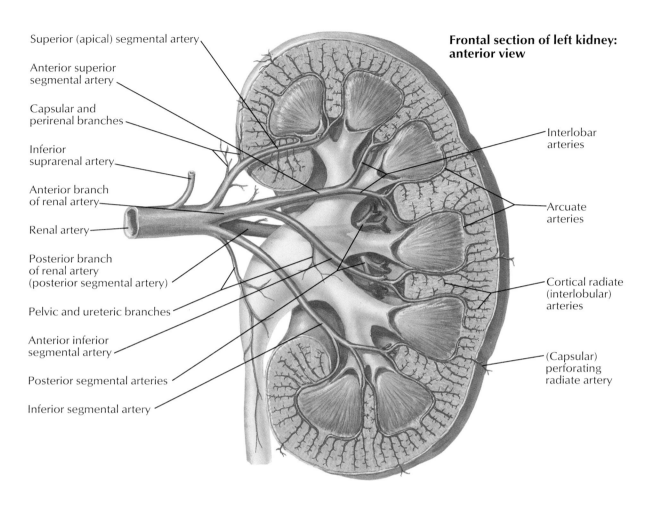

Superior (apical) segmental artery

Anterior superior segmental artery

Capsular and perirenal branches

Inferior suprarenal artery

Anterior branch of renal artery

Renal artery

Posterior branch of renal artery (posterior segmental artery)

Pelvic and ureteric branches

Anterior inferior segmental artery

Posterior segmental arteries

Inferior segmental artery

Frontal section of left kidney: anterior view

Interlobar arteries

Arcuate arteries

Cortical radiate (interlobular) arteries

(Capsular) perforating radiate artery

Vascular renal segments

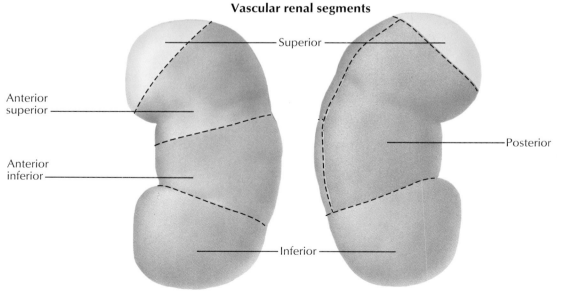

Superior

Anterior superior

Anterior inferior

Posterior

Inferior

Anterior surface of left kidney

Posterior surface of left kidney

Plate 312

Kidneys and Suprarenal Glands

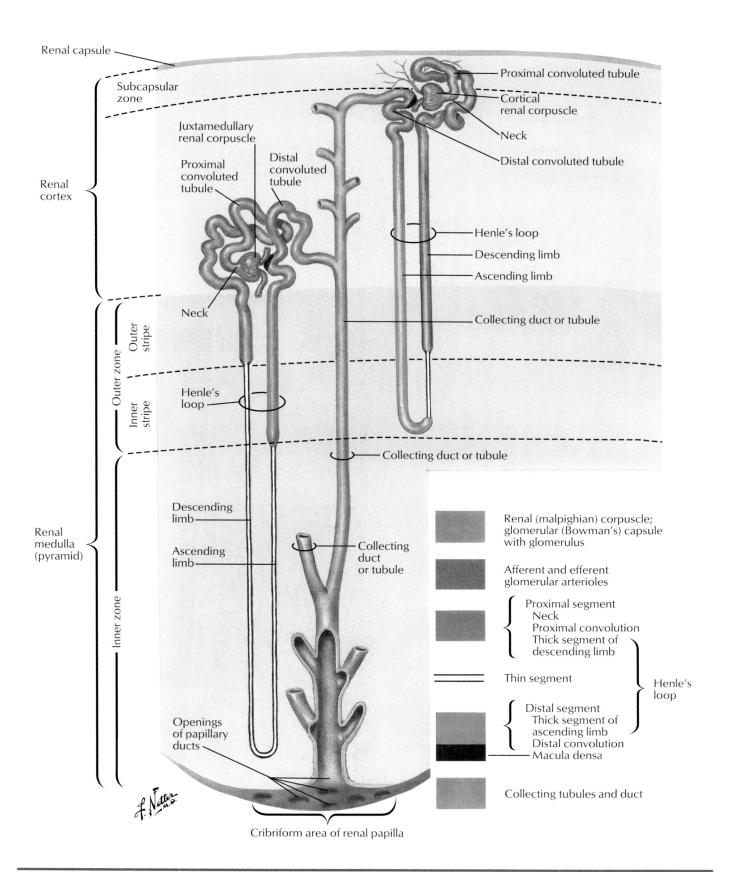

Renal capsule

Subcapsular zone

Renal cortex

Juxtamedullary renal corpuscle

Proximal convoluted tubule

Distal convoluted tubule

Proximal convoluted tubule

Cortical renal corpuscle

Neck

Distal convoluted tubule

Henle's loop

Descending limb

Ascending limb

Neck

Collecting duct or tubule

Outer zone

Outer stripe

Inner stripe

Henle's loop

Collecting duct or tubule

Renal medulla (pyramid)

Inner zone

Descending limb

Ascending limb

Collecting duct or tubule

Openings of papillary ducts

Cribriform area of renal papilla

Renal (malpighian) corpuscle; glomerular (Bowman's) capsule with glomerulus

Afferent and efferent glomerular arterioles

Proximal segment
Neck
Proximal convolution
Thick segment of descending limb

Thin segment

Henle's loop

Distal segment
Thick segment of ascending limb
Distal convolution
Macula densa

Collecting tubules and duct

Blood Vessels in Parenchyma of Kidney: Schema

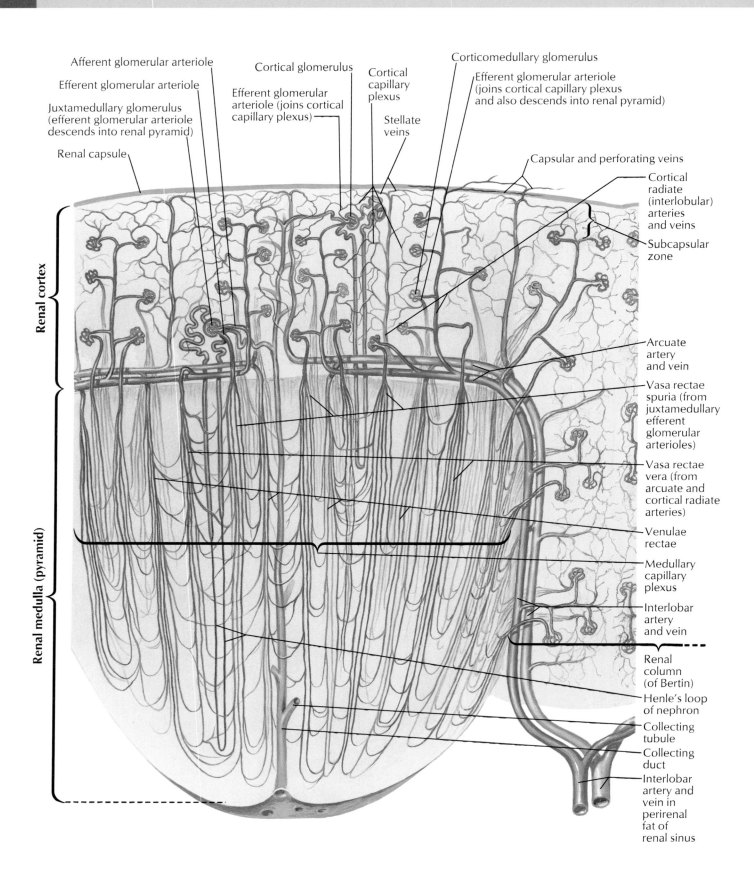

Afferent glomerular arteriole

Efferent glomerular arteriole

Juxtamedullary glomerulus
(efferent glomerular arteriole
descends into renal pyramid)

Renal capsule

Cortical glomerulus

Efferent glomerular
arteriole (joins cortical
capillary plexus)

Cortical
capillary
plexus

Stellate
veins

Corticomedullary glomerulus

Efferent glomerular arteriole
(joins cortical capillary plexus
and also descends into renal pyramid)

Capsular and perforating veins

Cortical
radiate
(interlobular)
arteries
and veins

Subcapsular
zone

Renal cortex

Renal medulla (pyramid)

Arcuate
artery
and vein

Vasa rectae
spuria (from
juxtamedullary
efferent
glomerular
arterioles)

Vasa rectae
vera (from
arcuate and
cortical radiate
arteries)

Venulae
rectae

Medullary
capillary
plexus

Interlobar
artery
and vein

Renal
column
(of Bertin)

Henle's loop
of nephron

Collecting
tubule

Collecting
duct

Interlobar
artery and
vein in
perirenal
fat of
renal sinus

Plate 314   **Kidneys and Suprarenal Glands**

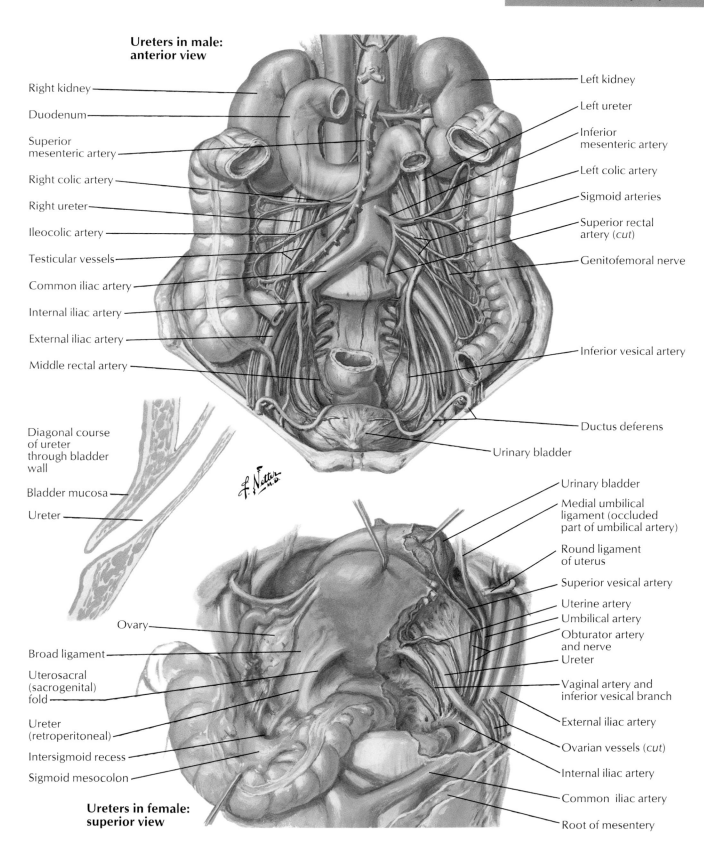

Ureters in male: anterior view

Right kidney

Duodenum

Superior mesenteric artery

Right colic artery

Right ureter

Ileocolic artery

Testicular vessels

Common iliac artery

Internal iliac artery

External iliac artery

Middle rectal artery

Left kidney

Left ureter

Inferior mesenteric artery

Left colic artery

Sigmoid arteries

Superior rectal artery (*cut*)

Genitofemoral nerve

Inferior vesical artery

Ductus deferens

Urinary bladder

Diagonal course of ureter through bladder wall

Bladder mucosa

Ureter

Urinary bladder

Medial umbilical ligament (occluded part of umbilical artery)

Round ligament of uterus

Superior vesical artery

Uterine artery

Umbilical artery

Obturator artery and nerve

Ureter

Vaginal artery and inferior vesical branch

External iliac artery

Ovarian vessels (*cut*)

Internal iliac artery

Common iliac artery

Root of mesentery

Ovary

Broad ligament

Uterosacral (sacrogenital) fold

Ureter (retroperitoneal)

Intersigmoid recess

Sigmoid mesocolon

Ureters in female: superior view

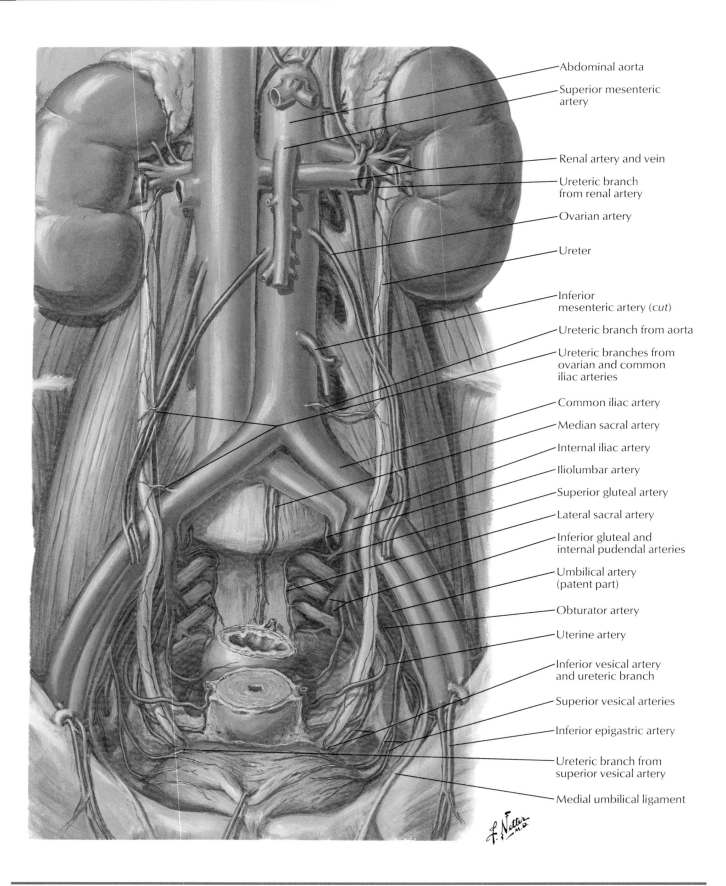

Abdominal aorta

Superior mesenteric artery

Renal artery and vein

Ureteric branch from renal artery

Ovarian artery

Ureter

Inferior mesenteric artery (*cut*)

Ureteric branch from aorta

Ureteric branches from ovarian and common iliac arteries

Common iliac artery

Median sacral artery

Internal iliac artery

Iliolumbar artery

Superior gluteal artery

Lateral sacral artery

Inferior gluteal and internal pudendal arteries

Umbilical artery (patent part)

Obturator artery

Uterine artery

Inferior vesical artery and ureteric branch

Superior vesical arteries

Inferior epigastric artery

Ureteric branch from superior vesical artery

Medial umbilical ligament

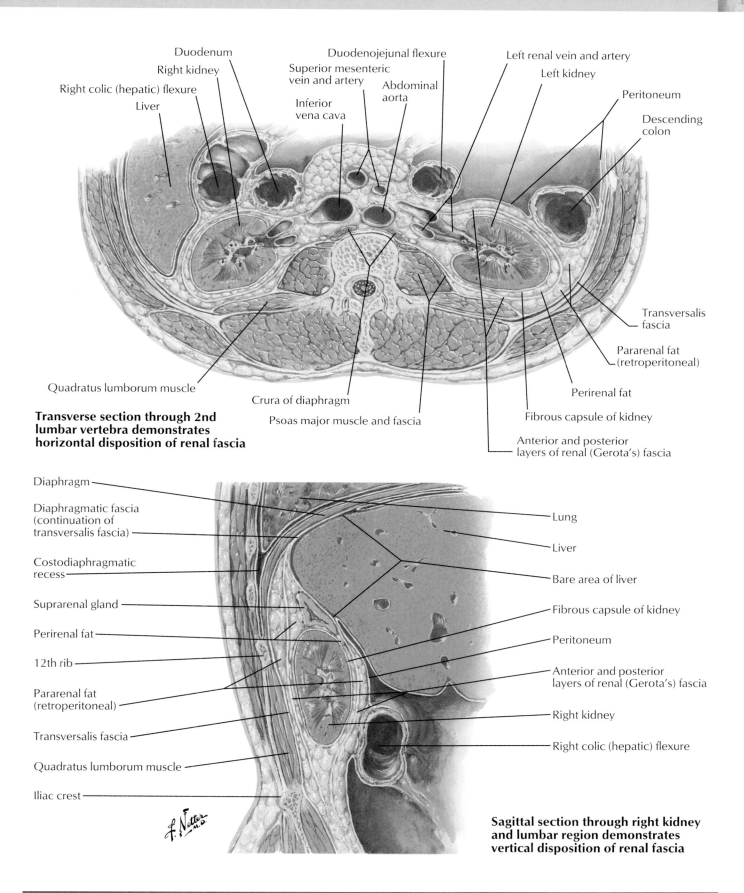

Duodenum

Right kidney

Right colic (hepatic) flexure

Liver

Duodenojejunal flexure

Superior mesenteric
vein and artery

Inferior
vena cava

Abdominal
aorta

Left renal vein and artery

Left kidney

Peritoneum

Descending
colon

Transversalis
fascia

Pararenal fat
(retroperitoneal)

Perirenal fat

Quadratus lumborum muscle

Crura of diaphragm

Psoas major muscle and fascia

Fibrous capsule of kidney

Anterior and posterior
layers of renal (Gerota's) fascia

**Transverse section through 2nd
lumbar vertebra demonstrates
horizontal disposition of renal fascia**

Diaphragm

Diaphragmatic fascia
(continuation of
transversalis fascia)

Costodiaphragmatic
recess

Suprarenal gland

Perirenal fat

12th rib

Pararenal fat
(retroperitoneal)

Transversalis fascia

Quadratus lumborum muscle

Iliac crest

Lung

Liver

Bare area of liver

Fibrous capsule of kidney

Peritoneum

Anterior and posterior
layers of renal (Gerota's) fascia

Right kidney

Right colic (hepatic) flexure

**Sagittal section through right kidney
and lumbar region demonstrates
vertical disposition of renal fascia**

Kidneys and Suprarenal Glands

Plate 317

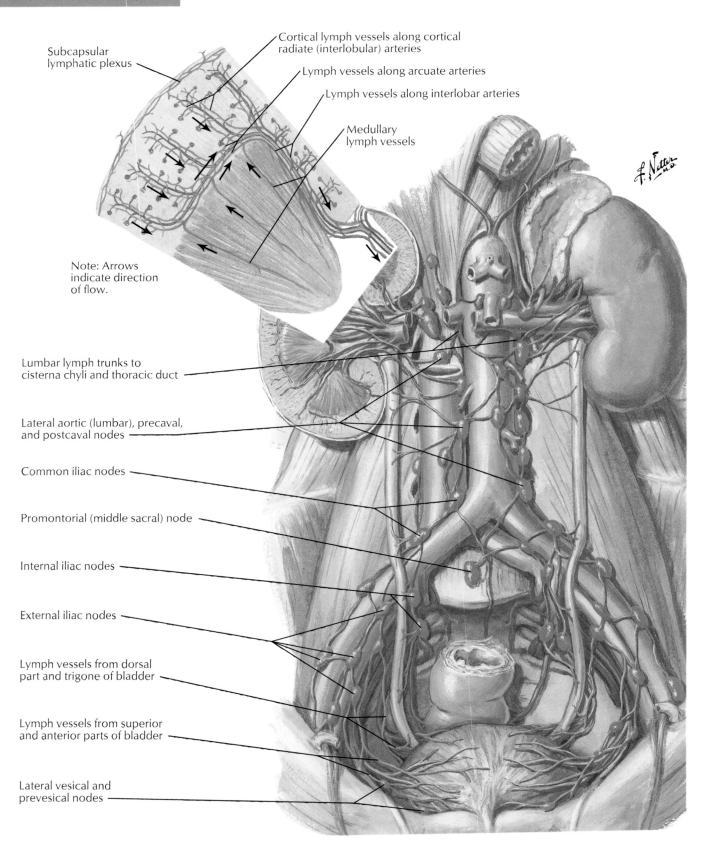

Subcapsular lymphatic plexus

Cortical lymph vessels along cortical radiate (interlobular) arteries

Lymph vessels along arcuate arteries

Lymph vessels along interlobar arteries

Medullary lymph vessels

Note: Arrows indicate direction of flow.

Lumbar lymph trunks to cisterna chyli and thoracic duct

Lateral aortic (lumbar), precaval, and postcaval nodes

Common iliac nodes

Promontorial (middle sacral) node

Internal iliac nodes

External iliac nodes

Lymph vessels from dorsal part and trigone of bladder

Lymph vessels from superior and anterior parts of bladder

Lateral vesical and prevesical nodes

Plate 318

Kidneys and Suprarenal Glands

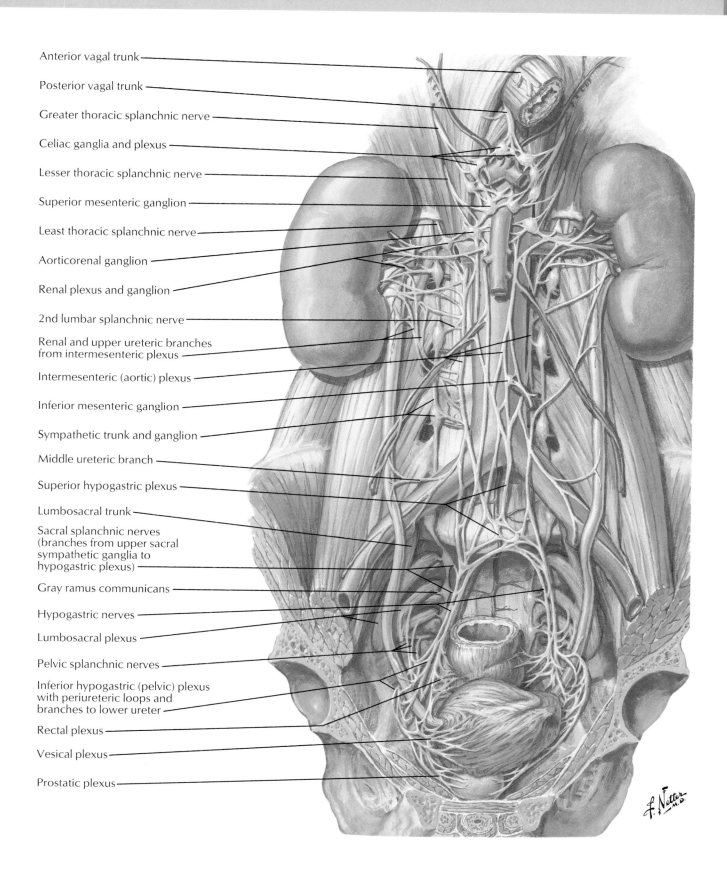

Anterior vagal trunk

Posterior vagal trunk

Greater thoracic splanchnic nerve

Celiac ganglia and plexus

Lesser thoracic splanchnic nerve

Superior mesenteric ganglion

Least thoracic splanchnic nerve

Aorticorenal ganglion

Renal plexus and ganglion

2nd lumbar splanchnic nerve

Renal and upper ureteric branches from intermesenteric plexus

Intermesenteric (aortic) plexus

Inferior mesenteric ganglion

Sympathetic trunk and ganglion

Middle ureteric branch

Superior hypogastric plexus

Lumbosacral trunk

Sacral splanchnic nerves (branches from upper sacral sympathetic ganglia to hypogastric plexus)

Gray ramus communicans

Hypogastric nerves

Lumbosacral plexus

Pelvic splanchnic nerves

Inferior hypogastric (pelvic) plexus with periureteric loops and branches to lower ureter

Rectal plexus

Vesical plexus

Prostatic plexus

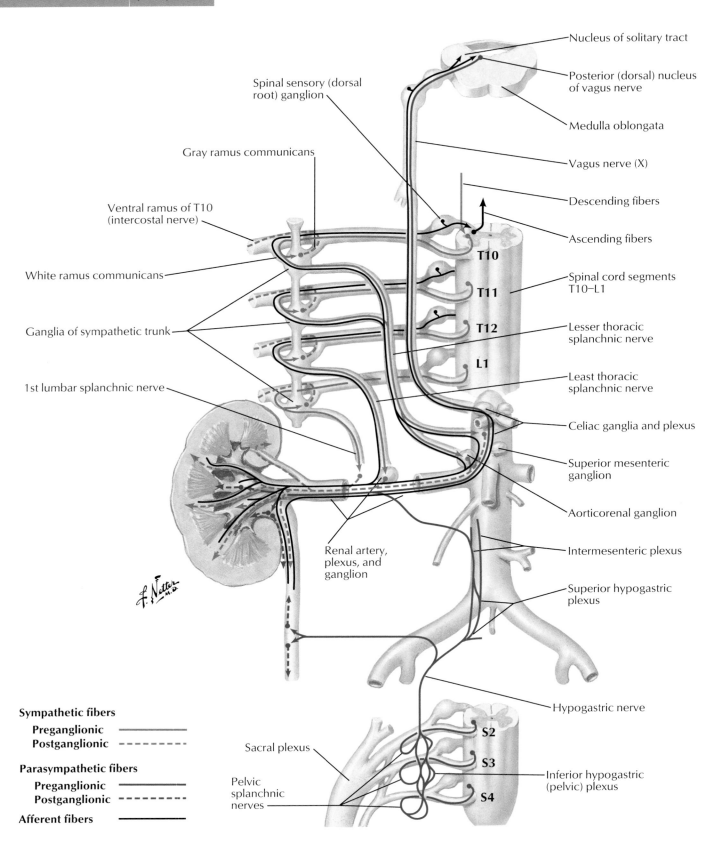

Nucleus of solitary tract

Spinal sensory (dorsal root) ganglion

Posterior (dorsal) nucleus of vagus nerve

Medulla oblongata

Gray ramus communicans

Vagus nerve (X)

Descending fibers

Ventral ramus of T10 (intercostal nerve)

Ascending fibers

T10

White ramus communicans

Spinal cord segments T10–L1

T11

T12

Lesser thoracic splanchnic nerve

Ganglia of sympathetic trunk

L1

Least thoracic splanchnic nerve

1st lumbar splanchnic nerve

Celiac ganglia and plexus

Superior mesenteric ganglion

Aorticorenal ganglion

Renal artery, plexus, and ganglion

Intermesenteric plexus

Superior hypogastric plexus

Hypogastric nerve

Sympathetic fibers
  Preganglionic ———
  Postganglionic - - - -

S2

Parasympathetic fibers
  Preganglionic ———
  Postganglionic - - - -

Sacral plexus

S3

Pelvic splanchnic nerves

Inferior hypogastric (pelvic) plexus

S4

Afferent fibers ———

Plate 320

Kidneys and Suprarenal Glands

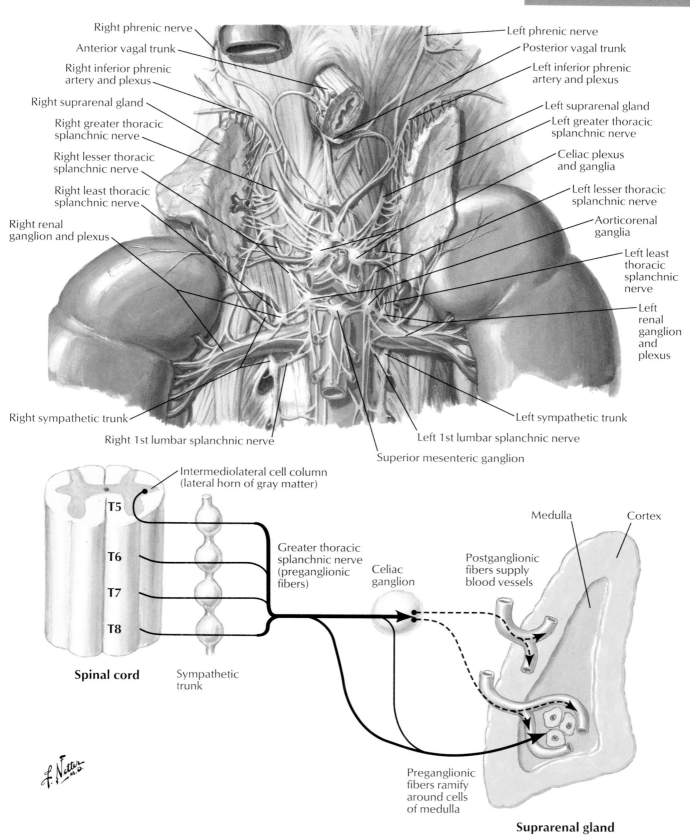

Right phrenic nerve
Anterior vagal trunk
Right inferior phrenic artery and plexus
Right suprarenal gland
Right greater thoracic splanchnic nerve
Right lesser thoracic splanchnic nerve
Right least thoracic splanchnic nerve
Right renal ganglion and plexus
Right sympathetic trunk

Left phrenic nerve
Posterior vagal trunk
Left inferior phrenic artery and plexus
Left suprarenal gland
Left greater thoracic splanchnic nerve
Celiac plexus and ganglia
Left lesser thoracic splanchnic nerve
Aorticorenal ganglia
Left least thoracic splanchnic nerve
Left renal ganglion and plexus
Left sympathetic trunk

Right 1st lumbar splanchnic nerve
Left 1st lumbar splanchnic nerve
Superior mesenteric ganglion

Intermediolateral cell column (lateral horn of gray matter)

T5
T6
T7
T8

Spinal cord

Sympathetic trunk

Greater thoracic splanchnic nerve (preganglionic fibers)

Celiac ganglion

Medulla   Cortex

Postganglionic fibers supply blood vessels

Preganglionic fibers ramify around cells of medulla

Suprarenal gland

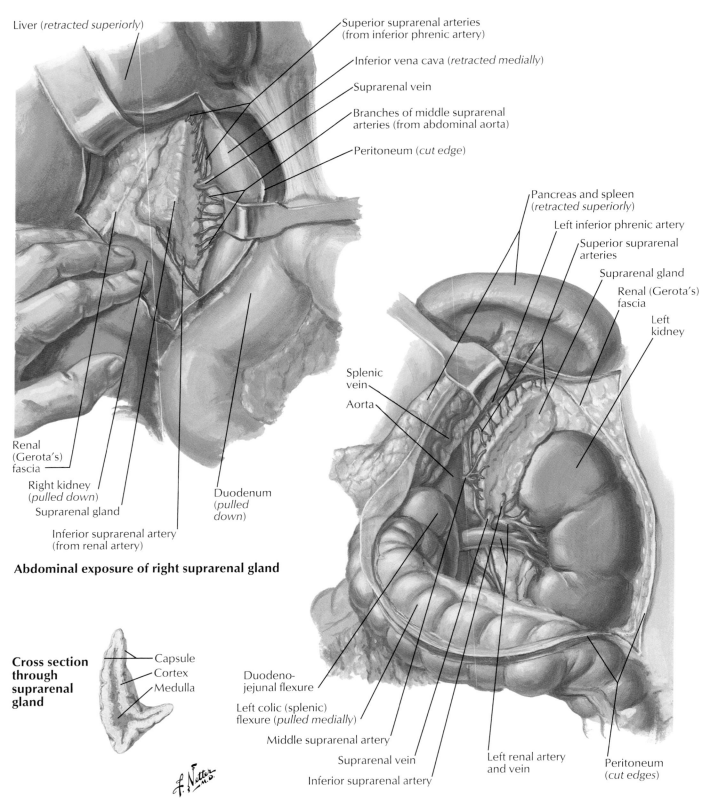

Liver (*retracted superiorly*)

Superior suprarenal arteries (from inferior phrenic artery)

Inferior vena cava (*retracted medially*)

Suprarenal vein

Branches of middle suprarenal arteries (from abdominal aorta)

Peritoneum (*cut edge*)

Pancreas and spleen (*retracted superiorly*)

Left inferior phrenic artery

Superior suprarenal arteries

Suprarenal gland

Renal (Gerota's) fascia

Left kidney

Splenic vein

Aorta

Renal (Gerota's) fascia

Right kidney (*pulled down*)

Suprarenal gland

Inferior suprarenal artery (from renal artery)

Duodenum (*pulled down*)

Abdominal exposure of right suprarenal gland

Cross section through suprarenal gland

Capsule

Cortex

Medulla

Duodeno-jejunal flexure

Left colic (splenic) flexure (*pulled medially*)

Middle suprarenal artery

Suprarenal vein

Inferior suprarenal artery

Left renal artery and vein

Peritoneum (*cut edges*)

Abdominal exposure of left suprarenal gland

Plate 322   **Kidneys and Suprarenal Glands**

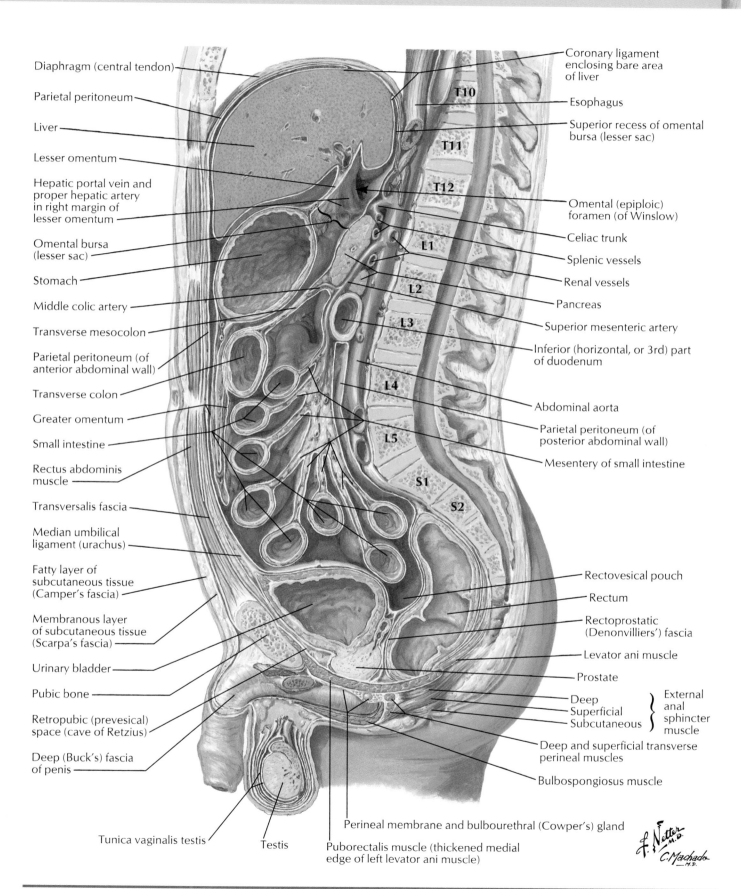

Diaphragm (central tendon)

Parietal peritoneum

Liver

Lesser omentum

Hepatic portal vein and proper hepatic artery in right margin of lesser omentum

Omental bursa (lesser sac)

Stomach

Middle colic artery

Transverse mesocolon

Parietal peritoneum (of anterior abdominal wall)

Transverse colon

Greater omentum

Small intestine

Rectus abdominis muscle

Transversalis fascia

Median umbilical ligament (urachus)

Fatty layer of subcutaneous tissue (Camper's fascia)

Membranous layer of subcutaneous tissue (Scarpa's fascia)

Urinary bladder

Pubic bone

Retropubic (prevesical) space (cave of Retzius)

Deep (Buck's) fascia of penis

Tunica vaginalis testis

Testis

Puborectalis muscle (thickened medial edge of left levator ani muscle)

Perineal membrane and bulbourethral (Cowper's) gland

T10

T11

T12

L1

L2

L3

L4

L5

S1

S2

Coronary ligament enclosing bare area of liver

Esophagus

Superior recess of omental bursa (lesser sac)

Omental (epiploic) foramen (of Winslow)

Celiac trunk

Splenic vessels

Renal vessels

Pancreas

Superior mesenteric artery

Inferior (horizontal, or 3rd) part of duodenum

Abdominal aorta

Parietal peritoneum (of posterior abdominal wall)

Mesentery of small intestine

Rectovesical pouch

Rectum

Rectoprostatic (Denonvilliers') fascia

Levator ani muscle

Prostate

Deep
Superficial
Subcutaneous
} External anal sphincter muscle

Deep and superficial transverse perineal muscles

Bulbospongiosus muscle

Series of abdominal axial CT images from superior (A) to inferior (D)

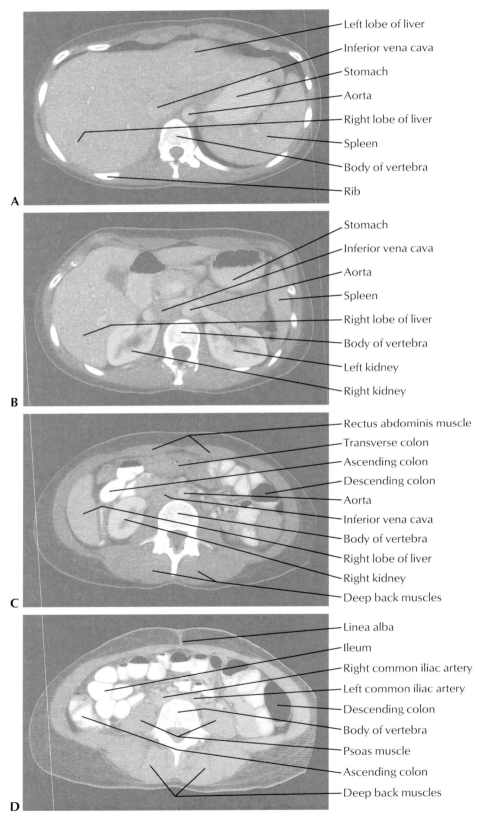

A
- Left lobe of liver
- Inferior vena cava
- Stomach
- Aorta
- Right lobe of liver
- Spleen
- Body of vertebra
- Rib

B
- Stomach
- Inferior vena cava
- Aorta
- Spleen
- Right lobe of liver
- Body of vertebra
- Left kidney
- Right kidney

C
- Rectus abdominis muscle
- Transverse colon
- Ascending colon
- Descending colon
- Aorta
- Inferior vena cava
- Body of vertebra
- Right lobe of liver
- Right kidney
- Deep back muscles

D
- Linea alba
- Ileum
- Right common iliac artery
- Left common iliac artery
- Descending colon
- Body of vertebra
- Psoas muscle
- Ascending colon
- Deep back muscles

Plate 324   **Cross-sectional Anatomy**

See also **Plates 326-329**

Transverse Section: Level of T10, Esophagogastric Junction

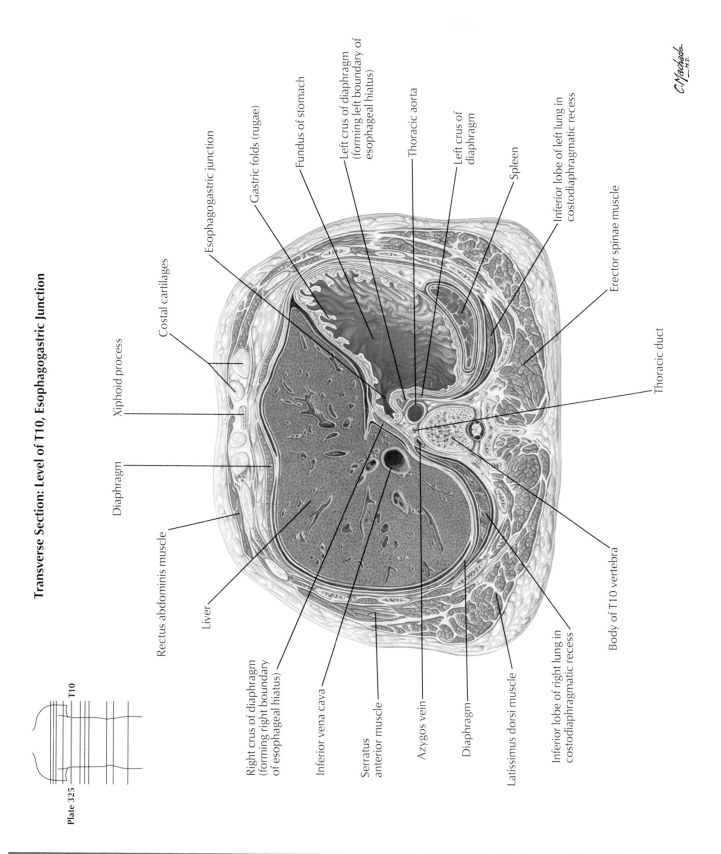

Esophagogastric junction

Gastric folds (rugae)

Fundus of stomach

Left crus of diaphragm (forming left boundary of esophageal hiatus)

Thoracic aorta

Left crus of diaphragm

Spleen

Inferior lobe of left lung in costodiaphragmatic recess

Erector spinae muscle

Costal cartilages

Xiphoid process

Diaphragm

Rectus abdominis muscle

Liver

Thoracic duct

Right crus of diaphragm (forming right boundary of esophageal hiatus)

Inferior vena cava

Serratus anterior muscle

Azygos vein

Diaphragm

Latissimus dorsi muscle

Inferior lobe of right lung in costodiaphragmatic recess

Body of T10 vertebra

T10

Plate 325

Transverse Section: Level of T12, Inferior to Xiphoid

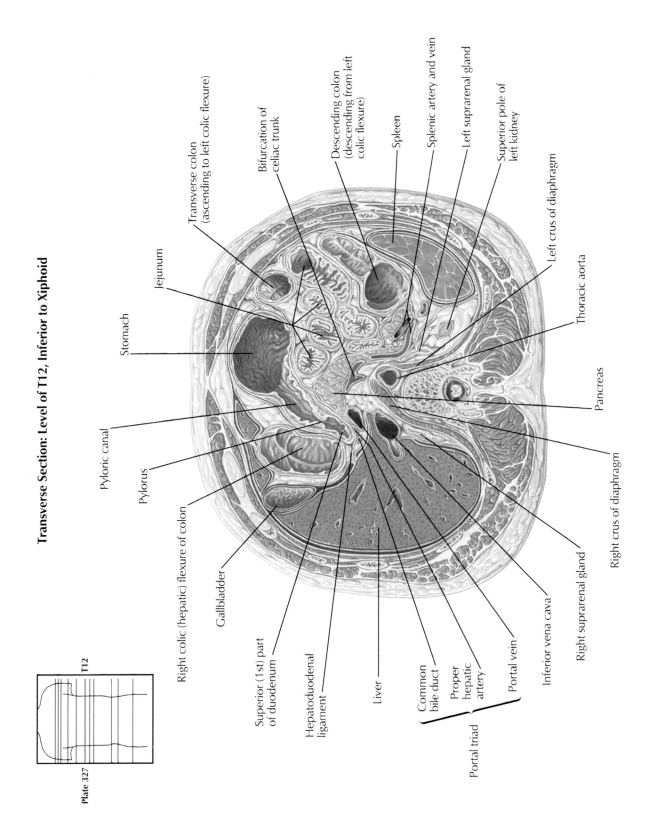

Transverse colon
(ascending to left colic flexure)

Bifurcation of
celiac trunk

Descending colon
(descending from left
colic flexure)

Spleen

Splenic artery and vein

Left suprarenal gland

Superior pole of
left kidney

Left crus of diaphragm

Thoracic aorta

Pancreas

Right crus of diaphragm

Right suprarenal gland

Inferior vena cava

Portal vein

Proper
hepatic
artery

Common
bile duct

Liver

Hepatoduodenal
ligament

Superior (1st) part
of duodenum

Gallbladder

Right colic (hepatic) flexure of colon

Pylorus

Pyloric canal

Stomach

Jejunum

Portal triad

T12

Plate 327

Plate 326   **Cross-sectional Anatomy**

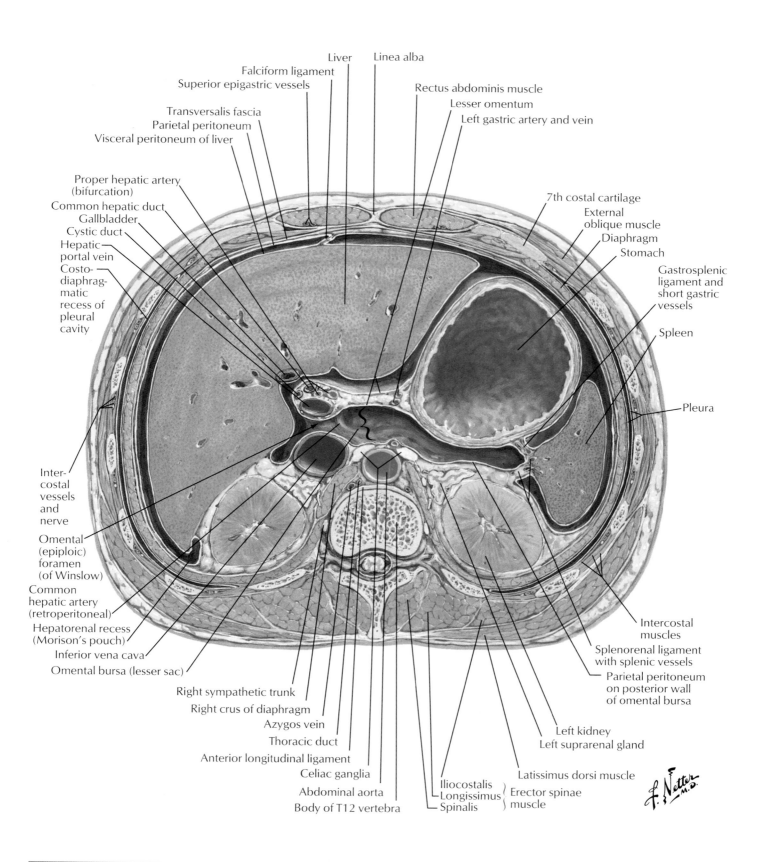

Liver

Linea alba

Falciform ligament

Superior epigastric vessels

Rectus abdominis muscle

Lesser omentum

Left gastric artery and vein

Transversalis fascia

Parietal peritoneum

Visceral peritoneum of liver

Proper hepatic artery
(bifurcation)

Common hepatic duct

Gallbladder

Cystic duct

Hepatic
portal vein

Costo-
diaphrag-
matic
recess
of pleural
cavity

7th costal cartilage

External
oblique muscle

Diaphragm

Stomach

Gastrosplenic
ligament and
short gastric
vessels

Spleen

Pleura

Inter-
costal
vessels
and
nerve

Omental
(epiploic)
foramen
(of Winslow)

Common
hepatic artery
(retroperitoneal)

Hepatorenal recess
(Morison's pouch)

Inferior vena cava

Omental bursa (lesser sac)

Right sympathetic trunk

Right crus of diaphragm

Azygos vein

Thoracic duct

Anterior longitudinal ligament

Celiac ganglia

Abdominal aorta

Body of T12 vertebra

Intercostal
muscles

Splenorenal ligament
with splenic vessels

Parietal peritoneum
on posterior wall
of omental bursa

Left kidney

Left suprarenal gland

Latissimus dorsi muscle

Iliocostalis
Longissimus
Spinalis
} Erector spinae
muscle

f. Netter
M.D.

Transverse Section: Level of T12–L1 Intervertebral Disc

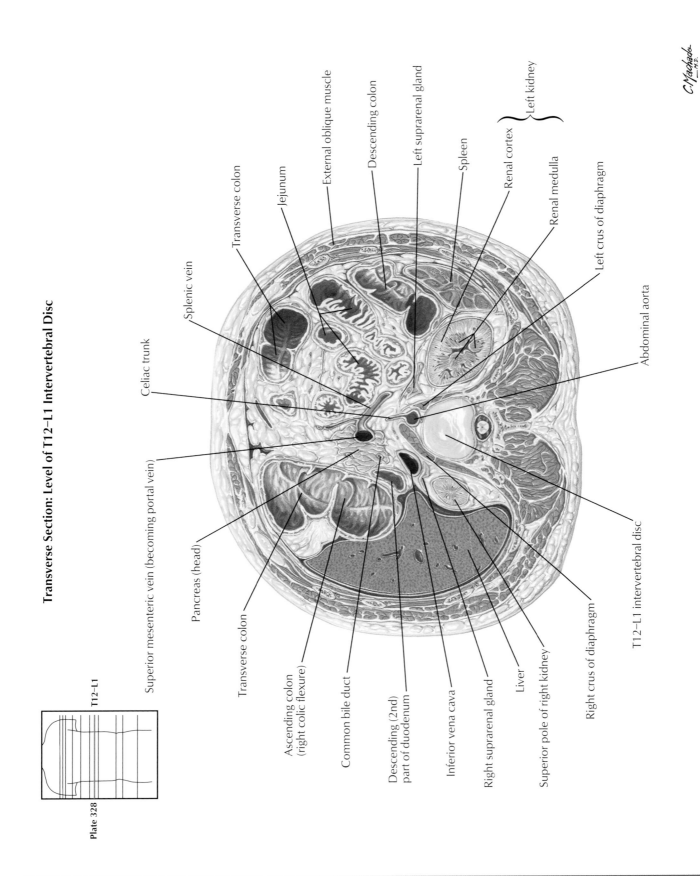

External oblique muscle

Descending colon

Left suprarenal gland

Spleen

Renal cortex

Renal medulla

Left kidney

Left crus of diaphragm

Jejunum

Transverse colon

Splenic vein

Abdominal aorta

Celiac trunk

Superior mesenteric vein (becoming portal vein)

Pancreas (head)

Transverse colon

T12–L1 intervertebral disc

Ascending colon (right colic flexure)

Common bile duct

Descending (2nd) part of duodenum

Inferior vena cava

Right suprarenal gland

Liver

Superior pole of right kidney

Right crus of diaphragm

T12–L1

Plate 328

Plate 328

Cross-sectional Anatomy

Transverse Section: Level of L1–2 Intervertebral Disc

Superior mesenteric artery

Transverse colon

Ileum

Jejunum

Perirenal fat

Ureteropelvic junction

Descending colon

Renal fascia

Left kidney

Major calyx and renal pelvis

Pararenal fat

Left renal artery

Left renal vein (entering inferior vena cava)

Left crus of diaphragm

Superior mesenteric vein

Abdominal aorta

Greater omentum

Pancreas with uncinate process

Transverse colon

Junction of 2nd and 3rd parts of duodenum

Ascending colon

Liver

Right renal vein (entering inferior vena cava)

Right kidney

Inferior vena cava

Right crus of diaphragm

Psoas major muscle

L1–2 intervertebral disc

Conus medullaris and cauda equina

C. Machado —M.D.

L1–2

Plate 329

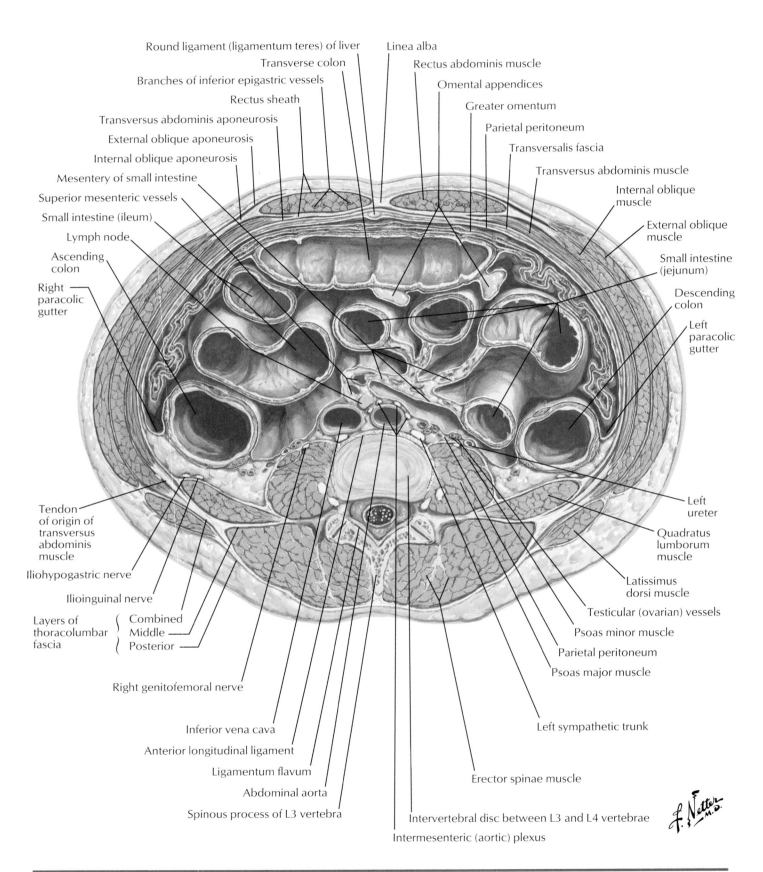

Round ligament (ligamentum teres) of liver

Transverse colon

Branches of inferior epigastric vessels

Rectus sheath

Transversus abdominis aponeurosis

External oblique aponeurosis

Internal oblique aponeurosis

Mesentery of small intestine

Superior mesenteric vessels

Small intestine (ileum)

Lymph node

Ascending colon

Right paracolic gutter

Linea alba

Rectus abdominis muscle

Omental appendices

Greater omentum

Parietal peritoneum

Transversalis fascia

Transversus abdominis muscle

Internal oblique muscle

External oblique muscle

Small intestine (jejunum)

Descending colon

Left paracolic gutter

Left ureter

Quadratus lumborum muscle

Latissimus dorsi muscle

Testicular (ovarian) vessels

Psoas minor muscle

Parietal peritoneum

Psoas major muscle

Left sympathetic trunk

Erector spinae muscle

Tendon of origin of transversus abdominis muscle

Iliohypogastric nerve

Ilioinguinal nerve

Layers of thoracolumbar fascia { Combined / Middle / Posterior

Right genitofemoral nerve

Inferior vena cava

Anterior longitudinal ligament

Ligamentum flavum

Abdominal aorta

Spinous process of L3 vertebra

Intervertebral disc between L3 and L4 vertebrae

Intermesenteric (aortic) plexus

Plate 330   **Cross-sectional Anatomy**

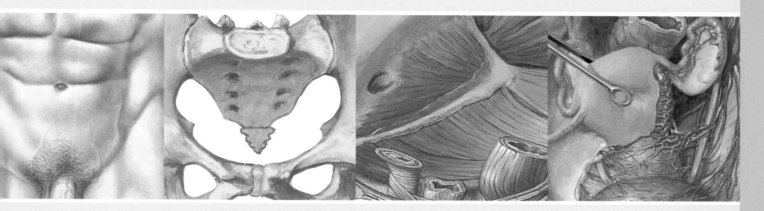

Section 5 PELVIS AND PERINEUM

Topographic Anatomy
Plate 331

331 Pelvis and Perineum

Bones and Ligaments
Plates 332-336

332 Bony Framework of Pelvis

333 Radiographs of Male and Female Pelvis

334 Sex Differences of Pelvis: Measurements

335 Bones and Ligaments of Pelvis

336 Bones and Ligaments of Pelvis (continued)

Pelvic Floor and Contents
Plates 337-347

337 Pelvic Diaphragm: Female

338 Pelvic Diaphragm: Female (continued)

339 Pelvic Diaphragm: Female (continued)

340 Pelvic Diaphragm: Male

341 Pelvic Diaphragm: Male (continued)

342 Pelvic Viscera and Perineum: Female

343 Pelvic Contents: Female

344 Pelvic Viscera: Female

345 Endopelvic Fascia and Potential Spaces

346 Pelvic Viscera and Perineum: Male

347 Pelvic Contents: Male

Urinary Bladder
Plates 348-351

348 Urinary Bladder: Orientation and Supports

349 Sphincters

350 Urinary Bladder: Female and Male

351 Male and Female Cystourethrograms

Uterus, Vagina, and Supporting Structures
Plates 352-355

352 Uterus, Vagina, and Supporting Structures

353 Uterus: Fascial Ligaments

354 Pelvic Ligaments

355 Uterus and Adnexa

Perineum and External Genitalia: Female
Plates 356-359

356 Female Perineum and External Genitalia (Pudendum or Vulva)

357 Female Perineum (Superficial Dissection)

358 Female Perineum and Deep Perineum

359 Female Perineal Spaces

Perineum and External Genitalia: Male
Plates 360-367

360 Male Perineum and External Genitalia (Superficial Dissection)

361 Male Perineum and External Genitalia (Deeper Dissection)

362 Penis

363 Male Perineal Spaces

364 Prostate and Seminal Vesicles

365 Urethra

366 Descent of Testis

367 Scrotum and Contents

Homologues of Genitalia
Plates 368-369

368 Homologues of External Genitalia

369 Homologues of Internal Genitalia

Testis, Epididymis, and Ductus Deferens
Plate 370

370 Testis, Epididymis, and Ductus Deferens

Rectum
Plates 371-376

371 Rectum in Situ: Female and Male

372 Ischioanal Fossae

373 Rectum and Anal Canal

374 Anorectal Musculature

375 External Anal Sphincter Muscle: Perineal Views

376 Actual and Potential Perineopelvic Spaces

Regional Scans
Plate 377

377 Pelvic Scans: Sagittal MR Images

Vasculature
Plate 378-388

378 Arteries of Rectum and Anal Canal: Male

379 Veins of Rectum and Anal Canal: Female

380 Arteries and Veins of Pelvic Organs: Female

381 Arteries and Veins of Testis

382 Arteries and Veins of Pelvis: Female

383 Arteries and Veins of Pelvis: Male

384 Arteries and Veins of Perineum and Uterus

385 Arteries and Veins of Perineum: Male

386 Lymph Vessels and Nodes of Pelvis and Genitalia: Female

387 Lymph Vessels and Nodes of Perineum: Female

388 Lymph Vessels and Nodes of Pelvis and Genitalia: Male

Innervation
Plates 389-397

389   Nerves of External Genitalia: Male

390   Nerves of Pelvic Viscera: Male

391   Nerves of Perineum: Male

392   Nerves of Pelvic Viscera: Female

393   Nerves of Perineum and External Genitalia: Female

394   Neuropathways in Parturition

395   Innervation of Female Reproductive Organs: Schema

396   Innervation of Male Reproductive Organs: Schema

397   Innervation of Urinary Bladder and Lower Ureter: Schema

Cross-sectional Anatomy
Plates 398-399

398   Male Pelvis: Bladder-Prostate Junction

399   Female Pelvis: Vagina-Urethra

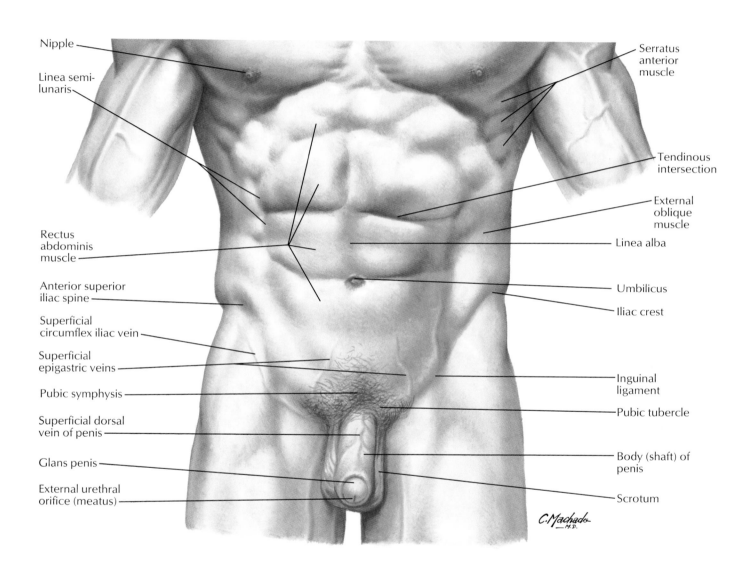

Nipple

Linea semi-lunaris

Rectus abdominis muscle

Anterior superior iliac spine

Superficial circumflex iliac vein

Superficial epigastric veins

Pubic symphysis

Superficial dorsal vein of penis

Glans penis

External urethral orifice (meatus)

Serratus anterior muscle

Tendinous intersection

External oblique muscle

Linea alba

Umbilicus

Iliac crest

Inguinal ligament

Pubic tubercle

Body (shaft) of penis

Scrotum

C. Machado
_M.D.

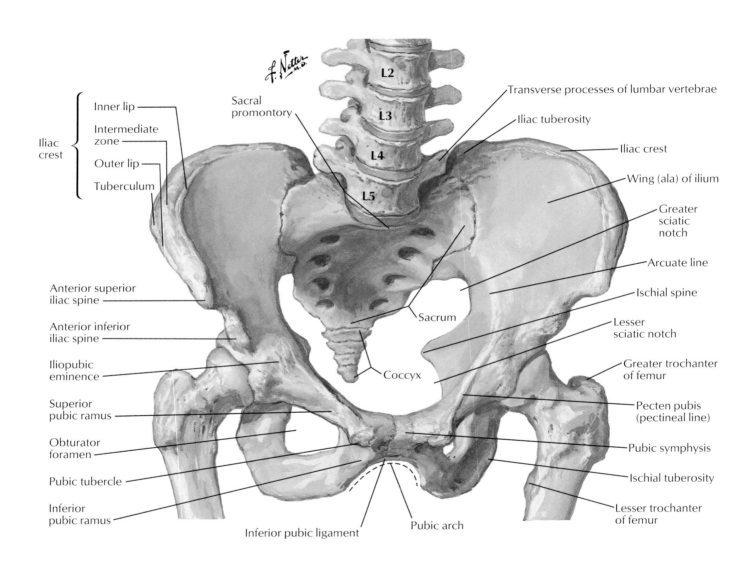

Iliac crest
- Inner lip
- Intermediate zone
- Outer lip
- Tuberculum

L2

L3

L4

L5

Sacral promontory

Transverse processes of lumbar vertebrae

Iliac tuberosity

Iliac crest

Wing (ala) of ilium

Greater sciatic notch

Arcuate line

Ischial spine

Lesser sciatic notch

Greater trochanter of femur

Pecten pubis (pectineal line)

Pubic symphysis

Ischial tuberosity

Lesser trochanter of femur

Anterior superior iliac spine

Anterior inferior iliac spine

Iliopubic eminence

Superior pubic ramus

Obturator foramen

Pubic tubercle

Inferior pubic ramus

Sacrum

Coccyx

Inferior pubic ligament

Pubic arch

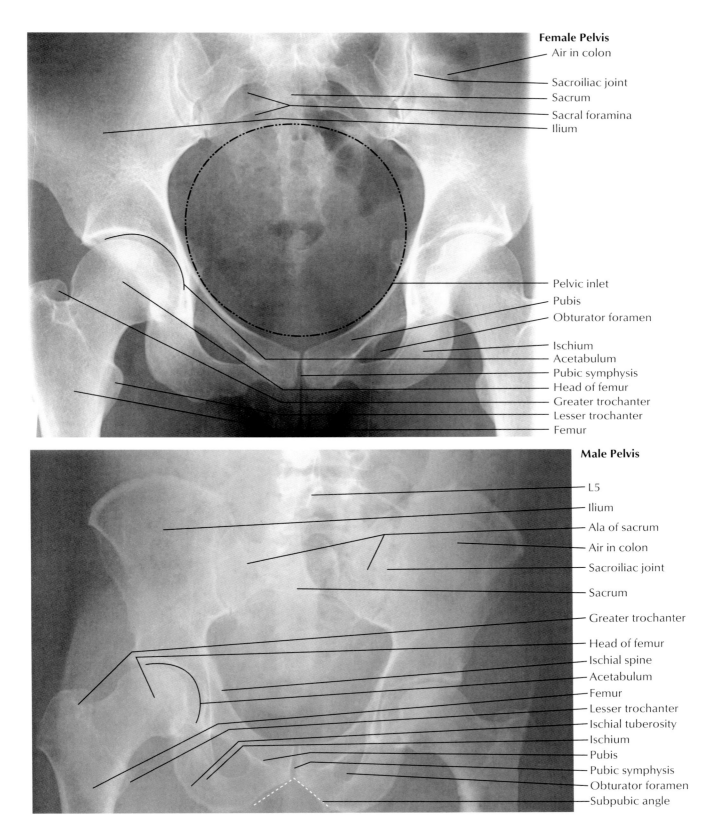

Female Pelvis
- Air in colon
- Sacroiliac joint
- Sacrum
- Sacral foramina
- Ilium

- Pelvic inlet
- Pubis
- Obturator foramen
- Ischium
- Acetabulum
- Pubic symphysis
- Head of femur
- Greater trochanter
- Lesser trochanter
- Femur

Male Pelvis
- L5
- Ilium
- Ala of sacrum
- Air in colon
- Sacroiliac joint
- Sacrum
- Greater trochanter
- Head of femur
- Ischial spine
- Acetabulum
- Femur
- Lesser trochanter
- Ischial tuberosity
- Ischium
- Pubis
- Pubic symphysis
- Obturator foramen
- Subpubic angle

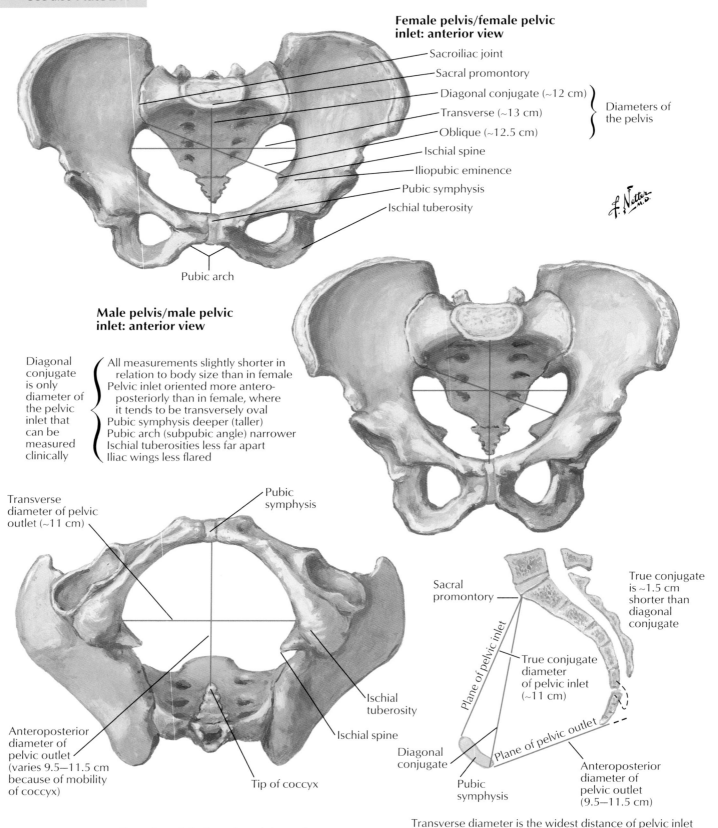

Female pelvis/female pelvic inlet: anterior view

Sacroiliac joint

Sacral promontory

Diagonal conjugate (~12 cm)

Transverse (~13 cm)

Oblique (~12.5 cm)

} Diameters of the pelvis

Ischial spine

Iliopubic eminence

Pubic symphysis

Ischial tuberosity

Pubic arch

F. Netter M.D.

Male pelvis/male pelvic inlet: anterior view

Diagonal conjugate is only diameter of the pelvic inlet that can be measured clinically
{
All measurements slightly shorter in relation to body size than in female
Pelvic inlet oriented more antero-posteriorly than in female, where it tends to be transversely oval
Pubic symphysis deeper (taller)
Pubic arch (subpubic angle) narrower
Ischial tuberosities less far apart
Iliac wings less flared

Transverse diameter of pelvic outlet (~11 cm)

Pubic symphysis

Anteroposterior diameter of pelvic outlet (varies 9.5—11.5 cm because of mobility of coccyx)

Ischial tuberosity

Ischial spine

Tip of coccyx

Female pelvis/female pelvic outlet: inferior view

Sacral promontory

True conjugate is ~1.5 cm shorter than diagonal conjugate

Plane of pelvic inlet

True conjugate diameter of pelvic inlet (~11 cm)

Plane of pelvic outlet

Diagonal conjugate

Pubic symphysis

Anteroposterior diameter of pelvic outlet (9.5—11.5 cm)

Transverse diameter is the widest distance of pelvic inlet

Female: sagittal section

Plate 334

Bones and Ligaments

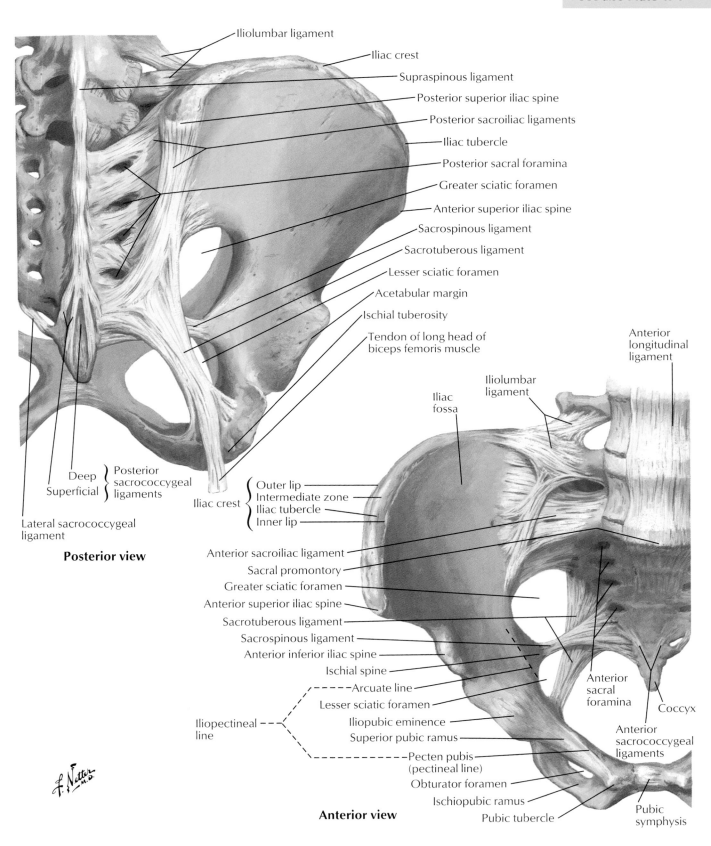

Iliolumbar ligament

Iliac crest

Supraspinous ligament

Posterior superior iliac spine

Posterior sacroiliac ligaments

Iliac tubercle

Posterior sacral foramina

Greater sciatic foramen

Anterior superior iliac spine

Sacrospinous ligament

Sacrotuberous ligament

Lesser sciatic foramen

Acetabular margin

Ischial tuberosity

Tendon of long head of biceps femoris muscle

Deep ⎫
Superficial ⎬ Posterior sacrococcygeal ligaments

Iliac crest

Lateral sacrococcygeal ligament

Posterior view

Anterior longitudinal ligament

Iliolumbar ligament

Iliac fossa

Outer lip
Intermediate zone
Iliac tubercle
Inner lip

Iliac crest

Anterior sacroiliac ligament

Sacral promontory

Greater sciatic foramen

Anterior superior iliac spine

Sacrotuberous ligament

Sacrospinous ligament

Anterior inferior iliac spine

Ischial spine

Arcuate line

Lesser sciatic foramen

Iliopectineal line

Iliopubic eminence

Superior pubic ramus

Pecten pubis (pectineal line)

Obturator foramen

Ischiopubic ramus

Pubic tubercle

Anterior sacral foramina

Coccyx

Anterior sacrococcygeal ligaments

Pubic symphysis

Anterior view

Median (sagittal) section

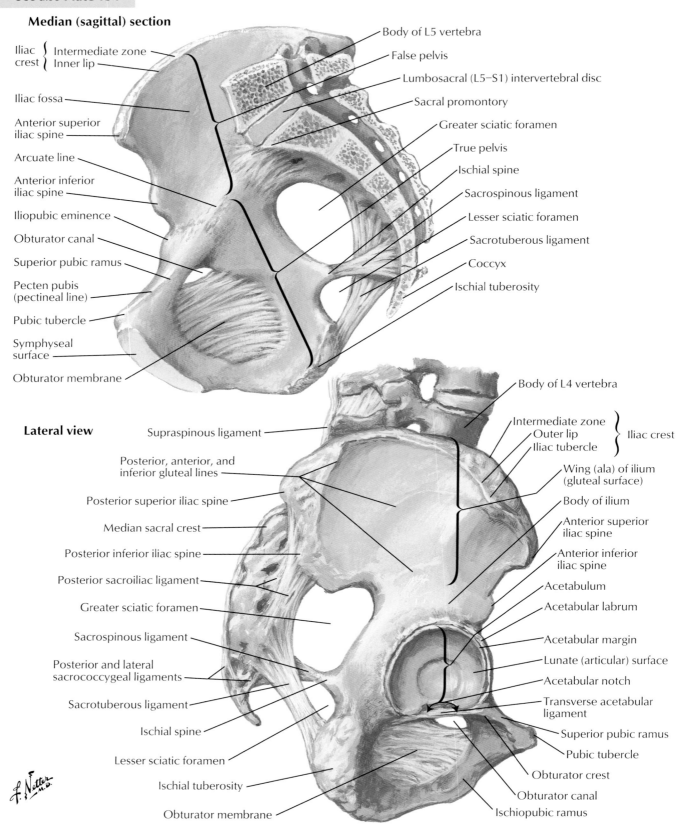

Iliac crest { Intermediate zone / Inner lip

Iliac fossa

Anterior superior iliac spine

Arcuate line

Anterior inferior iliac spine

Iliopubic eminence

Obturator canal

Superior pubic ramus

Pecten pubis (pectineal line)

Pubic tubercle

Symphyseal surface

Obturator membrane

Body of L5 vertebra

False pelvis

Lumbosacral (L5–S1) intervertebral disc

Sacral promontory

Greater sciatic foramen

True pelvis

Ischial spine

Sacrospinous ligament

Lesser sciatic foramen

Sacrotuberous ligament

Coccyx

Ischial tuberosity

Lateral view

Supraspinous ligament

Posterior, anterior, and inferior gluteal lines

Posterior superior iliac spine

Median sacral crest

Posterior inferior iliac spine

Posterior sacroiliac ligament

Greater sciatic foramen

Sacrospinous ligament

Posterior and lateral sacrococcygeal ligaments

Sacrotuberous ligament

Ischial spine

Lesser sciatic foramen

Ischial tuberosity

Obturator membrane

Body of L4 vertebra

Intermediate zone / Outer lip / Iliac tubercle } Iliac crest

Wing (ala) of ilium (gluteal surface)

Body of ilium

Anterior superior iliac spine

Anterior inferior iliac spine

Acetabulum

Acetabular labrum

Acetabular margin

Lunate (articular) surface

Acetabular notch

Transverse acetabular ligament

Superior pubic ramus

Pubic tubercle

Obturator crest

Obturator canal

Ischiopubic ramus

Plate 336   **Bones and Ligaments**

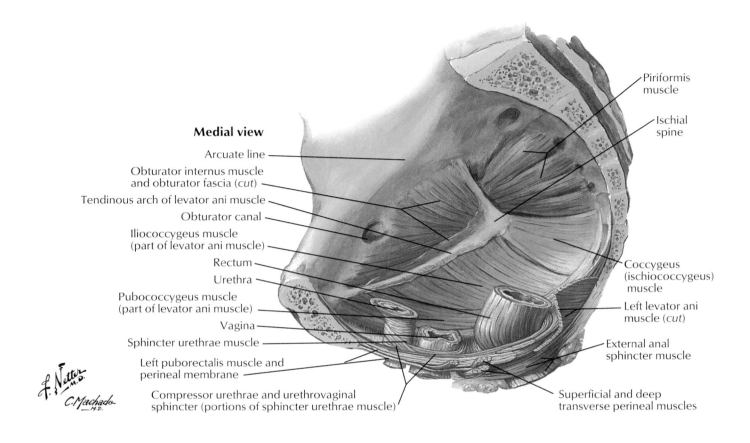

Medial view

- Arcuate line
- Obturator internus muscle and obturator fascia (*cut*)
- Tendinous arch of levator ani muscle
- Obturator canal
- Iliococcygeus muscle (part of levator ani muscle)
- Rectum
- Urethra
- Pubococcygeus muscle (part of levator ani muscle)
- Vagina
- Sphincter urethrae muscle
- Left puborectalis muscle and perineal membrane
- Compressor urethrae and urethrovaginal sphincter (portions of sphincter urethrae muscle)

- Piriformis muscle
- Ischial spine
- Coccygeus (ischiococcygeus) muscle
- Left levator ani muscle (*cut*)
- External anal sphincter muscle
- Superficial and deep transverse perineal muscles

F. Netter M.D.
C. Machado M.D.

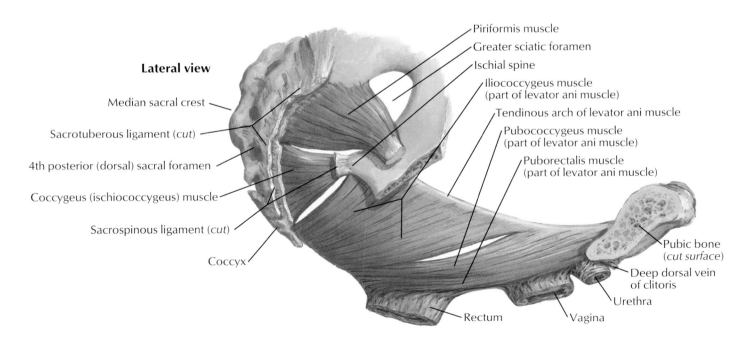

Lateral view

- Median sacral crest
- Sacrotuberous ligament (*cut*)
- 4th posterior (dorsal) sacral foramen
- Coccygeus (ischiococcygeus) muscle
- Sacrospinous ligament (*cut*)
- Coccyx

- Piriformis muscle
- Greater sciatic foramen
- Ischial spine
- Iliococcygeus muscle (part of levator ani muscle)
- Tendinous arch of levator ani muscle
- Pubococcygeus muscle (part of levator ani muscle)
- Puborectalis muscle (part of levator ani muscle)
- Pubic bone (*cut surface*)
- Deep dorsal vein of clitoris
- Urethra
- Vagina
- Rectum

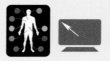

Medial view

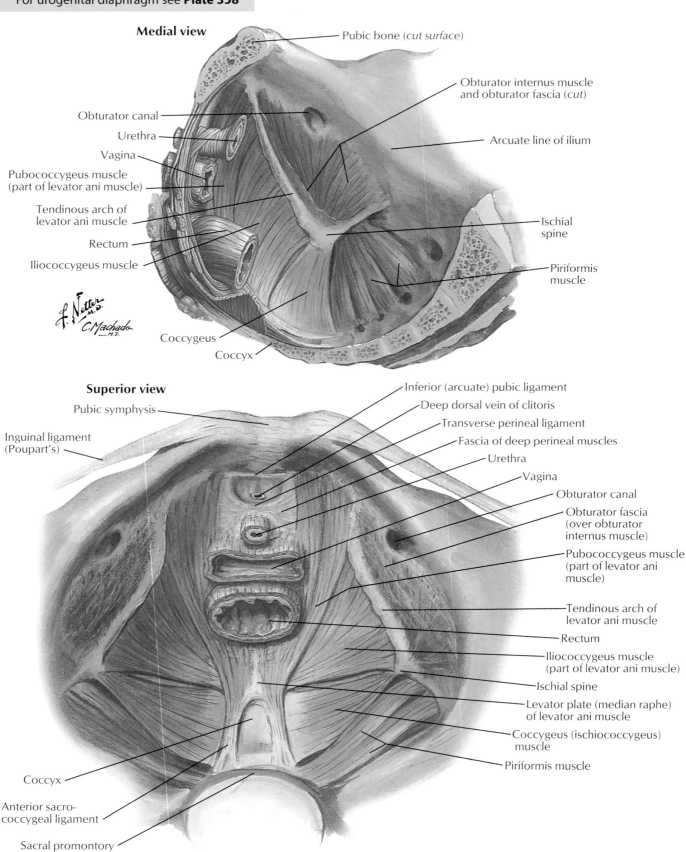

Pubic bone (*cut surface*)

Obturator internus muscle and obturator fascia (*cut*)

Obturator canal

Urethra

Vagina

Pubococcygeus muscle (part of levator ani muscle)

Tendinous arch of levator ani muscle

Rectum

Iliococcygeus muscle

Arcuate line of ilium

Ischial spine

Piriformis muscle

Coccygeus

Coccyx

Superior view

Pubic symphysis

Inguinal ligament (Poupart's)

Inferior (arcuate) pubic ligament

Deep dorsal vein of clitoris

Transverse perineal ligament

Fascia of deep perineal muscles

Urethra

Vagina

Obturator canal

Obturator fascia (over obturator internus muscle)

Pubococcygeus muscle (part of levator ani muscle)

Tendinous arch of levator ani muscle

Rectum

Iliococcygeus muscle (part of levator ani muscle)

Ischial spine

Levator plate (median raphe) of levator ani muscle

Coccygeus (ischiococcygeus) muscle

Piriformis muscle

Coccyx

Anterior sacro-coccygeal ligament

Sacral promontory

Plate 338

Pelvic Floor and Contents

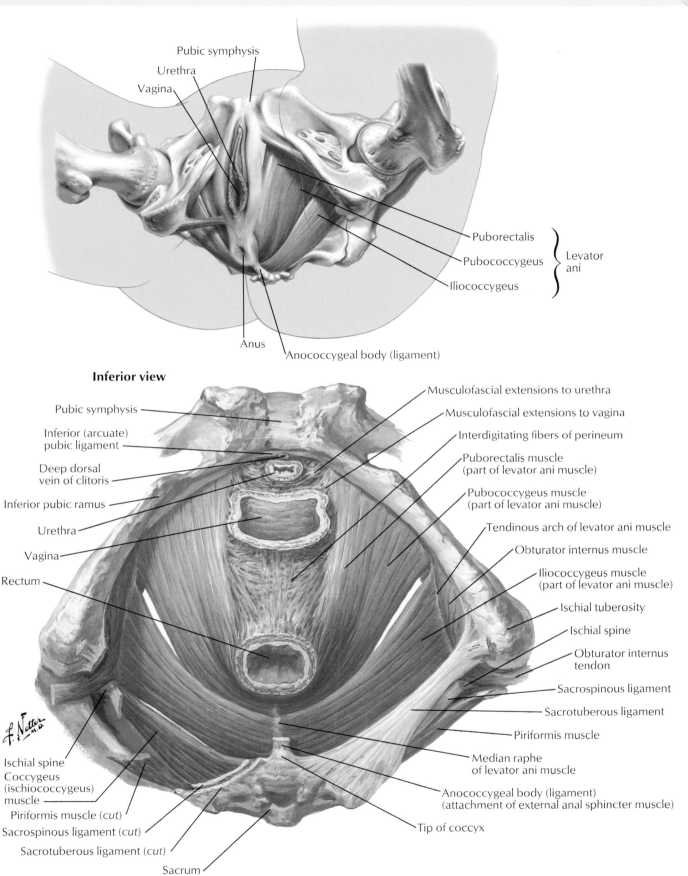

Pubic symphysis

Urethra

Vagina

Puborectalis ⎫
Pubococcygeus ⎬ Levator ani
Iliococcygeus ⎭

Anus

Anococcygeal body (ligament)

Inferior view

Pubic symphysis

Inferior (arcuate) pubic ligament

Deep dorsal vein of clitoris

Inferior pubic ramus

Urethra

Vagina

Rectum

Ischial spine

Coccygeus (ischiococcygeus) muscle

Piriformis muscle (*cut*)

Sacrospinous ligament (*cut*)

Sacrotuberous ligament (*cut*)

Sacrum

Musculofascial extensions to urethra

Musculofascial extensions to vagina

Interdigitating fibers of perineum

Puborectalis muscle (part of levator ani muscle)

Pubococcygeus muscle (part of levator ani muscle)

Tendinous arch of levator ani muscle

Obturator internus muscle

Iliococcygeus muscle (part of levator ani muscle)

Ischial tuberosity

Ischial spine

Obturator internus tendon

Sacrospinous ligament

Sacrotuberous ligament

Piriformis muscle

Median raphe of levator ani muscle

Anococcygeal body (ligament) (attachment of external anal sphincter muscle)

Tip of coccyx

Pelvic Diaphragm: Male

See also **Plates 256, 259, 372**

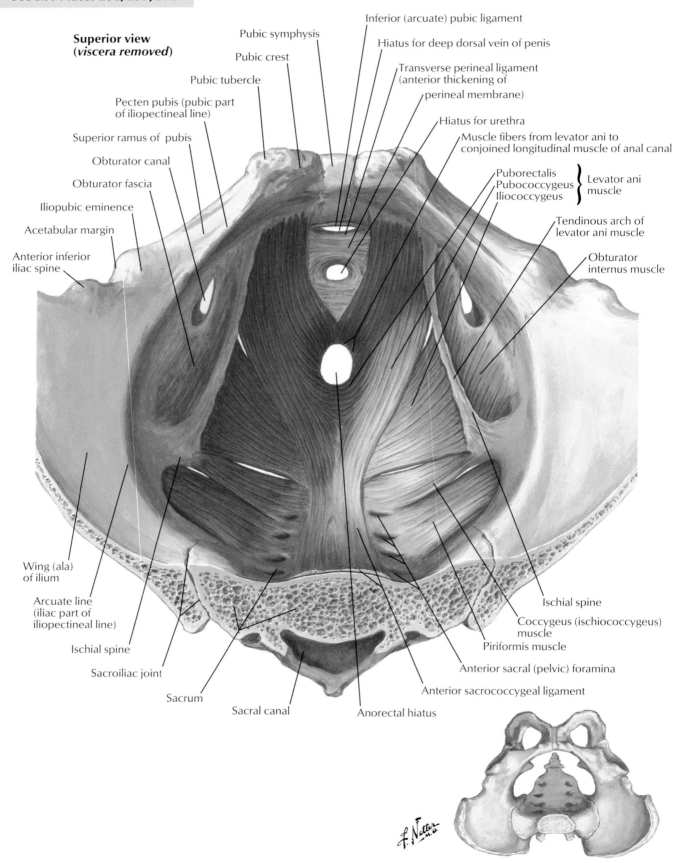

Superior view
(*viscera removed*)

Pubic symphysis

Pubic crest

Pubic tubercle

Pecten pubis (pubic part of iliopectineal line)

Superior ramus of pubis

Obturator canal

Obturator fascia

Iliopubic eminence

Acetabular margin

Anterior inferior iliac spine

Inferior (arcuate) pubic ligament

Hiatus for deep dorsal vein of penis

Transverse perineal ligament (anterior thickening of perineal membrane)

Hiatus for urethra

Muscle fibers from levator ani to conjoined longitudinal muscle of anal canal

Puborectalis
Pubococcygeus } Levator ani muscle
Iliococcygeus

Tendinous arch of levator ani muscle

Obturator internus muscle

Wing (ala) of ilium

Arcuate line (iliac part of iliopectineal line)

Ischial spine

Sacroiliac joint

Sacrum

Sacral canal

Anorectal hiatus

Anterior sacrococcygeal ligament

Anterior sacral (pelvic) foramina

Piriformis muscle

Coccygeus (ischiococcygeus) muscle

Ischial spine

Plate 340

Pelvic Floor and Contents

For urogenital diaphragm see **Plate 363**

Inferior view

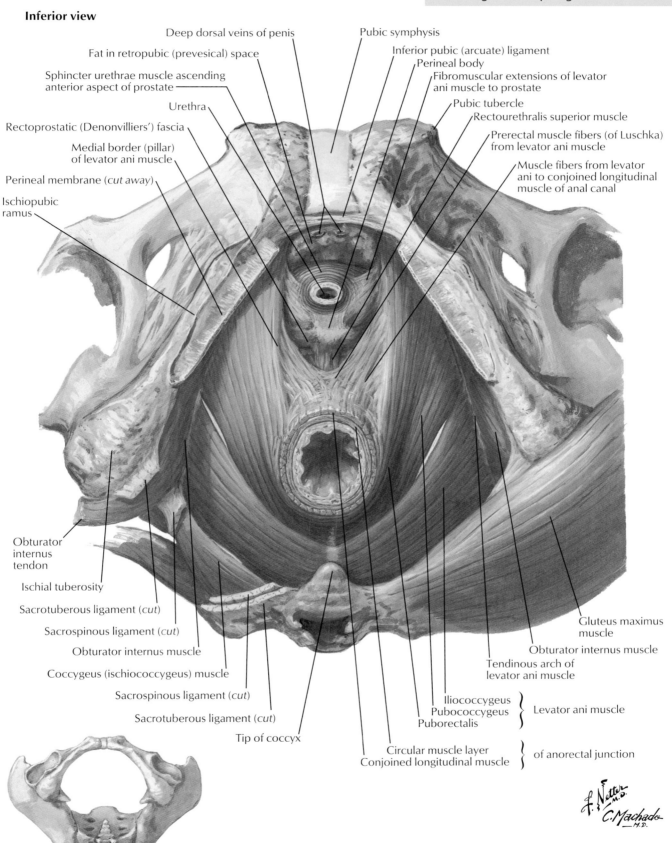

Deep dorsal veins of penis

Fat in retropubic (prevesical) space

Sphincter urethrae muscle ascending anterior aspect of prostate

Urethra

Rectoprostatic (Denonvilliers') fascia

Medial border (pillar) of levator ani muscle

Perineal membrane (*cut away*)

Ischiopubic ramus

Obturator internus tendon

Ischial tuberosity

Sacrotuberous ligament (*cut*)

Sacrospinous ligament (*cut*)

Obturator internus muscle

Coccygeus (ischiococcygeus) muscle

Sacrospinous ligament (*cut*)

Sacrotuberous ligament (*cut*)

Tip of coccyx

Pubic symphysis

Inferior pubic (arcuate) ligament

Perineal body

Fibromuscular extensions of levator ani muscle to prostate

Pubic tubercle

Rectourethralis superior muscle

Prerectal muscle fibers (of Luschka) from levator ani muscle

Muscle fibers from levator ani to conjoined longitudinal muscle of anal canal

Gluteus maximus muscle

Obturator internus muscle

Tendinous arch of levator ani muscle

Iliococcygeus }
Pubococcygeus } Levator ani muscle
Puborectalis }

Circular muscle layer } of anorectal junction
Conjoined longitudinal muscle }

Paramedian (sagittal) dissection

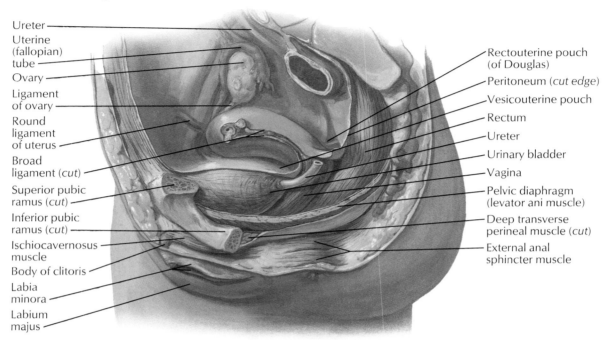

Ureter

Uterine (fallopian) tube

Ovary

Ligament of ovary

Round ligament of uterus

Broad ligament (cut)

Superior pubic ramus (cut)

Inferior pubic ramus (cut)

Ischiocavernosus muscle

Body of clitoris

Labia minora

Labium majus

Rectouterine pouch (of Douglas)

Peritoneum (cut edge)

Vesicouterine pouch

Rectum

Ureter

Urinary bladder

Vagina

Pelvic diaphragm (levator ani muscle)

Deep transverse perineal muscle (cut)

External anal sphincter muscle

Median (sagittal) section

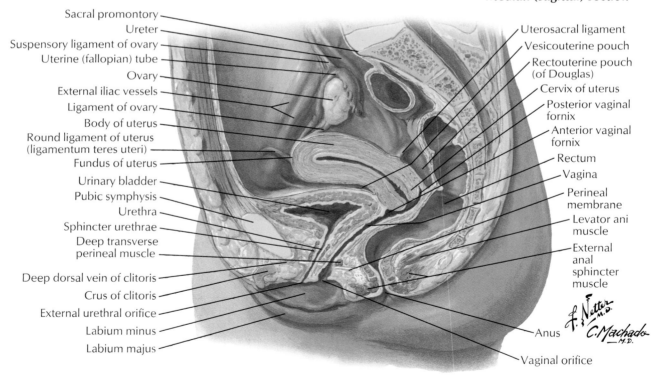

Sacral promontory

Ureter

Suspensory ligament of ovary

Uterine (fallopian) tube

Ovary

External iliac vessels

Ligament of ovary

Body of uterus

Round ligament of uterus (ligamentum teres uteri)

Fundus of uterus

Urinary bladder

Pubic symphysis

Urethra

Sphincter urethrae

Deep transverse perineal muscle

Deep dorsal vein of clitoris

Crus of clitoris

External urethral orifice

Labium minus

Labium majus

Uterosacral ligament

Vesicouterine pouch

Rectouterine pouch (of Douglas)

Cervix of uterus

Posterior vaginal fornix

Anterior vaginal fornix

Rectum

Vagina

Perineal membrane

Levator ani muscle

External anal sphincter muscle

Anus

Vaginal orifice

Plate 342   **Pelvic Floor and Contents**

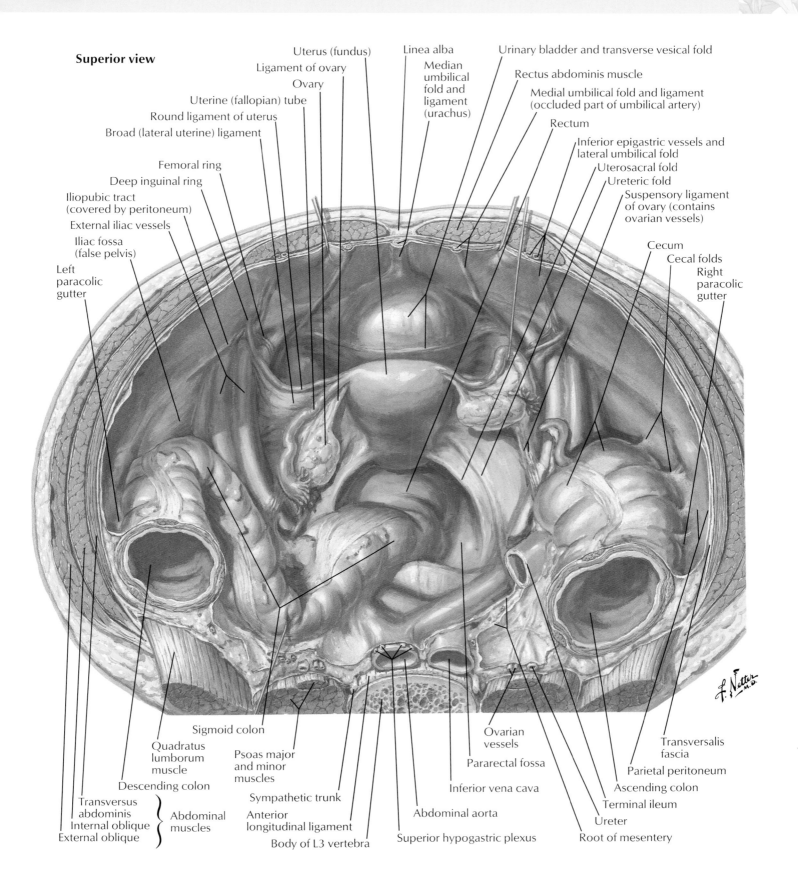

Superior view

Uterus (fundus)

Ligament of ovary

Ovary

Uterine (fallopian) tube

Round ligament of uterus

Broad (lateral uterine) ligament

Femoral ring

Deep inguinal ring

Iliopubic tract
(covered by peritoneum)

External iliac vessels

Iliac fossa
(false pelvis)

Left
paracolic
gutter

Linea alba

Median
umbilical
fold and
ligament
(urachus)

Urinary bladder and transverse vesical fold

Rectus abdominis muscle

Medial umbilical fold and ligament
(occluded part of umbilical artery)

Rectum

Inferior epigastric vessels and
lateral umbilical fold

Uterosacral fold

Ureteric fold

Suspensory ligament
of ovary (contains
ovarian vessels)

Cecum

Cecal folds

Right
paracolic
gutter

Sigmoid colon

Quadratus
lumborum
muscle

Psoas major
and minor
muscles

Descending colon

Sympathetic trunk

Transversus
abdominis

Internal oblique

External oblique

} Abdominal
muscles

Anterior
longitudinal ligament

Body of L3 vertebra

Ovarian
vessels

Pararectal fossa

Inferior vena cava

Abdominal aorta

Superior hypogastric plexus

Abdominal aorta

Transversalis
fascia

Parietal peritoneum

Ascending colon

Terminal ileum

Ureter

Root of mesentery

Superior view with peritoneum intact

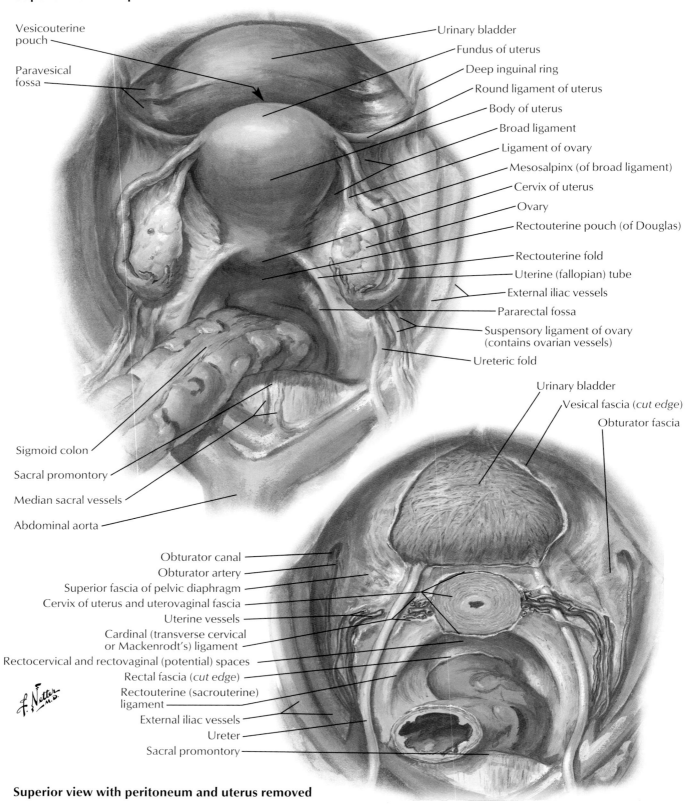

Vesicouterine pouch

Paravesical fossa

Urinary bladder

Fundus of uterus

Deep inguinal ring

Round ligament of uterus

Body of uterus

Broad ligament

Ligament of ovary

Mesosalpinx (of broad ligament)

Cervix of uterus

Ovary

Rectouterine pouch (of Douglas)

Rectouterine fold

Uterine (fallopian) tube

External iliac vessels

Pararectal fossa

Suspensory ligament of ovary (contains ovarian vessels)

Ureteric fold

Sigmoid colon

Sacral promontory

Median sacral vessels

Abdominal aorta

Urinary bladder

Vesical fascia (*cut edge*)

Obturator fascia

Obturator canal

Obturator artery

Superior fascia of pelvic diaphragm

Cervix of uterus and uterovaginal fascia

Uterine vessels

Cardinal (transverse cervical or Mackenrodt's) ligament

Rectocervical and rectovaginal (potential) spaces

Rectal fascia (*cut edge*)

Rectouterine (sacrouterine) ligament

External iliac vessels

Ureter

Sacral promontory

Superior view with peritoneum and uterus removed

Plate 344   **Pelvic Floor and Contents**

Female: superior view (peritoneum and loose areolar tissue removed)

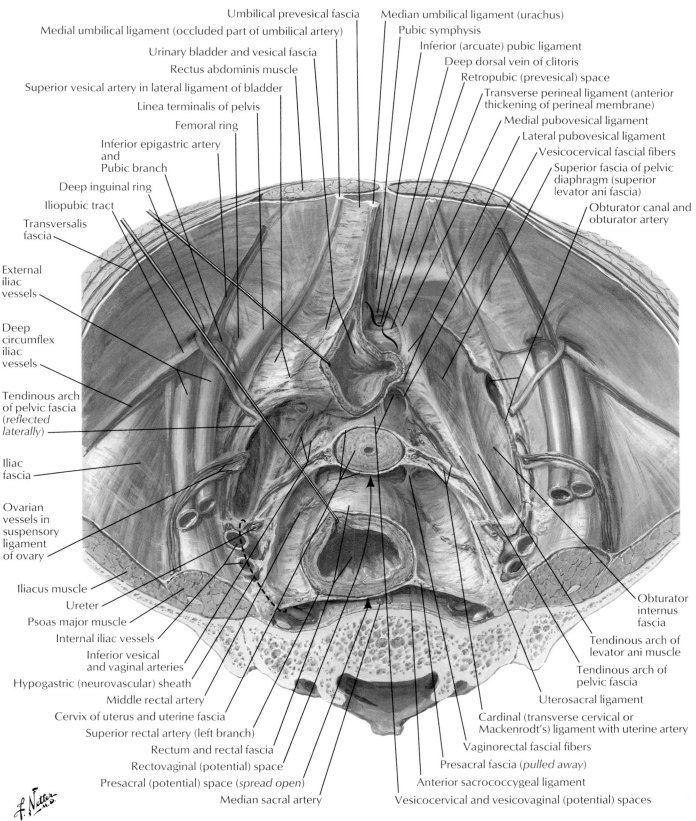

Umbilical prevesical fascia

Medial umbilical ligament (occluded part of umbilical artery)

Urinary bladder and vesical fascia

Rectus abdominis muscle

Superior vesical artery in lateral ligament of bladder

Linea terminalis of pelvis

Femoral ring

Inferior epigastric artery and Pubic branch

Deep inguinal ring

Iliopubic tract

Transversalis fascia

External iliac vessels

Deep circumflex iliac vessels

Tendinous arch of pelvic fascia (*reflected laterally*)

Iliac fascia

Ovarian vessels in suspensory ligament of ovary

Iliacus muscle

Ureter

Psoas major muscle

Internal iliac vessels

Inferior vesical and vaginal arteries

Hypogastric (neurovascular) sheath

Middle rectal artery

Cervix of uterus and uterine fascia

Superior rectal artery (left branch)

Rectum and rectal fascia

Rectovaginal (potential) space

Presacral (potential) space (*spread open*)

Median sacral artery

Median umbilical ligament (urachus)

Pubic symphysis

Inferior (arcuate) pubic ligament

Deep dorsal vein of clitoris

Retropubic (prevesical) space

Transverse perineal ligament (anterior thickening of perineal membrane)

Medial pubovesical ligament

Lateral pubovesical ligament

Vesicocervical fascial fibers

Superior fascia of pelvic diaphragm (superior levator ani fascia)

Obturator canal and obturator artery

Obturator internus fascia

Tendinous arch of levator ani muscle

Tendinous arch of pelvic fascia

Uterosacral ligament

Cardinal (transverse cervical or Mackenrodt's) ligament with uterine artery

Vaginorectal fascial fibers

Presacral fascia (*pulled away*)

Anterior sacrococcygeal ligament

Vesicocervical and vesicovaginal (potential) spaces

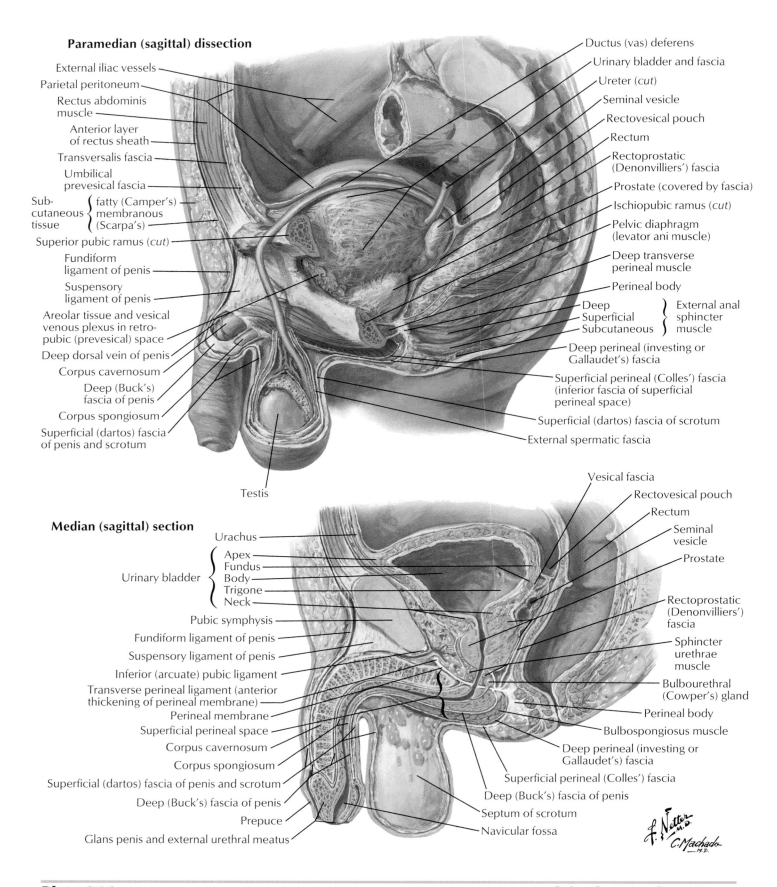

Paramedian (sagittal) dissection

External iliac vessels

Parietal peritoneum

Rectus abdominis muscle

Anterior layer of rectus sheath

Transversalis fascia

Umbilical prevesical fascia

Sub-cutaneous tissue { fatty (Camper's) / membranous (Scarpa's)

Superior pubic ramus (cut)

Fundiform ligament of penis

Suspensory ligament of penis

Areolar tissue and vesical venous plexus in retro-pubic (prevesical) space

Deep dorsal vein of penis

Corpus cavernosum

Deep (Buck's) fascia of penis

Corpus spongiosum

Superficial (dartos) fascia of penis and scrotum

Testis

Ductus (vas) deferens

Urinary bladder and fascia

Ureter (cut)

Seminal vesicle

Rectovesical pouch

Rectum

Rectoprostatic (Denonvilliers') fascia

Prostate (covered by fascia)

Ischiopubic ramus (cut)

Pelvic diaphragm (levator ani muscle)

Deep transverse perineal muscle

Perineal body

Deep / Superficial / Subcutaneous } External anal sphincter muscle

Deep perineal (investing or Gallaudet's) fascia

Superficial perineal (Colles') fascia (inferior fascia of superficial perineal space)

Superficial (dartos) fascia of scrotum

External spermatic fascia

Median (sagittal) section

Urachus

Urinary bladder { Apex / Fundus / Body / Trigone / Neck

Pubic symphysis

Fundiform ligament of penis

Suspensory ligament of penis

Inferior (arcuate) pubic ligament

Transverse perineal ligament (anterior thickening of perineal membrane)

Perineal membrane

Superficial perineal space

Corpus cavernosum

Corpus spongiosum

Superficial (dartos) fascia of penis and scrotum

Deep (Buck's) fascia of penis

Prepuce

Glans penis and external urethral meatus

Vesical fascia

Rectovesical pouch

Rectum

Seminal vesicle

Prostate

Rectoprostatic (Denonvilliers') fascia

Sphincter urethrae muscle

Bulbourethral (Cowper's) gland

Perineal body

Bulbospongiosus muscle

Deep perineal (investing or Gallaudet's) fascia

Superficial perineal (Colles') fascia

Deep (Buck's) fascia of penis

Septum of scrotum

Navicular fossa

F. Netter M.D.

C. Machado M.D.

Plate 346 **Pelvic Floor and Contents**

Superior view

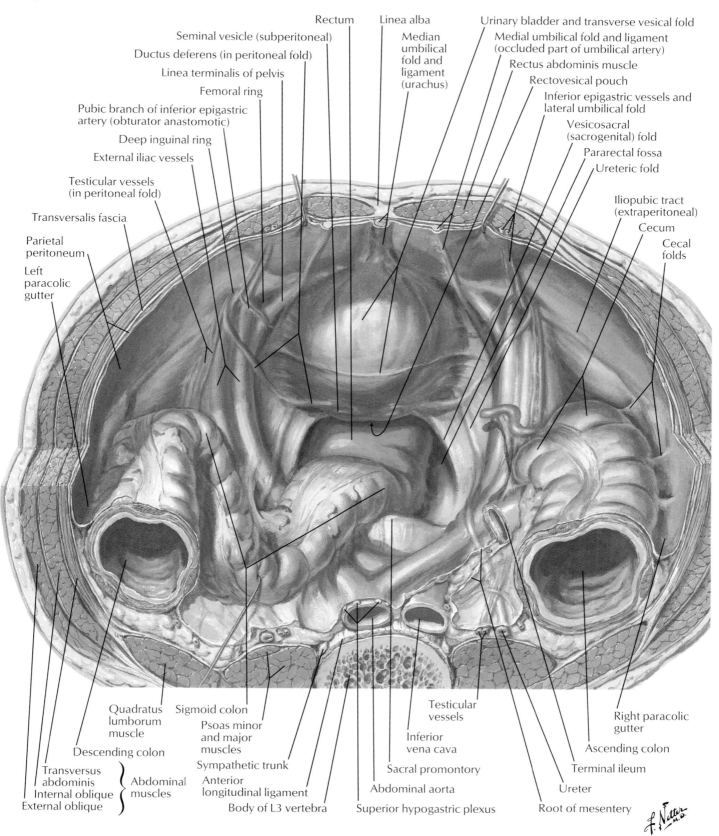

Rectum

Linea alba

Urinary bladder and transverse vesical fold

Seminal vesicle (subperitoneal)

Median umbilical fold and ligament (urachus)

Medial umbilical fold and ligament (occluded part of umbilical artery)

Ductus deferens (in peritoneal fold)

Rectus abdominis muscle

Linea terminalis of pelvis

Rectovesical pouch

Femoral ring

Inferior epigastric vessels and lateral umbilical fold

Pubic branch of inferior epigastric artery (obturator anastomotic)

Vesicosacral (sacrogenital) fold

Deep inguinal ring

Pararectal fossa

External iliac vessels

Ureteric fold

Testicular vessels (in peritoneal fold)

Iliopubic tract (extraperitoneal)

Transversalis fascia

Cecum

Parietal peritoneum

Cecal folds

Left paracolic gutter

Quadratus lumborum muscle

Sigmoid colon

Psoas minor and major muscles

Descending colon

Sympathetic trunk

Transversus abdominis

Internal oblique

External oblique

} Abdominal muscles

Anterior longitudinal ligament

Body of L3 vertebra

Inferior vena cava

Sacral promontory

Abdominal aorta

Superior hypogastric plexus

Testicular vessels

Right paracolic gutter

Ascending colon

Terminal ileum

Ureter

Root of mesentery

F. Netter M.D.

Female: midsagittal section

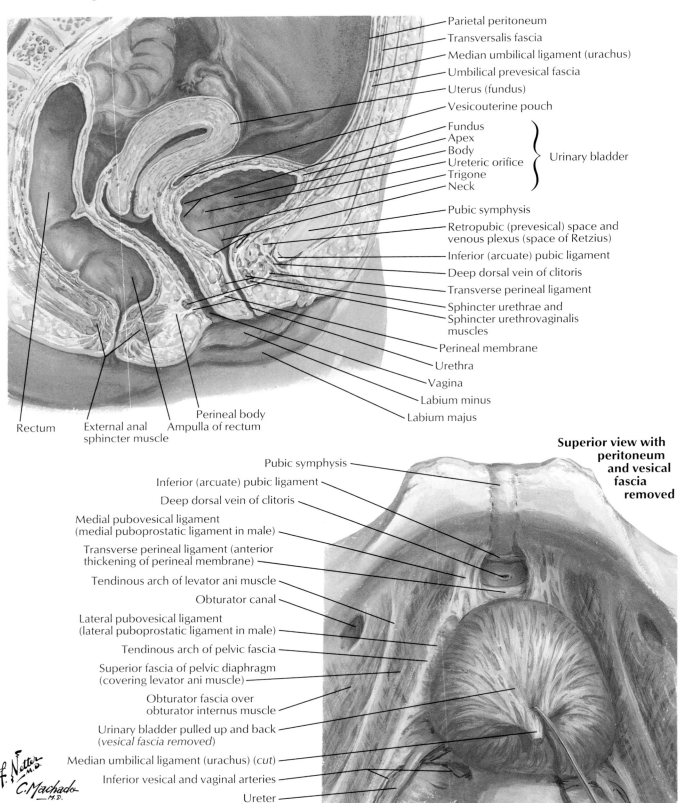

Parietal peritoneum
Transversalis fascia
Median umbilical ligament (urachus)
Umbilical prevesical fascia
Uterus (fundus)
Vesicouterine pouch
Fundus
Apex
Body
Ureteric orifice
Trigone
Neck
} Urinary bladder
Pubic symphysis
Retropubic (prevesical) space and venous plexus (space of Retzius)
Inferior (arcuate) pubic ligament
Deep dorsal vein of clitoris
Transverse perineal ligament
Sphincter urethrae and Sphincter urethrovaginalis muscles
Perineal membrane
Urethra
Vagina
Labium minus
Labium majus

Rectum
External anal sphincter muscle
Ampulla of rectum
Perineal body

Superior view with peritoneum and vesical fascia removed

Pubic symphysis
Inferior (arcuate) pubic ligament
Deep dorsal vein of clitoris
Medial pubovesical ligament (medial puboprostatic ligament in male)
Transverse perineal ligament (anterior thickening of perineal membrane)
Tendinous arch of levator ani muscle
Obturator canal
Lateral pubovesical ligament (lateral puboprostatic ligament in male)
Tendinous arch of pelvic fascia
Superior fascia of pelvic diaphragm (covering levator ani muscle)
Obturator fascia over obturator internus muscle
Urinary bladder pulled up and back (vesical fascia removed)
Median umbilical ligament (urachus) (cut)
Inferior vesical and vaginal arteries
Ureter

Plate 348 **Urinary Bladder**

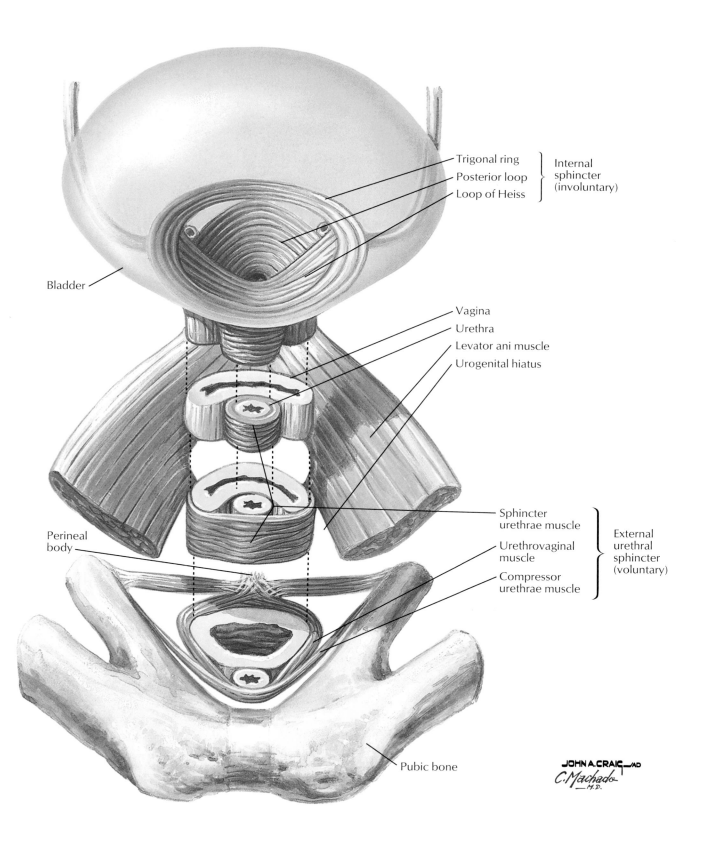

Trigonal ring
Posterior loop
Loop of Heiss
} Internal sphincter (involuntary)

Bladder

Vagina
Urethra
Levator ani muscle
Urogenital hiatus

Sphincter urethrae muscle
Urethrovaginal muscle
Compressor urethrae muscle
} External urethral sphincter (voluntary)

Perineal body

Pubic bone

JOHN A. CRAIG _AD
C. Machado
_M.D._

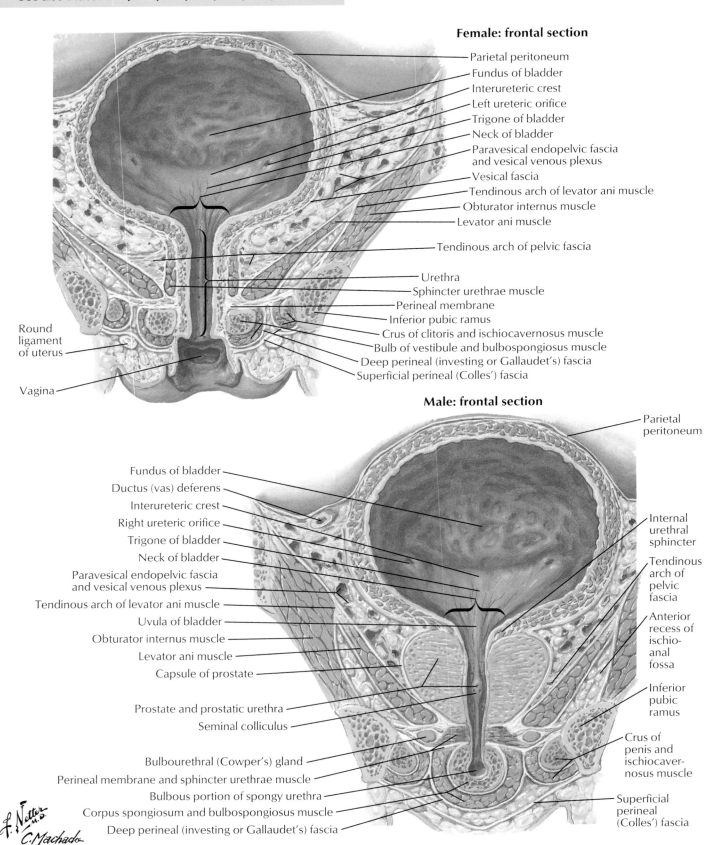

Female: frontal section

Parietal peritoneum
Fundus of bladder
Interureteric crest
Left ureteric orifice
Trigone of bladder
Neck of bladder
Paravesical endopelvic fascia and vesical venous plexus
Vesical fascia
Tendinous arch of levator ani muscle
Obturator internus muscle
Levator ani muscle
Tendinous arch of pelvic fascia
Urethra
Sphincter urethrae muscle
Perineal membrane
Inferior pubic ramus
Crus of clitoris and ischiocavernosus muscle
Bulb of vestibule and bulbospongiosus muscle
Deep perineal (investing or Gallaudet's) fascia
Superficial perineal (Colles') fascia

Round ligament of uterus

Vagina

Male: frontal section

Fundus of bladder
Ductus (vas) deferens
Interureteric crest
Right ureteric orifice
Trigone of bladder
Neck of bladder
Paravesical endopelvic fascia and vesical venous plexus
Tendinous arch of levator ani muscle
Uvula of bladder
Obturator internus muscle
Levator ani muscle
Capsule of prostate
Prostate and prostatic urethra
Seminal colliculus
Bulbourethral (Cowper's) gland
Perineal membrane and sphincter urethrae muscle
Bulbous portion of spongy urethra
Corpus spongiosum and bulbospongiosus muscle
Deep perineal (investing or Gallaudet's) fascia

Parietal peritoneum
Internal urethral sphincter
Tendinous arch of pelvic fascia
Anterior recess of ischio-anal fossa
Inferior pubic ramus
Crus of penis and ischiocavernosus muscle
Superficial perineal (Colles') fascia

Plate 350

Urinary Bladder

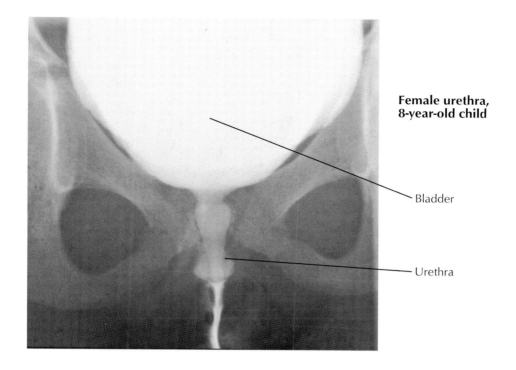

Female urethra,
8-year-old child

Bladder

Urethra

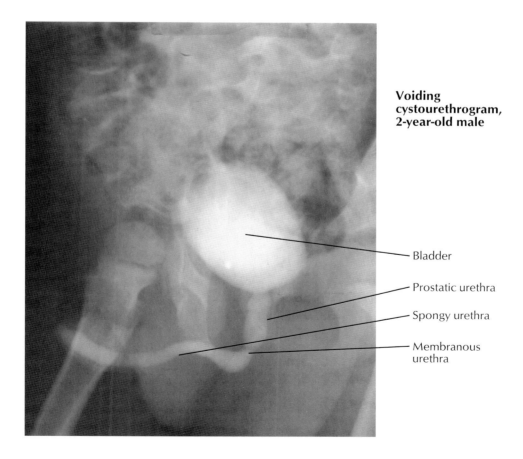

Voiding
cystourethrogram,
2-year-old male

Bladder

Prostatic urethra

Spongy urethra

Membranous
urethra

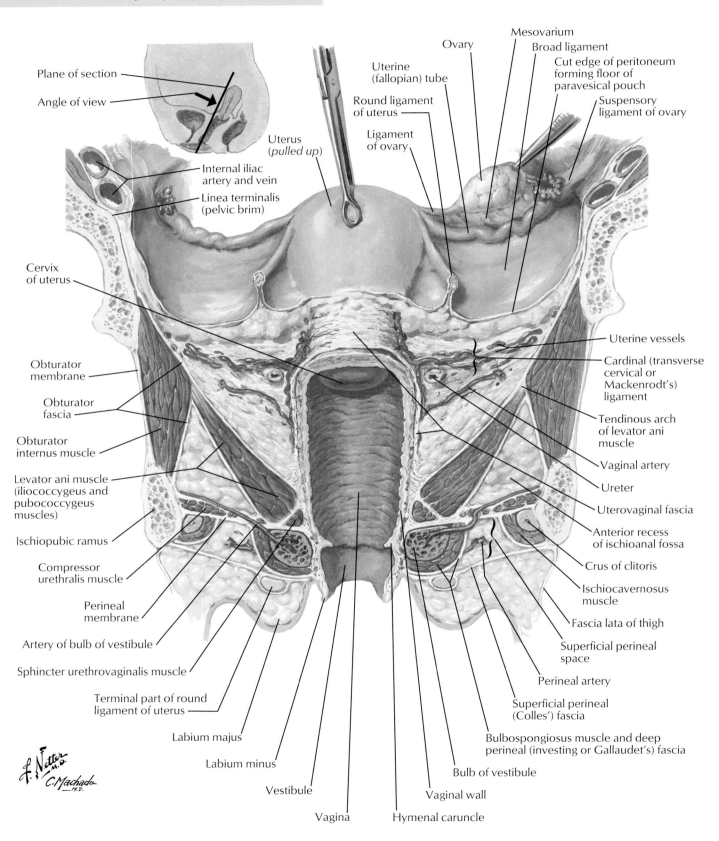

Plane of section

Angle of view

Uterus
(*pulled up*)

Internal iliac
artery and vein

Linea terminalis
(pelvic brim)

Cervix
of uterus

Obturator
membrane

Obturator
fascia

Obturator
internus muscle

Levator ani muscle
(iliococcygeus and
pubococcygeus
muscles)

Ischiopubic ramus

Compressor
urethralis muscle

Perineal
membrane

Artery of bulb of vestibule

Sphincter urethrovaginalis muscle

Terminal part of round
ligament of uterus

Labium majus

Labium minus

Vestibule

Vagina

Hymenal caruncle

Vaginal wall

Bulb of vestibule

Bulbospongiosus muscle and deep
perineal (investing or Gallaudet's) fascia

Superficial perineal
(Colles') fascia

Perineal artery

Superficial perineal
space

Fascia lata of thigh

Ischiocavernosus
muscle

Crus of clitoris

Anterior recess
of ischioanal fossa

Uterovaginal fascia

Ureter

Vaginal artery

Tendinous arch
of levator ani
muscle

Cardinal (transverse
cervical or
Mackenrodt's)
ligament

Uterine vessels

Ovary

Mesovarium

Broad ligament

Cut edge of peritoneum
forming floor of
paravesical pouch

Suspensory
ligament of ovary

Uterine
(fallopian) tube

Round ligament
of uterus

Ligament
of ovary

Plate 352   **Uterus, Vagina, and Supporting Structures**

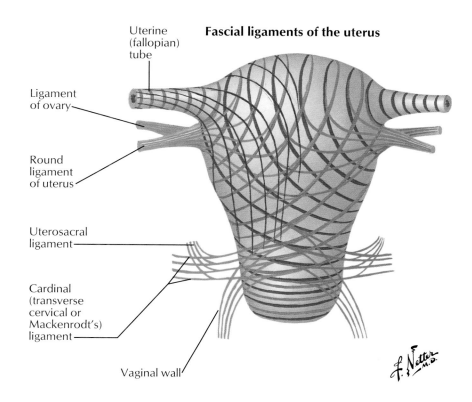

Uterine (fallopian) tube

Fascial ligaments of the uterus

Ligament of ovary

Round ligament of uterus

Uterosacral ligament

Cardinal (transverse cervical or Mackenrodt's) ligament

Vaginal wall

Pelvic fascia and ligaments

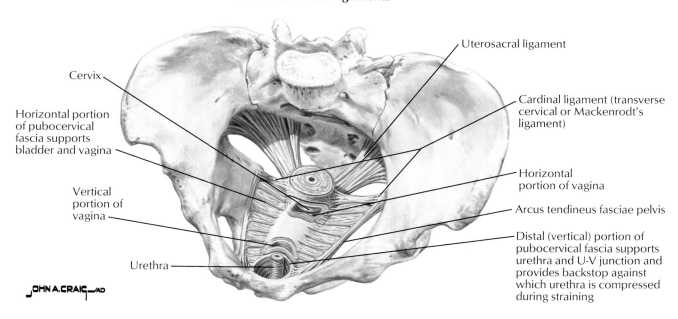

Cervix

Horizontal portion of pubocervical fascia supports bladder and vagina

Vertical portion of vagina

Urethra

Uterosacral ligament

Cardinal ligament (transverse cervical or Mackenrodt's ligament)

Horizontal portion of vagina

Arcus tendineus fasciae pelvis

Distal (vertical) portion of pubocervical fascia supports urethra and U-V junction and provides backstop against which urethra is compressed during straining

JOHN A.CRAIG—AD

Uterus, Vagina, and Supporting Structures

Plate 353

Anterior

Posterior

Subdivisions and contents of the broad ligament

Suspensory ligament of the ovary (containing the ovarian vessels)

Infundibulum of uterine tube

External iliac vessels

Fimbriae of uterine tube

Ampulla of uterine tube

Round ligament

Right ovary

Right ureter

Laminae of the mesosalpinx

Obliterated umbilical artery

Laminae of the mesovarium

Ovarian branches of uterine vessels

Posterior lamina of broad ligament

Round ligament

Anterior lamina of broad ligament

Transverse vesical fold

Vesicouterine (uterovesical) pouch

Uterine artery and venous plexus

Vaginal artery

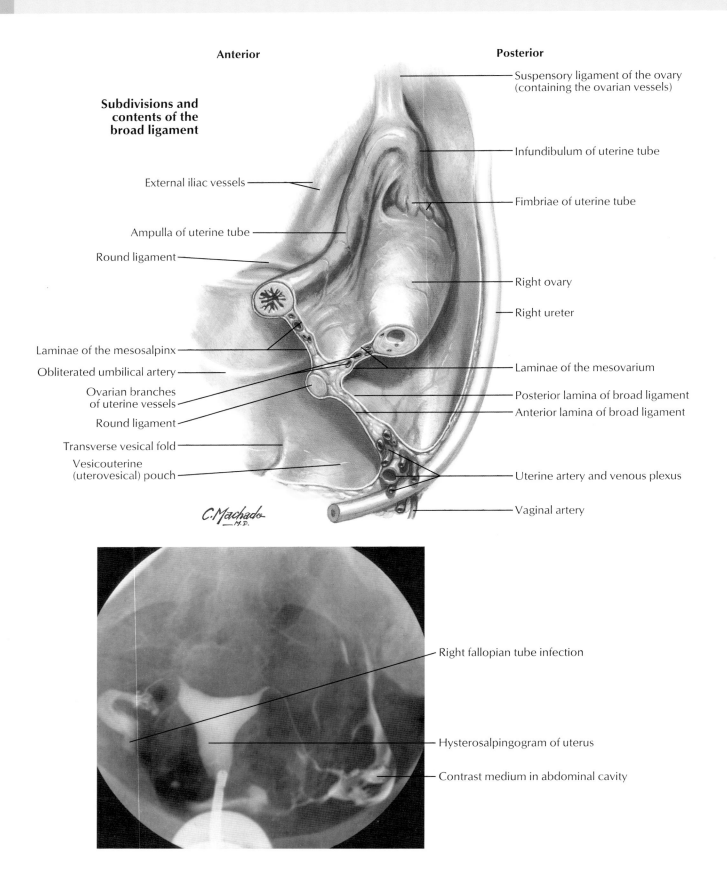

Right fallopian tube infection

Hysterosalpingogram of uterus

Contrast medium in abdominal cavity

Plate 354

Uterus, Vagina, and Supporting Structures

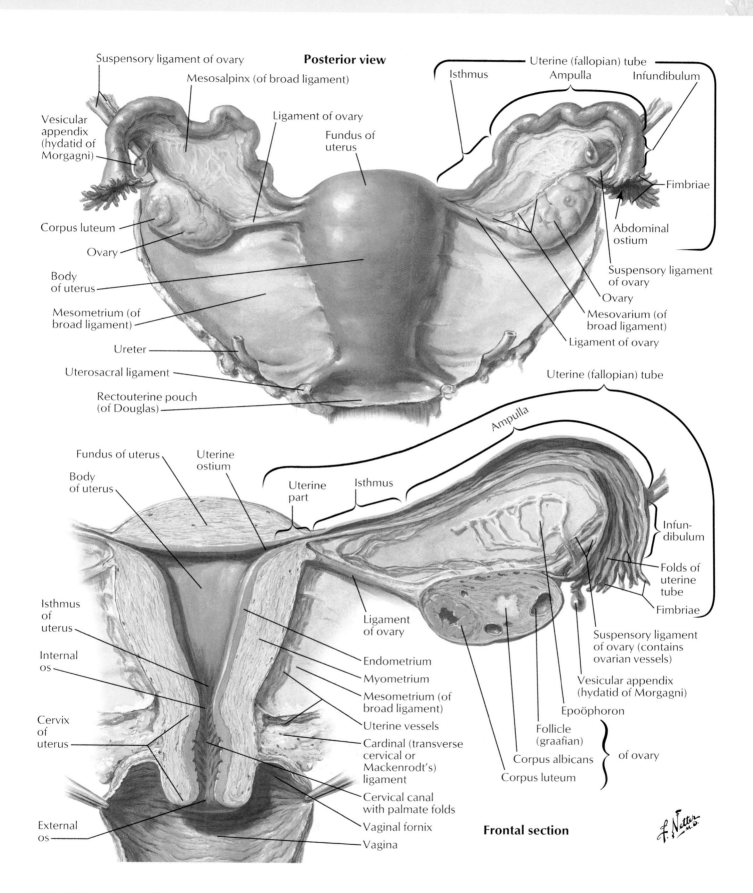

Posterior view

Suspensory ligament of ovary

Mesosalpinx (of broad ligament)

Ligament of ovary

Fundus of uterus

Vesicular appendix (hydatid of Morgagni)

Corpus luteum

Ovary

Body of uterus

Mesometrium (of broad ligament)

Ureter

Uterosacral ligament

Rectouterine pouch (of Douglas)

Isthmus

Uterine (fallopian) tube

Ampulla

Infundibulum

Fimbriae

Abdominal ostium

Suspensory ligament of ovary

Ovary

Mesovarium (of broad ligament)

Ligament of ovary

Uterine (fallopian) tube

Ampulla

Fundus of uterus

Body of uterus

Uterine ostium

Uterine part

Isthmus

Infundibulum

Folds of uterine tube

Fimbriae

Suspensory ligament of ovary (contains ovarian vessels)

Vesicular appendix (hydatid of Morgagni)

Epoöphoron

Follicle (graafian)

Corpus albicans

Corpus luteum

of ovary

Isthmus of uterus

Internal os

Cervix of uterus

External os

Ligament of ovary

Endometrium

Myometrium

Mesometrium (of broad ligament)

Uterine vessels

Cardinal (transverse cervical or Mackenrodt's) ligament

Cervical canal with palmate folds

Vaginal fornix

Vagina

Frontal section

f. Netter M.D.

Uterus, Vagina, and Supporting Structures

Plate 355

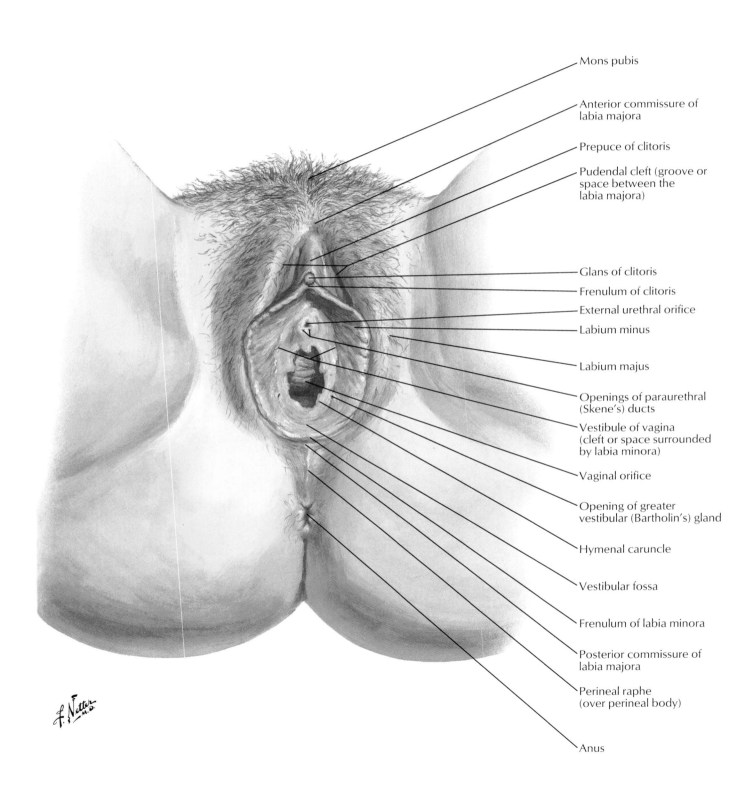

Mons pubis

Anterior commissure of labia majora

Prepuce of clitoris

Pudendal cleft (groove or space between the labia majora)

Glans of clitoris

Frenulum of clitoris

External urethral orifice

Labium minus

Labium majus

Openings of paraurethral (Skene's) ducts

Vestibule of vagina (cleft or space surrounded by labia minora)

Vaginal orifice

Opening of greater vestibular (Bartholin's) gland

Hymenal caruncle

Vestibular fossa

Frenulum of labia minora

Posterior commissure of labia majora

Perineal raphe (over perineal body)

Anus

Plate 356

Perineum and External Genitalia: Female

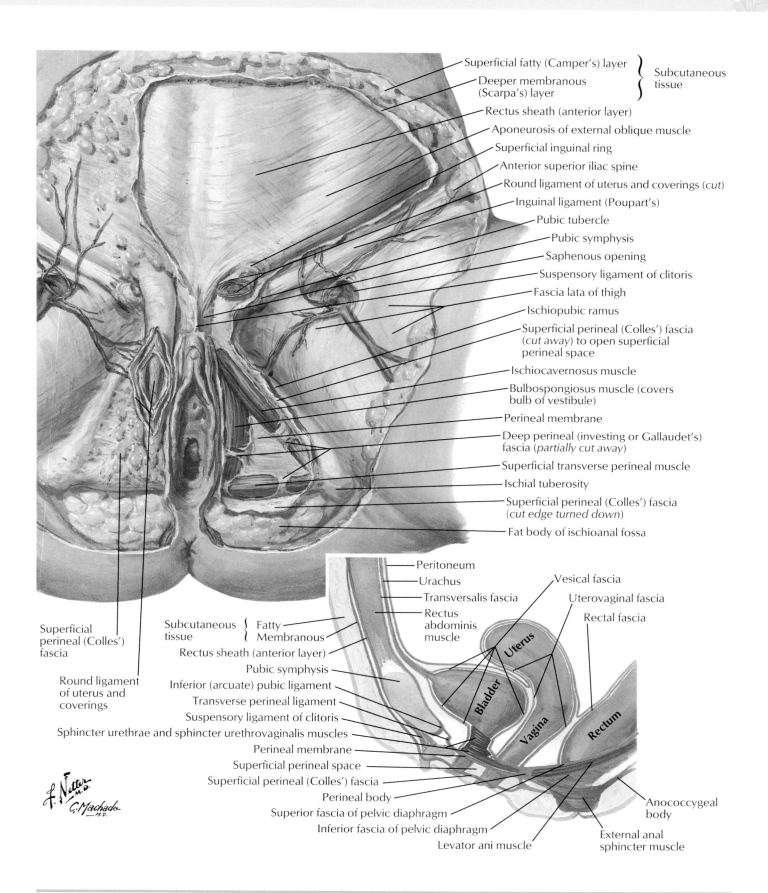

Superficial fatty (Camper's) layer ⎫
Deeper membranous ⎬ Subcutaneous
(Scarpa's) layer ⎭ tissue
Rectus sheath (anterior layer)
Aponeurosis of external oblique muscle
Superficial inguinal ring
Anterior superior iliac spine
Round ligament of uterus and coverings (cut)
Inguinal ligament (Poupart's)
Pubic tubercle
Pubic symphysis
Saphenous opening
Suspensory ligament of clitoris
Fascia lata of thigh
Ischiopubic ramus
Superficial perineal (Colles') fascia
(cut away) to open superficial
perineal space
Ischiocavernosus muscle
Bulbospongiosus muscle (covers
bulb of vestibule)
Perineal membrane
Deep perineal (investing or Gallaudet's)
fascia (partially cut away)
Superficial transverse perineal muscle
Ischial tuberosity
Superficial perineal (Colles') fascia
(cut edge turned down)
Fat body of ischioanal fossa

Superficial
perineal (Colles')
fascia

Round ligament
of uterus and
coverings

Peritoneum
Urachus
Transversalis fascia
Rectus
abdominis
muscle
Vesical fascia
Uterovaginal fascia
Rectal fascia

Subcutaneous ⎰ Fatty
tissue ⎱ Membranous
Rectus sheath (anterior layer)
Pubic symphysis
Inferior (arcuate) pubic ligament
Transverse perineal ligament
Suspensory ligament of clitoris
Sphincter urethrae and sphincter urethrovaginalis muscles
Perineal membrane
Superficial perineal space
Superficial perineal (Colles') fascia
Perineal body
Superior fascia of pelvic diaphragm
Inferior fascia of pelvic diaphragm
Levator ani muscle

Uterus
Bladder
Vagina
Rectum

Anococcygeal
body
External anal
sphincter muscle

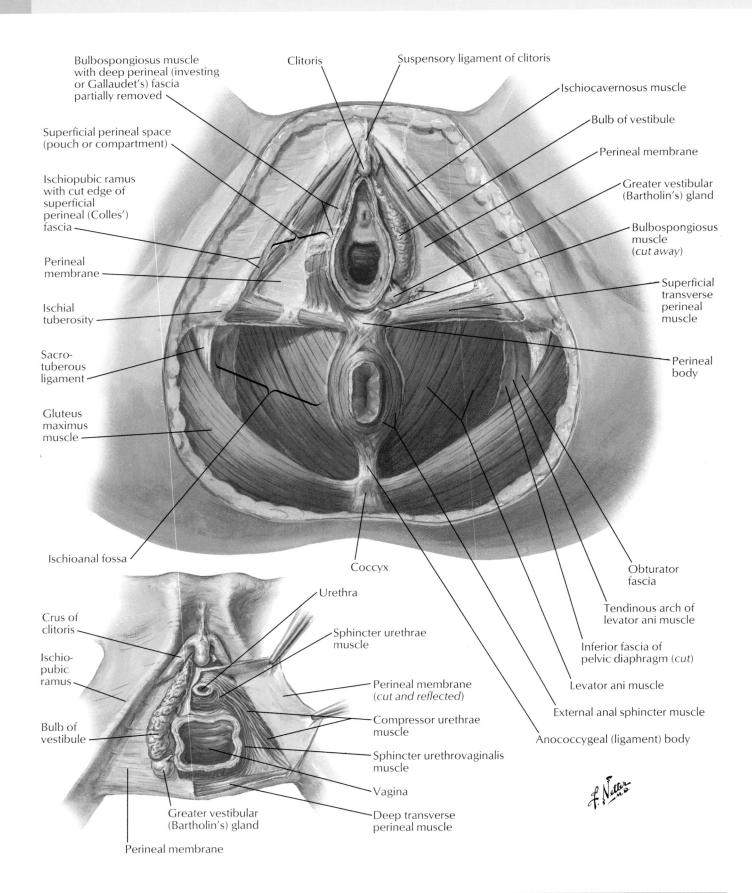

Bulbospongiosus muscle with deep perineal (investing or Gallaudet's) fascia partially removed

Superficial perineal space (pouch or compartment)

Ischiopubic ramus with cut edge of superficial perineal (Colles') fascia

Perineal membrane

Ischial tuberosity

Sacro-tuberous ligament

Gluteus maximus muscle

Ischioanal fossa

Clitoris

Suspensory ligament of clitoris

Ischiocavernosus muscle

Bulb of vestibule

Perineal membrane

Greater vestibular (Bartholin's) gland

Bulbospongiosus muscle (*cut away*)

Superficial transverse perineal muscle

Perineal body

Coccyx

Obturator fascia

Tendinous arch of levator ani muscle

Inferior fascia of pelvic diaphragm (*cut*)

Levator ani muscle

External anal sphincter muscle

Anococcygeal (ligament) body

Crus of clitoris

Ischio-pubic ramus

Bulb of vestibule

Urethra

Sphincter urethrae muscle

Perineal membrane (*cut and reflected*)

Compressor urethrae muscle

Sphincter urethrovaginalis muscle

Vagina

Deep transverse perineal muscle

Greater vestibular (Bartholin's) gland

Perineal membrane

F. Netter M.D.

Plate 358　　　**Perineum and External Genitalia: Female**

Superficial perineal space

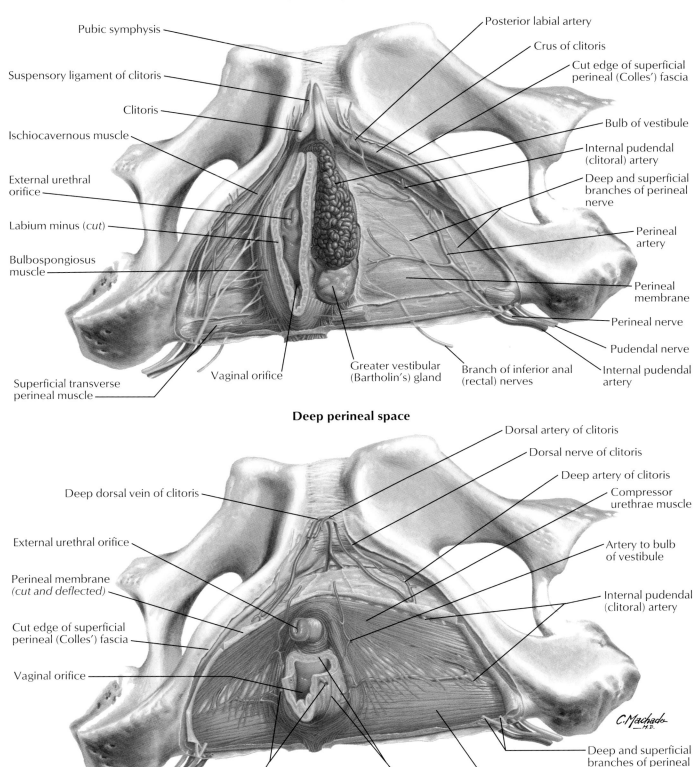

Pubic symphysis

Suspensory ligament of clitoris

Clitoris

Ischiocavernous muscle

External urethral orifice

Labium minus (*cut*)

Bulbospongiosus muscle

Superficial transverse perineal muscle

Vaginal orifice

Greater vestibular (Bartholin's) gland

Branch of inferior anal (rectal) nerves

Posterior labial artery

Crus of clitoris

Cut edge of superficial perineal (Colles') fascia

Bulb of vestibule

Internal pudendal (clitoral) artery

Deep and superficial branches of perineal nerve

Perineal artery

Perineal membrane

Perineal nerve

Pudendal nerve

Internal pudendal artery

Deep perineal space

Deep dorsal vein of clitoris

External urethral orifice

Perineal membrane (*cut and deflected*)

Cut edge of superficial perineal (Colles') fascia

Vaginal orifice

Greater vestibular (Bartholin's) glands

Vaginal wall

Deep transverse perineal muscle

Dorsal artery of clitoris

Dorsal nerve of clitoris

Deep artery of clitoris

Compressor urethrae muscle

Artery to bulb of vestibule

Internal pudendal (clitoral) artery

Deep and superficial branches of perineal nerve (*cut*)

C. Machado M.D.

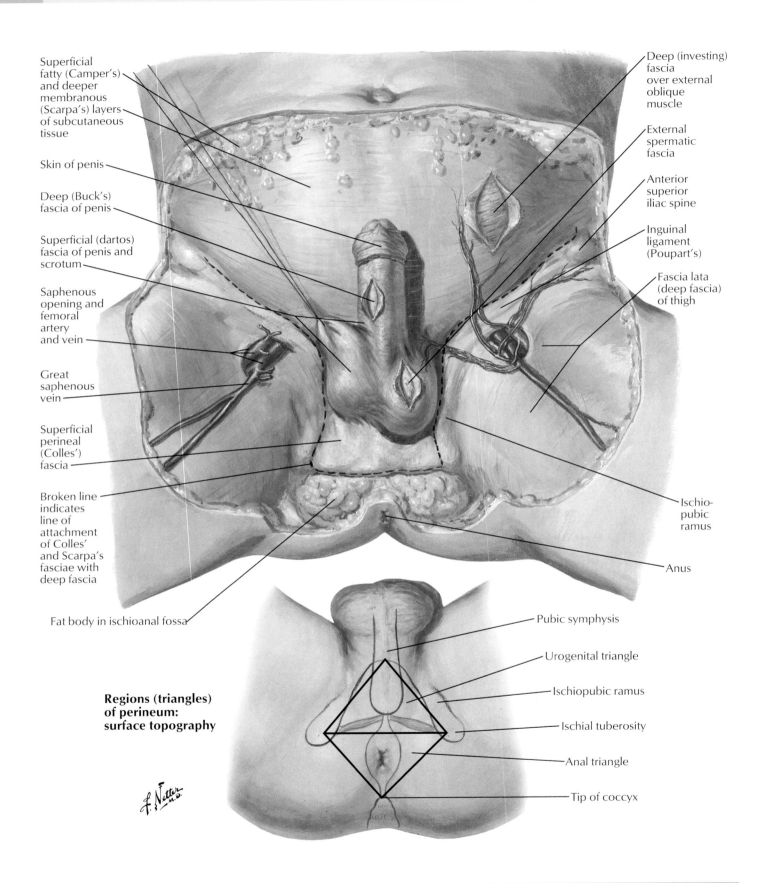

Superficial fatty (Camper's) and deeper membranous (Scarpa's) layers of subcutaneous tissue

Skin of penis

Deep (Buck's) fascia of penis

Superficial (dartos) fascia of penis and scrotum

Saphenous opening and femoral artery and vein

Great saphenous vein

Superficial perineal (Colles') fascia

Broken line indicates line of attachment of Colles' and Scarpa's fasciae with deep fascia

Fat body in ischioanal fossa

Deep (investing) fascia over external oblique muscle

External spermatic fascia

Anterior superior iliac spine

Inguinal ligament (Poupart's)

Fascia lata (deep fascia) of thigh

Ischio-pubic ramus

Anus

Regions (triangles) of perineum: surface topography

Pubic symphysis

Urogenital triangle

Ischiopubic ramus

Ischial tuberosity

Anal triangle

Tip of coccyx

f. Netter

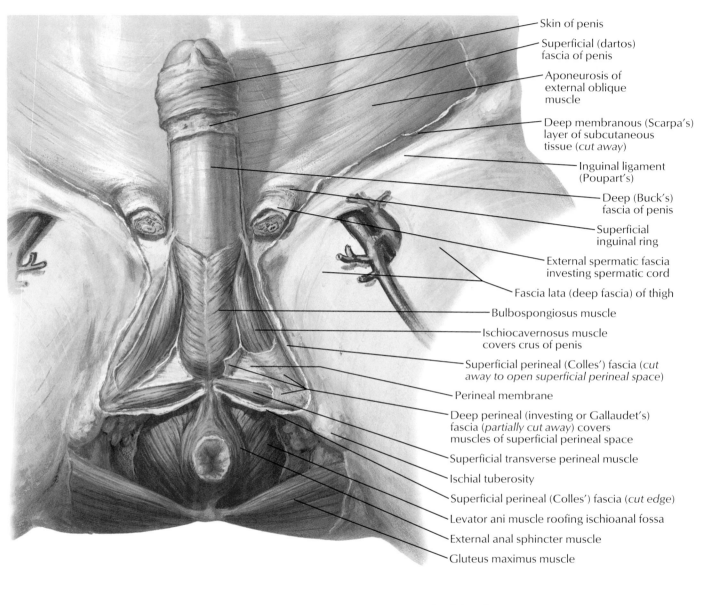

Skin of penis

Superficial (dartos) fascia of penis

Aponeurosis of external oblique muscle

Deep membranous (Scarpa's) layer of subcutaneous tissue (*cut away*)

Inguinal ligament (Poupart's)

Deep (Buck's) fascia of penis

Superficial inguinal ring

External spermatic fascia investing spermatic cord

Fascia lata (deep fascia) of thigh

Bulbospongiosus muscle

Ischiocavernosus muscle covers crus of penis

Superficial perineal (Colles') fascia (*cut away to open superficial perineal space*)

Perineal membrane

Deep perineal (investing or Gallaudet's) fascia (*partially cut away*) covers muscles of superficial perineal space

Superficial transverse perineal muscle

Ischial tuberosity

Superficial perineal (Colles') fascia (*cut edge*)

Levator ani muscle roofing ischioanal fossa

External anal sphincter muscle

Gluteus maximus muscle

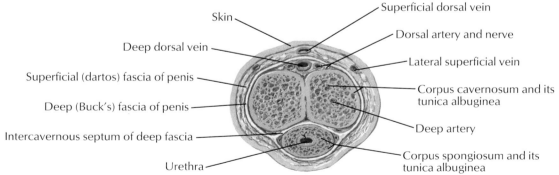

Skin

Superficial dorsal vein

Deep dorsal vein

Dorsal artery and nerve

Lateral superficial vein

Superficial (dartos) fascia of penis

Deep (Buck's) fascia of penis

Corpus cavernosum and its tunica albuginea

Intercavernous septum of deep fascia

Deep artery

Urethra

Corpus spongiosum and its tunica albuginea

Transverse section through body of penis

f. Netter
M.D.

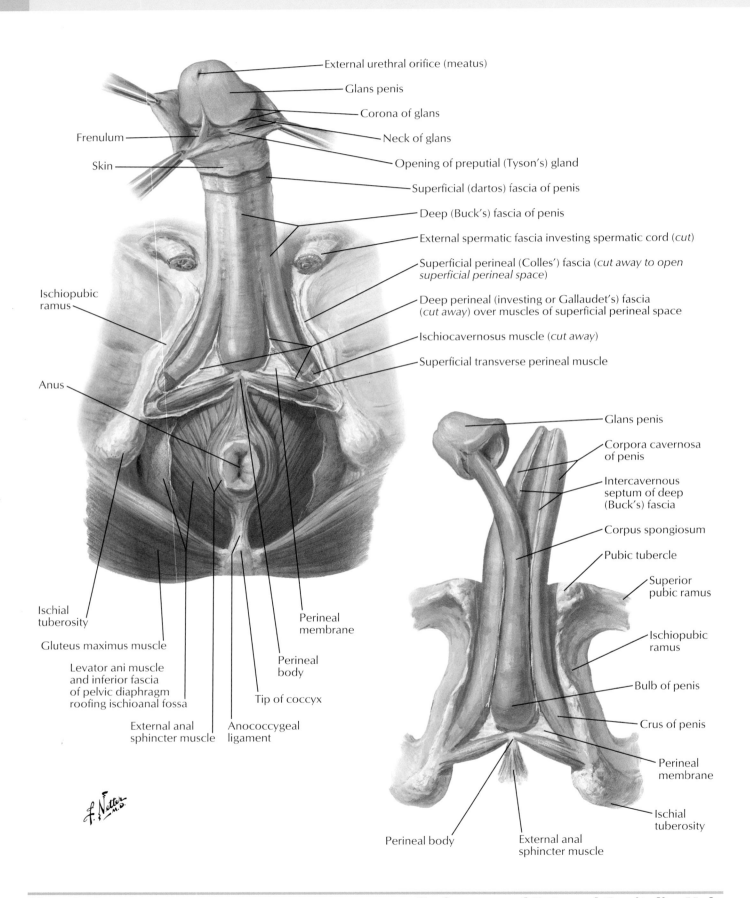

External urethral orifice (meatus)

Glans penis

Corona of glans

Neck of glans

Frenulum

Skin

Opening of preputial (Tyson's) gland

Superficial (dartos) fascia of penis

Deep (Buck's) fascia of penis

External spermatic fascia investing spermatic cord (*cut*)

Superficial perineal (Colles') fascia (*cut away to open superficial perineal space*)

Deep perineal (investing or Gallaudet's) fascia (*cut away*) over muscles of superficial perineal space

Ischiocavernosus muscle (*cut away*)

Superficial transverse perineal muscle

Ischiopubic ramus

Anus

Ischial tuberosity

Gluteus maximus muscle

Levator ani muscle and inferior fascia of pelvic diaphragm roofing ischioanal fossa

External anal sphincter muscle

Anococcygeal ligament

Tip of coccyx

Perineal body

Perineal membrane

Glans penis

Corpora cavernosa of penis

Intercavernous septum of deep (Buck's) fascia

Corpus spongiosum

Pubic tubercle

Superior pubic ramus

Ischiopubic ramus

Bulb of penis

Crus of penis

Perineal membrane

Ischial tuberosity

Perineal body

External anal sphincter muscle

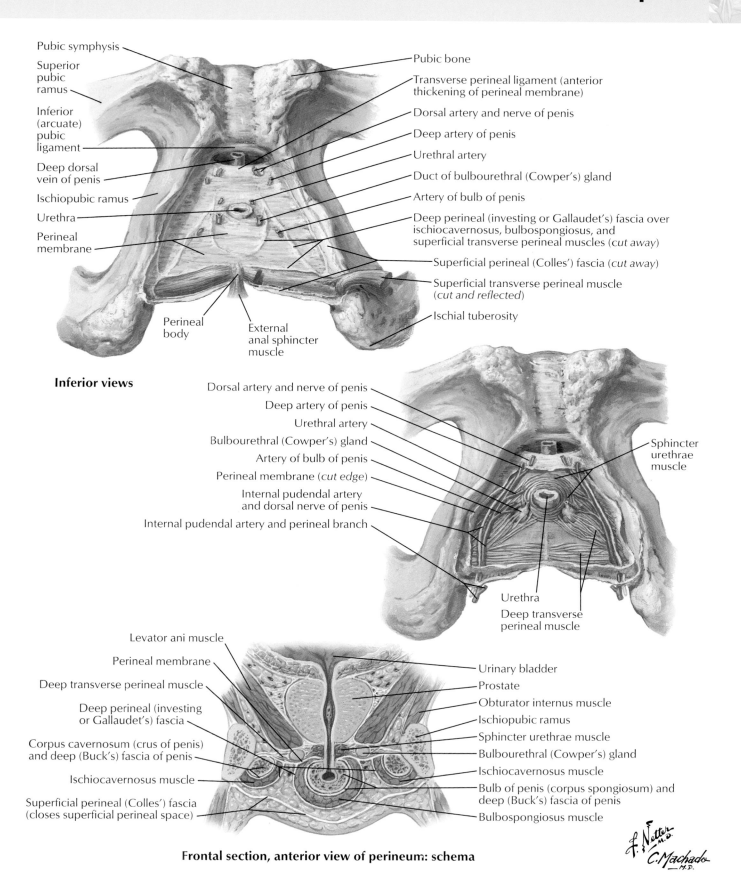

Pubic symphysis

Superior pubic ramus

Inferior (arcuate) pubic ligament

Deep dorsal vein of penis

Ischiopubic ramus

Urethra

Perineal membrane

Pubic bone

Transverse perineal ligament (anterior thickening of perineal membrane)

Dorsal artery and nerve of penis

Deep artery of penis

Urethral artery

Duct of bulbourethral (Cowper's) gland

Artery of bulb of penis

Deep perineal (investing or Gallaudet's) fascia over ischiocavernosus, bulbospongiosus, and superficial transverse perineal muscles (*cut away*)

Superficial perineal (Colles') fascia (*cut away*)

Superficial transverse perineal muscle (*cut and reflected*)

Ischial tuberosity

Perineal body

External anal sphincter muscle

Inferior views

Dorsal artery and nerve of penis

Deep artery of penis

Urethral artery

Bulbourethral (Cowper's) gland

Artery of bulb of penis

Perineal membrane (*cut edge*)

Internal pudendal artery and dorsal nerve of penis

Internal pudendal artery and perineal branch

Sphincter urethrae muscle

Urethra

Deep transverse perineal muscle

Levator ani muscle

Perineal membrane

Deep transverse perineal muscle

Deep perineal (investing or Gallaudet's) fascia

Corpus cavernosum (crus of penis) and deep (Buck's) fascia of penis

Ischiocavernosus muscle

Superficial perineal (Colles') fascia (closes superficial perineal space)

Urinary bladder

Prostate

Obturator internus muscle

Ischiopubic ramus

Sphincter urethrae muscle

Bulbourethral (Cowper's) gland

Ischiocavernosus muscle

Bulb of penis (corpus spongiosum) and deep (Buck's) fascia of penis

Bulbospongiosus muscle

Frontal section, anterior view of perineum: schema

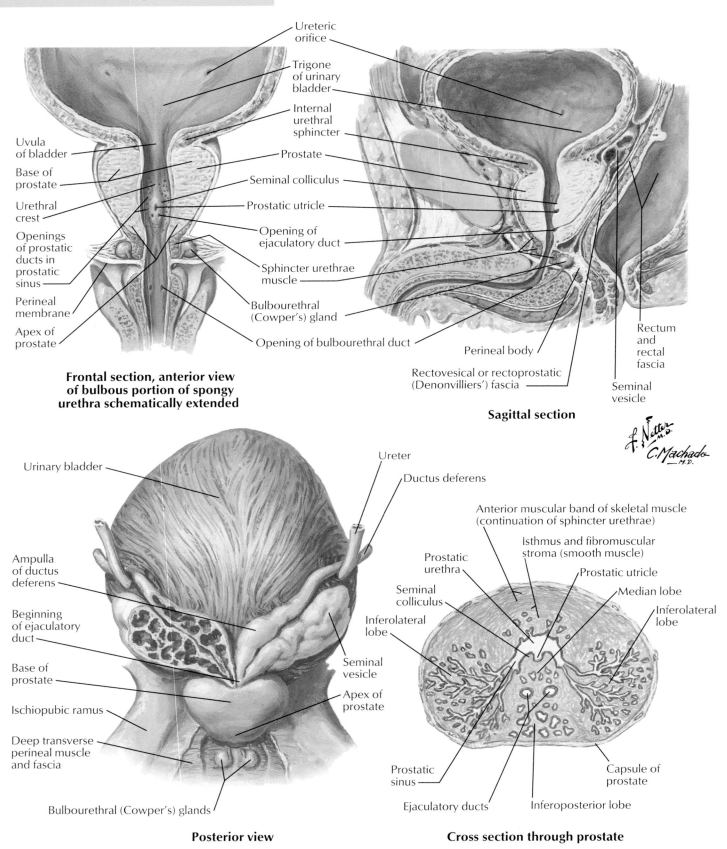

Ureteric orifice

Trigone of urinary bladder

Internal urethral sphincter

Prostate

Seminal colliculus

Prostatic utricle

Opening of ejaculatory duct

Sphincter urethrae muscle

Bulbourethral (Cowper's) gland

Opening of bulbourethral duct

Uvula of bladder

Base of prostate

Urethral crest

Openings of prostatic ducts in prostatic sinus

Perineal membrane

Apex of prostate

Frontal section, anterior view of bulbous portion of spongy urethra schematically extended

Rectum and rectal fascia

Seminal vesicle

Perineal body

Rectovesical or rectoprostatic (Denonvilliers') fascia

Sagittal section

Urinary bladder

Ureter

Ductus deferens

Ampulla of ductus deferens

Beginning of ejaculatory duct

Base of prostate

Ischiopubic ramus

Deep transverse perineal muscle and fascia

Seminal vesicle

Apex of prostate

Bulbourethral (Cowper's) glands

Posterior view

Anterior muscular band of skeletal muscle (continuation of sphincter urethrae)

Isthmus and fibromuscular stroma (smooth muscle)

Prostatic utricle

Median lobe

Inferolateral lobe

Prostatic urethra

Seminal colliculus

Inferolateral lobe

Capsule of prostate

Prostatic sinus

Ejaculatory ducts

Inferoposterior lobe

Cross section through prostate

Plate 364   **Perineum and External Genitalia: Male**

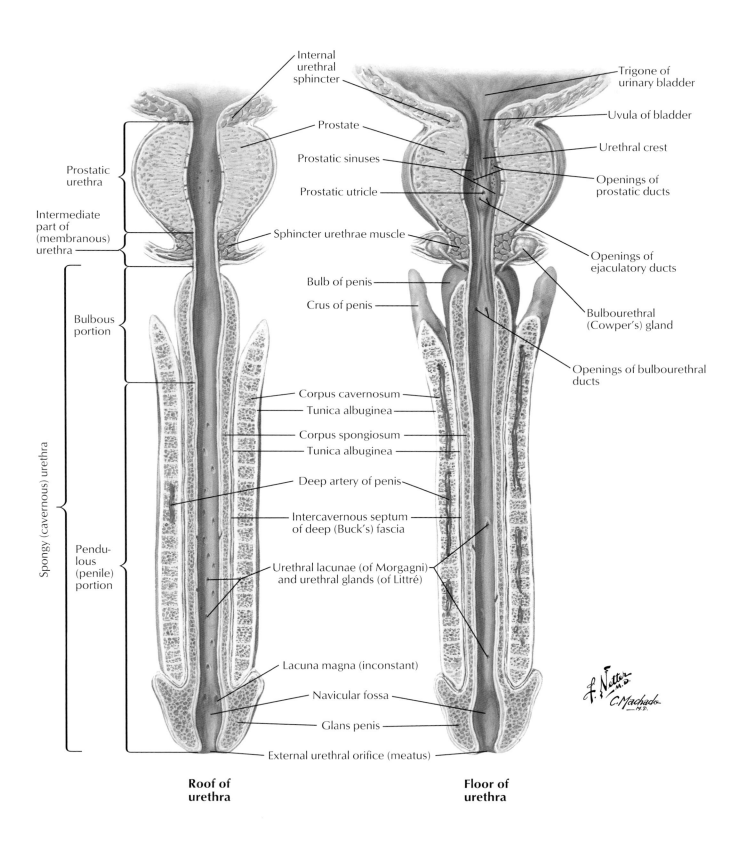

Internal urethral sphincter

Prostate

Prostatic sinuses

Prostatic utricle

Sphincter urethrae muscle

Bulb of penis

Crus of penis

Corpus cavernosum

Tunica albuginea

Corpus spongiosum

Tunica albuginea

Deep artery of penis

Intercavernous septum of deep (Buck's) fascia

Urethral lacunae (of Morgagni) and urethral glands (of Littré)

Lacuna magna (inconstant)

Navicular fossa

Glans penis

External urethral orifice (meatus)

Trigone of urinary bladder

Uvula of bladder

Urethral crest

Openings of prostatic ducts

Openings of ejaculatory ducts

Bulbourethral (Cowper's) gland

Openings of bulbourethral ducts

Prostatic urethra

Intermediate part of (membranous) urethra

Bulbous portion

Spongy (cavernous) urethra

Pendu-lous (penile) portion

Roof of urethra

Floor of urethra

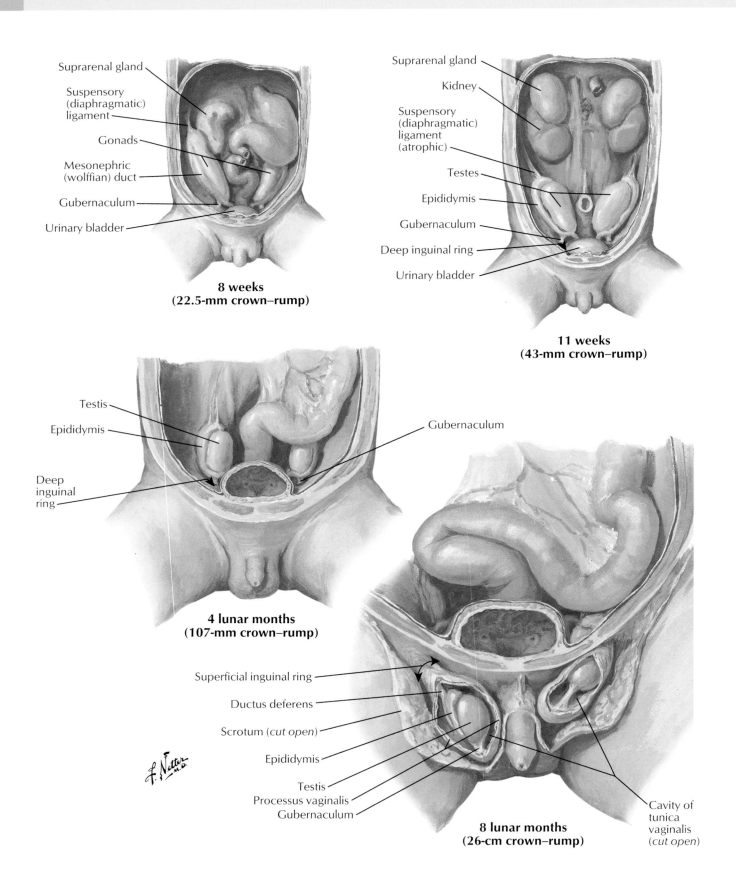

Suprarenal gland
Suspensory (diaphragmatic) ligament
Gonads
Mesonephric (wolffian) duct
Gubernaculum
Urinary bladder

8 weeks
(22.5-mm crown–rump)

Suprarenal gland
Kidney
Suspensory (diaphragmatic) ligament (atrophic)
Testes
Epididymis
Gubernaculum
Deep inguinal ring
Urinary bladder

11 weeks
(43-mm crown–rump)

Testis
Epididymis
Deep inguinal ring
Gubernaculum

4 lunar months
(107-mm crown–rump)

Superficial inguinal ring
Ductus deferens
Scrotum (*cut open*)
Epididymis
Testis
Processus vaginalis
Gubernaculum
Cavity of tunica vaginalis (*cut open*)

8 lunar months
(26-cm crown–rump)

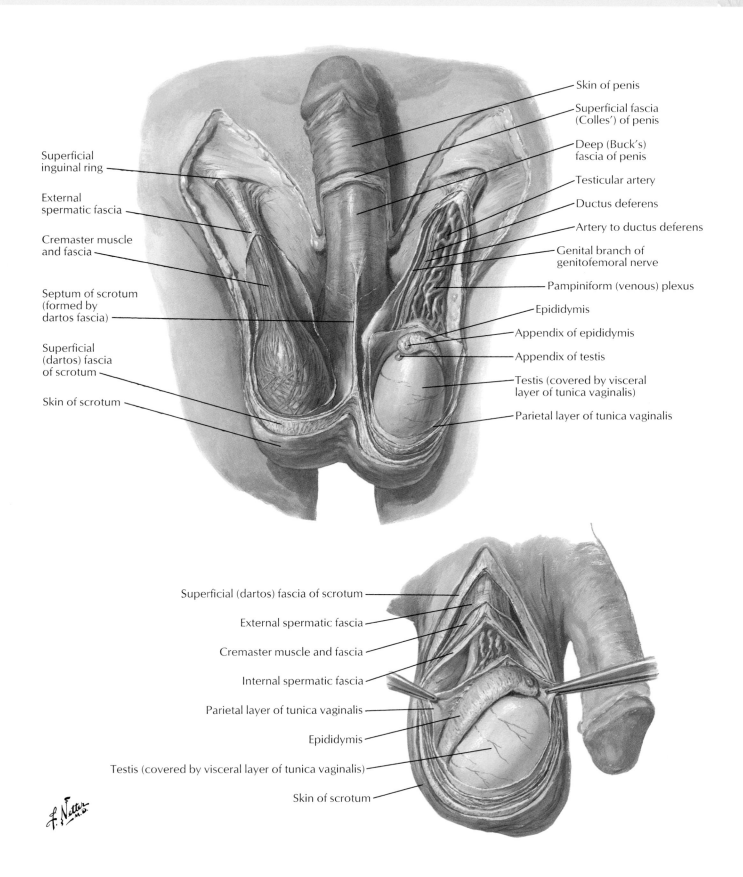

Skin of penis

Superficial fascia (Colles') of penis

Deep (Buck's) fascia of penis

Testicular artery

Ductus deferens

Artery to ductus deferens

Genital branch of genitofemoral nerve

Pampiniform (venous) plexus

Epididymis

Appendix of epididymis

Appendix of testis

Testis (covered by visceral layer of tunica vaginalis)

Parietal layer of tunica vaginalis

Superficial inguinal ring

External spermatic fascia

Cremaster muscle and fascia

Septum of scrotum (formed by dartos fascia)

Superficial (dartos) fascia of scrotum

Skin of scrotum

Superficial (dartos) fascia of scrotum

External spermatic fascia

Cremaster muscle and fascia

Internal spermatic fascia

Parietal layer of tunica vaginalis

Epididymis

Testis (covered by visceral layer of tunica vaginalis)

Skin of scrotum

Perineum and External Genitalia: Male

Plate 367

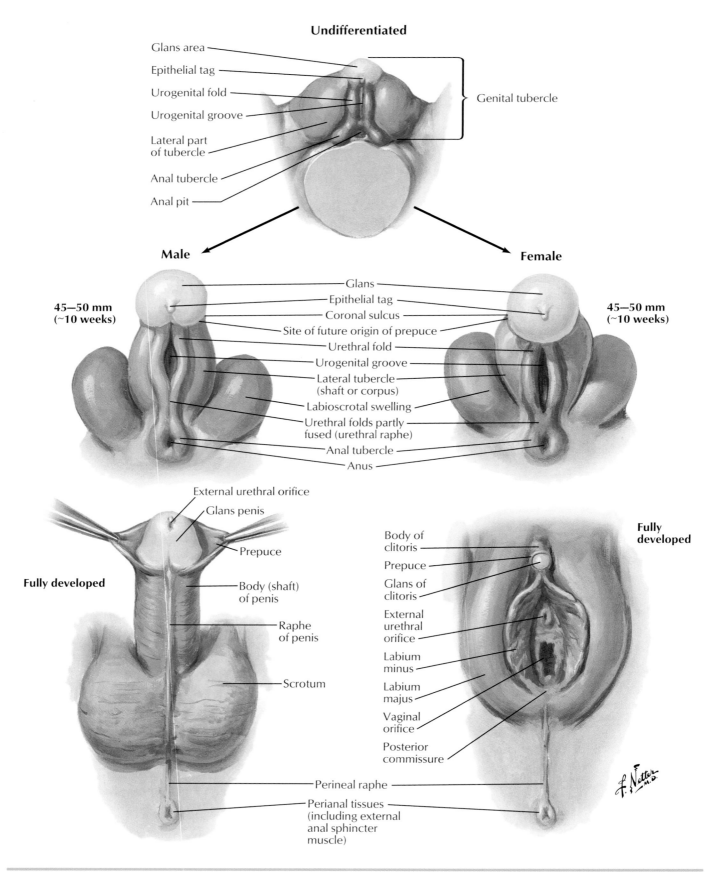

Undifferentiated

Glans area
Epithelial tag
Urogenital fold
Urogenital groove
Lateral part of tubercle
Anal tubercle
Anal pit

Genital tubercle

Male

Female

45–50 mm (~10 weeks)

45–50 mm (~10 weeks)

Glans
Epithelial tag
Coronal sulcus
Site of future origin of prepuce
Urethral fold
Urogenital groove
Lateral tubercle (shaft or corpus)
Labioscrotal swelling
Urethral folds partly fused (urethral raphe)
Anal tubercle
Anus

Fully developed

External urethral orifice
Glans penis
Prepuce
Body (shaft) of penis
Raphe of penis
Scrotum

Fully developed

Body of clitoris
Prepuce
Glans of clitoris
External urethral orifice
Labium minus
Labium majus
Vaginal orifice
Posterior commissure

Perineal raphe
Perianal tissues (including external anal sphincter muscle)

Plate 368   **Homologues of Genitalia**

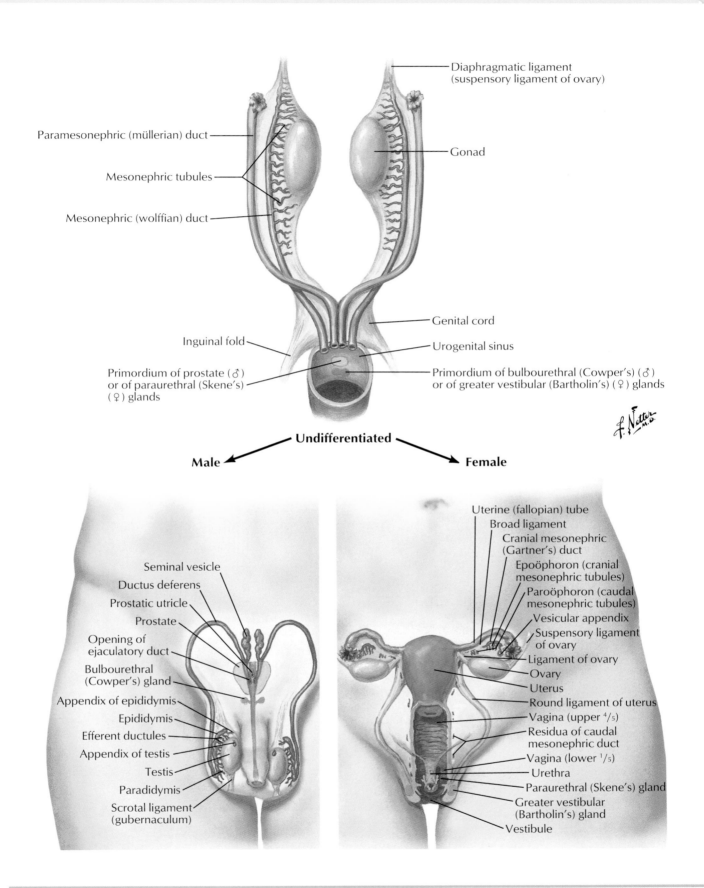

Diaphragmatic ligament
(suspensory ligament of ovary)

Paramesonephric (müllerian) duct

Mesonephric tubules

Mesonephric (wolffian) duct

Gonad

Genital cord

Inguinal fold

Urogenital sinus

Primordium of prostate (♂)
or of paraurethral (Skene's)
(♀) glands

Primordium of bulbourethral (Cowper's) (♂)
or of greater vestibular (Bartholin's) (♀) glands

Undifferentiated

Male

Female

Seminal vesicle

Ductus deferens

Prostatic utricle

Prostate

Opening of
ejaculatory duct

Bulbourethral
(Cowper's) gland

Appendix of epididymis

Epididymis

Efferent ductules

Appendix of testis

Testis

Paradidymis

Scrotal ligament
(gubernaculum)

Uterine (fallopian) tube

Broad ligament

Cranial mesonephric
(Gartner's) duct

Epoöphoron (cranial
mesonephric tubules)

Paroöphoron (caudal
mesonephric tubules)

Vesicular appendix

Suspensory ligament
of ovary

Ligament of ovary

Ovary

Uterus

Round ligament of uterus

Vagina (upper ⁴/₅)

Residua of caudal
mesonephric duct

Vagina (lower ¹/₅)

Urethra

Paraurethral (Skene's) gland

Greater vestibular
(Bartholin's) gland

Vestibule

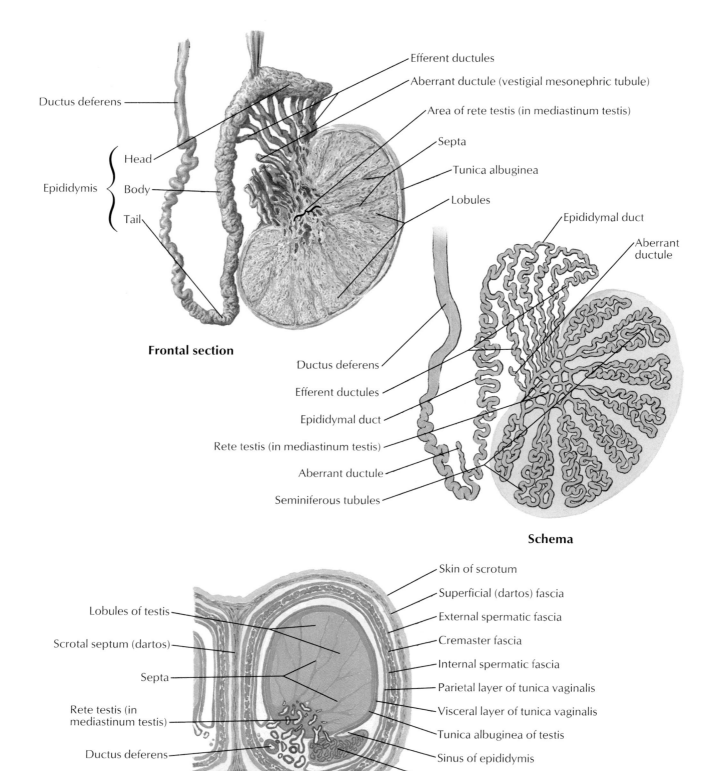

Ductus deferens

Epididymis
- Head
- Body
- Tail

Efferent ductules

Aberrant ductule (vestigial mesonephric tubule)

Area of rete testis (in mediastinum testis)

Septa

Tunica albuginea

Lobules

Frontal section

Epididymal duct

Aberrant ductule

Ductus deferens

Efferent ductules

Epididymal duct

Rete testis (in mediastinum testis)

Aberrant ductule

Seminiferous tubules

Schema

Lobules of testis

Scrotal septum (dartos)

Septa

Rete testis (in mediastinum testis)

Ductus deferens

Skin of scrotum

Superficial (dartos) fascia

External spermatic fascia

Cremaster fascia

Internal spermatic fascia

Parietal layer of tunica vaginalis

Visceral layer of tunica vaginalis

Tunica albuginea of testis

Sinus of epididymis

Epididymis

Cross section through scrotum and testis

Plate 370 **Testis, Epididymis, and Ductus Deferens**

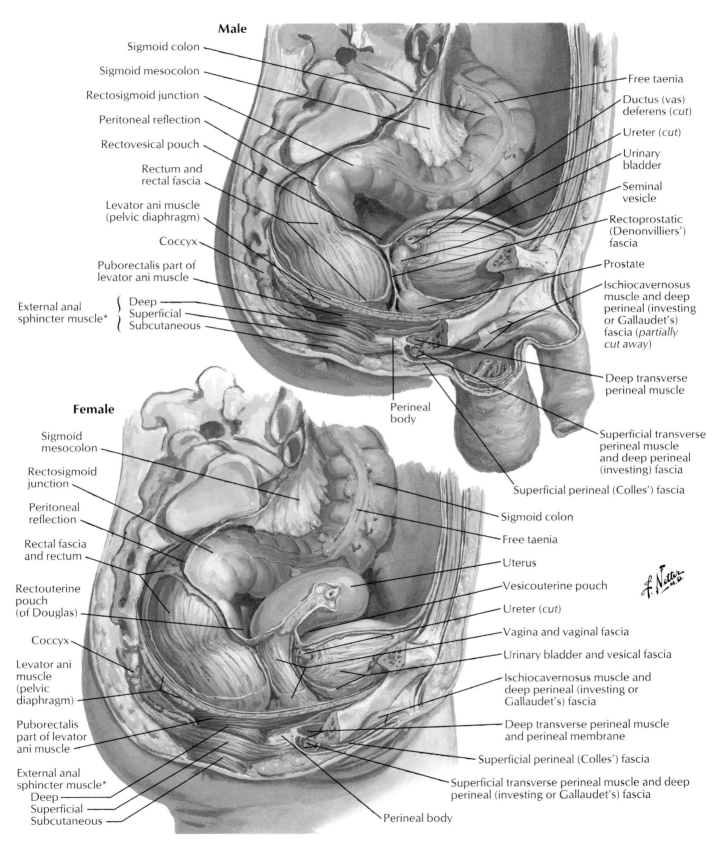

Male

Sigmoid colon

Sigmoid mesocolon

Rectosigmoid junction

Peritoneal reflection

Rectovesical pouch

Rectum and rectal fascia

Levator ani muscle (pelvic diaphragm)

Coccyx

Puborectalis part of levator ani muscle

External anal sphincter muscle*
{ Deep
Superficial
Subcutaneous

Free taenia

Ductus (vas) deferens (cut)

Ureter (cut)

Urinary bladder

Seminal vesicle

Rectoprostatic (Denonvilliers') fascia

Prostate

Ischiocavernosus muscle and deep perineal (investing or Gallaudet's) fascia (partially cut away)

Deep transverse perineal muscle

Superficial transverse perineal muscle and deep perineal (investing) fascia

Superficial perineal (Colles') fascia

Perineal body

Female

Sigmoid mesocolon

Rectosigmoid junction

Peritoneal reflection

Rectal fascia and rectum

Rectouterine pouch (of Douglas)

Coccyx

Levator ani muscle (pelvic diaphragm)

Puborectalis part of levator ani muscle

External anal sphincter muscle*
Deep
Superficial
Subcutaneous

Sigmoid colon

Free taenia

Uterus

Vesicouterine pouch

Ureter (cut)

Vagina and vaginal fascia

Urinary bladder and vesical fascia

Ischiocavernosus muscle and deep perineal (investing or Gallaudet's) fascia

Deep transverse perineal muscle and perineal membrane

Superficial perineal (Colles') fascia

Superficial transverse perineal muscle and deep perineal (investing or Gallaudet's) fascia

Perineal body

*Parts variable and often indistinct

Rectum

Plate 371

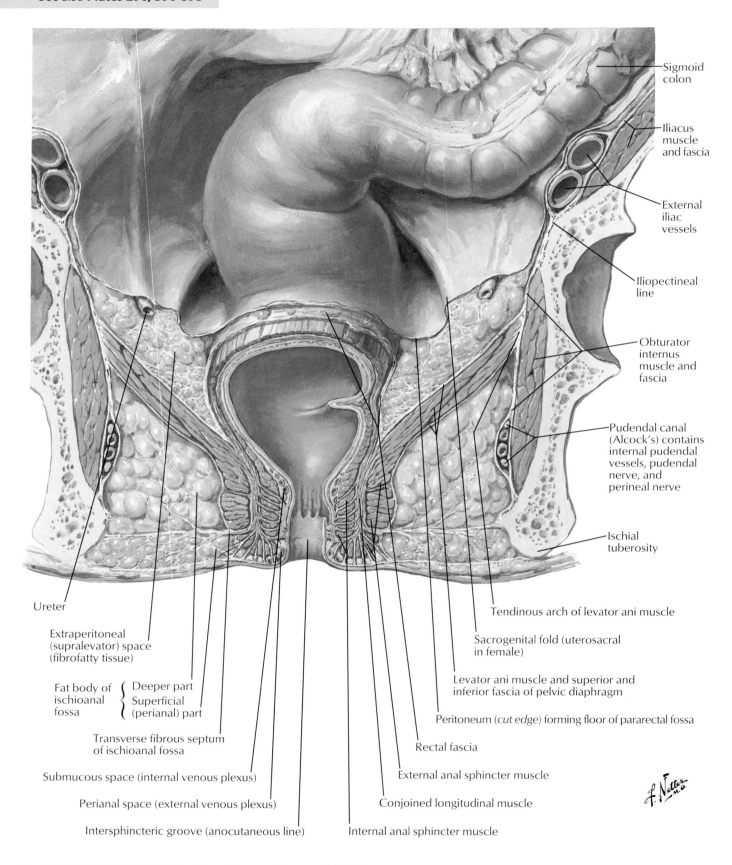

Sigmoid colon

Iliacus muscle and fascia

External iliac vessels

Iliopectineal line

Obturator internus muscle and fascia

Pudendal canal (Alcock's) contains internal pudendal vessels, pudendal nerve, and perineal nerve

Ischial tuberosity

Tendinous arch of levator ani muscle

Sacrogenital fold (uterosacral in female)

Levator ani muscle and superior and inferior fascia of pelvic diaphragm

Peritoneum (*cut edge*) forming floor of pararectal fossa

Rectal fascia

External anal sphincter muscle

Conjoined longitudinal muscle

Internal anal sphincter muscle

Ureter

Extraperitoneal (supralevator) space (fibrofatty tissue)

Fat body of ischioanal fossa { Deeper part / Superficial (perianal) part

Transverse fibrous septum of ischioanal fossa

Submucous space (internal venous plexus)

Perianal space (external venous plexus)

Intersphincteric groove (anocutaneous line)

F. Netter M.D.

Plate 372

Rectum

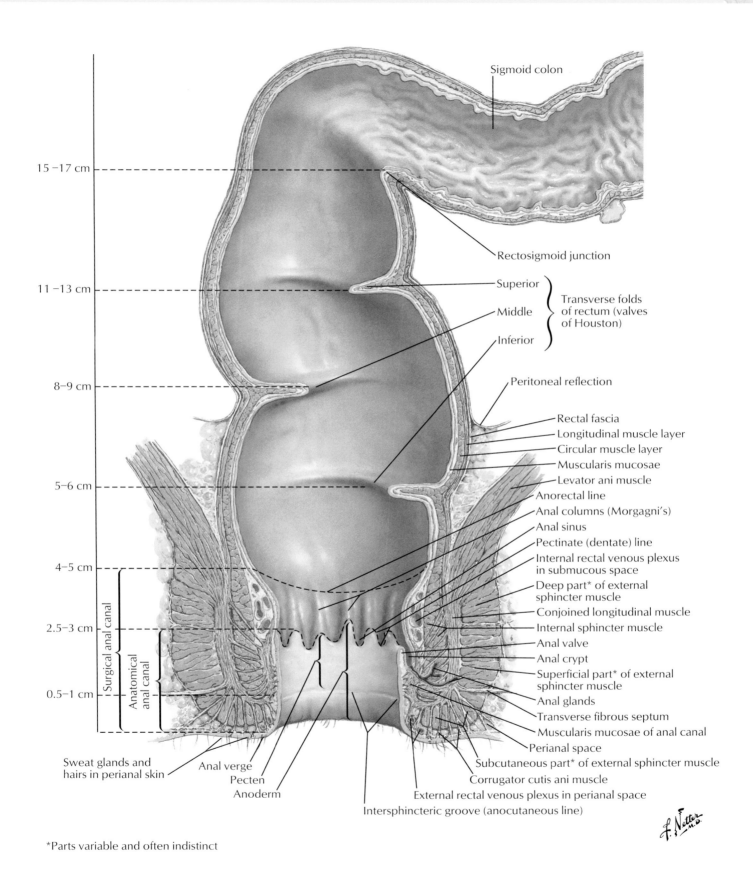

Sigmoid colon

Rectosigmoid junction

15–17 cm

11–13 cm

8–9 cm

5–6 cm

4–5 cm

2.5–3 cm

0.5–1 cm

Surgical anal canal

Anatomical anal canal

Superior
Middle
Inferior

Transverse folds of rectum (valves of Houston)

Peritoneal reflection

Rectal fascia
Longitudinal muscle layer
Circular muscle layer
Muscularis mucosae
Levator ani muscle
Anorectal line
Anal columns (Morgagni's)
Anal sinus
Pectinate (dentate) line
Internal rectal venous plexus in submucous space
Deep part* of external sphincter muscle
Conjoined longitudinal muscle
Internal sphincter muscle
Anal valve
Anal crypt
Superficial part* of external sphincter muscle
Anal glands
Transverse fibrous septum
Muscularis mucosae of anal canal
Perianal space
Subcutaneous part* of external sphincter muscle
Corrugator cutis ani muscle
External rectal venous plexus in perianal space
Intersphincteric groove (anocutaneous line)

Sweat glands and hairs in perianal skin
Anal verge
Pecten
Anoderm

*Parts variable and often indistinct

Rectum

Plate 373

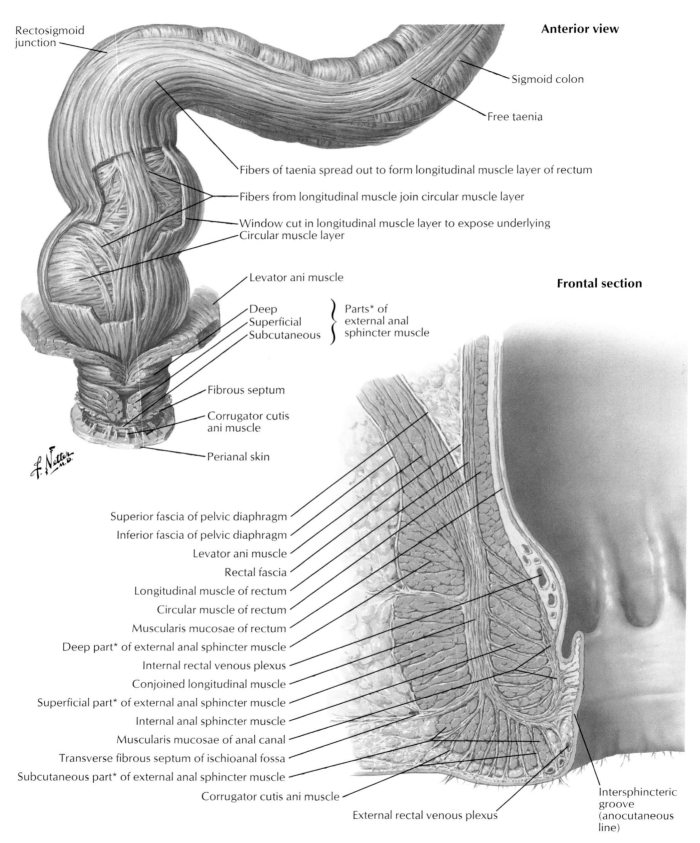

Anterior view

Rectosigmoid junction

Sigmoid colon

Free taenia

Fibers of taenia spread out to form longitudinal muscle layer of rectum

Fibers from longitudinal muscle join circular muscle layer

Window cut in longitudinal muscle layer to expose underlying Circular muscle layer

Levator ani muscle

Frontal section

Deep
Superficial
Subcutaneous
} Parts* of external anal sphincter muscle

Fibrous septum

Corrugator cutis ani muscle

Perianal skin

Superior fascia of pelvic diaphragm
Inferior fascia of pelvic diaphragm
Levator ani muscle
Rectal fascia
Longitudinal muscle of rectum
Circular muscle of rectum
Muscularis mucosae of rectum
Deep part* of external anal sphincter muscle
Internal rectal venous plexus
Conjoined longitudinal muscle
Superficial part* of external anal sphincter muscle
Internal anal sphincter muscle
Muscularis mucosae of anal canal
Transverse fibrous septum of ischioanal fossa
Subcutaneous part* of external anal sphincter muscle
Corrugator cutis ani muscle
External rectal venous plexus

Intersphincteric groove (anocutaneous line)

*Parts variable and often indistinct

Plate 374 | **Rectum**

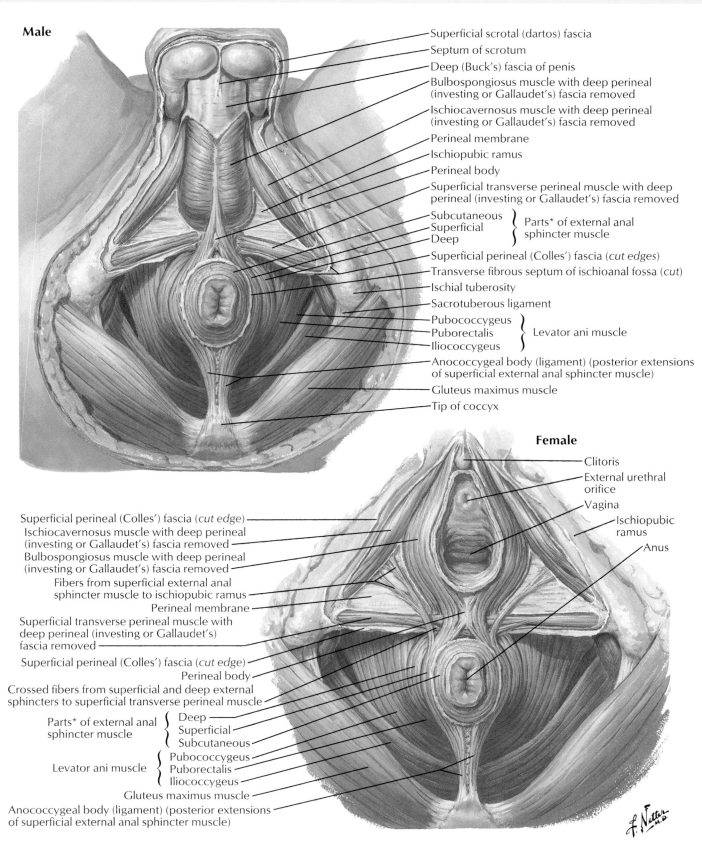

Male

Superficial scrotal (dartos) fascia

Septum of scrotum

Deep (Buck's) fascia of penis

Bulbospongiosus muscle with deep perineal (investing or Gallaudet's) fascia removed

Ischiocavernosus muscle with deep perineal (investing or Gallaudet's) fascia removed

Perineal membrane

Ischiopubic ramus

Perineal body

Superficial transverse perineal muscle with deep perineal (investing or Gallaudet's) fascia removed

Subcutaneous
Superficial
Deep } Parts* of external anal sphincter muscle

Superficial perineal (Colles') fascia (cut edges)

Transverse fibrous septum of ischioanal fossa (cut)

Ischial tuberosity

Sacrotuberous ligament

Pubococcygeus
Puborectalis
Iliococcygeus } Levator ani muscle

Anococcygeal body (ligament) (posterior extensions of superficial external anal sphincter muscle)

Gluteus maximus muscle

Tip of coccyx

Female

Clitoris

External urethral orifice

Vagina

Ischiopubic ramus

Anus

Superficial perineal (Colles') fascia (cut edge)

Ischiocavernosus muscle with deep perineal (investing or Gallaudet's) fascia removed

Bulbospongiosus muscle with deep perineal (investing or Gallaudet's) fascia removed

Fibers from superficial external anal sphincter muscle to ischiopubic ramus

Perineal membrane

Superficial transverse perineal muscle with deep perineal (investing or Gallaudet's) fascia removed

Superficial perineal (Colles') fascia (cut edge)

Perineal body

Crossed fibers from superficial and deep external sphincters to superficial transverse perineal muscle

Parts* of external anal sphincter muscle { Deep
Superficial
Subcutaneous

Levator ani muscle { Pubococcygeus
Puborectalis
Iliococcygeus

Gluteus maximus muscle

Anococcygeal body (ligament) (posterior extensions of superficial external anal sphincter muscle)

*Parts variable and often indistinct

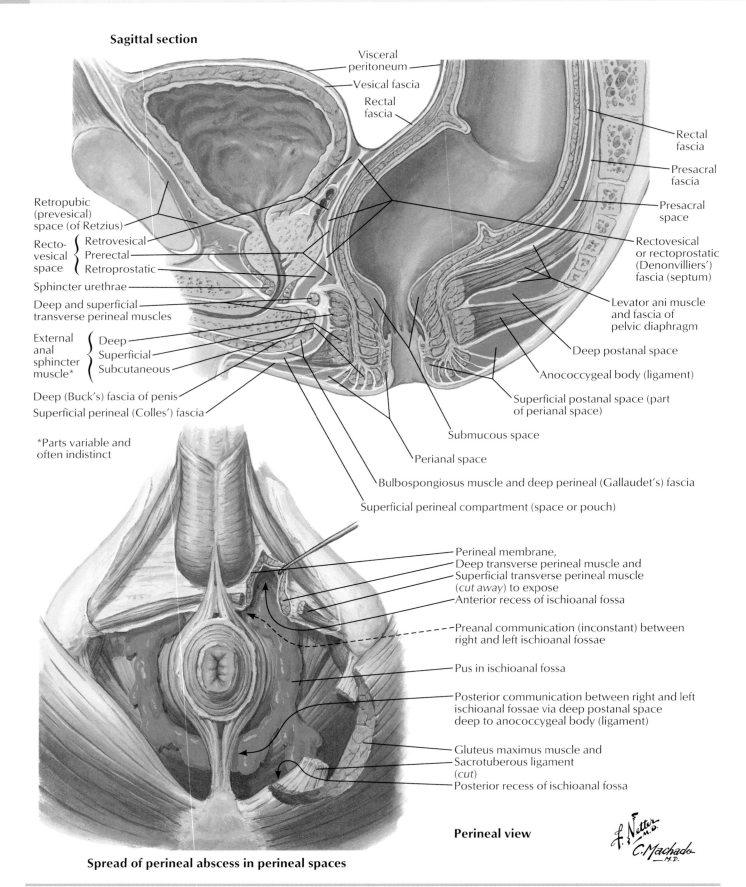

Sagittal section

Visceral peritoneum

Vesical fascia

Rectal fascia

Rectal fascia

Presacral fascia

Presacral space

Retropubic (prevesical) space (of Retzius)

Recto-vesical space { Retrovesical / Prerectal / Retroprostatic

Rectovesical or rectoprostatic (Denonvilliers') fascia (septum)

Sphincter urethrae

Deep and superficial transverse perineal muscles

Levator ani muscle and fascia of pelvic diaphragm

External anal sphincter muscle* { Deep / Superficial / Subcutaneous

Deep postanal space

Anococcygeal body (ligament)

Deep (Buck's) fascia of penis

Superficial perineal (Colles') fascia

Superficial postanal space (part of perianal space)

Submucous space

*Parts variable and often indistinct

Perianal space

Bulbospongiosus muscle and deep perineal (Gallaudet's) fascia

Superficial perineal compartment (space or pouch)

Perineal membrane,
Deep transverse perineal muscle and
Superficial transverse perineal muscle
(*cut away*) to expose
Anterior recess of ischioanal fossa

Preanal communication (inconstant) between right and left ischioanal fossae

Pus in ischioanal fossa

Posterior communication between right and left ischioanal fossae via deep postanal space deep to anococcygeal body (ligament)

Gluteus maximus muscle and
Sacrotuberous ligament
(*cut*)
Posterior recess of ischioanal fossa

Perineal view

Spread of perineal abscess in perineal spaces

Plate 376

Median (A) and paramedian (B) sagittal MR images of female pelvis

A   B

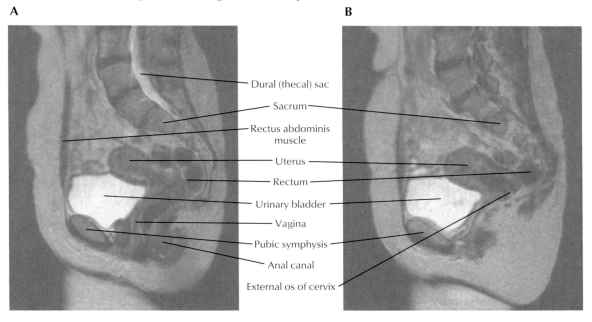

Dural (thecal) sac

Sacrum

Rectus abdominis muscle

Uterus

Rectum

Urinary bladder

Vagina

Pubic symphysis

Anal canal

External os of cervix

Median (C) and paramedian (D) sagittal MR images of male pelvis

C   D

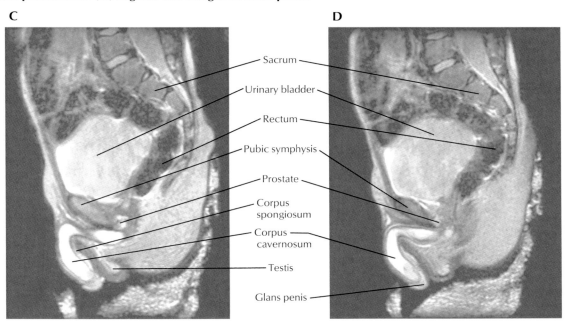

Sacrum

Urinary bladder

Rectum

Pubic symphysis

Prostate

Corpus spongiosum

Corpus cavernosum

Testis

Glans penis

Posterior view

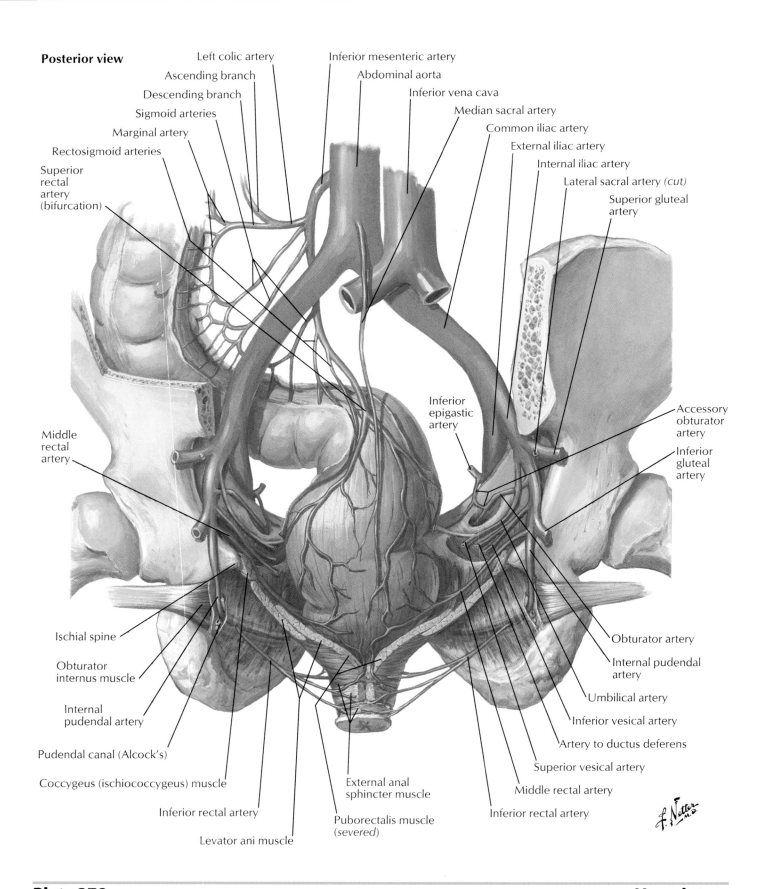

Left colic artery

Ascending branch

Descending branch

Sigmoid arteries

Marginal artery

Rectosigmoid arteries

Superior rectal artery (bifurcation)

Inferior mesenteric artery

Abdominal aorta

Inferior vena cava

Median sacral artery

Common iliac artery

External iliac artery

Internal iliac artery

Lateral sacral artery *(cut)*

Superior gluteal artery

Middle rectal artery

Inferior epigastric artery

Accessory obturator artery

Inferior gluteal artery

Ischial spine

Obturator internus muscle

Internal pudendal artery

Pudendal canal (Alcock's)

Coccygeus (ischiococcygeus) muscle

Inferior rectal artery

Levator ani muscle

External anal sphincter muscle

Puborectalis muscle *(severed)*

Obturator artery

Internal pudendal artery

Umbilical artery

Inferior vesical artery

Artery to ductus deferens

Superior vesical artery

Middle rectal artery

Inferior rectal artery

Plate 378 **Vasculature**

Anterior view

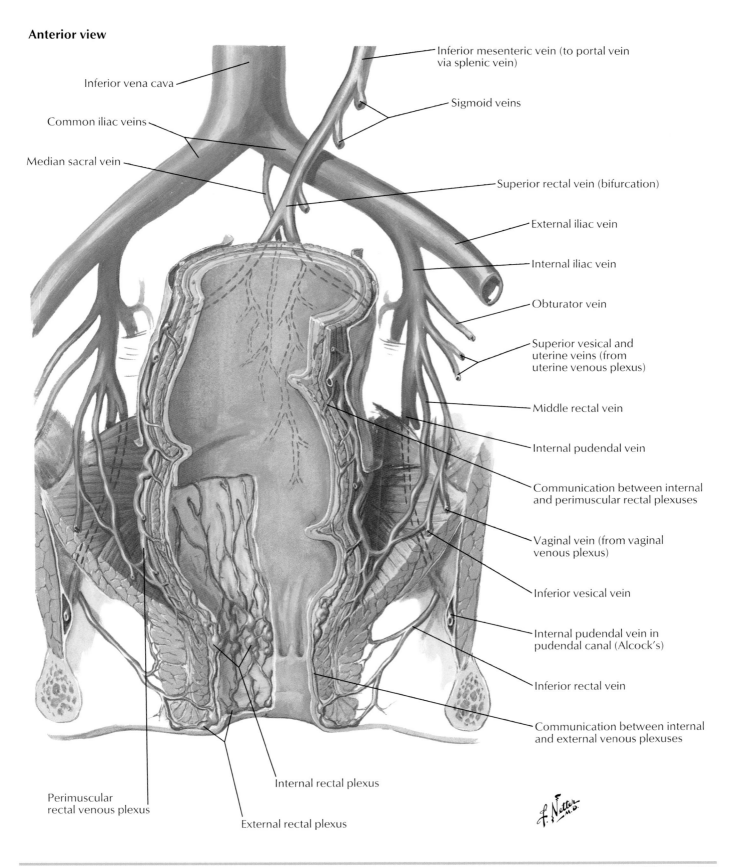

Inferior vena cava

Common iliac veins

Median sacral vein

Inferior mesenteric vein (to portal vein via splenic vein)

Sigmoid veins

Superior rectal vein (bifurcation)

External iliac vein

Internal iliac vein

Obturator vein

Superior vesical and uterine veins (from uterine venous plexus)

Middle rectal vein

Internal pudendal vein

Communication between internal and perimuscular rectal plexuses

Vaginal vein (from vaginal venous plexus)

Inferior vesical vein

Internal pudendal vein in pudendal canal (Alcock's)

Inferior rectal vein

Communication between internal and external venous plexuses

Perimuscular rectal venous plexus

Internal rectal plexus

External rectal plexus

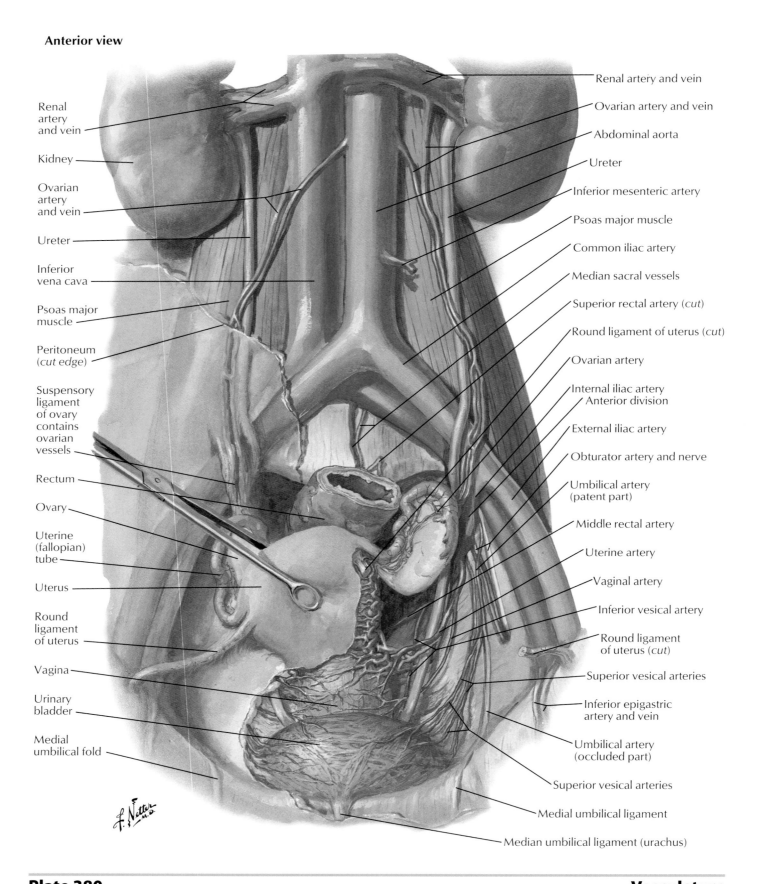

Anterior view

Renal artery and vein

Renal artery and vein

Ovarian artery and vein

Kidney

Abdominal aorta

Ovarian artery and vein

Ureter

Ureter

Inferior mesenteric artery

Inferior vena cava

Psoas major muscle

Psoas major muscle

Common iliac artery

Peritoneum (cut edge)

Median sacral vessels

Superior rectal artery (cut)

Suspensory ligament of ovary contains ovarian vessels

Round ligament of uterus (cut)

Ovarian artery

Rectum

Internal iliac artery Anterior division

Ovary

External iliac artery

Uterine (fallopian) tube

Obturator artery and nerve

Uterus

Umbilical artery (patent part)

Round ligament of uterus

Middle rectal artery

Uterine artery

Vagina

Vaginal artery

Urinary bladder

Inferior vesical artery

Medial umbilical fold

Round ligament of uterus (cut)

Superior vesical arteries

Inferior epigastric artery and vein

Umbilical artery (occluded part)

Superior vesical arteries

Medial umbilical ligament

Median umbilical ligament (urachus)

Plate 380

Vasculature

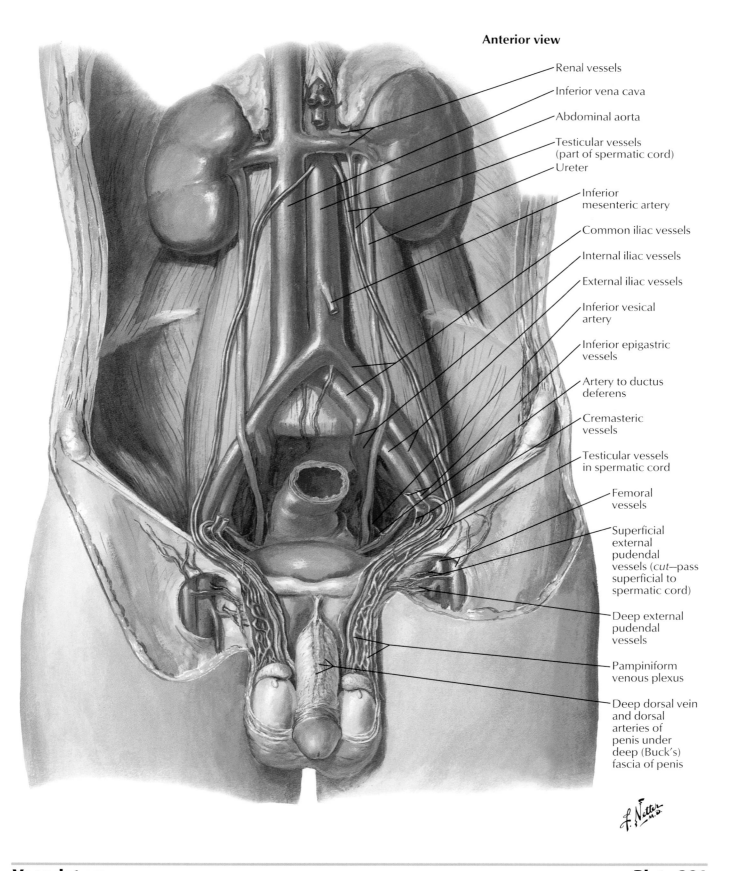

Anterior view

Renal vessels

Inferior vena cava

Abdominal aorta

Testicular vessels (part of spermatic cord)

Ureter

Inferior mesenteric artery

Common iliac vessels

Internal iliac vessels

External iliac vessels

Inferior vesical artery

Inferior epigastric vessels

Artery to ductus deferens

Cremasteric vessels

Testicular vessels in spermatic cord

Femoral vessels

Superficial external pudendal vessels (*cut*—pass superficial to spermatic cord)

Deep external pudendal vessels

Pampiniform venous plexus

Deep dorsal vein and dorsal arteries of penis under deep (Buck's) fascia of penis

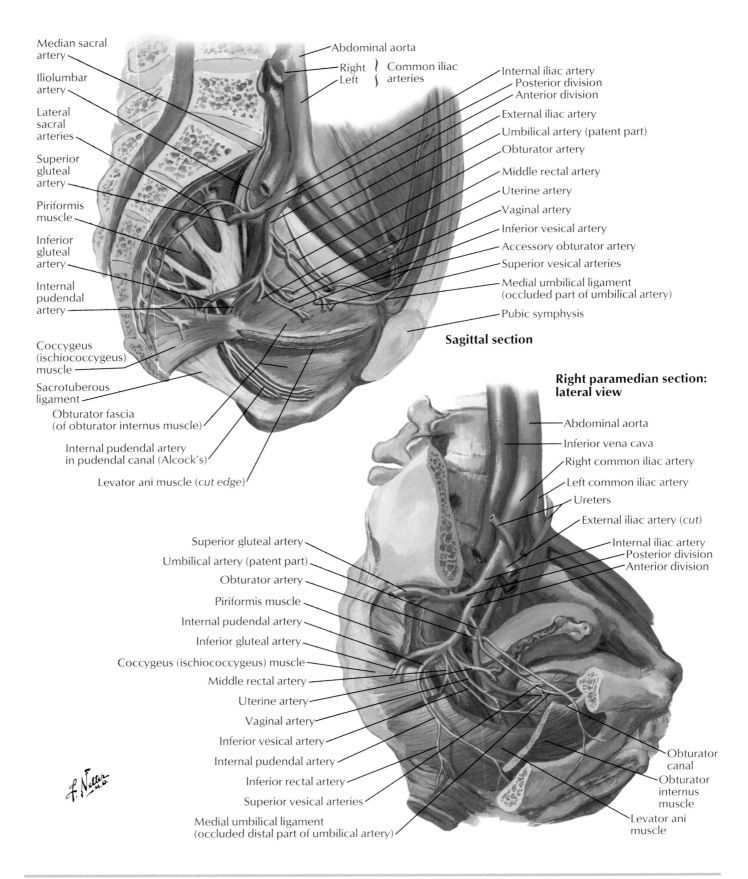

Median sacral artery

Iliolumbar artery

Lateral sacral arteries

Superior gluteal artery

Piriformis muscle

Inferior gluteal artery

Internal pudendal artery

Coccygeus (ischiococcygeus) muscle

Sacrotuberous ligament

Obturator fascia (of obturator internus muscle)

Internal pudendal artery in pudendal canal (Alcock's)

Levator ani muscle (*cut edge*)

Abdominal aorta

Right } Common iliac
Left } arteries

Internal iliac artery
Posterior division
Anterior division

External iliac artery

Umbilical artery (patent part)

Obturator artery

Middle rectal artery

Uterine artery

Vaginal artery

Inferior vesical artery

Accessory obturator artery

Superior vesical arteries

Medial umbilical ligament (occluded part of umbilical artery)

Pubic symphysis

Sagittal section

Right paramedian section: lateral view

Abdominal aorta

Inferior vena cava

Right common iliac artery

Left common iliac artery

Ureters

External iliac artery (*cut*)

Internal iliac artery
Posterior division
Anterior division

Superior gluteal artery

Umbilical artery (patent part)

Obturator artery

Piriformis muscle

Internal pudendal artery

Inferior gluteal artery

Coccygeus (ischiococcygeus) muscle

Middle rectal artery

Uterine artery

Vaginal artery

Inferior vesical artery

Internal pudendal artery

Inferior rectal artery

Superior vesical arteries

Medial umbilical ligament (occluded distal part of umbilical artery)

Obturator canal

Obturator internus muscle

Levator ani muscle

Plate 382   **Vasculature**

**Left paramedian section:
lateral view**

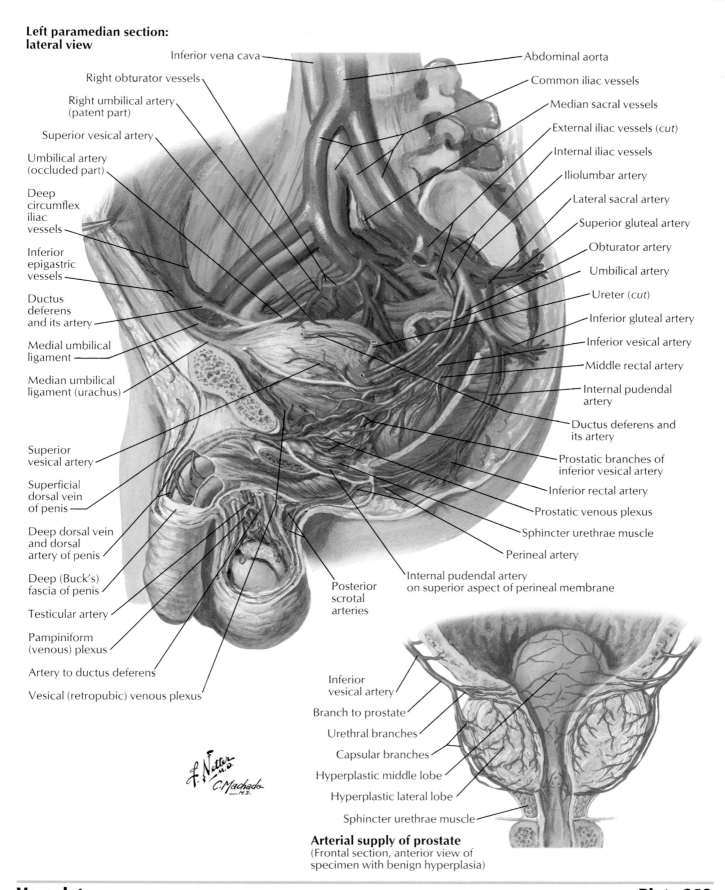

Inferior vena cava

Right obturator vessels

Right umbilical artery
(patent part)

Superior vesical artery

Umbilical artery
(occluded part)

Deep
circumflex
iliac
vessels

Inferior
epigastric
vessels

Ductus
deferens
and its artery

Medial umbilical
ligament

Median umbilical
ligament (urachus)

Superior
vesical artery

Superficial
dorsal vein
of penis

Deep dorsal vein
and dorsal
artery of penis

Deep (Buck's)
fascia of penis

Testicular artery

Pampiniform
(venous) plexus

Artery to ductus deferens

Vesical (retropubic) venous plexus

Abdominal aorta

Common iliac vessels

Median sacral vessels

External iliac vessels (*cut*)

Internal iliac vessels

Iliolumbar artery

Lateral sacral artery

Superior gluteal artery

Obturator artery

Umbilical artery

Ureter (*cut*)

Inferior gluteal artery

Inferior vesical artery

Middle rectal artery

Internal pudendal
artery

Ductus deferens and
its artery

Prostatic branches of
inferior vesical artery

Inferior rectal artery

Prostatic venous plexus

Sphincter urethrae muscle

Perineal artery

Internal pudendal artery
on superior aspect of perineal membrane

Posterior
scrotal
arteries

Inferior
vesical artery

Branch to prostate

Urethral branches

Capsular branches

Hyperplastic middle lobe

Hyperplastic lateral lobe

Sphincter urethrae muscle

Arterial supply of prostate
(Frontal section, anterior view of
specimen with benign hyperplasia)

Vasculature

Plate 383

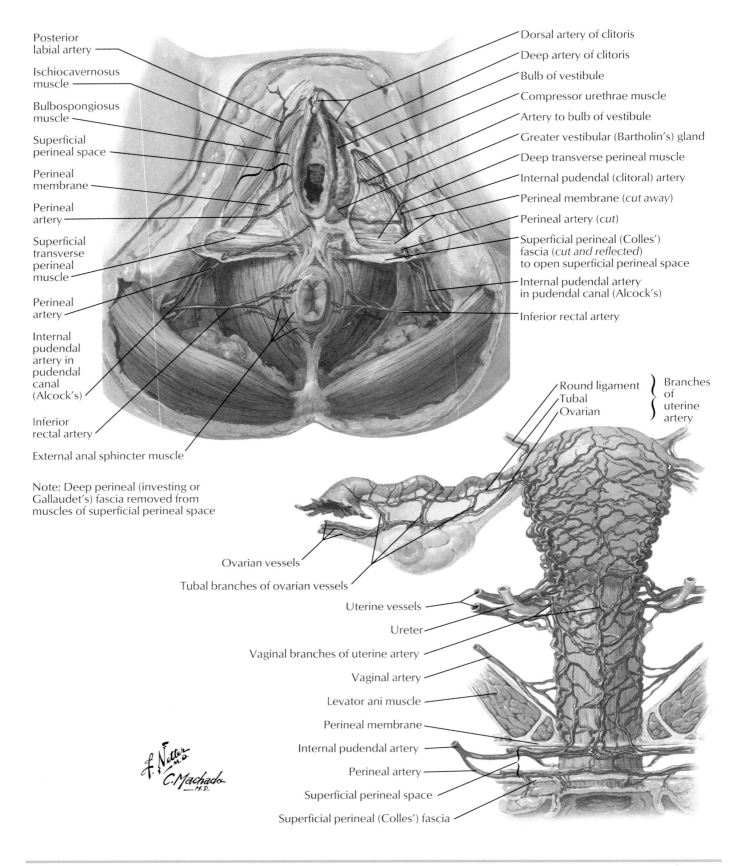

Posterior labial artery

Ischiocavernosus muscle

Bulbospongiosus muscle

Superficial perineal space

Perineal membrane

Perineal artery

Superficial transverse perineal muscle

Perineal artery

Internal pudendal artery in pudendal canal (Alcock's)

Inferior rectal artery

External anal sphincter muscle

Note: Deep perineal (investing or Gallaudet's) fascia removed from muscles of superficial perineal space

Dorsal artery of clitoris

Deep artery of clitoris

Bulb of vestibule

Compressor urethrae muscle

Artery to bulb of vestibule

Greater vestibular (Bartholin's) gland

Deep transverse perineal muscle

Internal pudendal (clitoral) artery

Perineal membrane (*cut away*)

Perineal artery (*cut*)

Superficial perineal (Colles') fascia (*cut and reflected*) to open superficial perineal space

Internal pudendal artery in pudendal canal (Alcock's)

Inferior rectal artery

Round ligament
Tubal
Ovarian
} Branches of uterine artery

Ovarian vessels

Tubal branches of ovarian vessels

Uterine vessels

Ureter

Vaginal branches of uterine artery

Vaginal artery

Levator ani muscle

Perineal membrane

Internal pudendal artery

Perineal artery

Superficial perineal space

Superficial perineal (Colles') fascia

Plate 384   **Vasculature**

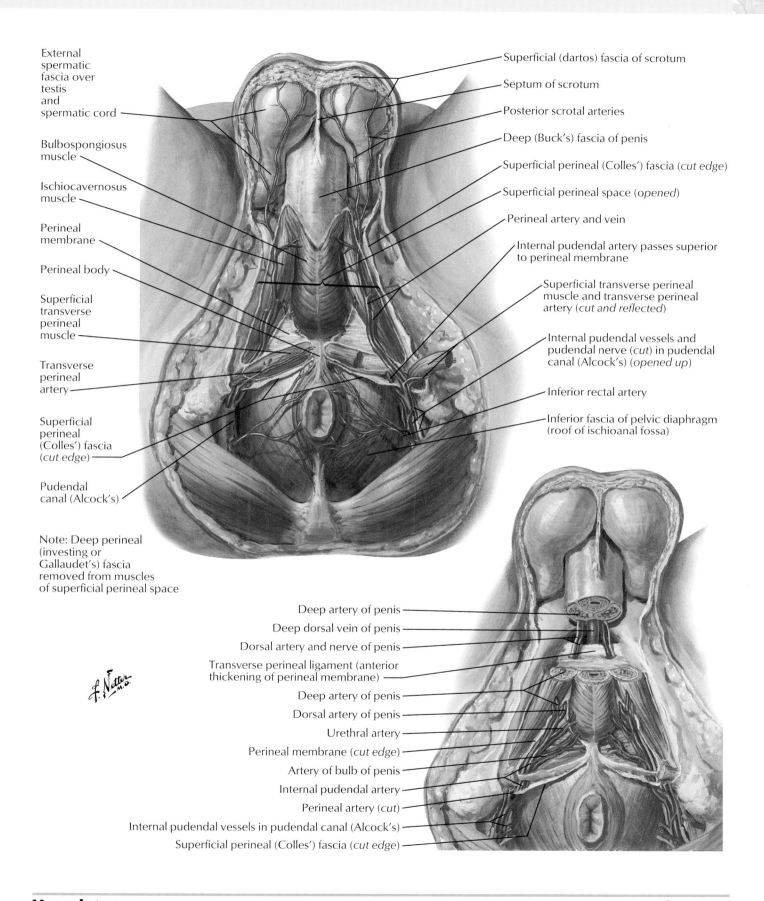

External spermatic fascia over testis and spermatic cord

Bulbospongiosus muscle

Ischiocavernosus muscle

Perineal membrane

Perineal body

Superficial transverse perineal muscle

Transverse perineal artery

Superficial perineal (Colles') fascia (cut edge)

Pudendal canal (Alcock's)

Note: Deep perineal (investing or Gallaudet's) fascia removed from muscles of superficial perineal space

Superficial (dartos) fascia of scrotum

Septum of scrotum

Posterior scrotal arteries

Deep (Buck's) fascia of penis

Superficial perineal (Colles') fascia (cut edge)

Superficial perineal space (opened)

Perineal artery and vein

Internal pudendal artery passes superior to perineal membrane

Superficial transverse perineal muscle and transverse perineal artery (cut and reflected)

Internal pudendal vessels and pudendal nerve (cut) in pudendal canal (Alcock's) (opened up)

Inferior rectal artery

Inferior fascia of pelvic diaphragm (roof of ischioanal fossa)

Deep artery of penis

Deep dorsal vein of penis

Dorsal artery and nerve of penis

Transverse perineal ligament (anterior thickening of perineal membrane)

Deep artery of penis

Dorsal artery of penis

Urethral artery

Perineal membrane (cut edge)

Artery of bulb of penis

Internal pudendal artery

Perineal artery (cut)

Internal pudendal vessels in pudendal canal (Alcock's)

Superficial perineal (Colles') fascia (cut edge)

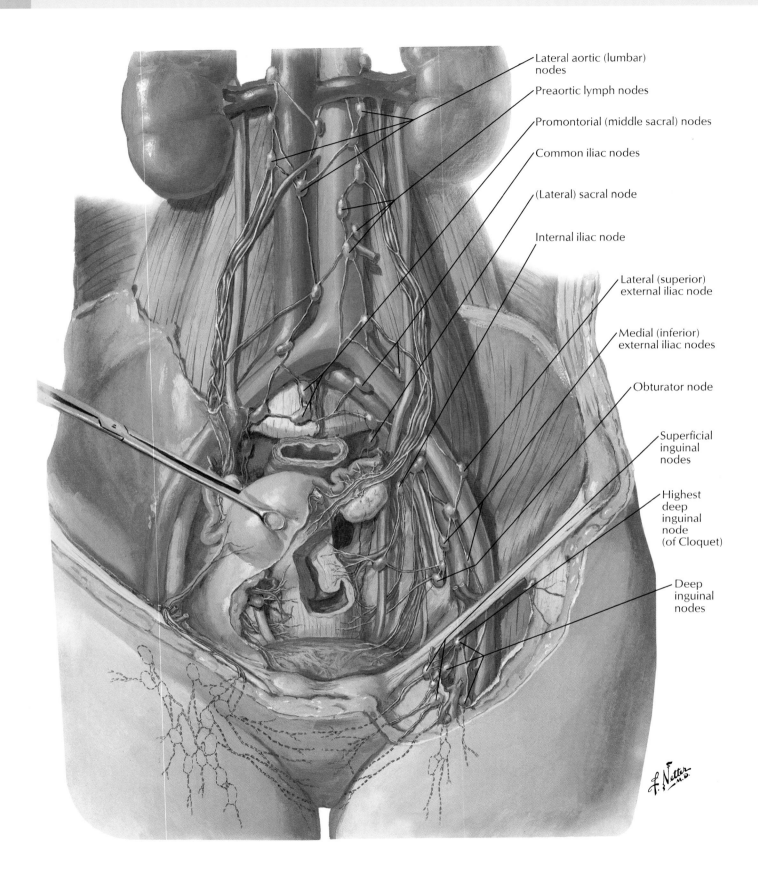

Lateral aortic (lumbar) nodes

Preaortic lymph nodes

Promontorial (middle sacral) nodes

Common iliac nodes

(Lateral) sacral node

Internal iliac node

Lateral (superior) external iliac node

Medial (inferior) external iliac nodes

Obturator node

Superficial inguinal nodes

Highest deep inguinal node (of Cloquet)

Deep inguinal nodes

Plate 386 **Vasculature**

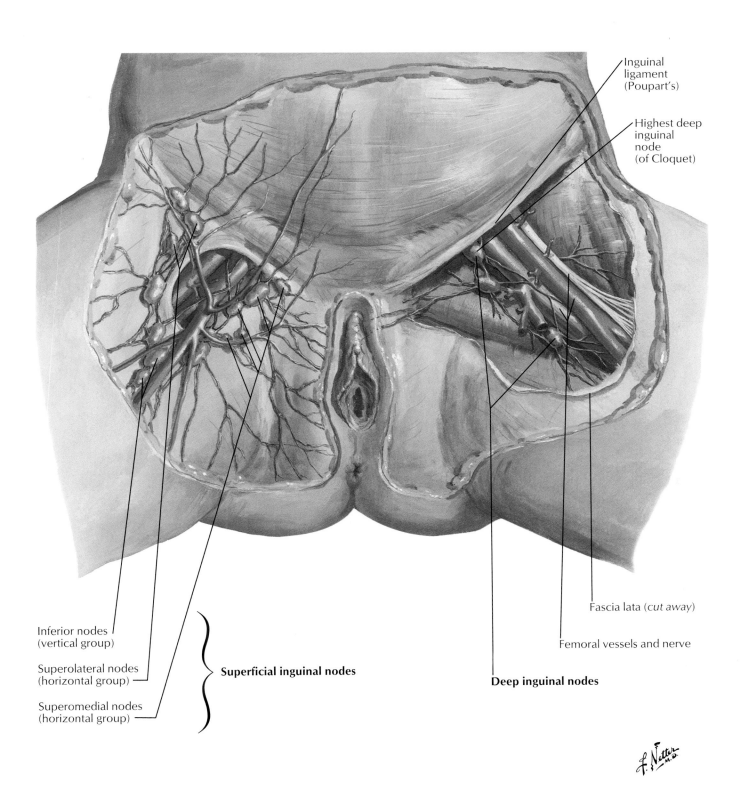

Inguinal ligament (Poupart's)

Highest deep inguinal node (of Cloquet)

Fascia lata (*cut away*)

Femoral vessels and nerve

Deep inguinal nodes

Inferior nodes (vertical group)

Superolateral nodes (horizontal group)

Superomedial nodes (horizontal group)

Superficial inguinal nodes

Lymph Vessels and Nodes of Pelvis and Genitalia: Male

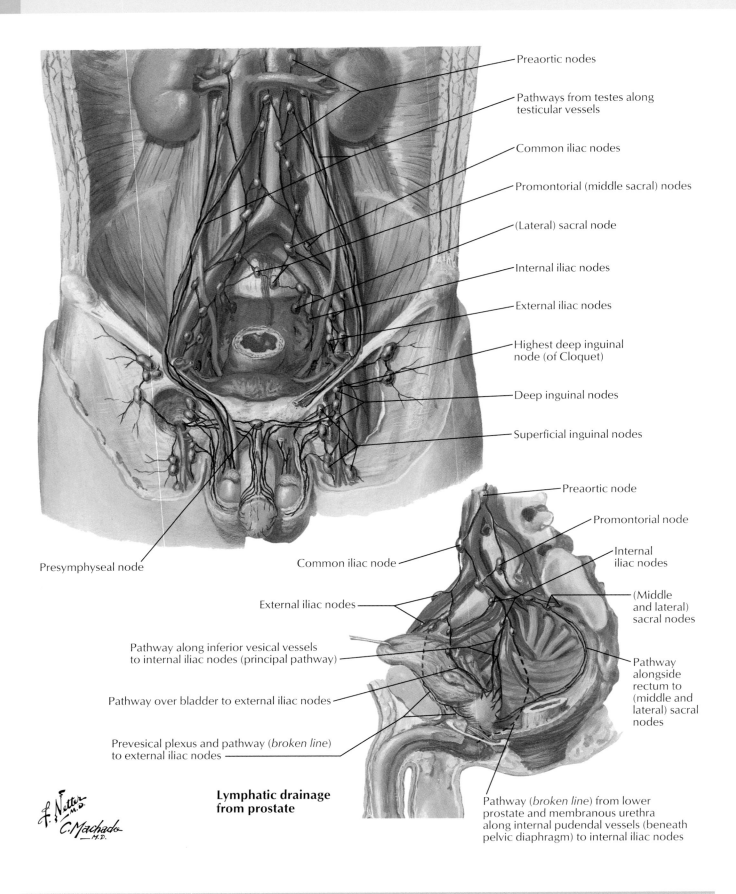

Preaortic nodes

Pathways from testes along testicular vessels

Common iliac nodes

Promontorial (middle sacral) nodes

(Lateral) sacral node

Internal iliac nodes

External iliac nodes

Highest deep inguinal node (of Cloquet)

Deep inguinal nodes

Superficial inguinal nodes

Preaortic node

Promontorial node

Internal iliac nodes

(Middle and lateral) sacral nodes

Common iliac node

Pathway alongside rectum to (middle and lateral) sacral nodes

External iliac nodes

Presymphyseal node

Pathway along inferior vesical vessels to internal iliac nodes (principal pathway)

Pathway over bladder to external iliac nodes

Prevesical plexus and pathway (*broken line*) to external iliac nodes

Lymphatic drainage from prostate

Pathway (*broken line*) from lower prostate and membranous urethra along internal pudendal vessels (beneath pelvic diaphragm) to internal iliac nodes

Plate 388   **Vasculature**

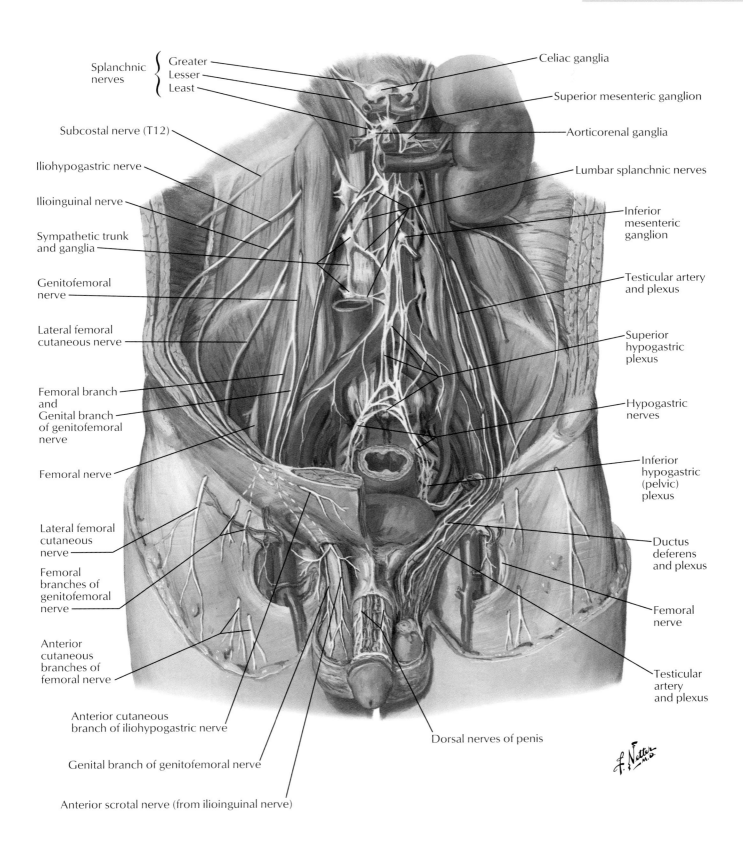

Splanchnic nerves { Greater — Lesser — Least —

Celiac ganglia

Superior mesenteric ganglion

Subcostal nerve (T12)

Aorticorenal ganglia

Iliohypogastric nerve

Lumbar splanchnic nerves

Ilioinguinal nerve

Inferior mesenteric ganglion

Sympathetic trunk and ganglia

Genitofemoral nerve

Testicular artery and plexus

Lateral femoral cutaneous nerve

Superior hypogastric plexus

Femoral branch and Genital branch of genitofemoral nerve

Hypogastric nerves

Femoral nerve

Inferior hypogastric (pelvic) plexus

Lateral femoral cutaneous nerve

Femoral branches of genitofemoral nerve

Ductus deferens and plexus

Anterior cutaneous branches of femoral nerve

Femoral nerve

Anterior cutaneous branch of iliohypogastric nerve

Testicular artery and plexus

Genital branch of genitofemoral nerve

Dorsal nerves of penis

Anterior scrotal nerve (from ilioinguinal nerve)

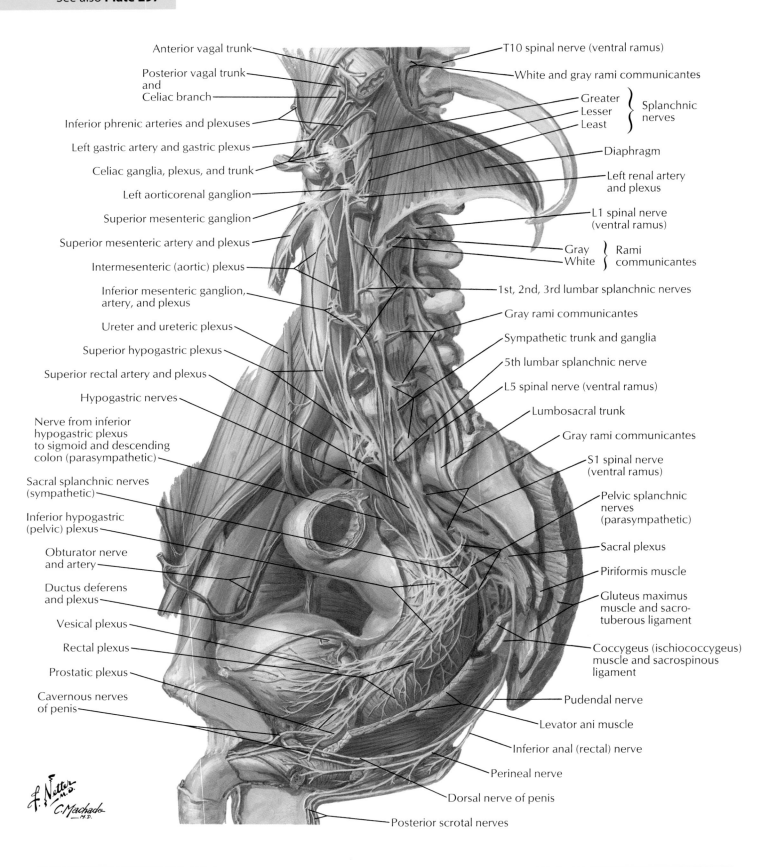

Anterior vagal trunk

Posterior vagal trunk and Celiac branch

Inferior phrenic arteries and plexuses

Left gastric artery and gastric plexus

Celiac ganglia, plexus, and trunk

Left aorticorenal ganglion

Superior mesenteric ganglion

Superior mesenteric artery and plexus

Intermesenteric (aortic) plexus

Inferior mesenteric ganglion, artery, and plexus

Ureter and ureteric plexus

Superior hypogastric plexus

Superior rectal artery and plexus

Hypogastric nerves

Nerve from inferior hypogastric plexus to sigmoid and descending colon (parasympathetic)

Sacral splanchnic nerves (sympathetic)

Inferior hypogastric (pelvic) plexus

Obturator nerve and artery

Ductus deferens and plexus

Vesical plexus

Rectal plexus

Prostatic plexus

Cavernous nerves of penis

T10 spinal nerve (ventral ramus)

White and gray rami communicantes

Greater
Lesser } Splanchnic
Least } nerves

Diaphragm

Left renal artery and plexus

L1 spinal nerve (ventral ramus)

Gray } Rami
White } communicantes

1st, 2nd, 3rd lumbar splanchnic nerves

Gray rami communicantes

Sympathetic trunk and ganglia

5th lumbar splanchnic nerve

L5 spinal nerve (ventral ramus)

Lumbosacral trunk

Gray rami communicantes

S1 spinal nerve (ventral ramus)

Pelvic splanchnic nerves (parasympathetic)

Sacral plexus

Piriformis muscle

Gluteus maximus muscle and sacro-tuberous ligament

Coccygeus (ischiococcygeus) muscle and sacrospinous ligament

Pudendal nerve

Levator ani muscle

Inferior anal (rectal) nerve

Perineal nerve

Dorsal nerve of penis

Posterior scrotal nerves

Plate 390

Innervation

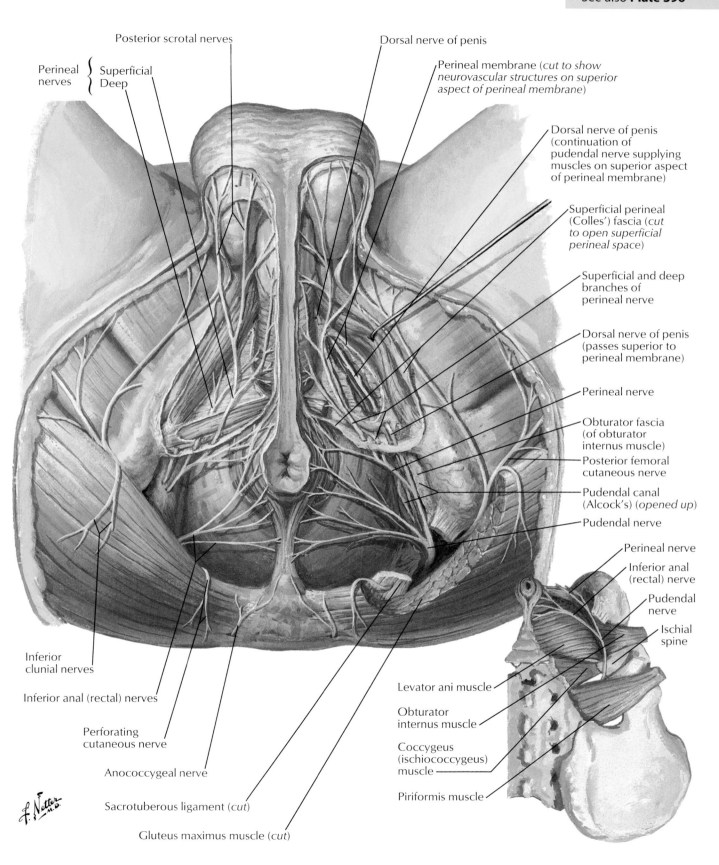

Posterior scrotal nerves

Dorsal nerve of penis

Perineal nerves { Superficial / Deep }

Perineal membrane (*cut to show neurovascular structures on superior aspect of perineal membrane*)

Dorsal nerve of penis (continuation of pudendal nerve supplying muscles on superior aspect of perineal membrane)

Superficial perineal (Colles') fascia (*cut to open superficial perineal space*)

Superficial and deep branches of perineal nerve

Dorsal nerve of penis (passes superior to perineal membrane)

Perineal nerve

Obturator fascia (of obturator internus muscle)

Posterior femoral cutaneous nerve

Pudendal canal (Alcock's) (*opened up*)

Pudendal nerve

Perineal nerve

Inferior anal (rectal) nerve

Pudendal nerve

Ischial spine

Inferior clunial nerves

Inferior anal (rectal) nerves

Perforating cutaneous nerve

Anococcygeal nerve

Sacrotuberous ligament (*cut*)

Gluteus maximus muscle (*cut*)

Levator ani muscle

Obturator internus muscle

Coccygeus (ischiococcygeus) muscle

Piriformis muscle

Innervation

Plate 391

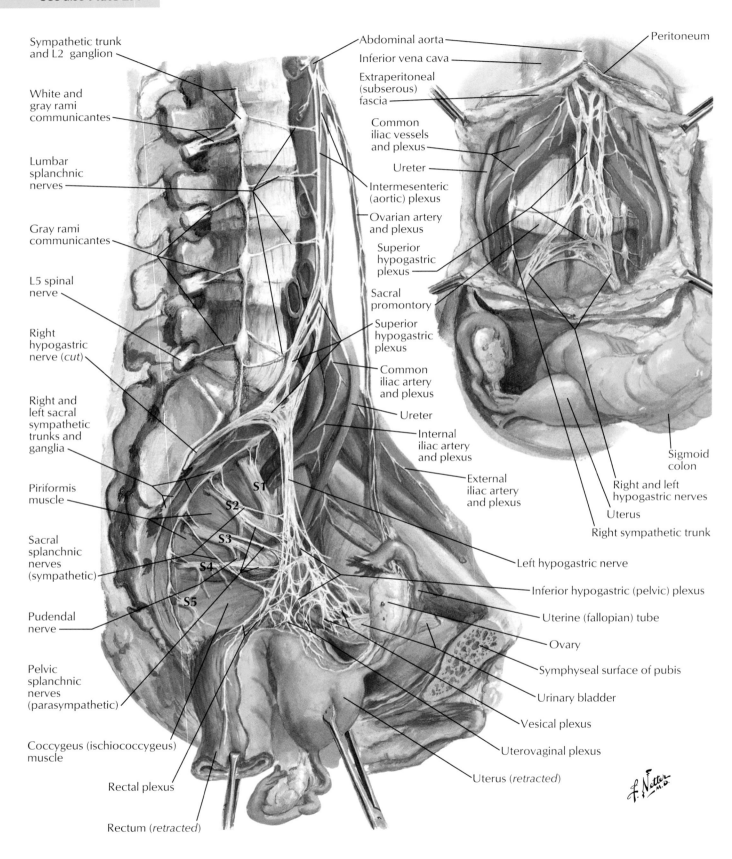

Sympathetic trunk and L2 ganglion

White and gray rami communicantes

Lumbar splanchnic nerves

Gray rami communicantes

L5 spinal nerve

Right hypogastric nerve (*cut*)

Right and left sacral sympathetic trunks and ganglia

Piriformis muscle

Sacral splanchnic nerves (sympathetic)

Pudendal nerve

Pelvic splanchnic nerves (parasympathetic)

Coccygeus (ischiococcygeus) muscle

Rectal plexus

Rectum (*retracted*)

Abdominal aorta

Inferior vena cava

Extraperitoneal (subserous) fascia

Common iliac vessels and plexus

Ureter

Intermesenteric (aortic) plexus

Ovarian artery and plexus

Superior hypogastric plexus

Sacral promontory

Superior hypogastric plexus

Common iliac artery and plexus

Ureter

Internal iliac artery and plexus

External iliac artery and plexus

Peritoneum

Sigmoid colon

Right and left hypogastric nerves

Uterus

Right sympathetic trunk

Left hypogastric nerve

Inferior hypogastric (pelvic) plexus

Uterine (fallopian) tube

Ovary

Symphyseal surface of pubis

Urinary bladder

Vesical plexus

Uterovaginal plexus

Uterus (*retracted*)

S1

S2

S3

S4

S5

Plate 392

Innervation

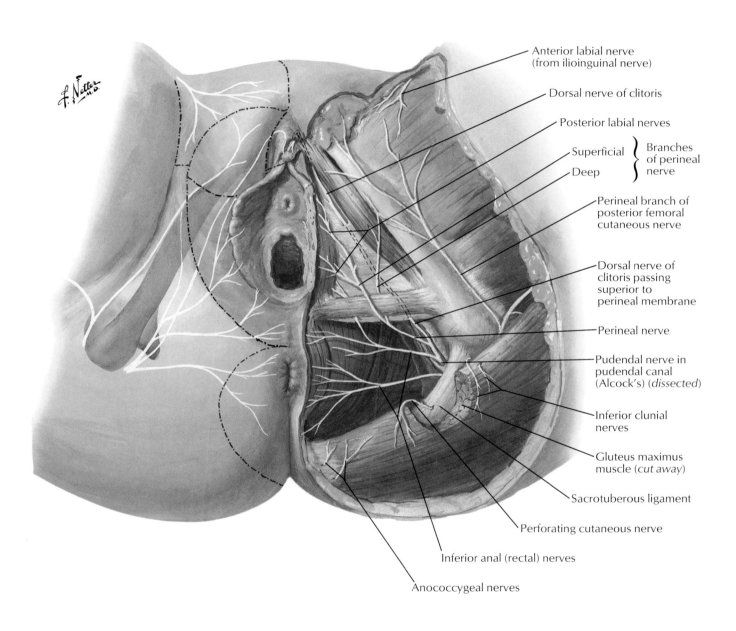

Anterior labial nerve
(from ilioinguinal nerve)

Dorsal nerve of clitoris

Posterior labial nerves

Superficial ⎫ Branches
          ⎬ of perineal
Deep   ⎭ nerve

Perineal branch of
posterior femoral
cutaneous nerve

Dorsal nerve of
clitoris passing
superior to
perineal membrane

Perineal nerve

Pudendal nerve in
pudendal canal
(Alcock's) (*dissected*)

Inferior clunial
nerves

Gluteus maximus
muscle (*cut away*)

Sacrotuberous ligament

Perforating cutaneous nerve

Inferior anal (rectal) nerves

Anococcygeal nerves

Neuropathways in Parturition

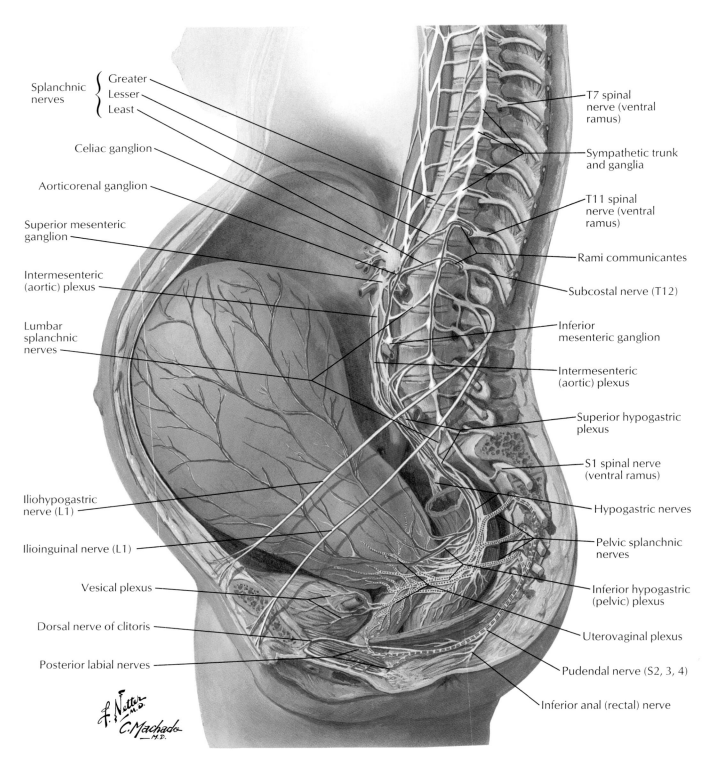

Splanchnic nerves
{ Greater
Lesser
Least

Celiac ganglion

Aorticorenal ganglion

Superior mesenteric ganglion

Intermesenteric (aortic) plexus

Lumbar splanchnic nerves

Iliohypogastric nerve (L1)

Ilioinguinal nerve (L1)

Vesical plexus

Dorsal nerve of clitoris

Posterior labial nerves

T7 spinal nerve (ventral ramus)

Sympathetic trunk and ganglia

T11 spinal nerve (ventral ramus)

Rami communicantes

Subcostal nerve (T12)

Inferior mesenteric ganglion

Intermesenteric (aortic) plexus

Superior hypogastric plexus

S1 spinal nerve (ventral ramus)

Hypogastric nerves

Pelvic splanchnic nerves

Inferior hypogastric (pelvic) plexus

Uterovaginal plexus

Pudendal nerve (S2, 3, 4)

Inferior anal (rectal) nerve

——— Sensory fibers from uterine body and fundus accompany sympathetic fibers via hypogastric plexuses to T11, 12 (L1?)

——— Motor fibers to uterine body and fundus (sympathetic)

··········· Sensory fibers from cervix and upper vagina accompany pelvic splanchnic nerves (parasympathetic) to S2, 3, 4

··········· Motor fibers to lower uterine segment, cervix, and upper vagina (parasympathetic)

– – – Sensory fibers from lower vagina and perineum accompany somatic fibers via pudendal nerve to S2, 3, 4

– – – – Motor fibers to lower vagina and perineum via pudendal nerve (somatic)

Plate 394

Innervation

See also **Plates 160, 161**

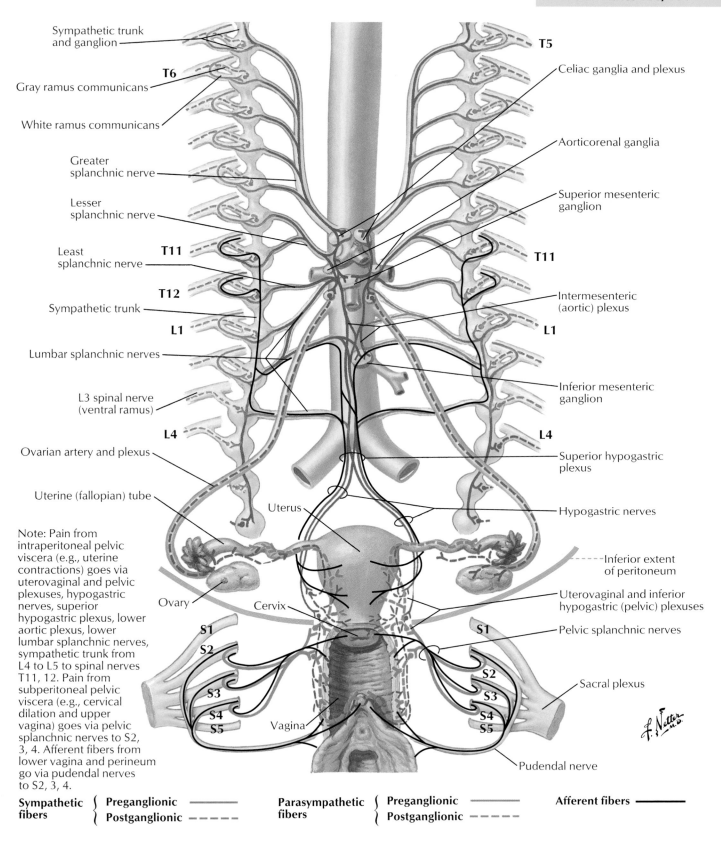

Sympathetic trunk and ganglion

T6

Gray ramus communicans

White ramus communicans

Greater splanchnic nerve

Lesser splanchnic nerve

Least splanchnic nerve — T11

T12

Sympathetic trunk

L1

Lumbar splanchnic nerves

L3 spinal nerve (ventral ramus)

L4

Ovarian artery and plexus

Uterine (fallopian) tube

Note: Pain from intraperitoneal pelvic viscera (e.g., uterine contractions) goes via uterovaginal and pelvic plexuses, hypogastric nerves, superior hypogastric plexus, lower aortic plexus, lower lumbar splanchnic nerves, sympathetic trunk from L4 to L5 to spinal nerves T11, 12. Pain from subperitoneal pelvic viscera (e.g., cervical dilation and upper vagina) goes via pelvic splanchnic nerves to S2, 3, 4. Afferent fibers from lower vagina and perineum go via pudendal nerves to S2, 3, 4.

Ovary

Cervix

S1

S2

S3

S4

S5

Vagina

T5

Celiac ganglia and plexus

Aorticorenal ganglia

Superior mesenteric ganglion

T11

Intermesenteric (aortic) plexus

L1

Inferior mesenteric ganglion

L4

Superior hypogastric plexus

Hypogastric nerves

Inferior extent of peritoneum

Uterovaginal and inferior hypogastric (pelvic) plexuses

Pelvic splanchnic nerves

S1

S2

Sacral plexus

S3

S4

S5

Pudendal nerve

Uterus

| Sympathetic fibers | Preganglionic ———— | Parasympathetic fibers | Preganglionic ———— | Afferent fibers ———— |
| | Postganglionic – – – – | | Postganglionic – – – – | |

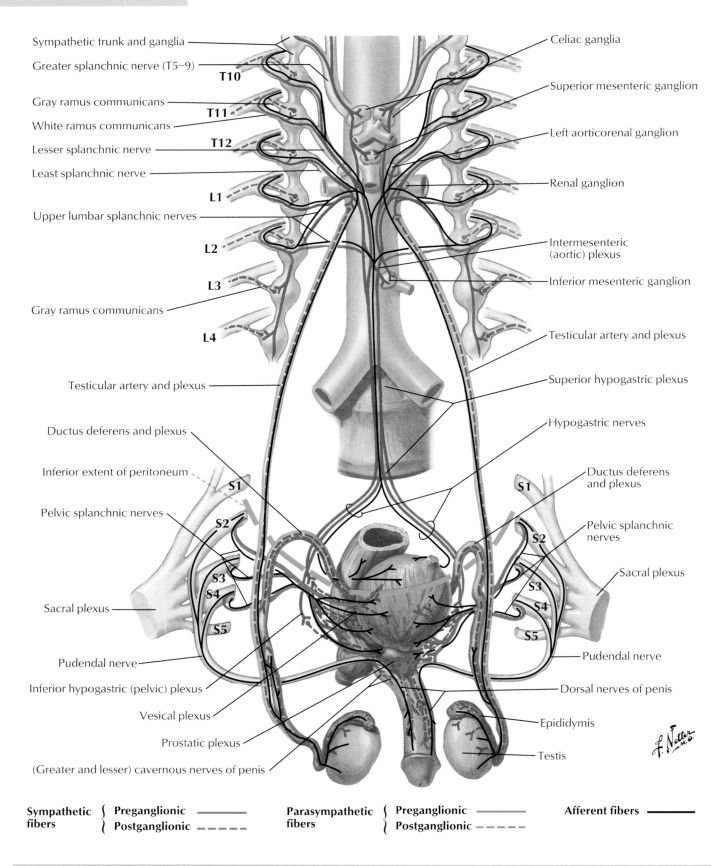

Sympathetic trunk and ganglia

Greater splanchnic nerve (T5–9)

T10

Gray ramus communicans

T11

White ramus communicans

Lesser splanchnic nerve

T12

Least splanchnic nerve

L1

Upper lumbar splanchnic nerves

L2

L3

Gray ramus communicans

L4

Testicular artery and plexus

Ductus deferens and plexus

Inferior extent of peritoneum

S1

Pelvic splanchnic nerves

S2

S3

S4

Sacral plexus

S5

Pudendal nerve

Inferior hypogastric (pelvic) plexus

Vesical plexus

Prostatic plexus

(Greater and lesser) cavernous nerves of penis

Celiac ganglia

Superior mesenteric ganglion

Left aorticorenal ganglion

Renal ganglion

Intermesenteric (aortic) plexus

Inferior mesenteric ganglion

Testicular artery and plexus

Superior hypogastric plexus

Hypogastric nerves

Ductus deferens and plexus

S1

Pelvic splanchnic nerves

S2

Sacral plexus

S3

S4

S5

Pudendal nerve

Dorsal nerves of penis

Epididymis

Testis

| Sympathetic fibers | Preganglionic ———— | Parasympathetic fibers | Preganglionic ———— | Afferent fibers ———— |
| | Postganglionic – – – – | | Postganglionic – – – – | |

Plate 396

Innervation

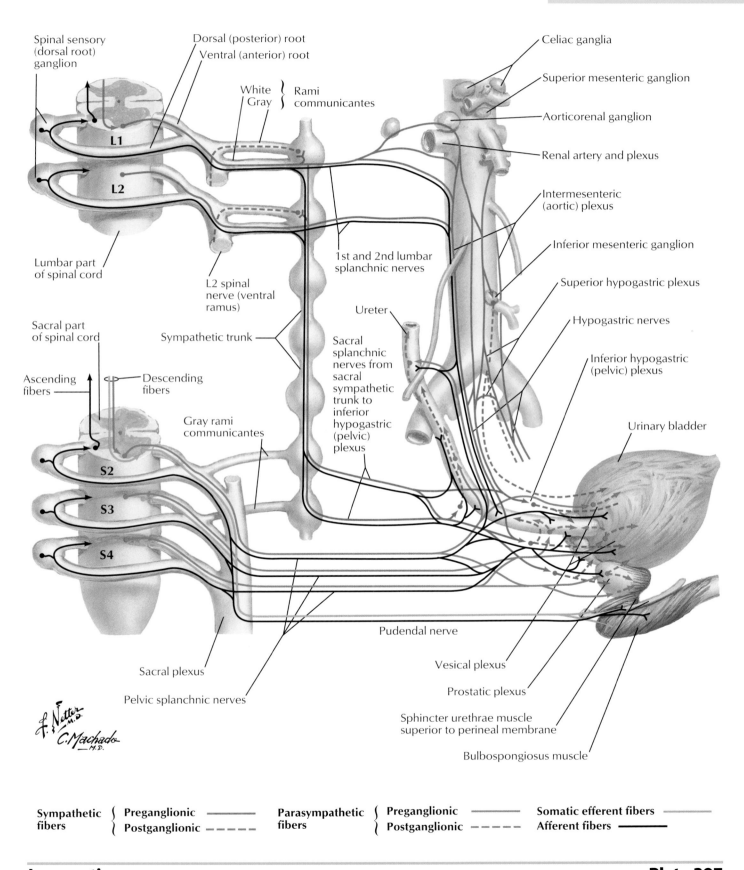

Spinal sensory (dorsal root) ganglion

Dorsal (posterior) root

Ventral (anterior) root

White
Gray } Rami communicantes

Celiac ganglia

Superior mesenteric ganglion

Aorticorenal ganglion

Renal artery and plexus

L1

L2

Lumbar part of spinal cord

L2 spinal nerve (ventral ramus)

Sympathetic trunk

1st and 2nd lumbar splanchnic nerves

Intermesenteric (aortic) plexus

Inferior mesenteric ganglion

Superior hypogastric plexus

Hypogastric nerves

Inferior hypogastric (pelvic) plexus

Sacral part of spinal cord

Ascending fibers

Descending fibers

Gray rami communicantes

Ureter

Sacral splanchnic nerves from sacral sympathetic trunk to inferior hypogastric (pelvic) plexus

Urinary bladder

S2

S3

S4

Pudendal nerve

Sacral plexus

Pelvic splanchnic nerves

Vesical plexus

Prostatic plexus

Sphincter urethrae muscle superior to perineal membrane

Bulbospongiosus muscle

Sympathetic fibers { **Preganglionic** ——— **Postganglionic** – – –

Parasympathetic fibers { **Preganglionic** ——— **Postganglionic** – – –

Somatic efferent fibers ———
Afferent fibers ———

Transverse Section: Pubic Crest, Femoral Heads, Coccyx

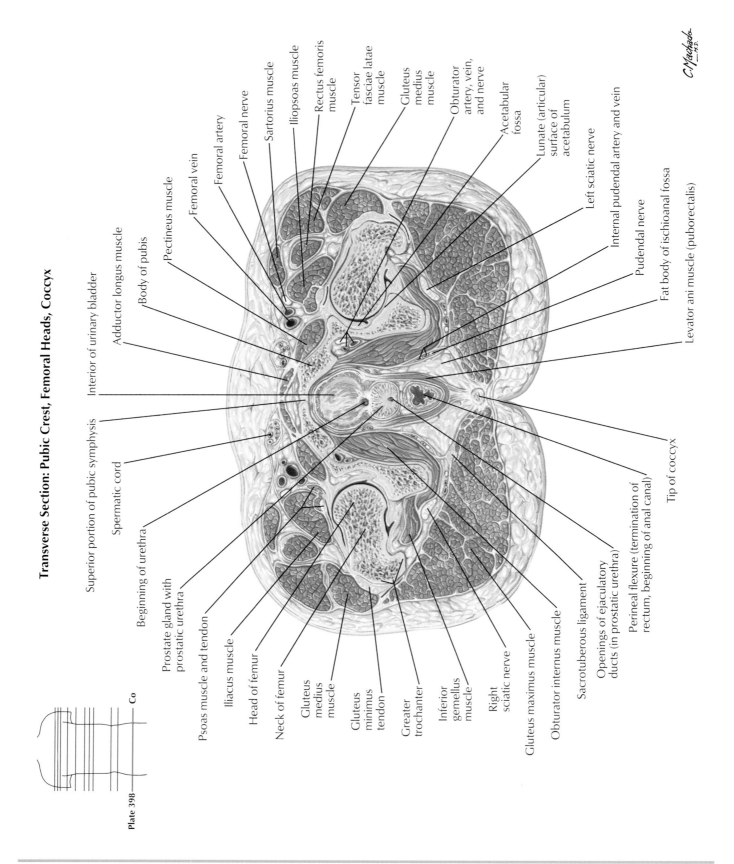

Femoral nerve

Sartorius muscle

Iliopsoas muscle

Rectus femoris muscle

Tensor fasciae latae muscle

Gluteus medius muscle

Obturator artery, vein, and nerve

Acetabular fossa

Lunate (articular) surface of acetabulum

Left sciatic nerve

Internal pudendal artery and vein

Pudendal nerve

Fat body of ischioanal fossa

Levator ani muscle (puborectalis)

Femoral artery

Femoral vein

Pectineus muscle

Body of pubis

Adductor longus muscle

Interior of urinary bladder

Superior portion of pubic symphysis

Spermatic cord

Beginning of urethra

Prostate gland with prostatic urethra

Psoas muscle and tendon

Iliacus muscle

Head of femur

Neck of femur

Gluteus medius muscle

Gluteus minimus tendon

Greater trochanter

Inferior gemellus muscle

Right sciatic nerve

Gluteus maximus muscle

Obturator internus muscle

Sacrotuberous ligament

Openings of ejaculatory ducts (in prostatic urethra)

Perineal flexure (termination of rectum, beginning of anal canal)

Tip of coccyx

Co

Plate 398

Plate 398 **Cross-sectional Anatomy**

Transverse Section: Vagina and Urethra

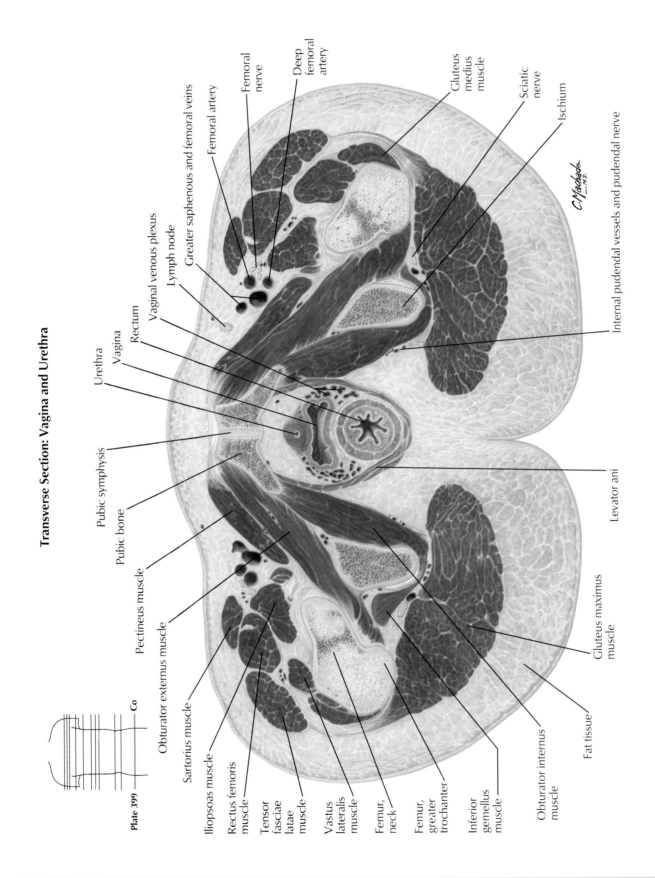

C.Machado

Plate 399

Co

Femoral nerve

Deep femoral artery

Greater saphenous and femoral veins

Femoral artery

Gluteus medius muscle

Sciatic nerve

Ischium

Internal pudendal vessels and pudendal nerve

Vaginal venous plexus

Lymph node

Vaginal venous plexus

Rectum

Vagina

Urethra

Pubic symphysis

Pubic bone

Pectineus muscle

Obturator externus muscle

Sartorius muscle

Iliopsoas muscle

Rectus femoris muscle

Tensor fasciae latae muscle

Vastus lateralis muscle

Femur, neck

Femur, greater trochanter

Inferior gemellus muscle

Obturator internus muscle

Fat tissue

Gluteus maximus muscle

Levator ani

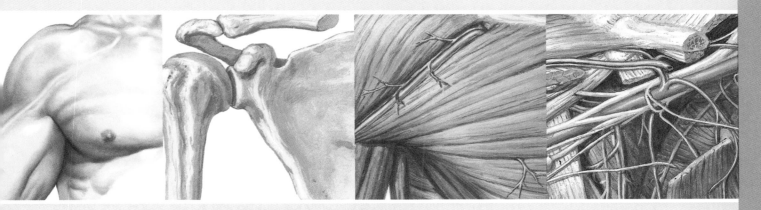

Section 6 **UPPER LIMB**

Topographic Anatomy
Plate 400

400 Upper Limb

Cutaneous Anatomy
Plates 401-405

401 Dermatomes of Upper Limb

402 Cutaneous Innervation of Upper Limb

403 Cutaneous Nerves and Superficial Veins of Shoulder and Arm

404 Cutaneous Nerves and Superficial Veins of Forearm

405 Lymph Vessels and Nodes of Upper Limb

Shoulder and Axilla
Plates 406-418

406 Clavicle and Sternoclavicular Joint

407 Humerus and Scapula: Anterior Views

408 Humerus and Scapula: Posterior View

409 Shoulder: Anteroposterior Radiograph

410 Shoulder (Glenohumeral Joint)

411 Muscles of Shoulder

412 Axilla: Posterior Wall and Cord

413 Muscles of Rotator Cuff

414 Scapulothoracic and Scapulohumeral Dissection

415 Axillary Artery and Anastomoses around Scapula

416 Pectoral, Clavipectoral, and Axillary Fasciae

417 Axilla (Dissection): Anterior View

418 Brachial Plexus: Schema

Arm
Plates 419-423

419 Muscles of Arm: Anterior Views

420 Muscles of Arm: Posterior Views

421 Brachial Artery in Situ

422 Brachial Artery and Anastomoses around Elbow

423 Arm: Serial Cross Sections

Elbow and Forearm
Plates 424-439

424 Bones of Elbow

425 Elbow: Radiographs

426 Ligaments of Elbow

427 Bones of Forearm

428 Individual Muscles of Forearm: Rotators of Radius

429 Individual Muscles of Forearm: Extensors of Wrist and Digits

430 Individual Muscles of Forearm: Flexors of Wrist

431 Individual Muscles of Forearm: Flexors of Digits

432 Muscles of Forearm (Superficial Layer): Posterior View

433 Muscles of Forearm (Deep Layer): Posterior View

434 Muscles of Forearm (Superficial Layer): Anterior View

435 Muscles of Forearm (Intermediate Layer): Anterior View

436 Muscles of Forearm (Deep Layer): Anterior View

437 Forearm: Serial Cross Sections

438 Attachments of Muscles of Forearm: Anterior View

439 Attachments of Muscles of Forearm: Posterior View

Wrist and Hand
Plates 440-459

440 Carpal Bones

441 Movements of Wrist

442 Ligaments of Wrist

443 Ligaments of Wrist (continued)

444 Bones of Wrist and Hand

445 Wrist and Hand: Radiographs

446 Metacarpophalangeal and Interphalangeal Ligaments

447 Wrist and Hand: Superficial Palmar Dissections

448 Wrist and Hand: Deeper Palmar Dissections

449 Flexor Tendons, Arteries, and Nerves at Wrist

450 Bursae, Spaces, and Tendon Sheaths of Hand

451 Lumbrical Muscles and Bursae, Spaces, and Sheaths: Schema

452 Flexor and Extensor Tendons in Fingers

453 Intrinsic Muscles of Hand

454 Arteries and Nerves of Hand: Palmar Views

455 Wrist and Hand: Superficial Radial Dissection

456 Wrist and Hand: Superficial Dorsal Dissection

457 Wrist and Hand: Deep Dorsal Dissection

458 Extensor Tendons at Wrist

459 Fingers

Neurovasculature
Plates 460-467

460 Cutaneous Innervation of Wrist and Hand

461 Arteries and Nerves of Upper Limb

462 Musculocutaneous Nerve

463 Median Nerve

464 Ulnar Nerve

465 Radial Nerve in Arm and Nerves of Posterior Shoulder

466 Radial Nerve in Forearm

467 Nerves of Upper Limb

Regional Scans
Plate 468

468 Shoulder Arthrogram, MRI, and CT

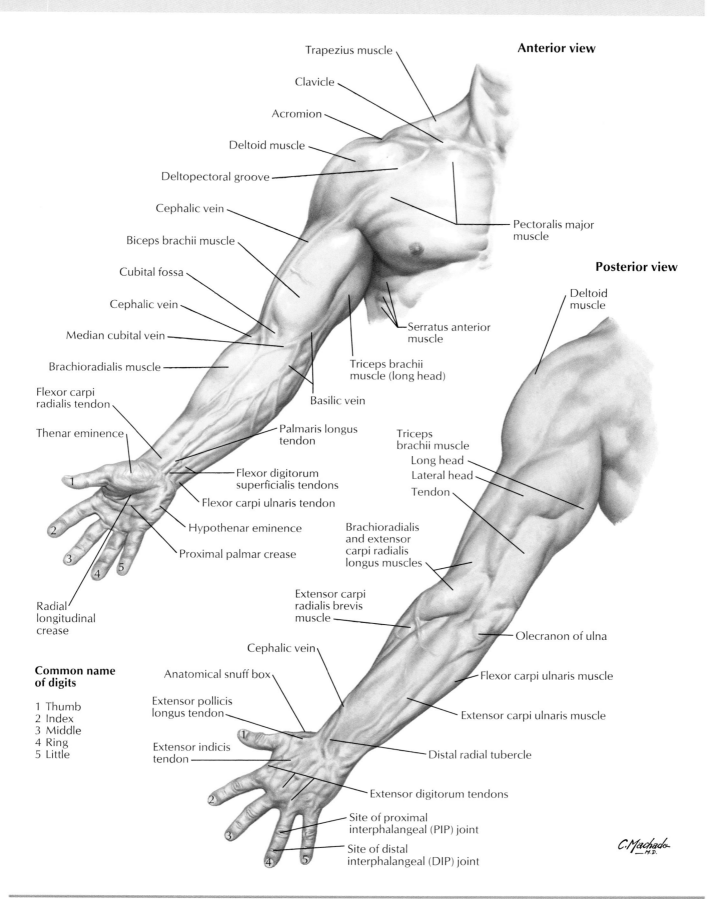

Anterior view

Trapezius muscle

Clavicle

Acromion

Deltoid muscle

Deltopectoral groove

Cephalic vein

Biceps brachii muscle

Cubital fossa

Cephalic vein

Median cubital vein

Brachioradialis muscle

Flexor carpi
radialis tendon

Thenar eminence

Palmaris longus
tendon

Flexor digitorum
superficialis tendons

Flexor carpi ulnaris tendon

Hypothenar eminence

Proximal palmar crease

Pectoralis major
muscle

Serratus anterior
muscle

Triceps brachii
muscle (long head)

Basilic vein

Posterior view

Deltoid
muscle

Triceps
brachii muscle

Long head

Lateral head

Tendon

Brachioradialis
and extensor
carpi radialis
longus muscles

Extensor carpi
radialis brevis
muscle

Cephalic vein

Anatomical snuff box

Extensor pollicis
longus tendon

Extensor indicis
tendon

Olecranon of ulna

Flexor carpi ulnaris muscle

Extensor carpi ulnaris muscle

Distal radial tubercle

Extensor digitorum tendons

Site of proximal
interphalangeal (PIP) joint

Site of distal
interphalangeal (DIP) joint

Radial
longitudinal
crease

**Common name
of digits**

1 Thumb
2 Index
3 Middle
4 Ring
5 Little

C. Machado
—M.D.

Dermatomes of Upper Limb

Note: Schematic demarcation of dermatomes (according to Keegan and Garrett) shown as distinct segments. There is actually considerable overlap between adjacent dermatomes. An alternative dermatome map is provided online.

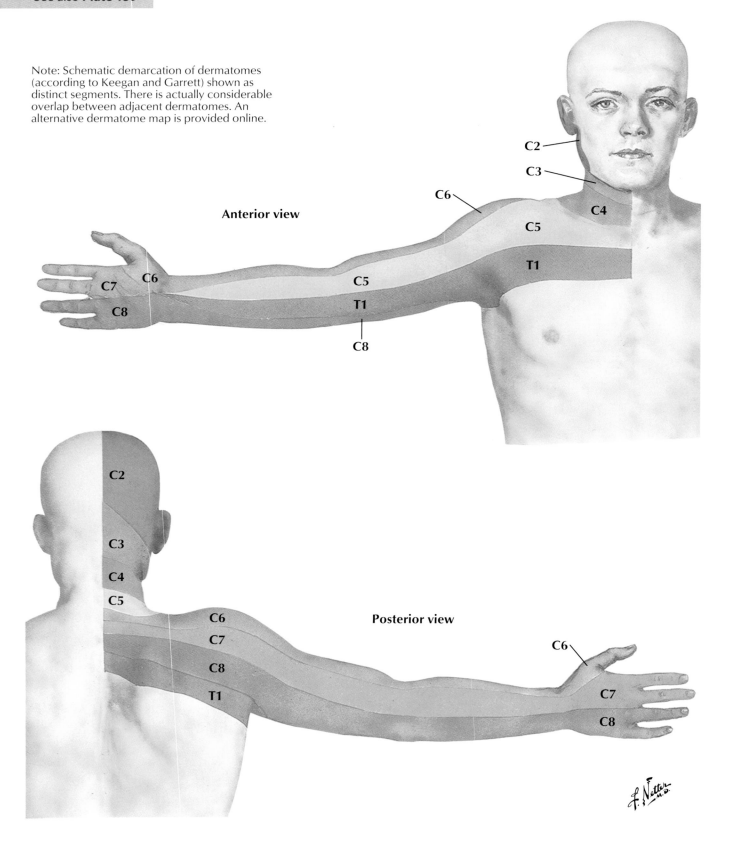

Anterior view

Posterior view

Plate 401

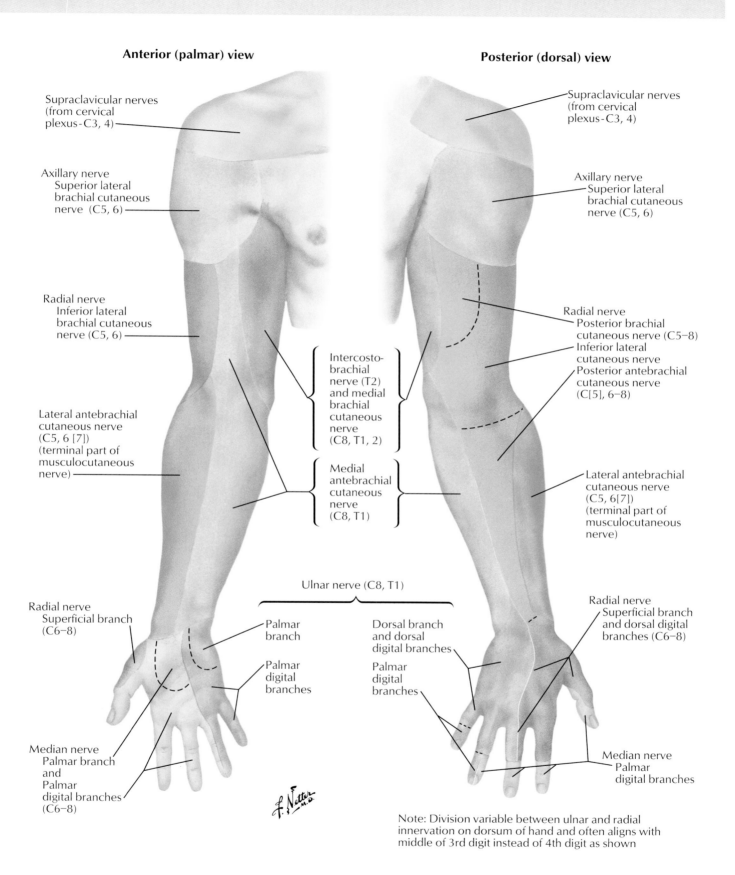

Anterior (palmar) view

Posterior (dorsal) view

Supraclavicular nerves (from cervical plexus - C3, 4)

Axillary nerve
Superior lateral brachial cutaneous nerve (C5, 6)

Radial nerve
Inferior lateral brachial cutaneous nerve (C5, 6)

Lateral antebrachial cutaneous nerve (C5, 6 [7]) (terminal part of musculocutaneous nerve)

Intercosto-brachial nerve (T2) and medial brachial cutaneous nerve (C8, T1, 2)

Medial antebrachial cutaneous nerve (C8, T1)

Supraclavicular nerves (from cervical plexus - C3, 4)

Axillary nerve
Superior lateral brachial cutaneous nerve (C5, 6)

Radial nerve
Posterior brachial cutaneous nerve (C5-8)
Inferior lateral cutaneous nerve
Posterior antebrachial cutaneous nerve (C[5], 6-8)

Lateral antebrachial cutaneous nerve (C5, 6[7]) (terminal part of musculocutaneous nerve)

Ulnar nerve (C8, T1)

Radial nerve
Superficial branch (C6-8)

Palmar branch

Palmar digital branches

Dorsal branch and dorsal digital branches

Palmar digital branches

Radial nerve
Superficial branch and dorsal digital branches (C6-8)

Median nerve
Palmar branch and Palmar digital branches (C6-8)

Median nerve
Palmar digital branches

Note: Division variable between ulnar and radial innervation on dorsum of hand and often aligns with middle of 3rd digit instead of 4th digit as shown

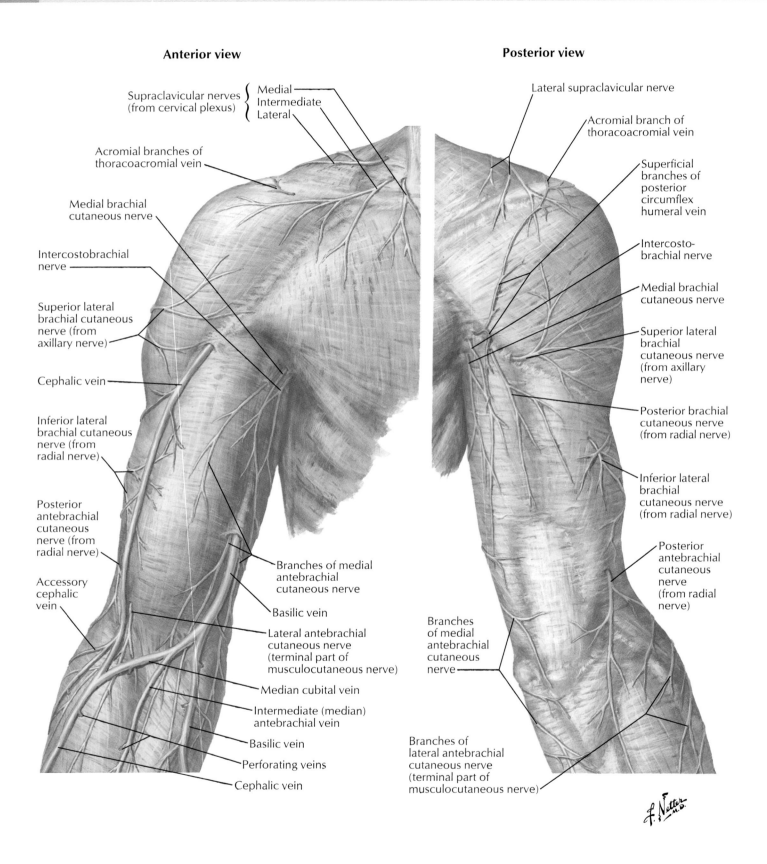

Anterior view

Posterior view

Supraclavicular nerves (from cervical plexus) { Medial / Intermediate / Lateral }

Acromial branches of thoracoacromial vein

Medial brachial cutaneous nerve

Intercostobrachial nerve

Superior lateral brachial cutaneous nerve (from axillary nerve)

Cephalic vein

Inferior lateral brachial cutaneous nerve (from radial nerve)

Posterior antebrachial cutaneous nerve (from radial nerve)

Accessory cephalic vein

Branches of medial antebrachial cutaneous nerve

Basilic vein

Lateral antebrachial cutaneous nerve (terminal part of musculocutaneous nerve)

Median cubital vein

Intermediate (median) antebrachial vein

Basilic vein

Perforating veins

Cephalic vein

Lateral supraclavicular nerve

Acromial branch of thoracoacromial vein

Superficial branches of posterior circumflex humeral vein

Intercosto-brachial nerve

Medial brachial cutaneous nerve

Superior lateral brachial cutaneous nerve (from axillary nerve)

Posterior brachial cutaneous nerve (from radial nerve)

Inferior lateral brachial cutaneous nerve (from radial nerve)

Posterior antebrachial cutaneous nerve (from radial nerve)

Branches of medial antebrachial cutaneous nerve

Branches of lateral antebrachial cutaneous nerve (terminal part of musculocutaneous nerve)

Plate 403   **Cutaneous Anatomy**

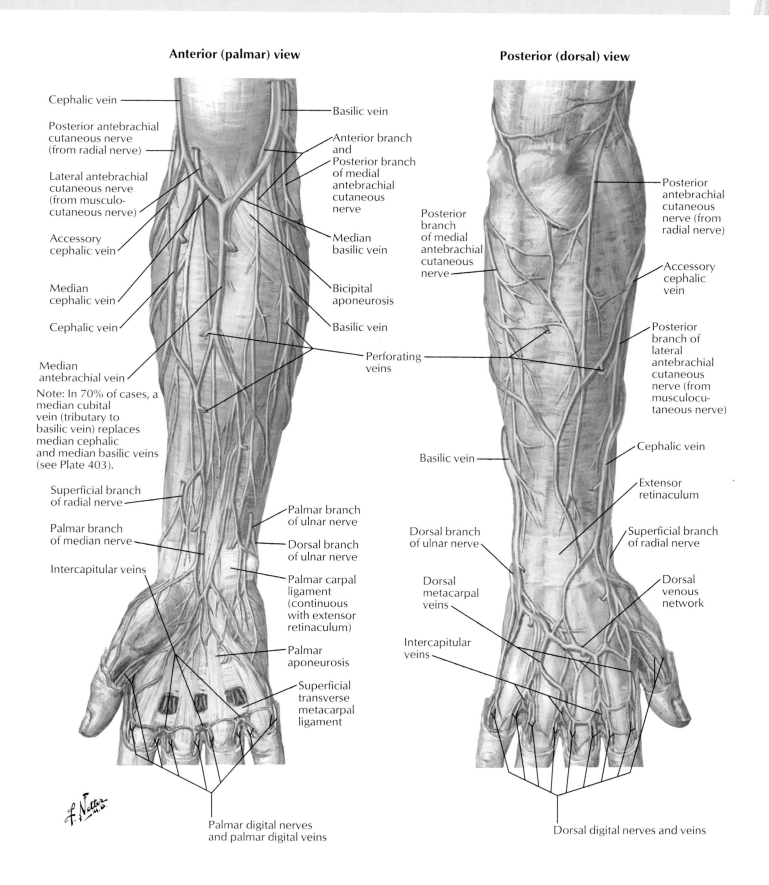

Anterior (palmar) view

Cephalic vein

Posterior antebrachial cutaneous nerve (from radial nerve)

Lateral antebrachial cutaneous nerve (from musculo-cutaneous nerve)

Accessory cephalic vein

Median cephalic vein

Cephalic vein

Median antebrachial vein

Note: In 70% of cases, a median cubital vein (tributary to basilic vein) replaces median cephalic and median basilic veins (see Plate 403).

Superficial branch of radial nerve

Palmar branch of median nerve

Intercapitular veins

Basilic vein

Anterior branch and Posterior branch of medial antebrachial cutaneous nerve

Median basilic vein

Bicipital aponeurosis

Basilic vein

Perforating veins

Palmar branch of ulnar nerve

Dorsal branch of ulnar nerve

Palmar carpal ligament (continuous with extensor retinaculum)

Palmar aponeurosis

Superficial transverse metacarpal ligament

Palmar digital nerves and palmar digital veins

Posterior (dorsal) view

Posterior branch of medial antebrachial cutaneous nerve

Posterior antebrachial cutaneous nerve (from radial nerve)

Accessory cephalic vein

Posterior branch of lateral antebrachial cutaneous nerve (from musculocutaneous nerve)

Cephalic vein

Extensor retinaculum

Superficial branch of radial nerve

Dorsal venous network

Basilic vein

Dorsal branch of ulnar nerve

Dorsal metacarpal veins

Intercapitular veins

Dorsal digital nerves and veins

Cutaneous Anatomy

Plate 404

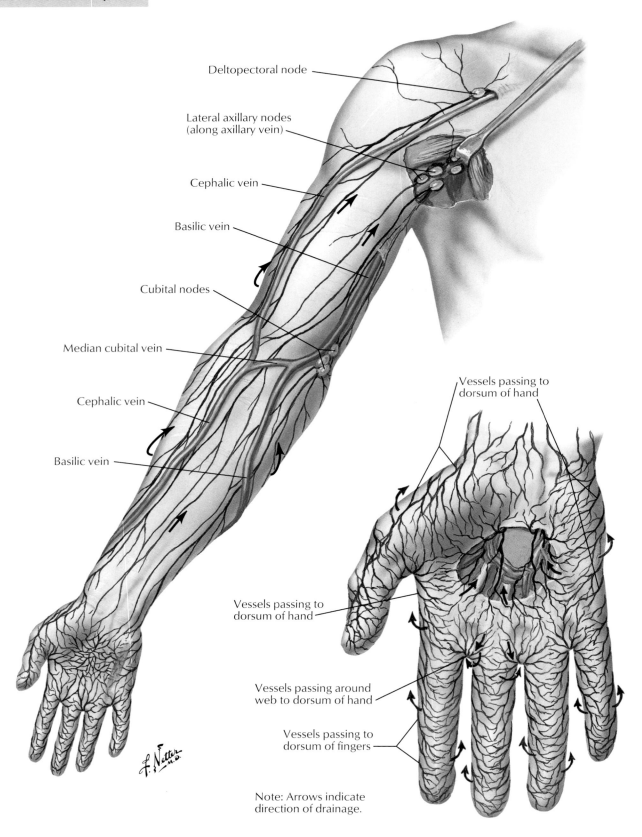

Deltopectoral node

Lateral axillary nodes
(along axillary vein)

Cephalic vein

Basilic vein

Cubital nodes

Median cubital vein

Cephalic vein

Basilic vein

Vessels passing to
dorsum of hand

Vessels passing to
dorsum of hand

Vessels passing around
web to dorsum of hand

Vessels passing to
dorsum of fingers

Note: Arrows indicate
direction of drainage.

Plate 405   **Cutaneous Anatomy**

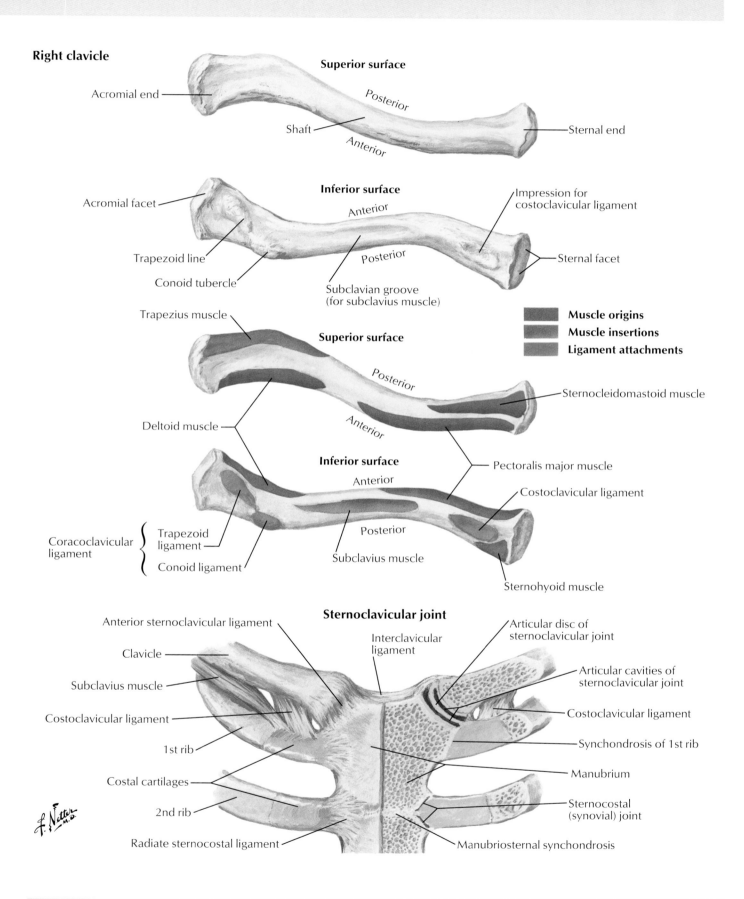

Right clavicle

Superior surface

Acromial end

Posterior

Shaft — Sternal end

Anterior

Inferior surface

Acromial facet

Impression for costoclavicular ligament

Anterior

Trapezoid line

Posterior

Conoid tubercle

Sternal facet

Subclavian groove (for subclavius muscle)

Trapezius muscle

Muscle origins
Muscle insertions
Ligament attachments

Superior surface

Posterior

Sternocleidomastoid muscle

Deltoid muscle

Anterior

Inferior surface

Anterior

Pectoralis major muscle

Costoclavicular ligament

Coracoclavicular ligament { Trapezoid ligament

Posterior

Conoid ligament

Subclavius muscle

Sternohyoid muscle

Sternoclavicular joint

Anterior sternoclavicular ligament

Interclavicular ligament

Articular disc of sternoclavicular joint

Clavicle

Articular cavities of sternoclavicular joint

Subclavius muscle

Costoclavicular ligament

Costoclavicular ligament

1st rib

Synchondrosis of 1st rib

Costal cartilages

Manubrium

2nd rib

Sternocostal (synovial) joint

Radiate sternocostal ligament

Manubriosternal synchondrosis

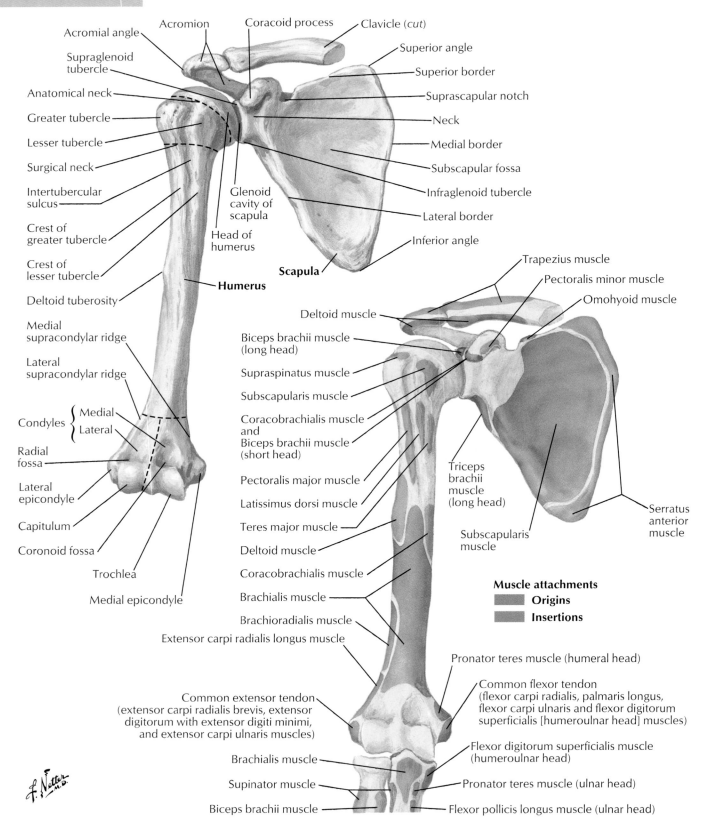

Acromial angle
Acromion
Coracoid process
Clavicle (*cut*)
Supraglenoid tubercle
Anatomical neck
Greater tubercle
Lesser tubercle
Surgical neck
Intertubercular sulcus
Crest of greater tubercle
Crest of lesser tubercle
Deltoid tuberosity
Medial supracondylar ridge
Lateral supracondylar ridge
Condyles { Medial / Lateral }
Radial fossa
Lateral epicondyle
Capitulum
Coronoid fossa
Trochlea
Medial epicondyle

Glenoid cavity of scapula
Head of humerus
Humerus

Superior angle
Superior border
Suprascapular notch
Neck
Medial border
Subscapular fossa
Infraglenoid tubercle
Lateral border
Inferior angle
Scapula

Deltoid muscle
Biceps brachii muscle (long head)
Supraspinatus muscle
Subscapularis muscle
Coracobrachialis muscle and Biceps brachii muscle (short head)
Pectoralis major muscle
Latissimus dorsi muscle
Teres major muscle
Deltoid muscle
Coracobrachialis muscle
Brachialis muscle
Brachioradialis muscle
Extensor carpi radialis longus muscle

Common extensor tendon (extensor carpi radialis brevis, extensor digitorum with extensor digiti minimi, and extensor carpi ulnaris muscles)
Brachialis muscle
Supinator muscle
Biceps brachii muscle

Trapezius muscle
Pectoralis minor muscle
Omohyoid muscle

Triceps brachii muscle (long head)
Subscapularis muscle
Serratus anterior muscle

Muscle attachments
█ **Origins**
█ **Insertions**

Pronator teres muscle (humeral head)
Common flexor tendon (flexor carpi radialis, palmaris longus, flexor carpi ulnaris and flexor digitorum superficialis [humeroulnar head] muscles)
Flexor digitorum superficialis muscle (humeroulnar head)
Pronator teres muscle (ulnar head)
Flexor pollicis longus muscle (ulnar head)

Plate 407   **Shoulder and Axilla**

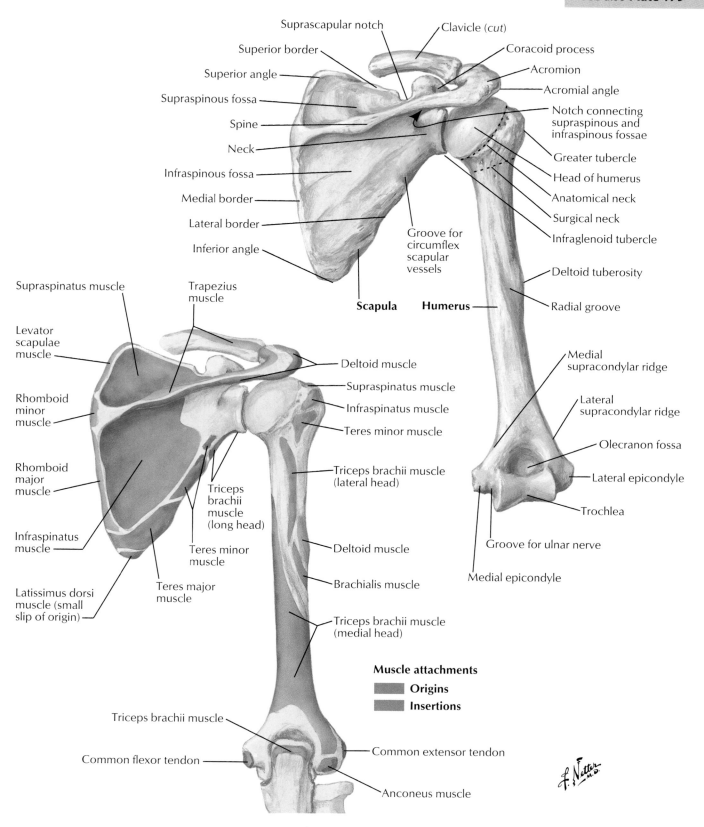

Suprascapular notch

Clavicle (*cut*)

Superior border

Coracoid process

Superior angle

Acromion

Supraspinous fossa

Acromial angle

Spine

Notch connecting supraspinous and infraspinous fossae

Neck

Greater tubercle

Infraspinous fossa

Head of humerus

Medial border

Anatomical neck

Lateral border

Surgical neck

Inferior angle

Infraglenoid tubercle

Groove for circumflex scapular vessels

Deltoid tuberosity

Scapula

Humerus

Radial groove

Supraspinatus muscle

Trapezius muscle

Levator scapulae muscle

Deltoid muscle

Supraspinatus muscle

Medial supracondylar ridge

Rhomboid minor muscle

Infraspinatus muscle

Lateral supracondylar ridge

Teres minor muscle

Olecranon fossa

Rhomboid major muscle

Triceps brachii muscle (lateral head)

Lateral epicondyle

Triceps brachii muscle (long head)

Trochlea

Infraspinatus muscle

Teres minor muscle

Deltoid muscle

Groove for ulnar nerve

Latissimus dorsi muscle (small slip of origin)

Teres major muscle

Brachialis muscle

Medial epicondyle

Triceps brachii muscle (medial head)

Muscle attachments

■ **Origins**

■ **Insertions**

Triceps brachii muscle

Common flexor tendon

Common extensor tendon

Anconeus muscle

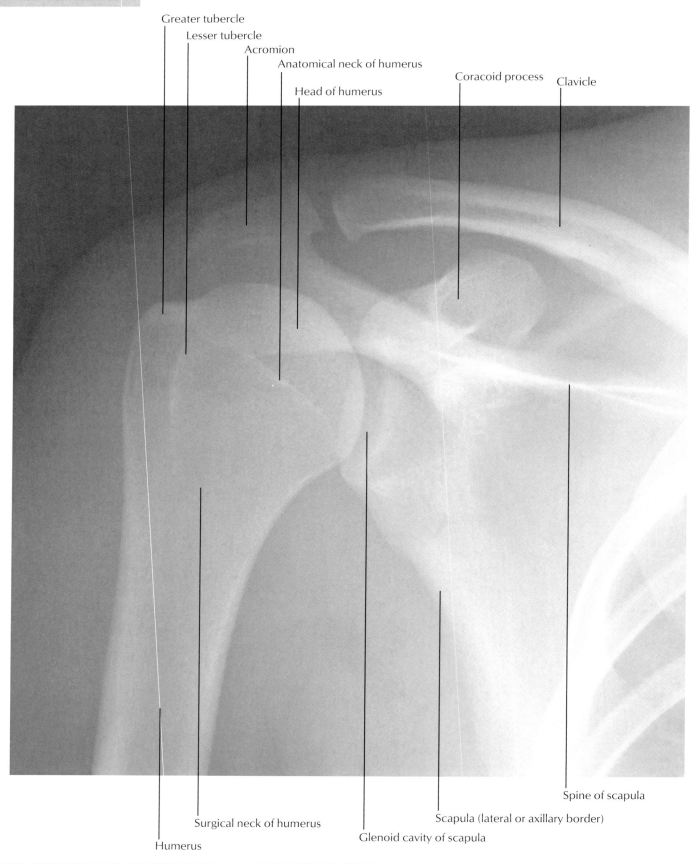

Greater tubercle

Lesser tubercle

Acromion

Anatomical neck of humerus

Head of humerus

Coracoid process

Clavicle

Humerus

Surgical neck of humerus

Glenoid cavity of scapula

Scapula (lateral or axillary border)

Spine of scapula

Plate 409

Shoulder and Axilla

Anterior view

Acromioclavicular joint capsule
(incorporating acromioclavicular ligament)

Acromion

Coracoacromial ligament

Supraspinatus tendon (*cut*)

Coracohumeral ligament

Greater tubercle and
Lesser tubercle
of humerus

Transverse humeral ligament

Intertubercular tendon sheath
(communicates with synovial cavity)

Subscapularis tendon (*cut*)

Biceps brachii tendon (long head)

Clavicle

Trapezoid
ligament

Conoid
ligament

} Coraco-
clavicular
ligament

Transverse scapular
ligament and
suprascapular foramen

Coracoid process

Communication of
subtendinous
bursa of subscapularis

Broken line indicates
position of subtendinous
bursa of subscapularis

Capsular
ligaments

**Anterior
view**

Deltoid
muscle
(*reflected*)

Capsular
ligament

Supraspinatus muscle

Subdeltoid bursa fused with
subacromial bursa

Subscapularis muscle

Acromion

Supraspinatus tendon
(fused to capsule)

Subdeltoid bursa

Infraspinatus tendon
(fused to capsule)

Glenoid cavity
(articular cartilage)

Teres minor tendon
(fused to capsule)

Synovial membrane (*cut edge*)

Opening of subtendinous
bursa of subscapularis

Coracoacromial ligament

Coracoid process

Coracohumeral ligament

Biceps brachii tendon
(long head)

Superior glenohumeral
ligament

Subscapularis tendon
(fused to capsule)

Middle glenohumeral
ligament

Inferior glenohumeral
ligament

Joint opened: lateral view

Subdeltoid bursa

Supraspinatus tendon

Capsular ligament

Synovial membrane

Acromion

Acromioclavicular
joint

Deltoid
muscle

Glenoid
labrum

Glenoid
cavity of
scapula

Axillary recess

Coronal section through joint

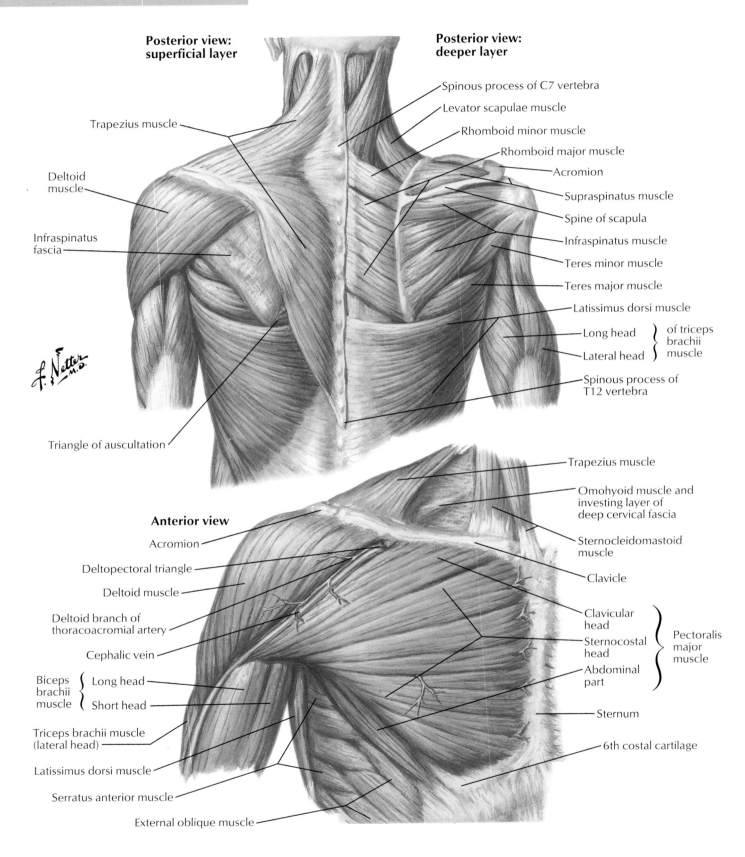

Posterior view: superficial layer

Trapezius muscle

Deltoid muscle

Infraspinatus fascia

Triangle of auscultation

Posterior view: deeper layer

Spinous process of C7 vertebra

Levator scapulae muscle

Rhomboid minor muscle

Rhomboid major muscle

Acromion

Supraspinatus muscle

Spine of scapula

Infraspinatus muscle

Teres minor muscle

Teres major muscle

Latissimus dorsi muscle

Long head } of triceps brachii
Lateral head } muscle

Spinous process of T12 vertebra

Trapezius muscle

Omohyoid muscle and investing layer of deep cervical fascia

Sternocleidomastoid muscle

Clavicle

Anterior view

Acromion

Deltopectoral triangle

Deltoid muscle

Deltoid branch of thoracoacromial artery

Cephalic vein

Biceps brachii muscle { Long head

Short head

Triceps brachii muscle (lateral head)

Latissimus dorsi muscle

Serratus anterior muscle

External oblique muscle

Clavicular head

Sternocostal head } Pectoralis major muscle

Abdominal part

Sternum

6th costal cartilage

Plate 411

Shoulder and Axilla

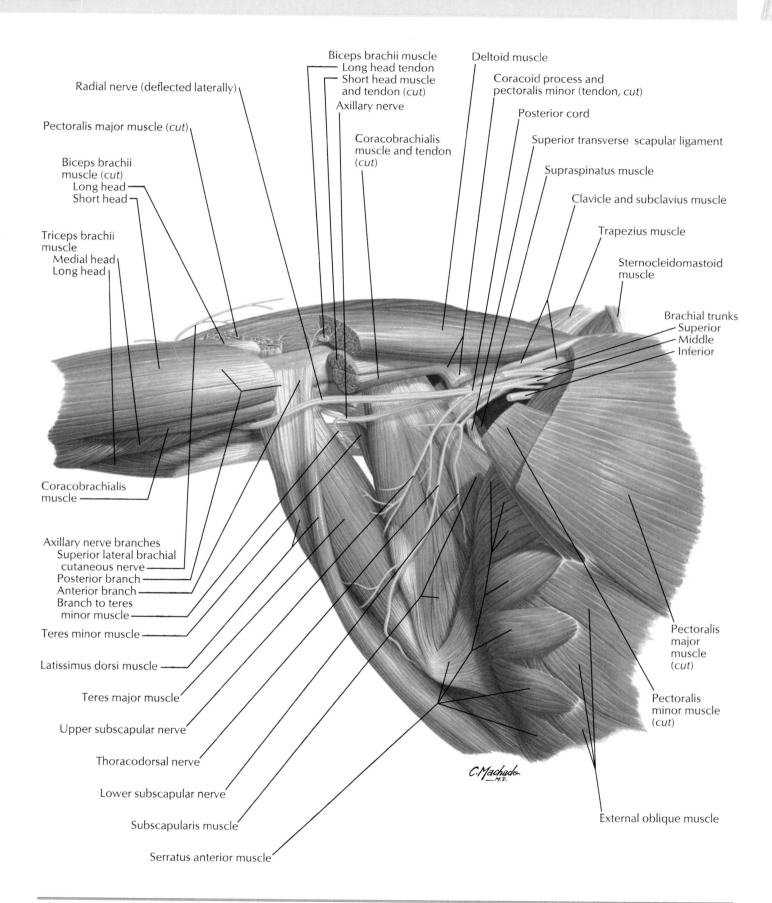

Biceps brachii muscle
— Long head tendon
— Short head muscle and tendon (*cut*)
Axillary nerve

Deltoid muscle

Coracoid process and pectoralis minor (tendon, *cut*)

Posterior cord

Radial nerve (deflected laterally)

Coracobrachialis muscle and tendon (*cut*)

Superior transverse scapular ligament

Pectoralis major muscle (*cut*)

Supraspinatus muscle

Biceps brachii muscle (*cut*)
Long head
Short head

Clavicle and subclavius muscle

Trapezius muscle

Triceps brachii muscle
Medial head
Long head

Sternocleidomastoid muscle

Brachial trunks
Superior
Middle
Inferior

Coracobrachialis muscle

Axillary nerve branches
Superior lateral brachial cutaneous nerve
Posterior branch
Anterior branch
Branch to teres minor muscle

Teres minor muscle

Latissimus dorsi muscle

Teres major muscle

Upper subscapular nerve

Thoracodorsal nerve

Lower subscapular nerve

Subscapularis muscle

Serratus anterior muscle

Pectoralis major muscle (*cut*)

Pectoralis minor muscle (*cut*)

C. Machado
_M.D.

External oblique muscle

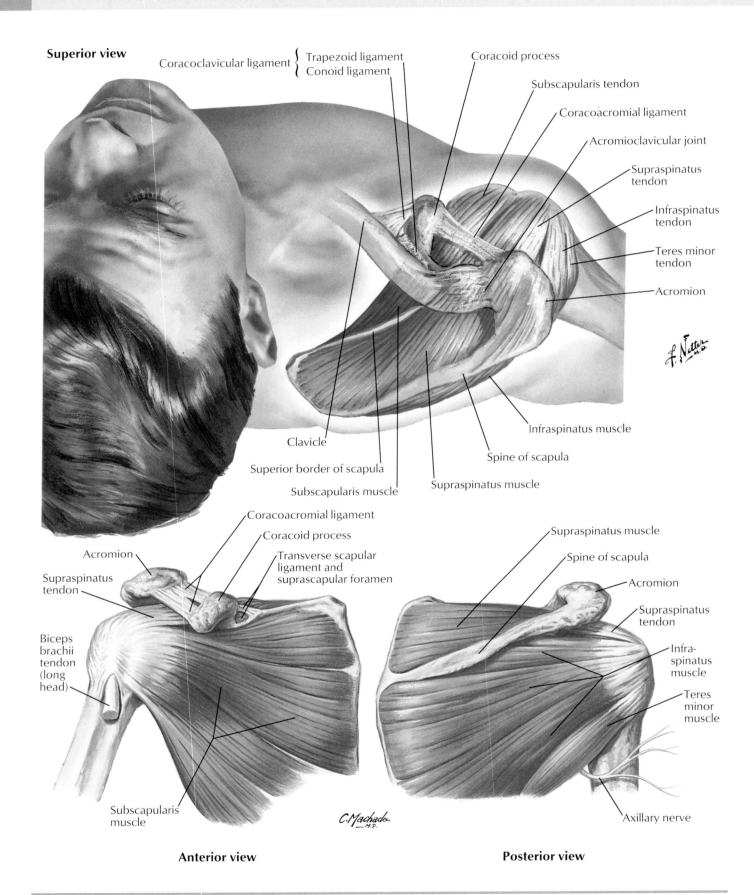

Superior view

Coracoclavicular ligament { Trapezoid ligament
Conoid ligament

Coracoid process

Subscapularis tendon

Coracoacromial ligament

Acromioclavicular joint

Supraspinatus tendon

Infraspinatus tendon

Teres minor tendon

Acromion

Infraspinatus muscle

Spine of scapula

Supraspinatus muscle

Clavicle

Superior border of scapula

Subscapularis muscle

Coracoacromial ligament

Coracoid process

Acromion

Supraspinatus tendon

Transverse scapular ligament and suprascapular foramen

Biceps brachii tendon (long head)

Subscapularis muscle

Supraspinatus muscle

Spine of scapula

Acromion

Supraspinatus tendon

Infra-spinatus muscle

Teres minor muscle

Axillary nerve

Anterior view

Posterior view

Plate 413

Shoulder and Axilla

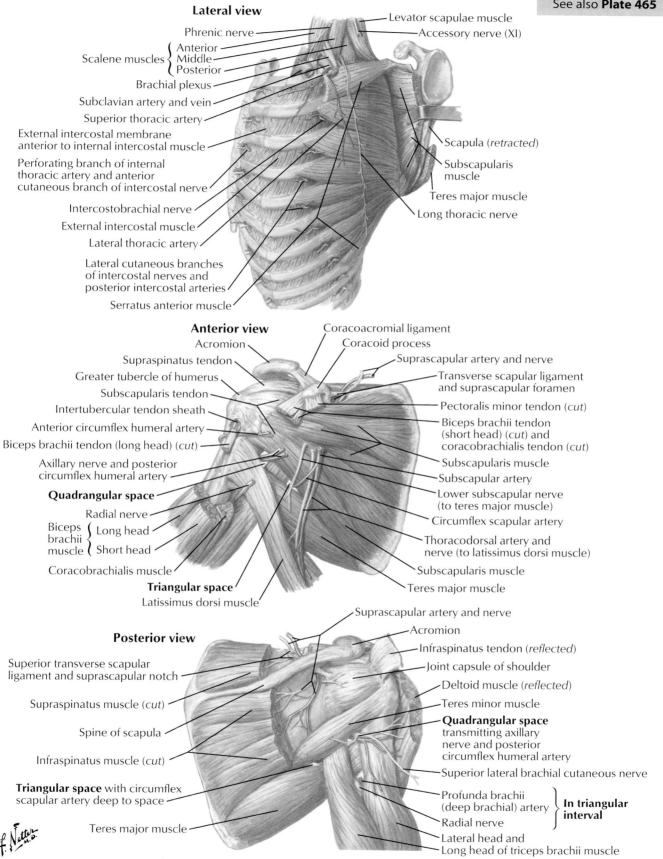

Lateral view

- Levator scapulae muscle
- Accessory nerve (XI)
- Phrenic nerve
- Scalene muscles { Anterior, Middle, Posterior }
- Brachial plexus
- Subclavian artery and vein
- Superior thoracic artery
- External intercostal membrane anterior to internal intercostal muscle
- Perforating branch of internal thoracic artery and anterior cutaneous branch of intercostal nerve
- Intercostobrachial nerve
- External intercostal muscle
- Lateral thoracic artery
- Lateral cutaneous branches of intercostal nerves and posterior intercostal arteries
- Serratus anterior muscle
- Scapula (*retracted*)
- Subscapularis muscle
- Teres major muscle
- Long thoracic nerve

Anterior view

- Coracoacromial ligament
- Coracoid process
- Acromion
- Supraspinatus tendon
- Greater tubercle of humerus
- Subscapularis tendon
- Intertubercular tendon sheath
- Anterior circumflex humeral artery
- Biceps brachii tendon (long head) (*cut*)
- Axillary nerve and posterior circumflex humeral artery
- **Quadrangular space**
- Radial nerve
- Biceps brachii muscle { Long head, Short head }
- Coracobrachialis muscle
- **Triangular space**
- Latissimus dorsi muscle
- Suprascapular artery and nerve
- Transverse scapular ligament and suprascapular foramen
- Pectoralis minor tendon (*cut*)
- Biceps brachii tendon (short head) (*cut*) and coracobrachialis tendon (*cut*)
- Subscapularis muscle
- Subscapular artery
- Lower subscapular nerve (to teres major muscle)
- Circumflex scapular artery
- Thoracodorsal artery and nerve (to latissimus dorsi muscle)
- Subscapularis muscle
- Teres major muscle

Posterior view

- Suprascapular artery and nerve
- Acromion
- Superior transverse scapular ligament and suprascapular notch
- Supraspinatus muscle (*cut*)
- Spine of scapula
- Infraspinatus muscle (*cut*)
- **Triangular space** with circumflex scapular artery deep to space
- Teres major muscle
- Infraspinatus tendon (*reflected*)
- Joint capsule of shoulder
- Deltoid muscle (*reflected*)
- Teres minor muscle
- **Quadrangular space** transmitting axillary nerve and posterior circumflex humeral artery
- Superior lateral brachial cutaneous nerve
- Profunda brachii (deep brachial) artery } **In triangular interval**
- Radial nerve
- Lateral head and Long head of triceps brachii muscle

F. Netter, M.D.

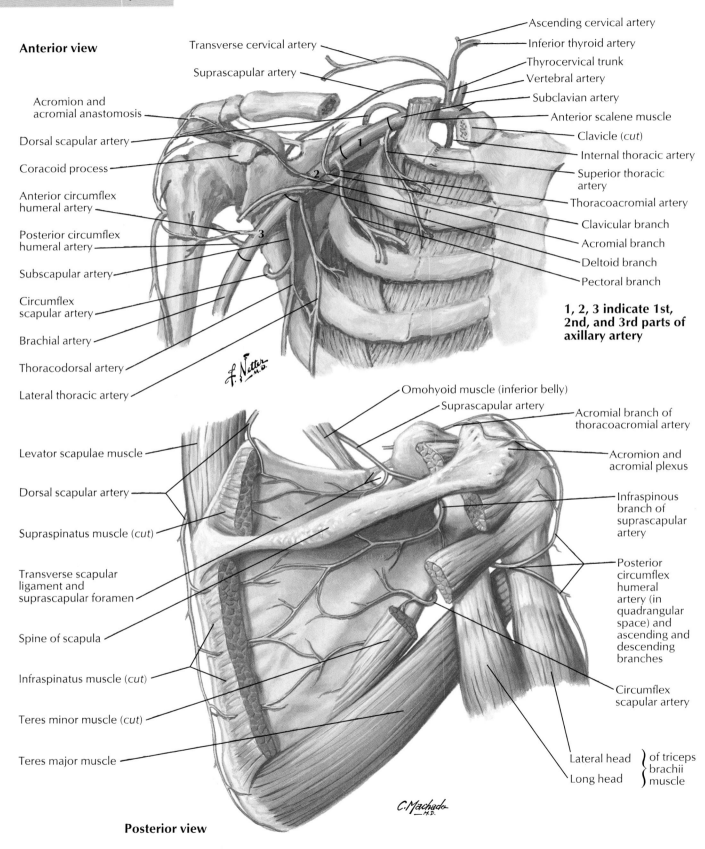

Anterior view

Transverse cervical artery

Suprascapular artery

Acromion and acromial anastomosis

Dorsal scapular artery

Coracoid process

Anterior circumflex humeral artery

Posterior circumflex humeral artery

Subscapular artery

Circumflex scapular artery

Brachial artery

Thoracodorsal artery

Lateral thoracic artery

Ascending cervical artery

Inferior thyroid artery

Thyrocervical trunk

Vertebral artery

Subclavian artery

Anterior scalene muscle

Clavicle (*cut*)

Internal thoracic artery

Superior thoracic artery

Thoracoacromial artery

Clavicular branch

Acromial branch

Deltoid branch

Pectoral branch

1, 2, 3 indicate 1st, 2nd, and 3rd parts of axillary artery

Omohyoid muscle (inferior belly)

Suprascapular artery

Levator scapulae muscle

Dorsal scapular artery

Suprascapular muscle (*cut*)

Transverse scapular ligament and suprascapular foramen

Spine of scapula

Infraspinatus muscle (*cut*)

Teres minor muscle (*cut*)

Teres major muscle

Acromial branch of thoracoacromial artery

Acromion and acromial plexus

Infraspinous branch of suprascapular artery

Posterior circumflex humeral artery (in quadrangular space) and ascending and descending branches

Circumflex scapular artery

Lateral head } of triceps brachii muscle
Long head }

Posterior view

Plate 415

Shoulder and Axilla

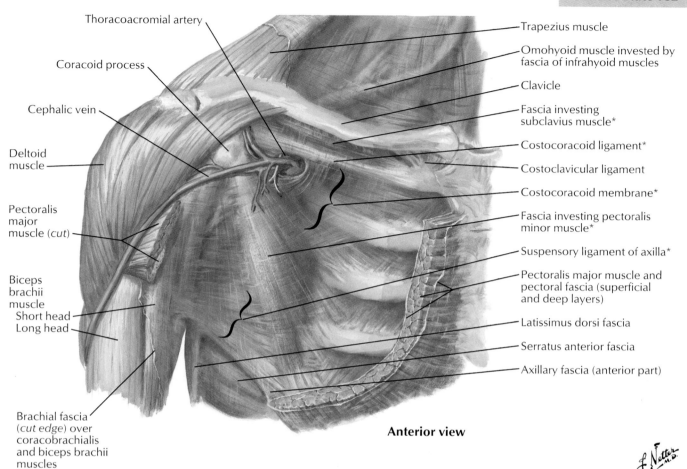

Thoracoacromial artery

Coracoid process

Cephalic vein

Deltoid muscle

Pectoralis major muscle (*cut*)

Biceps brachii muscle
Short head
Long head

Brachial fascia (*cut edge*) over coracobrachialis and biceps brachii muscles

Trapezius muscle

Omohyoid muscle invested by fascia of infrahyoid muscles

Clavicle

Fascia investing subclavius muscle*

Costocoracoid ligament*

Costoclavicular ligament

Costocoracoid membrane*

Fascia investing pectoralis minor muscle*

Suspensory ligament of axilla*

Pectoralis major muscle and pectoral fascia (superficial and deep layers)

Latissimus dorsi fascia

Serratus anterior fascia

Axillary fascia (anterior part)

Anterior view

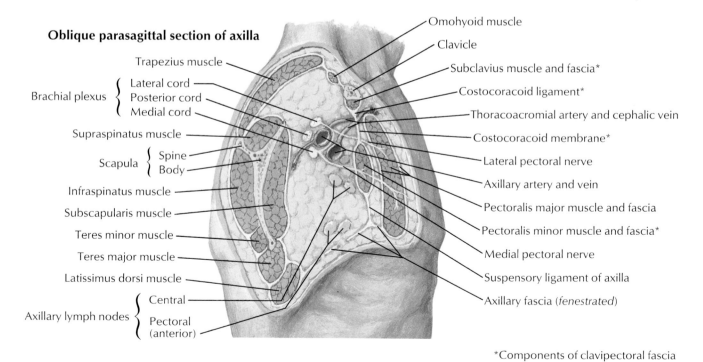

Oblique parasagittal section of axilla

Trapezius muscle

Brachial plexus
{ Lateral cord
Posterior cord
Medial cord

Supraspinatus muscle

Scapula { Spine
Body

Infraspinatus muscle

Subscapularis muscle

Teres minor muscle

Teres major muscle

Latissimus dorsi muscle

Axillary lymph nodes { Central
Pectoral (anterior)

Omohyoid muscle

Clavicle

Subclavius muscle and fascia*

Costocoracoid ligament*

Thoracoacromial artery and cephalic vein

Costocoracoid membrane*

Lateral pectoral nerve

Axillary artery and vein

Pectoralis major muscle and fascia

Pectoralis minor muscle and fascia*

Medial pectoral nerve

Suspensory ligament of axilla

Axillary fascia (*fenestrated*)

*Components of clavipectoral fascia

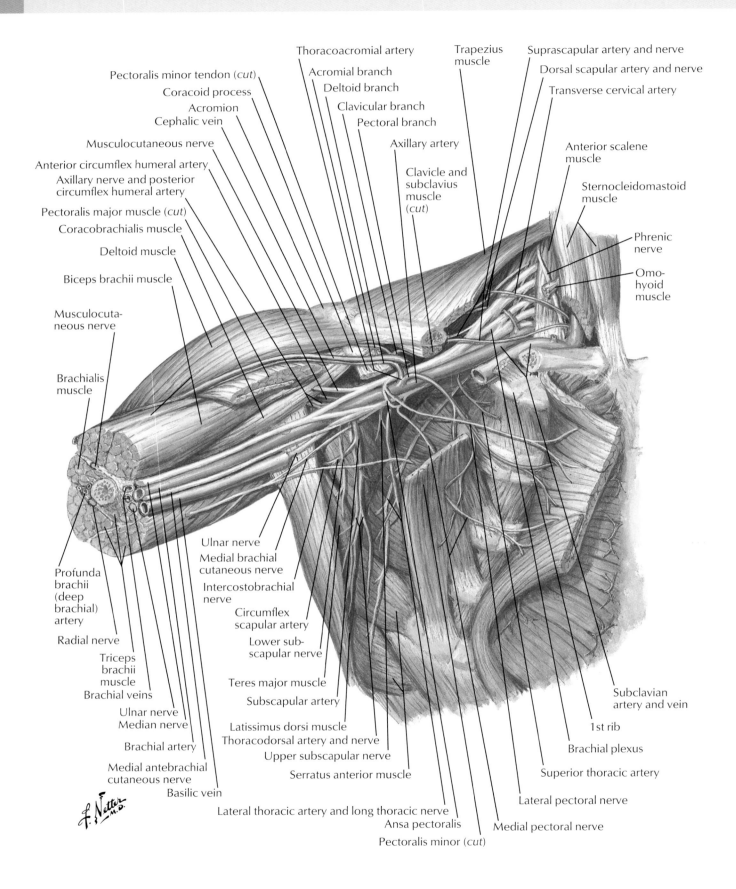

Thoracoacromial artery

Pectoralis minor tendon (*cut*)

Coracoid process

Acromion

Cephalic vein

Musculocutaneous nerve

Anterior circumflex humeral artery

Axillary nerve and posterior circumflex humeral artery

Pectoralis major muscle (*cut*)

Coracobrachialis muscle

Deltoid muscle

Biceps brachii muscle

Musculocutaneous nerve

Brachialis muscle

Acromial branch

Deltoid branch

Clavicular branch

Pectoral branch

Axillary artery

Clavicle and subclavius muscle (*cut*)

Trapezius muscle

Suprascapular artery and nerve

Dorsal scapular artery and nerve

Transverse cervical artery

Anterior scalene muscle

Sternocleidomastoid muscle

Phrenic nerve

Omo-hyoid muscle

Profunda brachii (deep brachial) artery

Radial nerve

Triceps brachii muscle

Brachial veins

Ulnar nerve

Median nerve

Brachial artery

Medial antebrachial cutaneous nerve

Basilic vein

Ulnar nerve

Medial brachial cutaneous nerve

Intercostobrachial nerve

Circumflex scapular artery

Lower sub-scapular nerve

Teres major muscle

Subscapular artery

Latissimus dorsi muscle

Thoracodorsal artery and nerve

Upper subscapular nerve

Serratus anterior muscle

Lateral thoracic artery and long thoracic nerve

Ansa pectoralis

Pectoralis minor (*cut*)

Subclavian artery and vein

1st rib

Brachial plexus

Superior thoracic artery

Lateral pectoral nerve

Medial pectoral nerve

f. Netter M.D.

Plate 417 **Shoulder and Axilla**

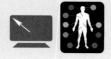

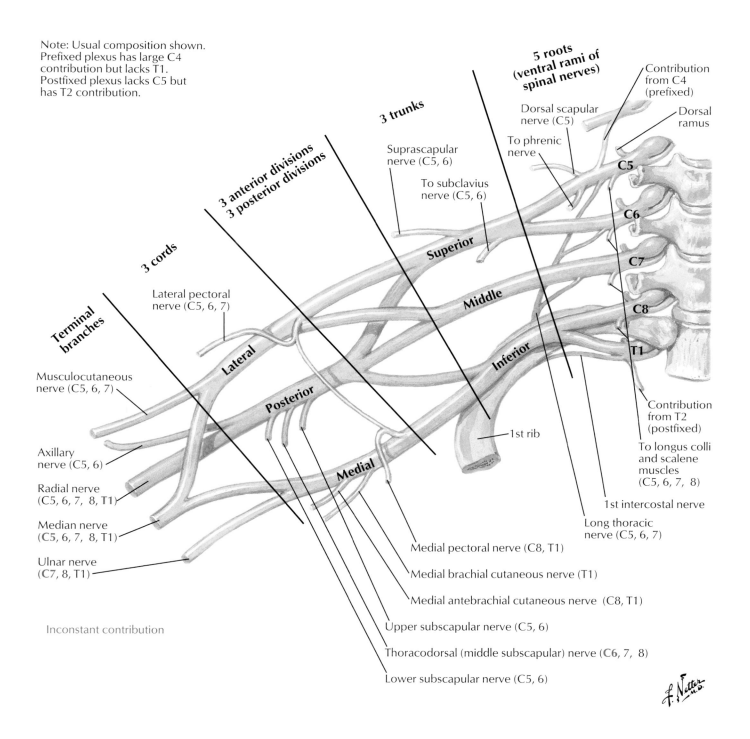

Note: Usual composition shown. Prefixed plexus has large C4 contribution but lacks T1. Postfixed plexus lacks C5 but has T2 contribution.

5 roots (ventral rami of spinal nerves)

Contribution from C4 (prefixed)

Dorsal scapular nerve (C5)

Dorsal ramus

3 trunks

Suprascapular nerve (C5, 6)

To phrenic nerve

C5

3 anterior divisions
3 posterior divisions

To subclavius nerve (C5, 6)

C6

Superior

C7

3 cords

Lateral pectoral nerve (C5, 6, 7)

Middle

C8

Lateral

Terminal branches

T1

Musculocutaneous nerve (C5, 6, 7)

Posterior

Inferior

Contribution from T2 (postfixed)

1st rib

To longus colli and scalene muscles (C5, 6, 7, 8)

Axillary nerve (C5, 6)

Medial

Radial nerve (C5, 6, 7, 8, **T1**)

1st intercostal nerve

Median nerve (**C5**, 6, 7, 8, T1)

Long thoracic nerve (C5, 6, 7)

Medial pectoral nerve (C8, T1)

Ulnar nerve (**C7**, 8, T1)

Medial brachial cutaneous nerve (T1)

Medial antebrachial cutaneous nerve (C8, T1)

Upper subscapular nerve (C5, 6)

Inconstant contribution

Thoracodorsal (middle subscapular) nerve (**C6**, 7, 8)

Lower subscapular nerve (C5, 6)

f. Netter M.D.

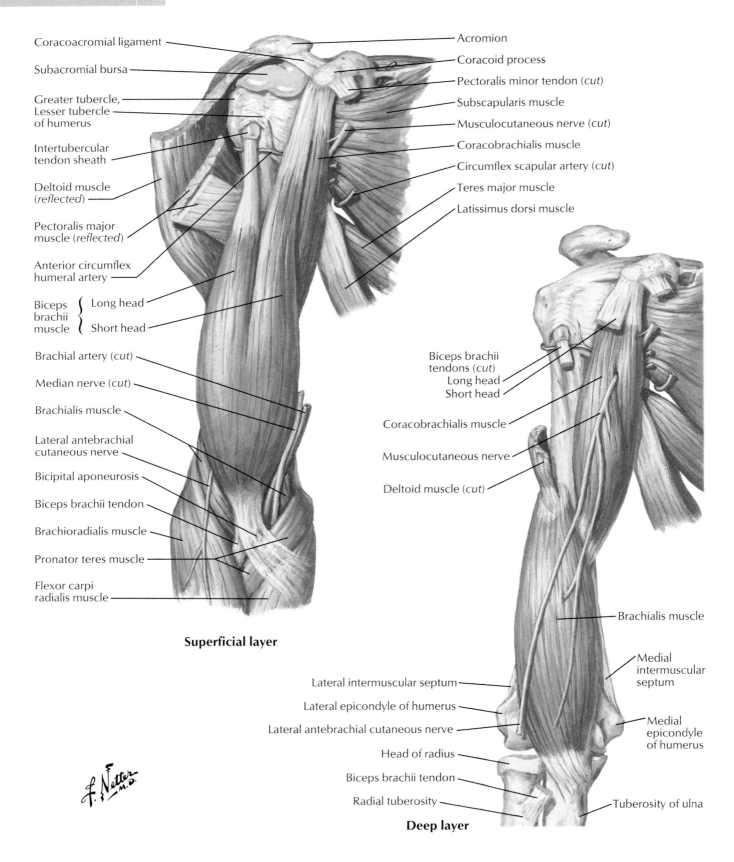

Coracoacromial ligament

Subacromial bursa

Greater tubercle,
Lesser tubercle
of humerus

Intertubercular
tendon sheath

Deltoid muscle
(reflected)

Pectoralis major
muscle (reflected)

Anterior circumflex
humeral artery

Biceps brachii muscle { Long head

Biceps brachii muscle { Short head

Brachial artery (cut)

Median nerve (cut)

Brachialis muscle

Lateral antebrachial
cutaneous nerve

Bicipital aponeurosis

Biceps brachii tendon

Brachioradialis muscle

Pronator teres muscle

Flexor carpi
radialis muscle

Acromion

Coracoid process

Pectoralis minor tendon (cut)

Subscapularis muscle

Musculocutaneous nerve (cut)

Coracobrachialis muscle

Circumflex scapular artery (cut)

Teres major muscle

Latissimus dorsi muscle

Superficial layer

Biceps brachii
tendons (cut)
Long head
Short head

Coracobrachialis muscle

Musculocutaneous nerve

Deltoid muscle (cut)

Brachialis muscle

Medial
intermuscular
septum

Lateral intermuscular septum

Lateral epicondyle of humerus

Lateral antebrachial cutaneous nerve

Head of radius

Biceps brachii tendon

Radial tuberosity

Medial
epicondyle
of humerus

Tuberosity of ulna

Deep layer

Plate 419

Arm

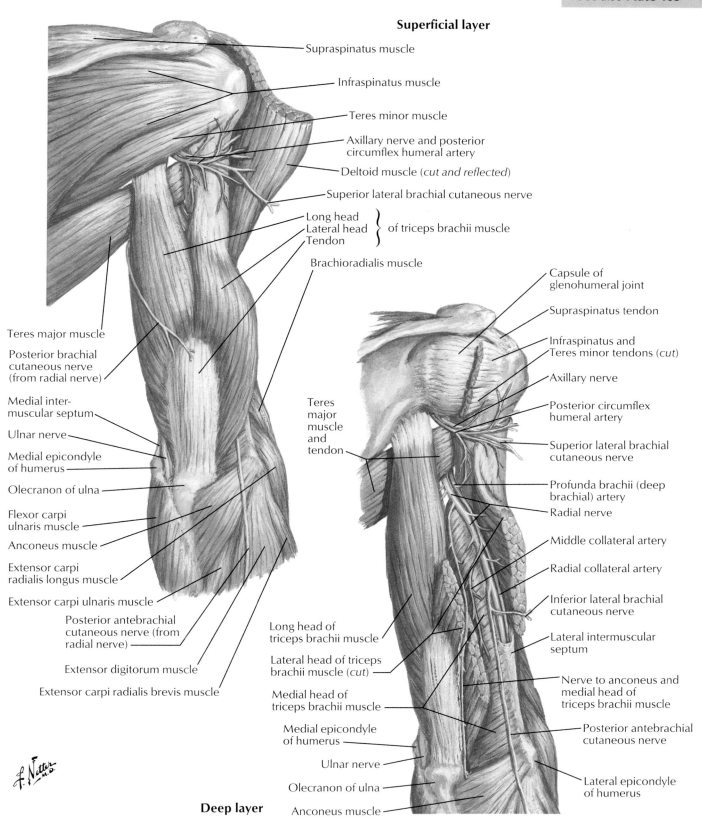

Superficial layer

Supraspinatus muscle

Infraspinatus muscle

Teres minor muscle

Axillary nerve and posterior circumflex humeral artery

Deltoid muscle (*cut and reflected*)

Superior lateral brachial cutaneous nerve

Long head
Lateral head } of triceps brachii muscle
Tendon

Brachioradialis muscle

Capsule of glenohumeral joint

Supraspinatus tendon

Infraspinatus and Teres minor tendons (*cut*)

Axillary nerve

Posterior circumflex humeral artery

Superior lateral brachial cutaneous nerve

Profunda brachii (deep brachial) artery

Radial nerve

Middle collateral artery

Radial collateral artery

Inferior lateral brachial cutaneous nerve

Lateral intermuscular septum

Nerve to anconeus and medial head of triceps brachii muscle

Posterior antebrachial cutaneous nerve

Lateral epicondyle of humerus

Teres major muscle

Posterior brachial cutaneous nerve (from radial nerve)

Medial intermuscular septum

Ulnar nerve

Medial epicondyle of humerus

Olecranon of ulna

Flexor carpi ulnaris muscle

Anconeus muscle

Extensor carpi radialis longus muscle

Extensor carpi ulnaris muscle

Posterior antebrachial cutaneous nerve (from radial nerve)

Extensor digitorum muscle

Extensor carpi radialis brevis muscle

Teres major muscle and tendon

Long head of triceps brachii muscle

Lateral head of triceps brachii muscle (*cut*)

Medial head of triceps brachii muscle

Medial epicondyle of humerus

Ulnar nerve

Olecranon of ulna

Anconeus muscle

Deep layer

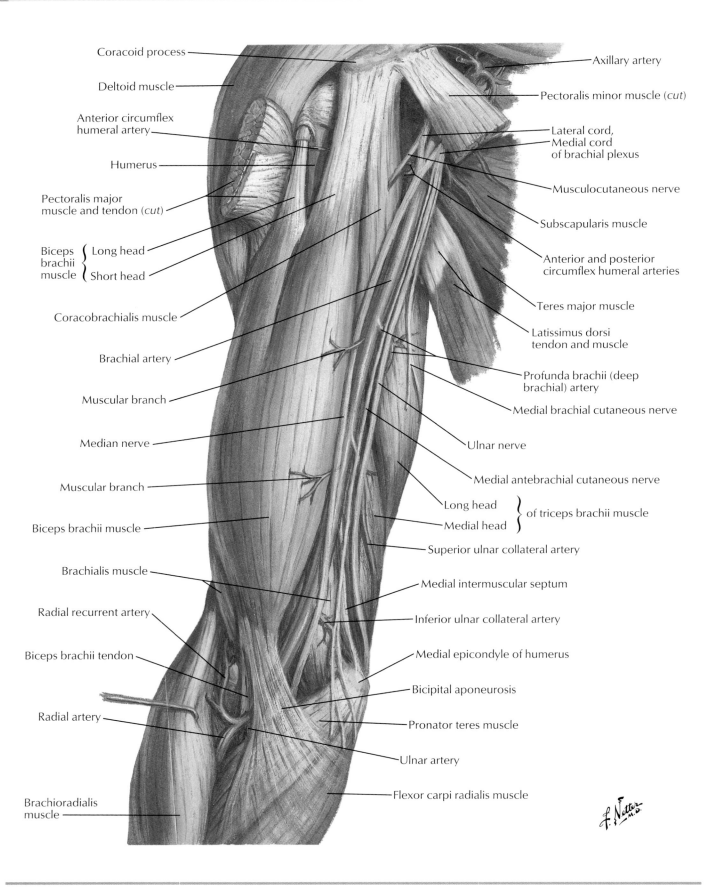

Coracoid process

Deltoid muscle

Anterior circumflex humeral artery

Humerus

Pectoralis major muscle and tendon (cut)

Biceps brachii muscle { Long head / Short head }

Coracobrachialis muscle

Brachial artery

Muscular branch

Median nerve

Muscular branch

Biceps brachii muscle

Brachialis muscle

Radial recurrent artery

Biceps brachii tendon

Radial artery

Brachioradialis muscle

Axillary artery

Pectoralis minor muscle (cut)

Lateral cord, Medial cord of brachial plexus

Musculocutaneous nerve

Subscapularis muscle

Anterior and posterior circumflex humeral arteries

Teres major muscle

Latissimus dorsi tendon and muscle

Profunda brachii (deep brachial) artery

Medial brachial cutaneous nerve

Ulnar nerve

Medial antebrachial cutaneous nerve

Long head / Medial head } of triceps brachii muscle

Superior ulnar collateral artery

Medial intermuscular septum

Inferior ulnar collateral artery

Medial epicondyle of humerus

Bicipital aponeurosis

Pronator teres muscle

Ulnar artery

Flexor carpi radialis muscle

Plate 421 **Arm**

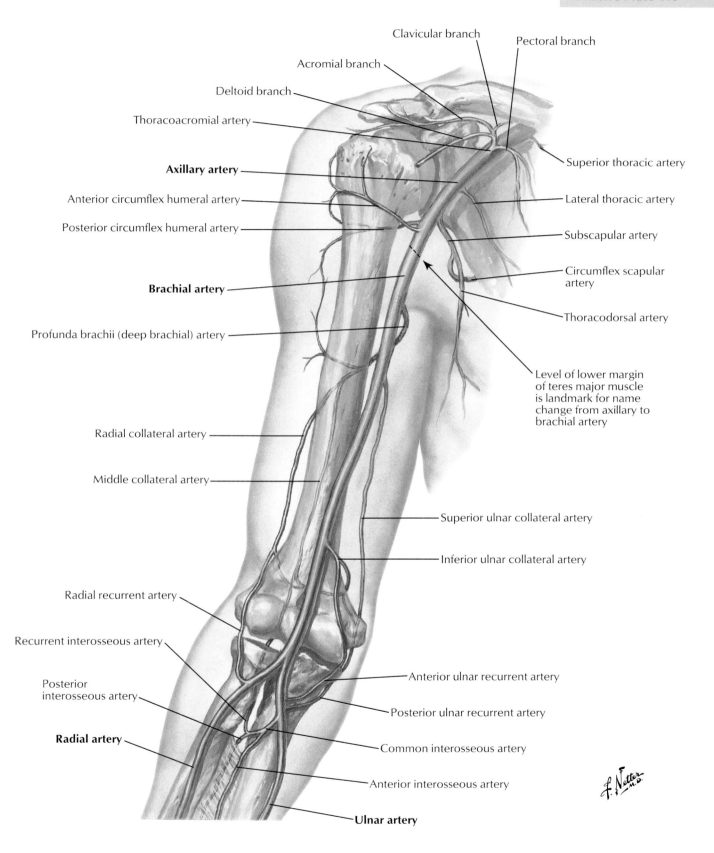

Clavicular branch

Pectoral branch

Acromial branch

Deltoid branch

Thoracoacromial artery

Axillary artery

Anterior circumflex humeral artery

Posterior circumflex humeral artery

Brachial artery

Profunda brachii (deep brachial) artery

Radial collateral artery

Middle collateral artery

Radial recurrent artery

Recurrent interosseous artery

Posterior interosseous artery

Radial artery

Superior thoracic artery

Lateral thoracic artery

Subscapular artery

Circumflex scapular artery

Thoracodorsal artery

Level of lower margin of teres major muscle is landmark for name change from axillary to brachial artery

Superior ulnar collateral artery

Inferior ulnar collateral artery

Anterior ulnar recurrent artery

Posterior ulnar recurrent artery

Common interosseous artery

Anterior interosseous artery

Ulnar artery

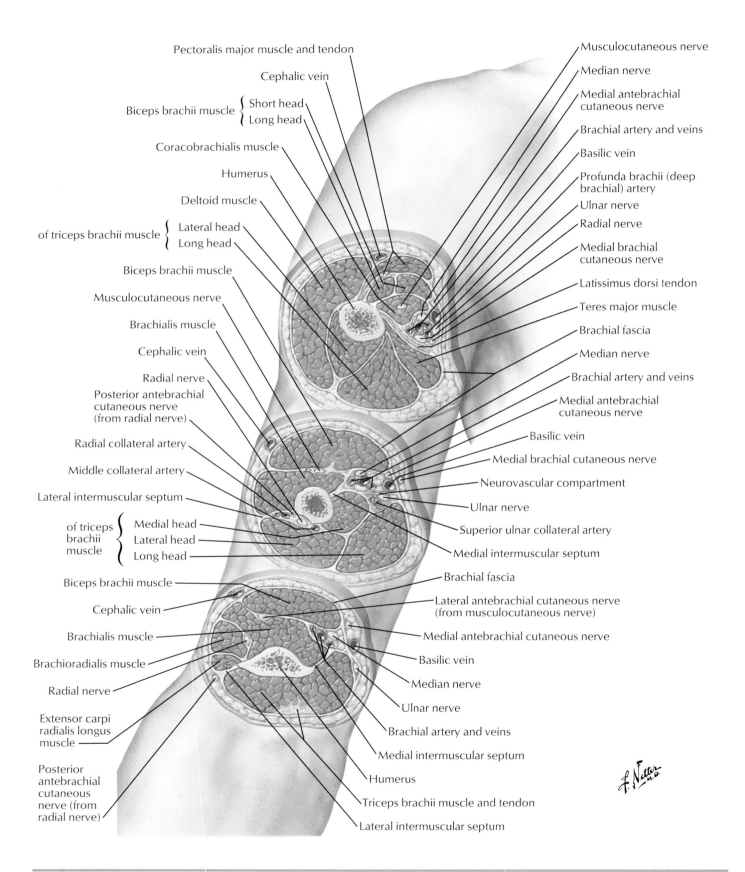

Pectoralis major muscle and tendon

Cephalic vein

Biceps brachii muscle { Short head / Long head

Coracobrachialis muscle

Humerus

Deltoid muscle

of triceps brachii muscle { Lateral head / Long head

Biceps brachii muscle

Musculocutaneous nerve

Brachialis muscle

Cephalic vein

Radial nerve

Posterior antebrachial cutaneous nerve (from radial nerve)

Radial collateral artery

Middle collateral artery

Lateral intermuscular septum

of triceps brachii muscle { Medial head / Lateral head / Long head

Biceps brachii muscle

Cephalic vein

Brachialis muscle

Brachioradialis muscle

Radial nerve

Extensor carpi radialis longus muscle

Posterior antebrachial cutaneous nerve (from radial nerve)

Musculocutaneous nerve

Median nerve

Medial antebrachial cutaneous nerve

Brachial artery and veins

Basilic vein

Profunda brachii (deep brachial) artery

Ulnar nerve

Radial nerve

Medial brachial cutaneous nerve

Latissimus dorsi tendon

Teres major muscle

Brachial fascia

Median nerve

Brachial artery and veins

Medial antebrachial cutaneous nerve

Basilic vein

Medial brachial cutaneous nerve

Neurovascular compartment

Ulnar nerve

Superior ulnar collateral artery

Medial intermuscular septum

Brachial fascia

Lateral antebrachial cutaneous nerve (from musculocutaneous nerve)

Medial antebrachial cutaneous nerve

Basilic vein

Median nerve

Ulnar nerve

Brachial artery and veins

Medial intermuscular septum

Humerus

Triceps brachii muscle and tendon

Lateral intermuscular septum

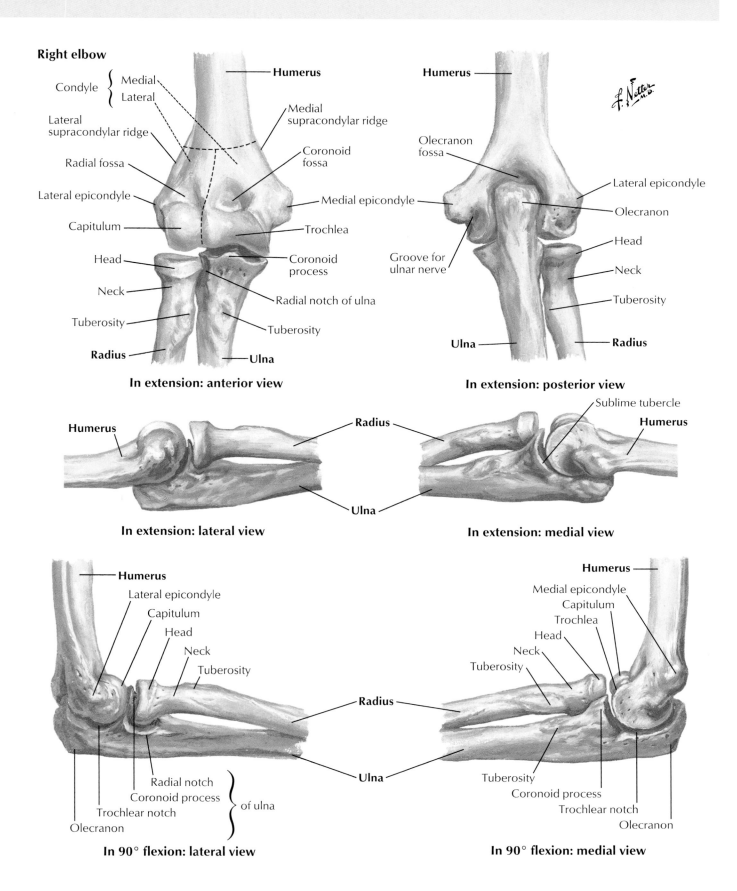

Right elbow

Condyle { Medial
Lateral

Lateral
supracondylar ridge

Radial fossa

Lateral epicondyle

Capitulum

Head

Neck

Tuberosity

Radius

Humerus

Medial
supracondylar ridge

Coronoid
fossa

Medial epicondyle

Trochlea

Coronoid
process

Radial notch of ulna

Tuberosity

Ulna

In extension: anterior view

Humerus

Olecranon
fossa

Groove for
ulnar nerve

Ulna

Lateral epicondyle

Olecranon

Head

Neck

Tuberosity

Radius

In extension: posterior view

Humerus

Radius

Ulna

In extension: lateral view

Sublime tubercle

Humerus

Radius

Ulna

In extension: medial view

Humerus

Lateral epicondyle

Capitulum

Head

Neck

Tuberosity

Radius

Radial notch
Coronoid process } of ulna
Trochlear notch

Olecranon

Ulna

In 90° flexion: lateral view

Humerus

Medial epicondyle

Capitulum

Trochlea

Head

Neck

Tuberosity

Radius

Tuberosity

Coronoid process

Trochlear notch

Olecranon

Ulna

In 90° flexion: medial view

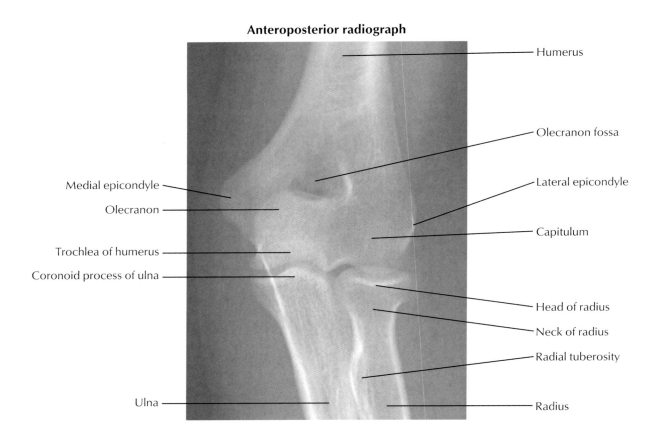

Anteroposterior radiograph

Humerus

Olecranon fossa

Medial epicondyle

Olecranon

Lateral epicondyle

Trochlea of humerus

Capitulum

Coronoid process of ulna

Head of radius

Neck of radius

Radial tuberosity

Ulna

Radius

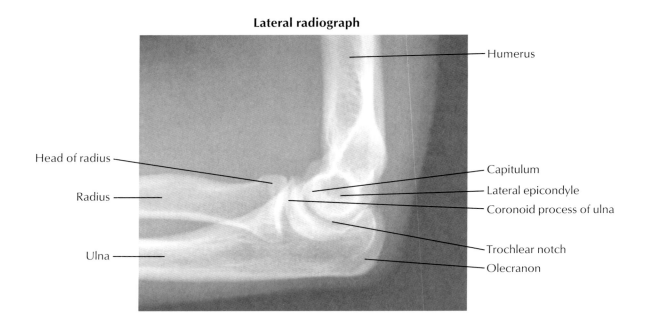

Lateral radiograph

Humerus

Head of radius

Radius

Capitulum

Lateral epicondyle

Coronoid process of ulna

Trochlear notch

Ulna

Olecranon

Plate 425   **Elbow and Forearm**

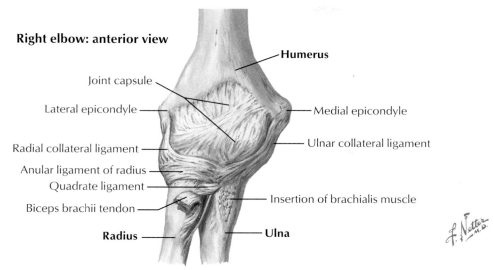

Right elbow: anterior view

Joint capsule

Humerus

Lateral epicondyle

Medial epicondyle

Radial collateral ligament

Ulnar collateral ligament

Anular ligament of radius

Quadrate ligament

Biceps brachii tendon

Insertion of brachialis muscle

Radius

Ulna

F. Netter M.D.

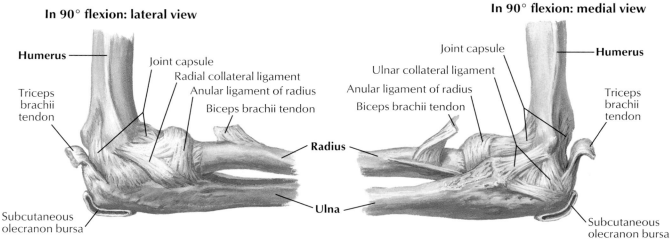

In 90° flexion: lateral view

Humerus

Joint capsule

Radial collateral ligament

Anular ligament of radius

Biceps brachii tendon

Triceps brachii tendon

Radius

Subcutaneous olecranon bursa

Ulna

In 90° flexion: medial view

Joint capsule

Ulnar collateral ligament

Anular ligament of radius

Biceps brachii tendon

Humerus

Triceps brachii tendon

Subcutaneous olecranon bursa

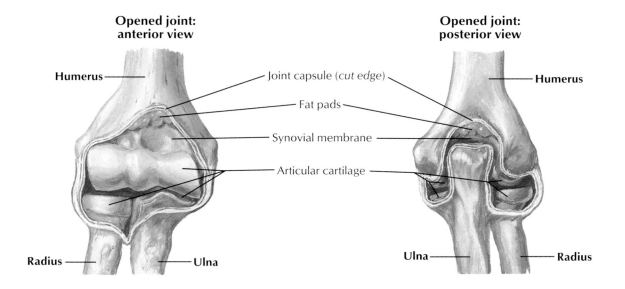

Opened joint: anterior view

Humerus

Joint capsule (*cut edge*)

Fat pads

Synovial membrane

Articular cartilage

Radius

Ulna

Opened joint: posterior view

Humerus

Ulna

Radius

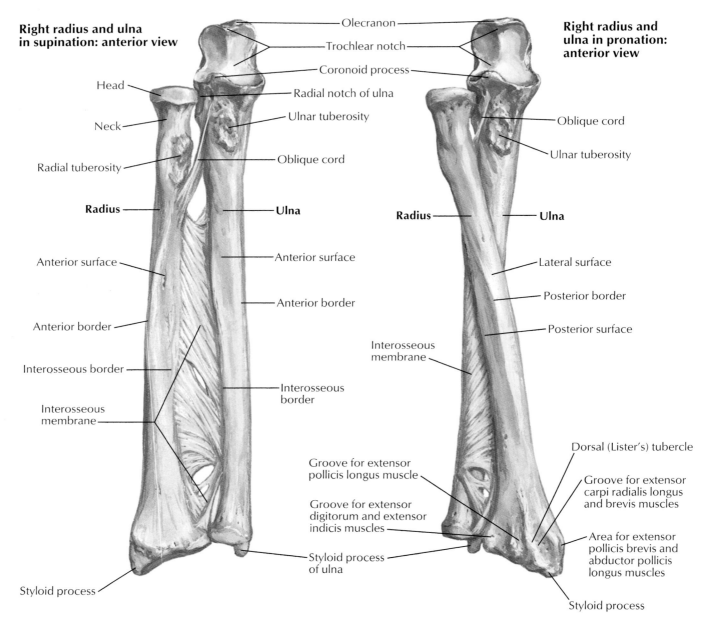

Right radius and ulna
in supination: anterior view

Right radius and
ulna in pronation:
anterior view

Olecranon

Trochlear notch

Coronoid process

Head

Radial notch of ulna

Neck

Ulnar tuberosity

Oblique cord

Radial tuberosity

Oblique cord

Ulnar tuberosity

Radius

Ulna

Radius

Ulna

Anterior surface

Anterior surface

Lateral surface

Anterior border

Posterior border

Anterior border

Posterior surface

Interosseous border

Interosseous
membrane

Interosseous
membrane

Interosseous
border

Dorsal (Lister's) tubercle

Groove for extensor
pollicis longus muscle

Groove for extensor
carpi radialis longus
and brevis muscles

Groove for extensor
digitorum and extensor
indicis muscles

Area for extensor
pollicis brevis and
abductor pollicis
longus muscles

Styloid process
of ulna

Styloid process

Styloid process

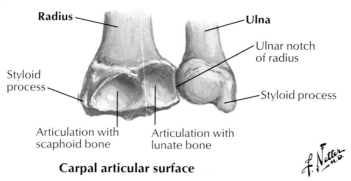

Radius

Ulna

Ulnar notch
of radius

Styloid
process

Styloid process

Articulation with
scaphoid bone

Articulation with
lunate bone

Carpal articular surface

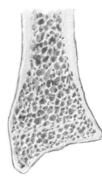

Coronal section of
radius demonstrates
how thickness of
cortical bone of
shaft diminishes
to thin layer over
cancellous bone
at distal end

f. Netter
M.D.

Plate 427

Elbow and Forearm

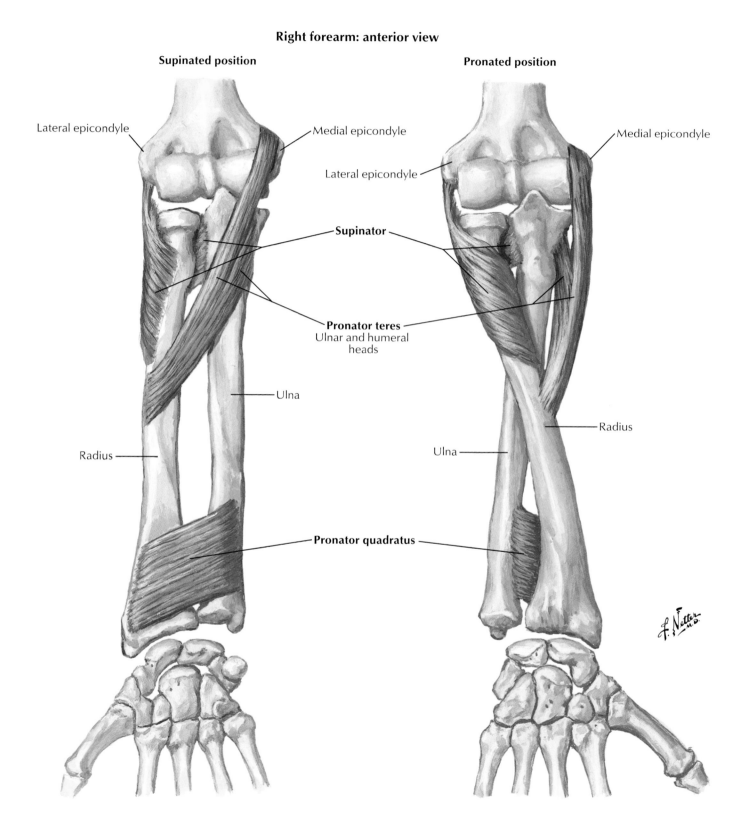

Right forearm: anterior view

Supinated position

Pronated position

Lateral epicondyle

Medial epicondyle

Medial epicondyle

Lateral epicondyle

Supinator

Pronator teres
Ulnar and humeral heads

Ulna

Radius

Ulna

Radius

Pronator quadratus

F. Netter
M.D.

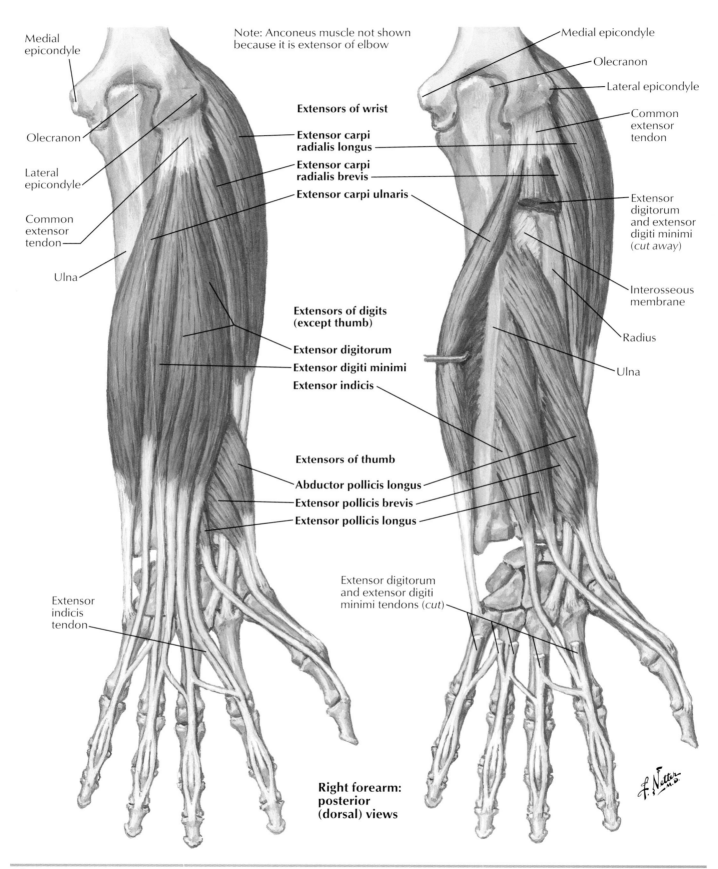

Medial epicondyle

Olecranon

Lateral epicondyle

Common extensor tendon

Ulna

Note: Anconeus muscle not shown because it is extensor of elbow

Extensors of wrist

Extensor carpi radialis longus

Extensor carpi radialis brevis

Extensor carpi ulnaris

Extensors of digits (except thumb)

Extensor digitorum

Extensor digiti minimi

Extensor indicis

Extensors of thumb

Abductor pollicis longus

Extensor pollicis brevis

Extensor pollicis longus

Extensor indicis tendon

Medial epicondyle

Olecranon

Lateral epicondyle

Common extensor tendon

Extensor digitorum and extensor digiti minimi (*cut away*)

Interosseous membrane

Radius

Ulna

Extensor digitorum and extensor digiti minimi tendons (*cut*)

Right forearm: posterior (dorsal) views

f. Netter M.D.

Plate 429

Elbow and Forearm

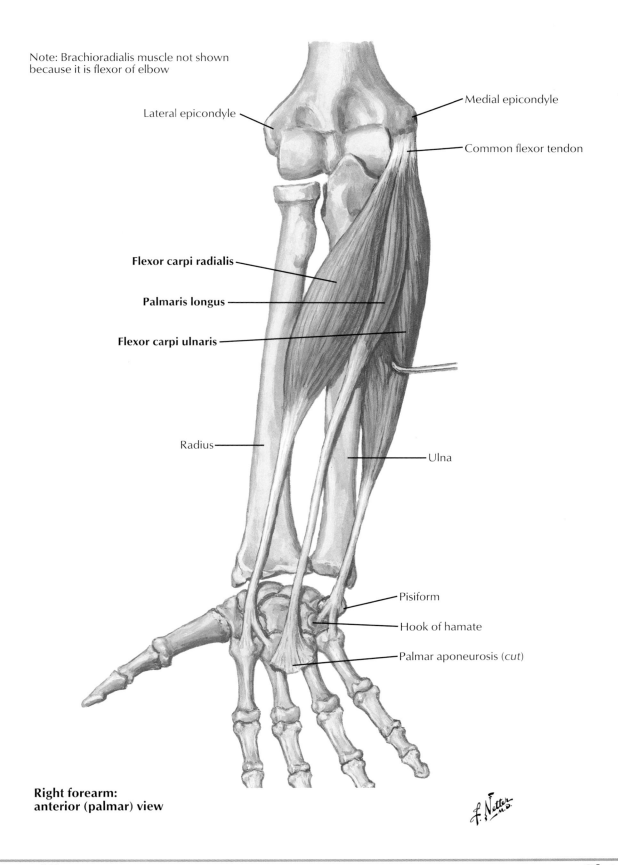

Note: Brachioradialis muscle not shown because it is flexor of elbow

Lateral epicondyle

Medial epicondyle

Common flexor tendon

Flexor carpi radialis

Palmaris longus

Flexor carpi ulnaris

Radius

Ulna

Pisiform

Hook of hamate

Palmar aponeurosis (*cut*)

**Right forearm:
anterior (palmar) view**

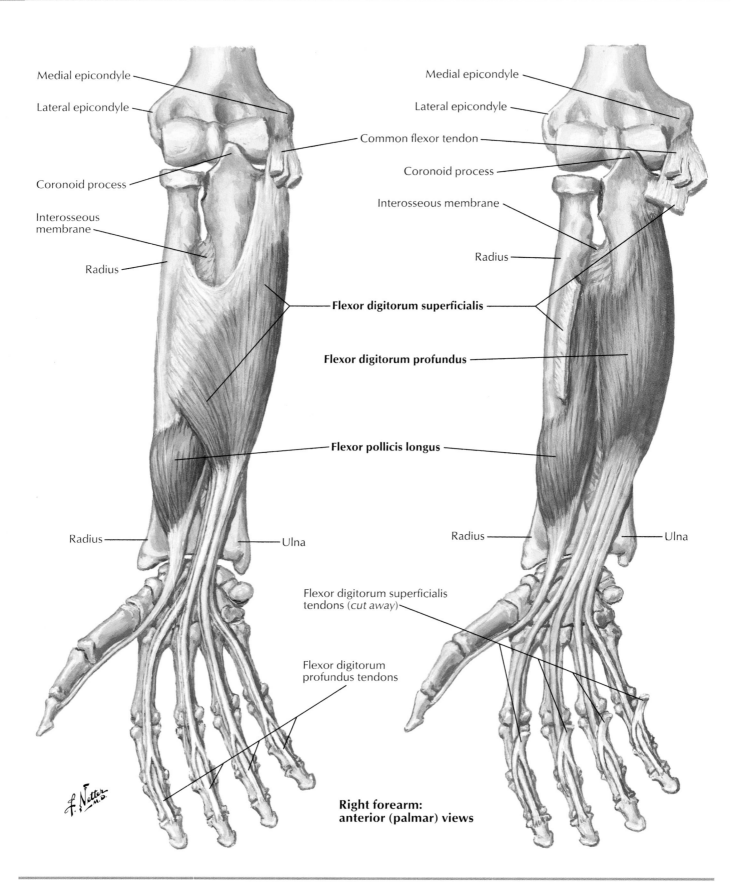

Medial epicondyle

Lateral epicondyle

Common flexor tendon

Coronoid process

Interosseous membrane

Radius

Medial epicondyle

Lateral epicondyle

Coronoid process

Interosseous membrane

Radius

Flexor digitorum superficialis

Flexor digitorum profundus

Flexor pollicis longus

Radius

Ulna

Radius

Ulna

Flexor digitorum superficialis tendons (*cut away*)

Flexor digitorum profundus tendons

Right forearm: anterior (palmar) views

Plate 431   **Elbow and Forearm**

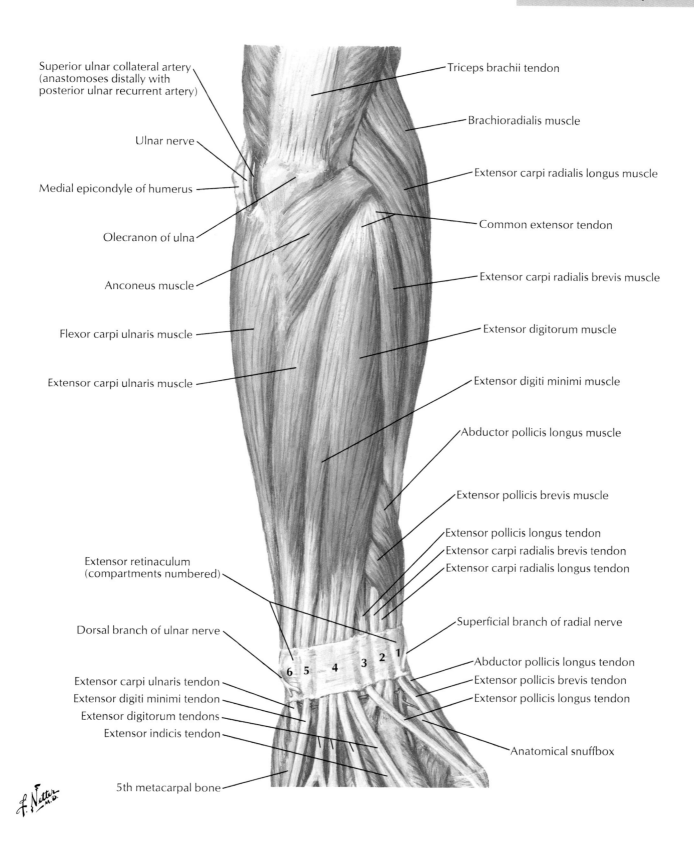

Superior ulnar collateral artery (anastomoses distally with posterior ulnar recurrent artery)

Ulnar nerve

Medial epicondyle of humerus

Olecranon of ulna

Anconeus muscle

Flexor carpi ulnaris muscle

Extensor carpi ulnaris muscle

Extensor retinaculum (compartments numbered)

Dorsal branch of ulnar nerve

Extensor carpi ulnaris tendon

Extensor digiti minimi tendon

Extensor digitorum tendons

Extensor indicis tendon

5th metacarpal bone

Triceps brachii tendon

Brachioradialis muscle

Extensor carpi radialis longus muscle

Common extensor tendon

Extensor carpi radialis brevis muscle

Extensor digitorum muscle

Extensor digiti minimi muscle

Abductor pollicis longus muscle

Extensor pollicis brevis muscle

Extensor pollicis longus tendon
Extensor carpi radialis brevis tendon
Extensor carpi radialis longus tendon

Superficial branch of radial nerve

Abductor pollicis longus tendon
Extensor pollicis brevis tendon
Extensor pollicis longus tendon

Anatomical snuffbox

6 5 4 3 2 1

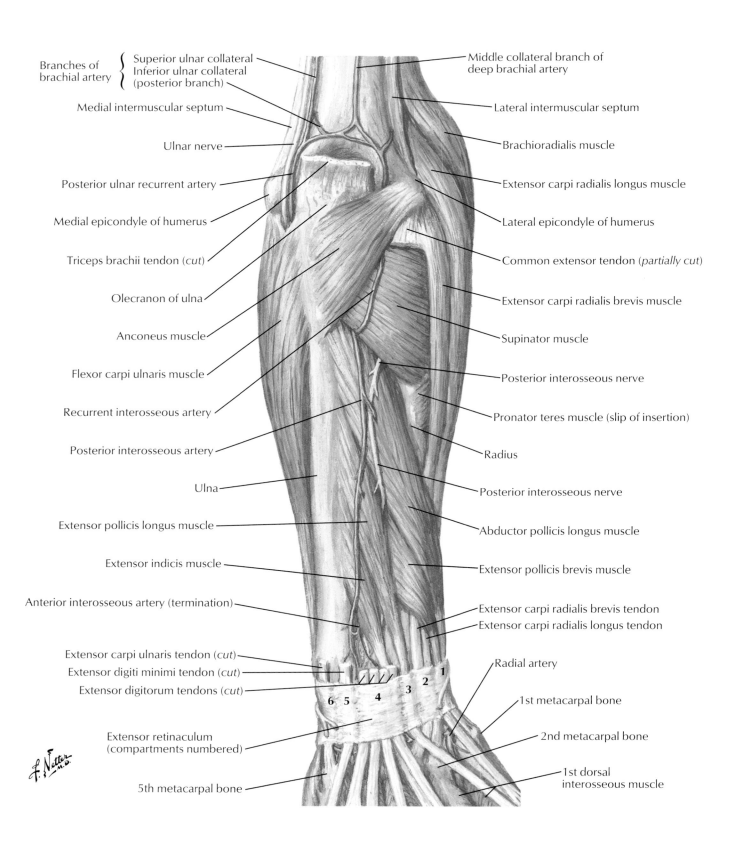

Branches of brachial artery { Superior ulnar collateral

Inferior ulnar collateral (posterior branch)

Middle collateral branch of deep brachial artery

Medial intermuscular septum

Lateral intermuscular septum

Ulnar nerve

Brachioradialis muscle

Posterior ulnar recurrent artery

Extensor carpi radialis longus muscle

Medial epicondyle of humerus

Lateral epicondyle of humerus

Triceps brachii tendon (*cut*)

Common extensor tendon (*partially cut*)

Olecranon of ulna

Extensor carpi radialis brevis muscle

Anconeus muscle

Supinator muscle

Flexor carpi ulnaris muscle

Posterior interosseous nerve

Recurrent interosseous artery

Pronator teres muscle (slip of insertion)

Posterior interosseous artery

Radius

Ulna

Posterior interosseous nerve

Extensor pollicis longus muscle

Abductor pollicis longus muscle

Extensor indicis muscle

Extensor pollicis brevis muscle

Anterior interosseous artery (termination)

Extensor carpi radialis brevis tendon

Extensor carpi radialis longus tendon

Extensor carpi ulnaris tendon (*cut*)

Extensor digiti minimi tendon (*cut*)

Extensor digitorum tendons (*cut*)

Radial artery

1st metacarpal bone

Extensor retinaculum (compartments numbered)

2nd metacarpal bone

1st dorsal interosseous muscle

5th metacarpal bone

Plate 433

Elbow and Forearm

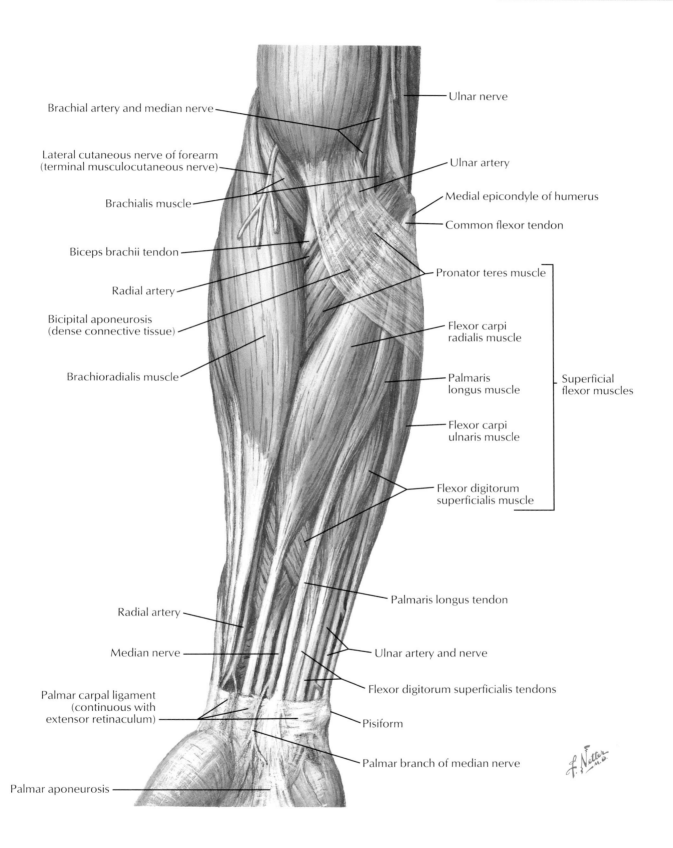

Brachial artery and median nerve

Lateral cutaneous nerve of forearm
(terminal musculocutaneous nerve)

Brachialis muscle

Biceps brachii tendon

Radial artery

Bicipital aponeurosis
(dense connective tissue)

Brachioradialis muscle

Radial artery

Median nerve

Palmar carpal ligament
(continuous with
extensor retinaculum)

Palmar aponeurosis

Ulnar nerve

Ulnar artery

Medial epicondyle of humerus

Common flexor tendon

Pronator teres muscle

Flexor carpi
radialis muscle

Palmaris
longus muscle

Flexor carpi
ulnaris muscle

Flexor digitorum
superficialis muscle

Superficial
flexor muscles

Palmaris longus tendon

Ulnar artery and nerve

Flexor digitorum superficialis tendons

Pisiform

Palmar branch of median nerve

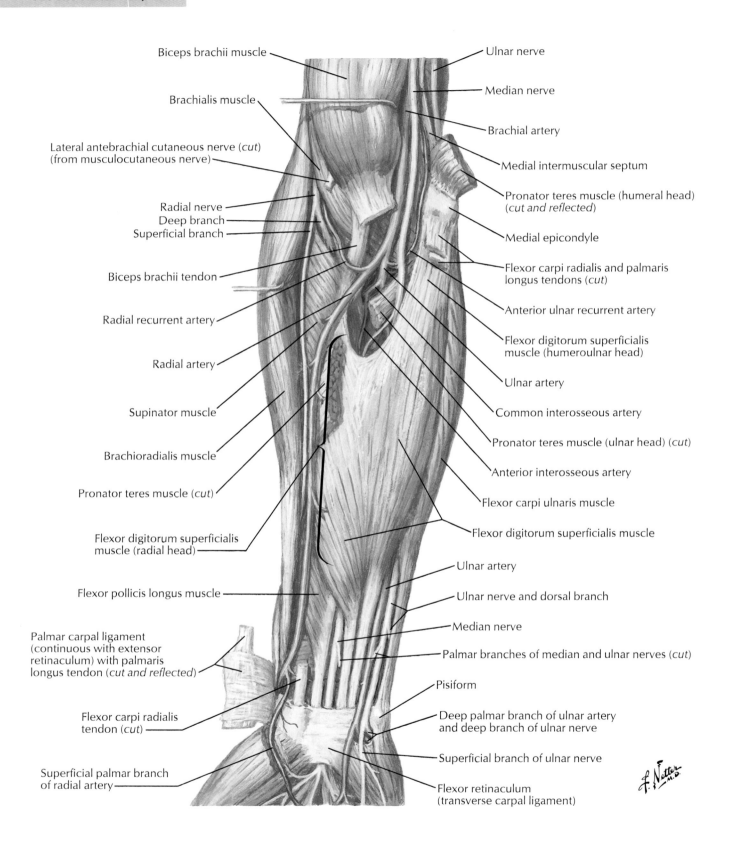

Biceps brachii muscle

Brachialis muscle

Lateral antebrachial cutaneous nerve (*cut*)
(from musculocutaneous nerve)

Radial nerve
Deep branch
Superficial branch

Biceps brachii tendon

Radial recurrent artery

Radial artery

Supinator muscle

Brachioradialis muscle

Pronator teres muscle (*cut*)

Flexor digitorum superficialis
muscle (radial head)

Flexor pollicis longus muscle

Palmar carpal ligament
(continuous with extensor
retinaculum) with palmaris
longus tendon (*cut and reflected*)

Flexor carpi radialis
tendon (*cut*)

Superficial palmar branch
of radial artery

Ulnar nerve

Median nerve

Brachial artery

Medial intermuscular septum

Pronator teres muscle (humeral head)
(*cut and reflected*)

Medial epicondyle

Flexor carpi radialis and palmaris
longus tendons (*cut*)

Anterior ulnar recurrent artery

Flexor digitorum superficialis
muscle (humeroulnar head)

Ulnar artery

Common interosseous artery

Pronator teres muscle (ulnar head) (*cut*)

Anterior interosseous artery

Flexor carpi ulnaris muscle

Flexor digitorum superficialis muscle

Ulnar artery

Ulnar nerve and dorsal branch

Median nerve

Palmar branches of median and ulnar nerves (*cut*)

Pisiform

Deep palmar branch of ulnar artery
and deep branch of ulnar nerve

Superficial branch of ulnar nerve

Flexor retinaculum
(transverse carpal ligament)

Plate 435

Elbow and Forearm

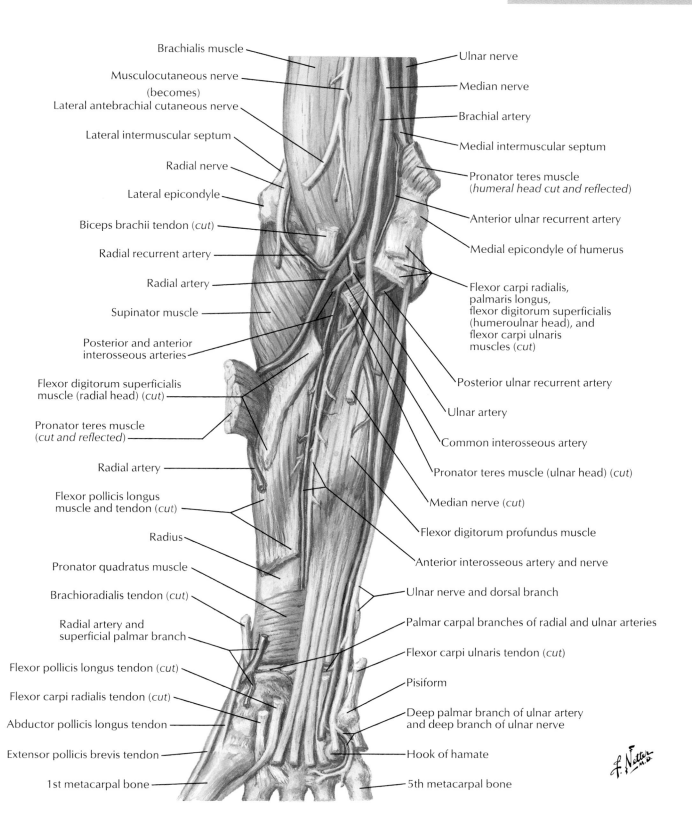

Brachialis muscle

Musculocutaneous nerve (becomes)

Lateral antebrachial cutaneous nerve

Lateral intermuscular septum

Radial nerve

Lateral epicondyle

Biceps brachii tendon (cut)

Radial recurrent artery

Radial artery

Supinator muscle

Posterior and anterior interosseous arteries

Flexor digitorum superficialis muscle (radial head) (cut)

Pronator teres muscle (cut and reflected)

Radial artery

Flexor pollicis longus muscle and tendon (cut)

Radius

Pronator quadratus muscle

Brachioradialis tendon (cut)

Radial artery and superficial palmar branch

Flexor pollicis longus tendon (cut)

Flexor carpi radialis tendon (cut)

Abductor pollicis longus tendon

Extensor pollicis brevis tendon

1st metacarpal bone

Ulnar nerve

Median nerve

Brachial artery

Medial intermuscular septum

Pronator teres muscle (humeral head cut and reflected)

Anterior ulnar recurrent artery

Medial epicondyle of humerus

Flexor carpi radialis, palmaris longus, flexor digitorum superficialis (humeroulnar head), and flexor carpi ulnaris muscles (cut)

Posterior ulnar recurrent artery

Ulnar artery

Common interosseous artery

Pronator teres muscle (ulnar head) (cut)

Median nerve (cut)

Flexor digitorum profundus muscle

Anterior interosseous artery and nerve

Ulnar nerve and dorsal branch

Palmar carpal branches of radial and ulnar arteries

Flexor carpi ulnaris tendon (cut)

Pisiform

Deep palmar branch of ulnar artery and deep branch of ulnar nerve

Hook of hamate

5th metacarpal bone

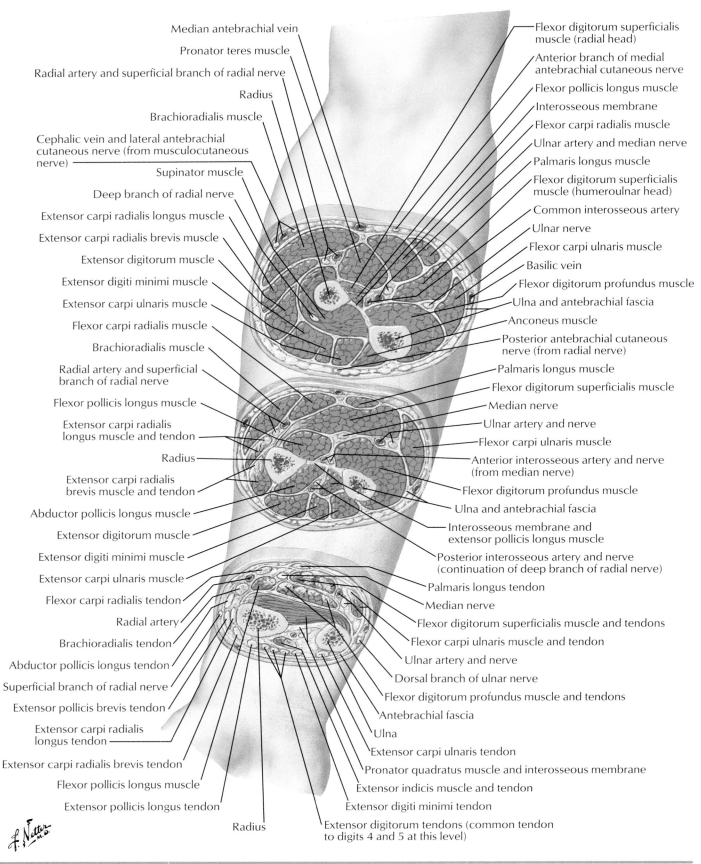

Median antebrachial vein

Pronator teres muscle

Radial artery and superficial branch of radial nerve

Radius

Brachioradialis muscle

Cephalic vein and lateral antebrachial cutaneous nerve (from musculocutaneous nerve)

Supinator muscle

Deep branch of radial nerve

Extensor carpi radialis longus muscle

Extensor carpi radialis brevis muscle

Extensor digitorum muscle

Extensor digiti minimi muscle

Extensor carpi ulnaris muscle

Flexor carpi radialis muscle

Brachioradialis muscle

Radial artery and superficial branch of radial nerve

Flexor pollicis longus muscle

Extensor carpi radialis longus muscle and tendon

Radius

Extensor carpi radialis brevis muscle and tendon

Abductor pollicis longus muscle

Extensor digitorum muscle

Extensor digiti minimi muscle

Extensor carpi ulnaris muscle

Flexor carpi radialis tendon

Radial artery

Brachioradialis tendon

Abductor pollicis longus tendon

Superficial branch of radial nerve

Extensor pollicis brevis tendon

Extensor carpi radialis longus tendon

Extensor carpi radialis brevis tendon

Flexor pollicis longus muscle

Extensor pollicis longus tendon

Radius

Flexor digitorum superficialis muscle (radial head)

Anterior branch of medial antebrachial cutaneous nerve

Flexor pollicis longus muscle

Interosseous membrane

Flexor carpi radialis muscle

Ulnar artery and median nerve

Palmaris longus muscle

Flexor digitorum superficialis muscle (humeroulnar head)

Common interosseous artery

Ulnar nerve

Flexor carpi ulnaris muscle

Basilic vein

Flexor digitorum profundus muscle

Ulna and antebrachial fascia

Anconeus muscle

Posterior antebrachial cutaneous nerve (from radial nerve)

Palmaris longus muscle

Flexor digitorum superficialis muscle

Median nerve

Ulnar artery and nerve

Flexor carpi ulnaris muscle

Anterior interosseous artery and nerve (from median nerve)

Flexor digitorum profundus muscle

Ulna and antebrachial fascia

Interosseous membrane and extensor pollicis longus muscle

Posterior interosseous artery and nerve (continuation of deep branch of radial nerve)

Palmaris longus tendon

Median nerve

Flexor digitorum superficialis muscle and tendons

Flexor carpi ulnaris muscle and tendon

Ulnar artery and nerve

Dorsal branch of ulnar nerve

Flexor digitorum profundus muscle and tendons

Antebrachial fascia

Ulna

Extensor carpi ulnaris tendon

Pronator quadratus muscle and interosseous membrane

Extensor indicis muscle and tendon

Extensor digiti minimi tendon

Extensor digitorum tendons (common tendon to digits 4 and 5 at this level)

Plate 437

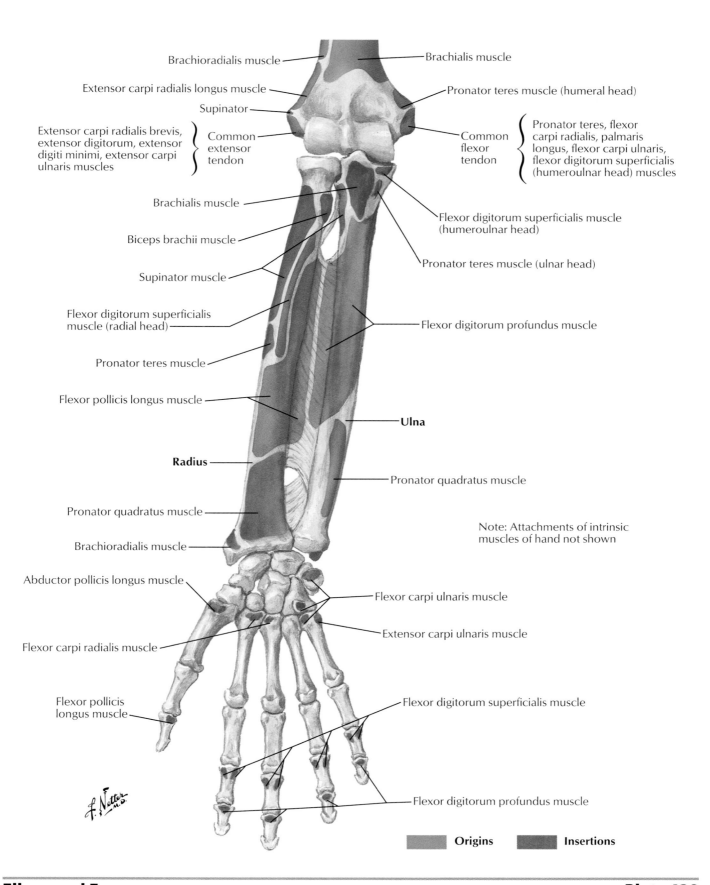

Brachioradialis muscle

Extensor carpi radialis longus muscle

Supinator

Extensor carpi radialis brevis, extensor digitorum, extensor digiti minimi, extensor carpi ulnaris muscles

Common extensor tendon

Brachialis muscle

Biceps brachii muscle

Supinator muscle

Flexor digitorum superficialis muscle (radial head)

Pronator teres muscle

Flexor pollicis longus muscle

Radius

Pronator quadratus muscle

Brachioradialis muscle

Abductor pollicis longus muscle

Flexor carpi radialis muscle

Flexor pollicis longus muscle

Brachialis muscle

Pronator teres muscle (humeral head)

Common flexor tendon

Pronator teres, flexor carpi radialis, palmaris longus, flexor carpi ulnaris, flexor digitorum superficialis (humeroulnar head) muscles

Flexor digitorum superficialis muscle (humeroulnar head)

Pronator teres muscle (ulnar head)

Flexor digitorum profundus muscle

Ulna

Pronator quadratus muscle

Note: Attachments of intrinsic muscles of hand not shown

Flexor carpi ulnaris muscle

Extensor carpi ulnaris muscle

Flexor digitorum superficialis muscle

Flexor digitorum profundus muscle

Origins   Insertions

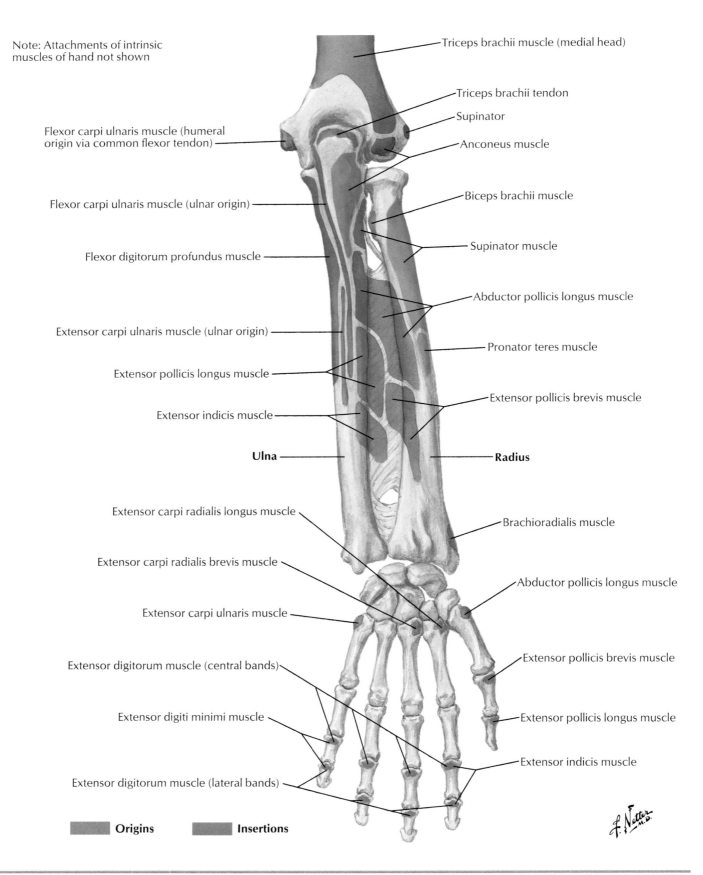

Note: Attachments of intrinsic muscles of hand not shown

Triceps brachii muscle (medial head)

Triceps brachii tendon

Supinator

Flexor carpi ulnaris muscle (humeral origin via common flexor tendon)

Anconeus muscle

Biceps brachii muscle

Flexor carpi ulnaris muscle (ulnar origin)

Supinator muscle

Flexor digitorum profundus muscle

Abductor pollicis longus muscle

Extensor carpi ulnaris muscle (ulnar origin)

Pronator teres muscle

Extensor pollicis longus muscle

Extensor pollicis brevis muscle

Extensor indicis muscle

Ulna

Radius

Extensor carpi radialis longus muscle

Brachioradialis muscle

Extensor carpi radialis brevis muscle

Abductor pollicis longus muscle

Extensor carpi ulnaris muscle

Extensor digitorum muscle (central bands)

Extensor pollicis brevis muscle

Extensor digiti minimi muscle

Extensor pollicis longus muscle

Extensor digitorum muscle (lateral bands)

Extensor indicis muscle

Origins   Insertions

Plate 439   **Elbow and Forearm**

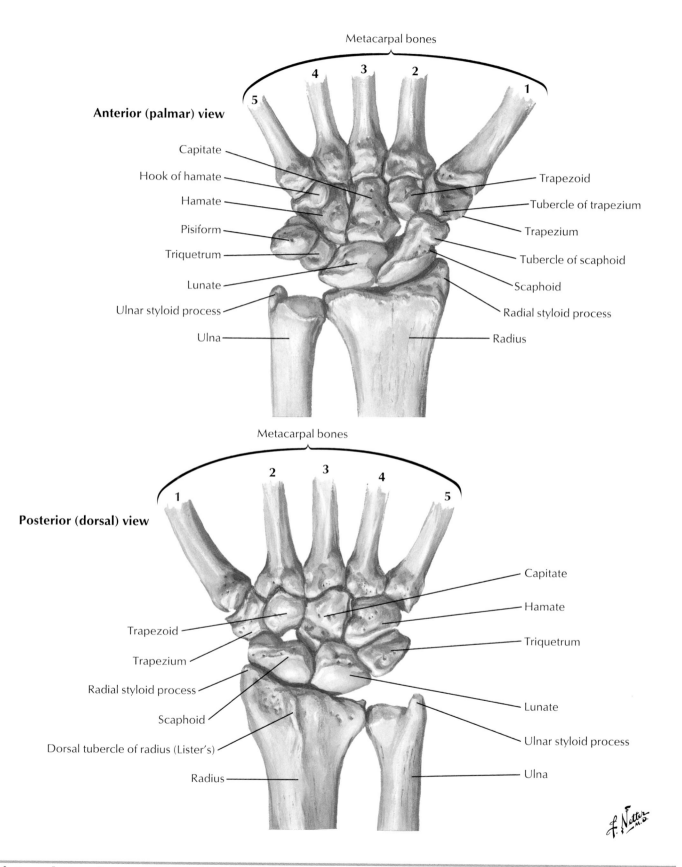

Metacarpal bones

5   4   3   2   1

Anterior (palmar) view

Capitate

Hook of hamate

Hamate

Pisiform

Triquetrum

Lunate

Ulnar styloid process

Ulna

Trapezoid

Tubercle of trapezium

Trapezium

Tubercle of scaphoid

Scaphoid

Radial styloid process

Radius

Metacarpal bones

1   2   3   4   5

Posterior (dorsal) view

Trapezoid

Trapezium

Radial styloid process

Scaphoid

Dorsal tubercle of radius (Lister's)

Radius

Capitate

Hamate

Triquetrum

Lunate

Ulnar styloid process

Ulna

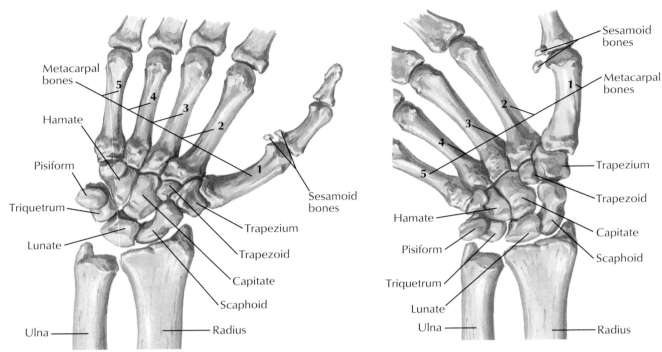

Position of carpal bones with hand in abduction: anterior (palmar) view

Position of carpal bones with hand in adduction: anterior (palmar) view

Metacarpal bones
5
4
3
2
Hamate
Pisiform
Triquetrum
Lunate
Ulna — Radius
Sesamoid bones
Trapezium
Trapezoid
Capitate
Scaphoid

Sesamoid bones
Metacarpal bones
1
2
3
4
5
Hamate
Pisiform
Triquetrum
Lunate
Ulna — Radius
Trapezium
Trapezoid
Capitate
Scaphoid

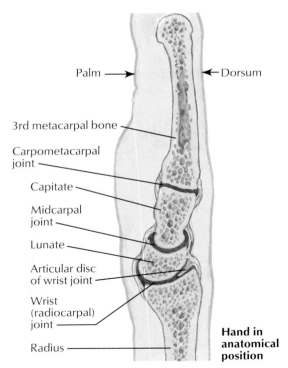

Palm → ← Dorsum

3rd metacarpal bone
Carpometacarpal joint
Capitate
Midcarpal joint
Lunate
Articular disc of wrist joint
Wrist (radiocarpal) joint
Radius

Hand in anatomical position

Sagittal sections through wrist and middle finger

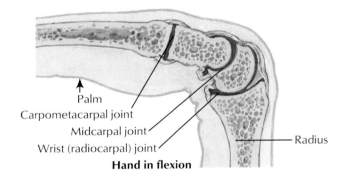

Palm
Carpometacarpal joint
Midcarpal joint
Wrist (radiocarpal) joint
Radius

Hand in flexion

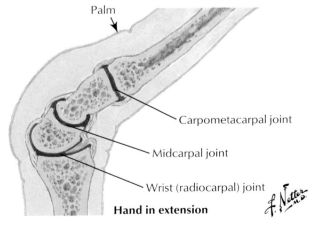

Palm
Carpometacarpal joint
Midcarpal joint
Wrist (radiocarpal) joint

Hand in extension

F. Netter M.D.

Plate 441   **Wrist and Hand**

Carpal tunnel: palmar view

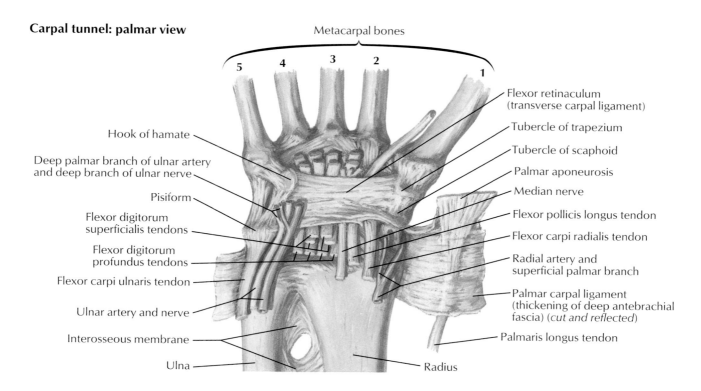

Metacarpal bones

5   4   3   2   1

Hook of hamate

Deep palmar branch of ulnar artery and deep branch of ulnar nerve

Pisiform

Flexor digitorum superficialis tendons

Flexor digitorum profundus tendons

Flexor carpi ulnaris tendon

Ulnar artery and nerve

Interosseous membrane

Ulna

Flexor retinaculum (transverse carpal ligament)

Tubercle of trapezium

Tubercle of scaphoid

Palmar aponeurosis

Median nerve

Flexor pollicis longus tendon

Flexor carpi radialis tendon

Radial artery and superficial palmar branch

Palmar carpal ligament (thickening of deep antebrachial fascia) (cut and reflected)

Palmaris longus tendon

Radius

Flexor retinaculum removed: palmar view

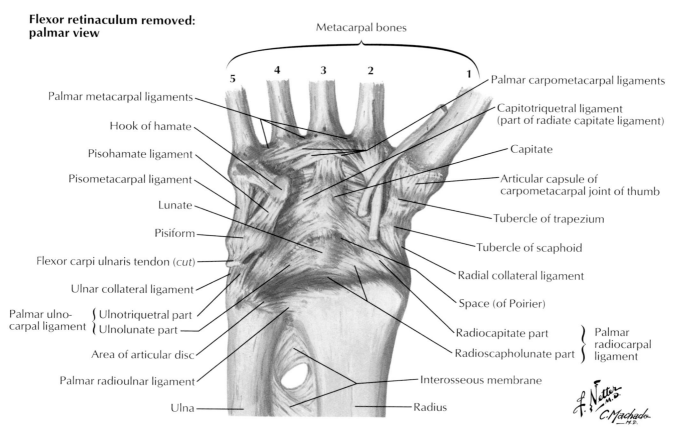

Metacarpal bones

5   4   3   2   1

Palmar metacarpal ligaments

Hook of hamate

Pisohamate ligament

Pisometacarpal ligament

Lunate

Pisiform

Flexor carpi ulnaris tendon (cut)

Ulnar collateral ligament

Palmar ulno-carpal ligament { Ulnotriquetral part / Ulnolunate part

Area of articular disc

Palmar radioulnar ligament

Ulna

Palmar carpometacarpal ligaments

Capitotriquetral ligament (part of radiate capitate ligament)

Capitate

Articular capsule of carpometacarpal joint of thumb

Tubercle of trapezium

Tubercle of scaphoid

Radial collateral ligament

Space (of Poirier)

Radiocapite part

Radioscapholunate part } Palmar radiocarpal ligament

Interosseous membrane

Radius

Posterior (dorsal) view

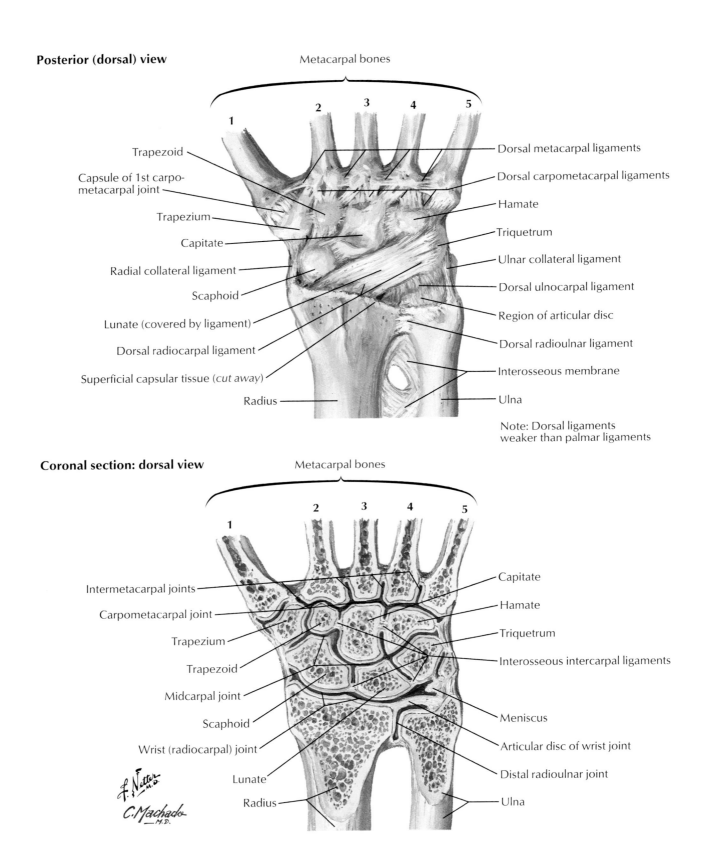

Metacarpal bones

1 2 3 4 5

Trapezoid

Capsule of 1st carpo-metacarpal joint

Trapezium

Capitate

Radial collateral ligament

Scaphoid

Lunate (covered by ligament)

Dorsal radiocarpal ligament

Superficial capsular tissue (*cut away*)

Radius

Dorsal metacarpal ligaments

Dorsal carpometacarpal ligaments

Hamate

Triquetrum

Ulnar collateral ligament

Dorsal ulnocarpal ligament

Region of articular disc

Dorsal radioulnar ligament

Interosseous membrane

Ulna

Note: Dorsal ligaments weaker than palmar ligaments

Coronal section: dorsal view

Metacarpal bones

1 2 3 4 5

Intermetacarpal joints

Carpometacarpal joint

Trapezium

Trapezoid

Midcarpal joint

Scaphoid

Wrist (radiocarpal) joint

Lunate

Radius

Capitate

Hamate

Triquetrum

Interosseous intercarpal ligaments

Meniscus

Articular disc of wrist joint

Distal radioulnar joint

Ulna

Plate 443

Wrist and Hand

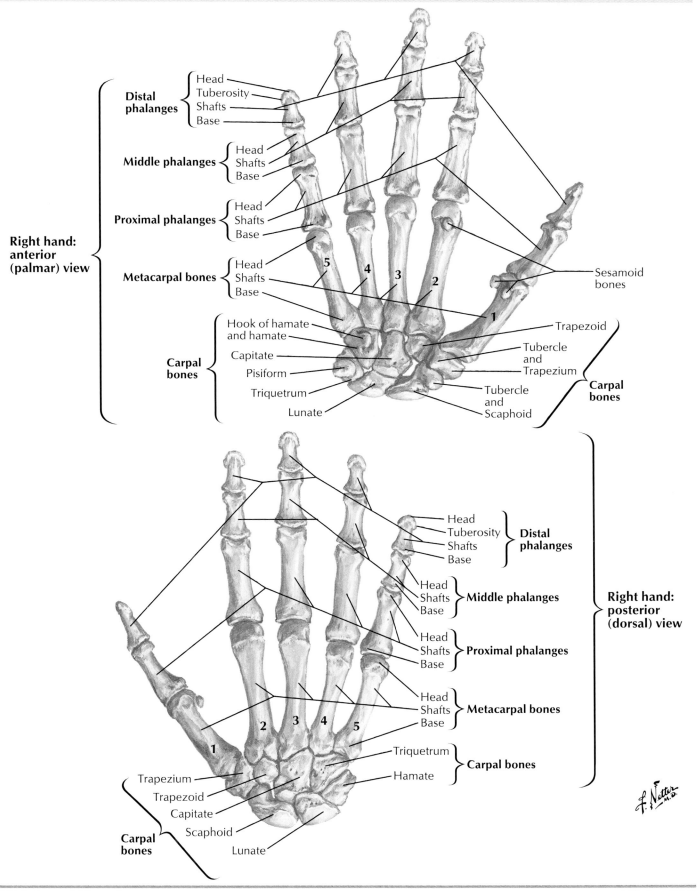

Right hand: anterior (palmar) view

Distal phalanges
- Head
- Tuberosity
- Shafts
- Base

Middle phalanges
- Head
- Shafts
- Base

Proximal phalanges
- Head
- Shafts
- Base

Metacarpal bones
- Head
- Shafts
- Base

5 4 3 2 1

Carpal bones
- Hook of hamate and hamate
- Capitate
- Pisiform
- Triquetrum
- Lunate

Sesamoid bones

Trapezoid

Tubercle and Trapezium

Tubercle and Scaphoid

Carpal bones

Distal phalanges
- Head
- Tuberosity
- Shafts
- Base

Middle phalanges
- Head
- Shafts
- Base

Proximal phalanges
- Head
- Shafts
- Base

Metacarpal bones
- Head
- Shafts
- Base

Right hand: posterior (dorsal) view

Carpal bones
- Triquetrum
- Hamate

2 3 4 5

1

Carpal bones
- Trapezium
- Trapezoid
- Capitate
- Scaphoid
- Lunate

F. Netter M.D.

See also **Plate 444**

Anteroposterior view

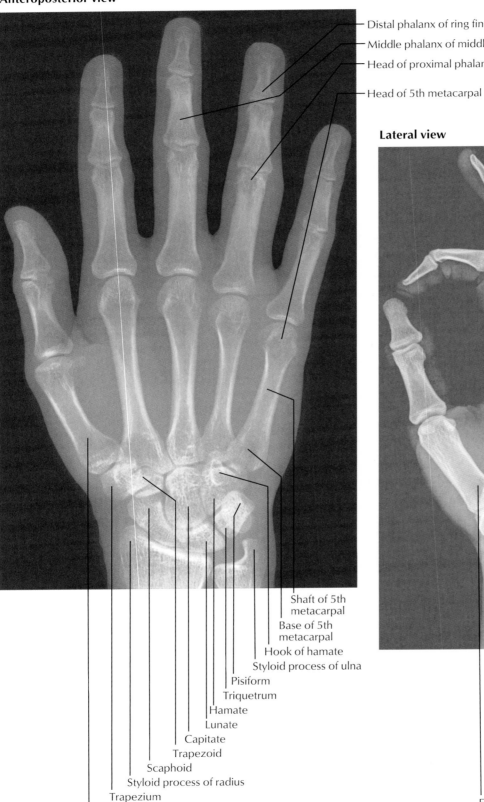

Distal phalanx of ring finger

Middle phalanx of middle finger

Head of proximal phalanx

Head of 5th metacarpal

Lateral view

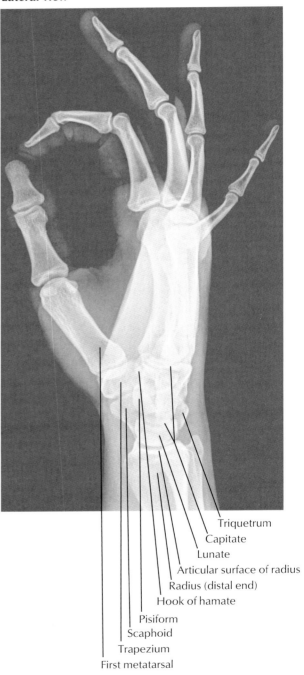

Shaft of 5th metacarpal

Base of 5th metacarpal

Hook of hamate

Styloid process of ulna

Pisiform

Triquetrum

Hamate

Lunate

Capitate

Trapezoid

Scaphoid

Styloid process of radius

Trapezium

Base of thumb metacarpal

Triquetrum

Capitate

Lunate

Articular surface of radius

Radius (distal end)

Hook of hamate

Pisiform

Scaphoid

Trapezium

First metatarsal

Plate 445

Wrist and Hand

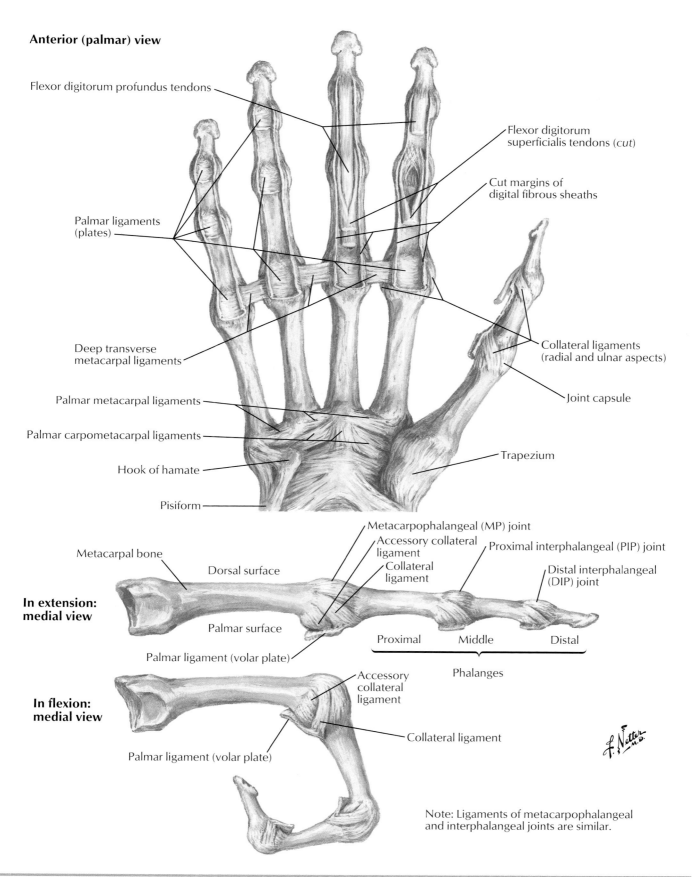

Anterior (palmar) view

Flexor digitorum profundus tendons

Flexor digitorum superficialis tendons (*cut*)

Cut margins of digital fibrous sheaths

Palmar ligaments (plates)

Collateral ligaments (radial and ulnar aspects)

Deep transverse metacarpal ligaments

Joint capsule

Palmar metacarpal ligaments

Palmar carpometacarpal ligaments

Hook of hamate

Trapezium

Pisiform

In extension: medial view

Metacarpal bone

Dorsal surface

Metacarpophalangeal (MP) joint

Accessory collateral ligament

Collateral ligament

Proximal interphalangeal (PIP) joint

Distal interphalangeal (DIP) joint

Palmar surface

Palmar ligament (volar plate)

Proximal   Middle   Distal

Phalanges

In flexion: medial view

Accessory collateral ligament

Collateral ligament

Palmar ligament (volar plate)

Note: Ligaments of metacarpophalangeal and interphalangeal joints are similar.

Anterior (palmar) views

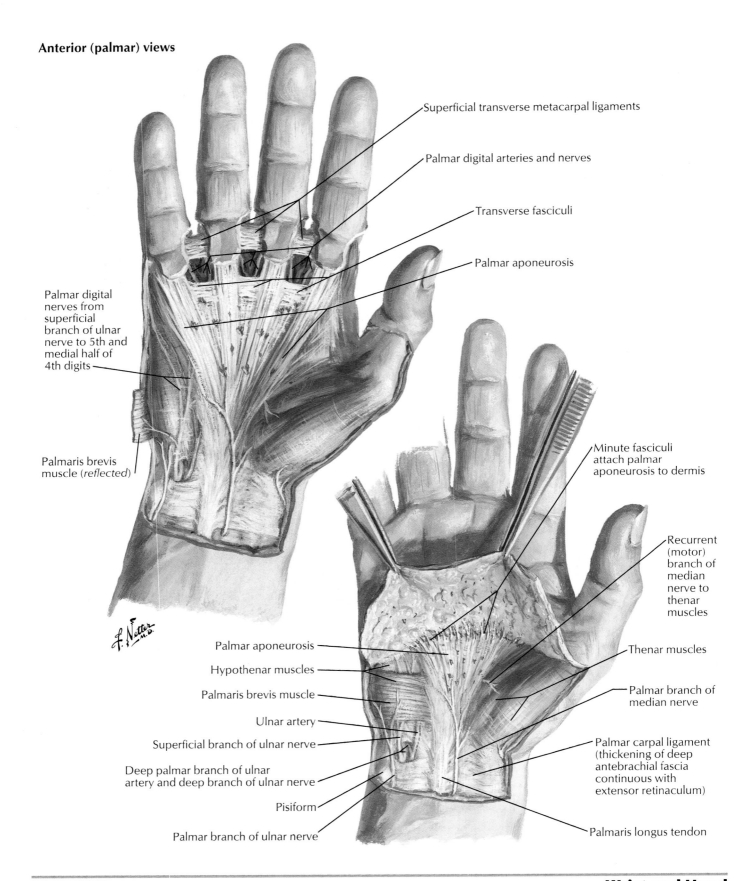

Superficial transverse metacarpal ligaments

Palmar digital arteries and nerves

Transverse fasciculi

Palmar aponeurosis

Palmar digital nerves from superficial branch of ulnar nerve to 5th and medial half of 4th digits

Palmaris brevis muscle (*reflected*)

Minute fasciculi attach palmar aponeurosis to dermis

Recurrent (motor) branch of median nerve to thenar muscles

Thenar muscles

Palmar branch of median nerve

Palmar carpal ligament (thickening of deep antebrachial fascia continuous with extensor retinaculum)

Palmaris longus tendon

Palmar aponeurosis

Hypothenar muscles

Palmaris brevis muscle

Ulnar artery

Superficial branch of ulnar nerve

Deep palmar branch of ulnar artery and deep branch of ulnar nerve

Pisiform

Palmar branch of ulnar nerve

Plate 447 **Wrist and Hand**

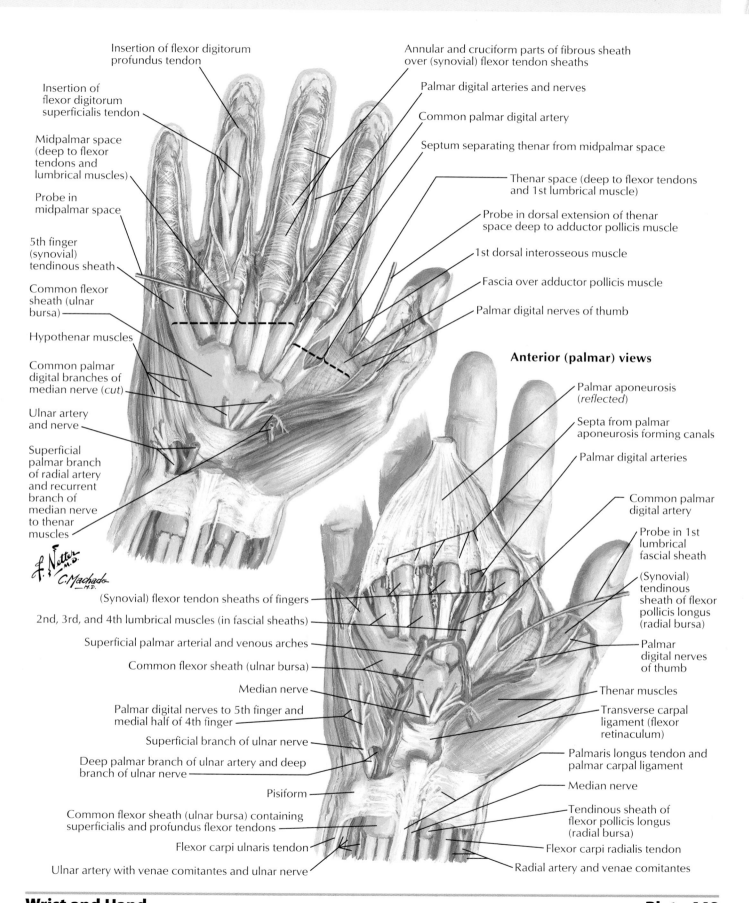

Insertion of flexor digitorum profundus tendon

Insertion of flexor digitorum superficialis tendon

Midpalmar space (deep to flexor tendons and lumbrical muscles)

Probe in midpalmar space

5th finger (synovial) tendinous sheath

Common flexor sheath (ulnar bursa)

Hypothenar muscles

Common palmar digital branches of median nerve (cut)

Ulnar artery and nerve

Superficial palmar branch of radial artery and recurrent branch of median nerve to thenar muscles

Annular and cruciform parts of fibrous sheath over (synovial) flexor tendon sheaths

Palmar digital arteries and nerves

Common palmar digital artery

Septum separating thenar from midpalmar space

Thenar space (deep to flexor tendons and 1st lumbrical muscle)

Probe in dorsal extension of thenar space deep to adductor pollicis muscle

1st dorsal interosseous muscle

Fascia over adductor pollicis muscle

Palmar digital nerves of thumb

Anterior (palmar) views

Palmar aponeurosis (*reflected*)

Septa from palmar aponeurosis forming canals

Palmar digital arteries

Common palmar digital artery

Probe in 1st lumbrical fascial sheath

(Synovial) tendinous sheath of flexor pollicis longus (radial bursa)

Palmar digital nerves of thumb

Thenar muscles

Transverse carpal ligament (flexor retinaculum)

Palmaris longus tendon and palmar carpal ligament

Median nerve

Tendinous sheath of flexor pollicis longus (radial bursa)

Flexor carpi radialis tendon

Radial artery and venae comitantes

(Synovial) flexor tendon sheaths of fingers

2nd, 3rd, and 4th lumbrical muscles (in fascial sheaths)

Superficial palmar arterial and venous arches

Common flexor sheath (ulnar bursa)

Median nerve

Palmar digital nerves to 5th finger and medial half of 4th finger

Superficial branch of ulnar nerve

Deep palmar branch of ulnar artery and deep branch of ulnar nerve

Pisiform

Common flexor sheath (ulnar bursa) containing superficialis and profundus flexor tendons

Flexor carpi ulnaris tendon

Ulnar artery with venae comitantes and ulnar nerve

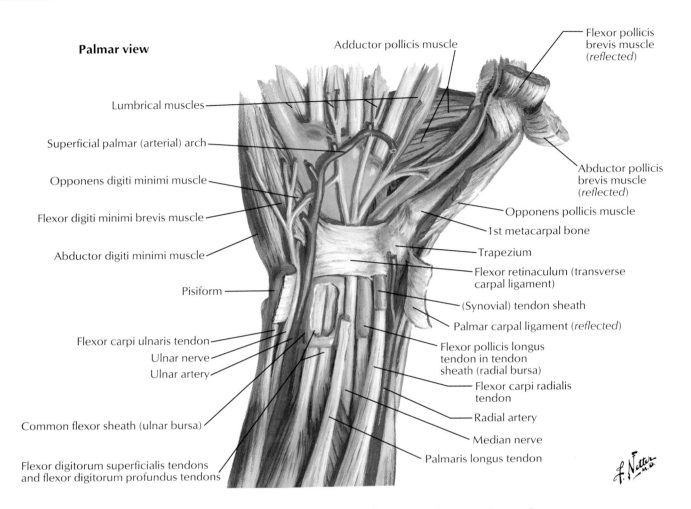

Palmar view

Adductor pollicis muscle

Flexor pollicis brevis muscle (*reflected*)

Lumbrical muscles

Superficial palmar (arterial) arch

Opponens digiti minimi muscle

Flexor digiti minimi brevis muscle

Abductor digiti minimi muscle

Abductor pollicis brevis muscle (*reflected*)

Opponens pollicis muscle

1st metacarpal bone

Trapezium

Flexor retinaculum (transverse carpal ligament)

(Synovial) tendon sheath

Palmar carpal ligament (*reflected*)

Flexor pollicis longus tendon in tendon sheath (radial bursa)

Flexor carpi radialis tendon

Radial artery

Median nerve

Palmaris longus tendon

Pisiform

Flexor carpi ulnaris tendon

Ulnar nerve

Ulnar artery

Common flexor sheath (ulnar bursa)

Flexor digitorum superficialis tendons and flexor digitorum profundus tendons

Transverse cross section of wrist demonstrating carpal tunnel

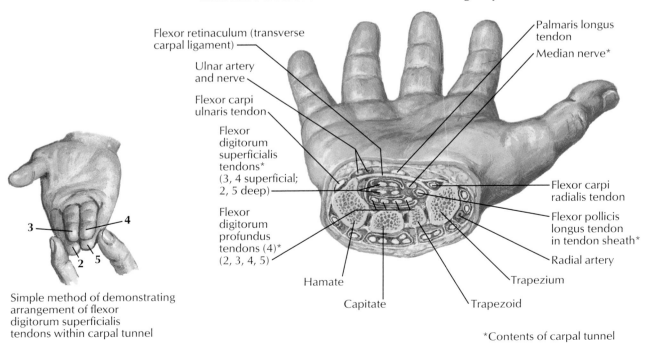

Flexor retinaculum (transverse carpal ligament)

Palmaris longus tendon

Median nerve*

Ulnar artery and nerve

Flexor carpi ulnaris tendon

Flexor digitorum superficialis tendons* (3, 4 superficial; 2, 5 deep)

Flexor digitorum profundus tendons (4)* (2, 3, 4, 5)

Flexor carpi radialis tendon

Flexor pollicis longus tendon in tendon sheath*

Radial artery

Trapezium

Trapezoid

Capitate

Hamate

3

4

2 5

Simple method of demonstrating arrangement of flexor digitorum superficialis tendons within carpal tunnel

*Contents of carpal tunnel

Plate 449

Wrist and Hand

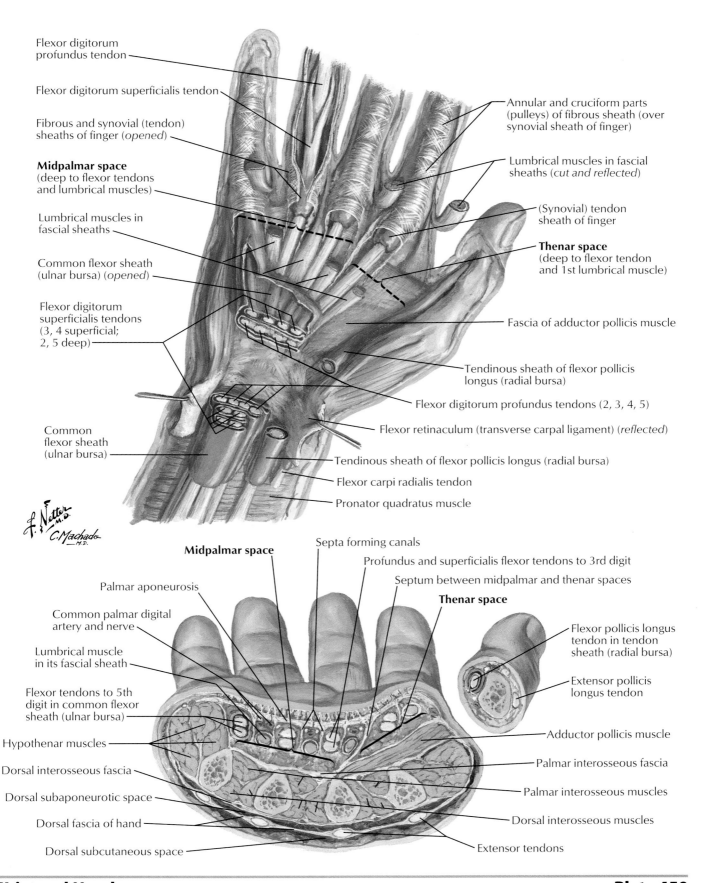

Flexor digitorum profundus tendon

Flexor digitorum superficialis tendon

Fibrous and synovial (tendon) sheaths of finger (*opened*)

Midpalmar space (deep to flexor tendons and lumbrical muscles)

Lumbrical muscles in fascial sheaths

Common flexor sheath (ulnar bursa) (*opened*)

Flexor digitorum superficialis tendons (3, 4 superficial; 2, 5 deep)

Common flexor sheath (ulnar bursa)

Annular and cruciform parts (pulleys) of fibrous sheath (over synovial sheath of finger)

Lumbrical muscles in fascial sheaths (*cut and reflected*)

(Synovial) tendon sheath of finger

Thenar space (deep to flexor tendon and 1st lumbrical muscle)

Fascia of adductor pollicis muscle

Tendinous sheath of flexor pollicis longus (radial bursa)

Flexor digitorum profundus tendons (2, 3, 4, 5)

Flexor retinaculum (transverse carpal ligament) (*reflected*)

Tendinous sheath of flexor pollicis longus (radial bursa)

Flexor carpi radialis tendon

Pronator quadratus muscle

Septa forming canals

Profundus and superficialis flexor tendons to 3rd digit

Septum between midpalmar and thenar spaces

Midpalmar space

Thenar space

Palmar aponeurosis

Common palmar digital artery and nerve

Lumbrical muscle in its fascial sheath

Flexor tendons to 5th digit in common flexor sheath (ulnar bursa)

Hypothenar muscles

Dorsal interosseous fascia

Dorsal subaponeurotic space

Dorsal fascia of hand

Dorsal subcutaneous space

Flexor pollicis longus tendon in tendon sheath (radial bursa)

Extensor pollicis longus tendon

Adductor pollicis muscle

Palmar interosseous fascia

Palmar interosseous muscles

Dorsal interosseous muscles

Extensor tendons

Lumbrical Muscles and Bursae, Spaces, and Sheaths: Schema

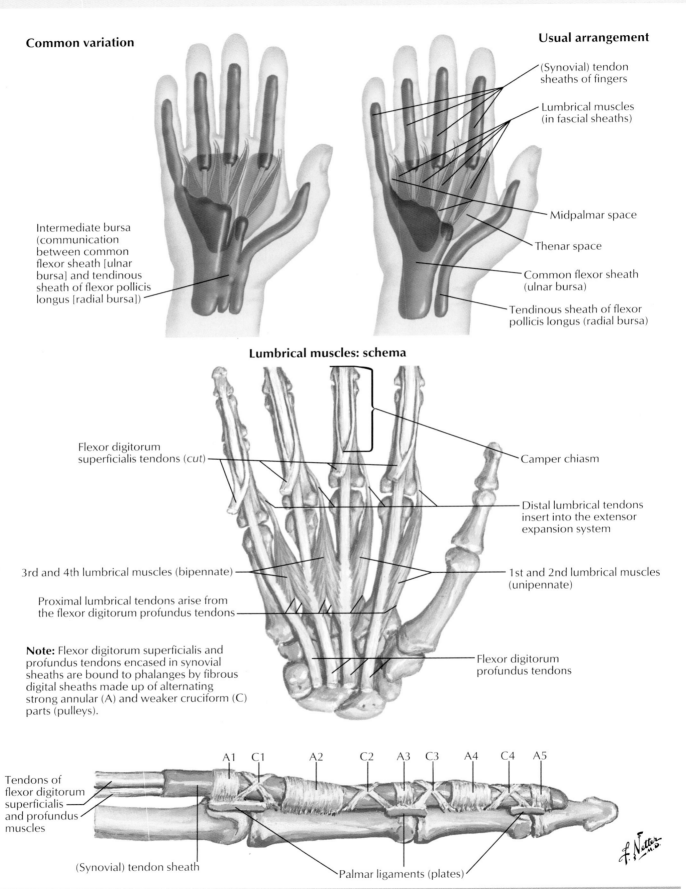

Common variation

Usual arrangement

(Synovial) tendon sheaths of fingers

Lumbrical muscles (in fascial sheaths)

Intermediate bursa (communication between common flexor sheath [ulnar bursa] and tendinous sheath of flexor pollicis longus [radial bursa])

Midpalmar space

Thenar space

Common flexor sheath (ulnar bursa)

Tendinous sheath of flexor pollicis longus (radial bursa)

Lumbrical muscles: schema

Flexor digitorum superficialis tendons (*cut*)

Camper chiasm

Distal lumbrical tendons insert into the extensor expansion system

3rd and 4th lumbrical muscles (bipennate)

1st and 2nd lumbrical muscles (unipennate)

Proximal lumbrical tendons arise from the flexor digitorum profundus tendons

Flexor digitorum profundus tendons

Note: Flexor digitorum superficialis and profundus tendons encased in synovial sheaths are bound to phalanges by fibrous digital sheaths made up of alternating strong annular (A) and weaker cruciform (C) parts (pulleys).

A1 C1 A2 C2 A3 C3 A4 C4 A5

Tendons of flexor digitorum superficialis and profundus muscles

(Synovial) tendon sheath

Palmar ligaments (plates)

f. Netter

Plate 451   **Wrist and Hand**

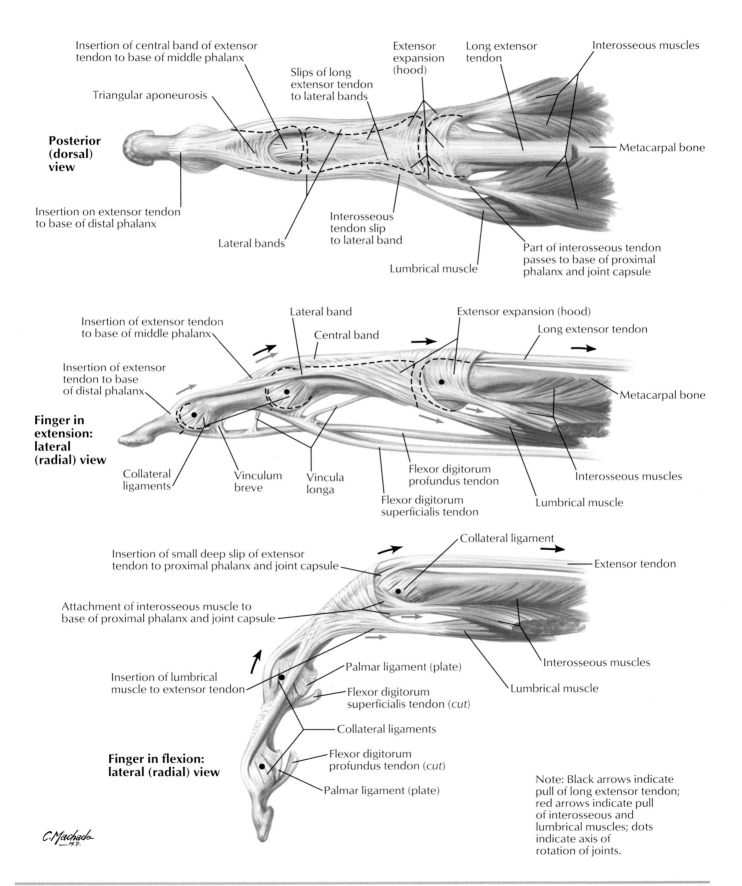

Posterior (dorsal) view

Insertion of central band of extensor tendon to base of middle phalanx

Triangular aponeurosis

Slips of long extensor tendon to lateral bands

Extensor expansion (hood)

Long extensor tendon

Interosseous muscles

Metacarpal bone

Insertion on extensor tendon to base of distal phalanx

Lateral bands

Interosseous tendon slip to lateral band

Lumbrical muscle

Part of interosseous tendon passes to base of proximal phalanx and joint capsule

Finger in extension: lateral (radial) view

Insertion of extensor tendon to base of middle phalanx

Insertion of extensor tendon to base of distal phalanx

Lateral band

Central band

Extensor expansion (hood)

Long extensor tendon

Metacarpal bone

Collateral ligaments

Vinculum breve

Vincula longa

Flexor digitorum profundus tendon

Flexor digitorum superficialis tendon

Interosseous muscles

Lumbrical muscle

Finger in flexion: lateral (radial) view

Insertion of small deep slip of extensor tendon to proximal phalanx and joint capsule

Attachment of interosseous muscle to base of proximal phalanx and joint capsule

Insertion of lumbrical muscle to extensor tendon

Collateral ligament

Extensor tendon

Palmar ligament (plate)

Flexor digitorum superficialis tendon (*cut*)

Collateral ligaments

Flexor digitorum profundus tendon (*cut*)

Palmar ligament (plate)

Interosseous muscles

Lumbrical muscle

Note: Black arrows indicate pull of long extensor tendon; red arrows indicate pull of interosseous and lumbrical muscles; dots indicate axis of rotation of joints.

C. Machado —M.D.

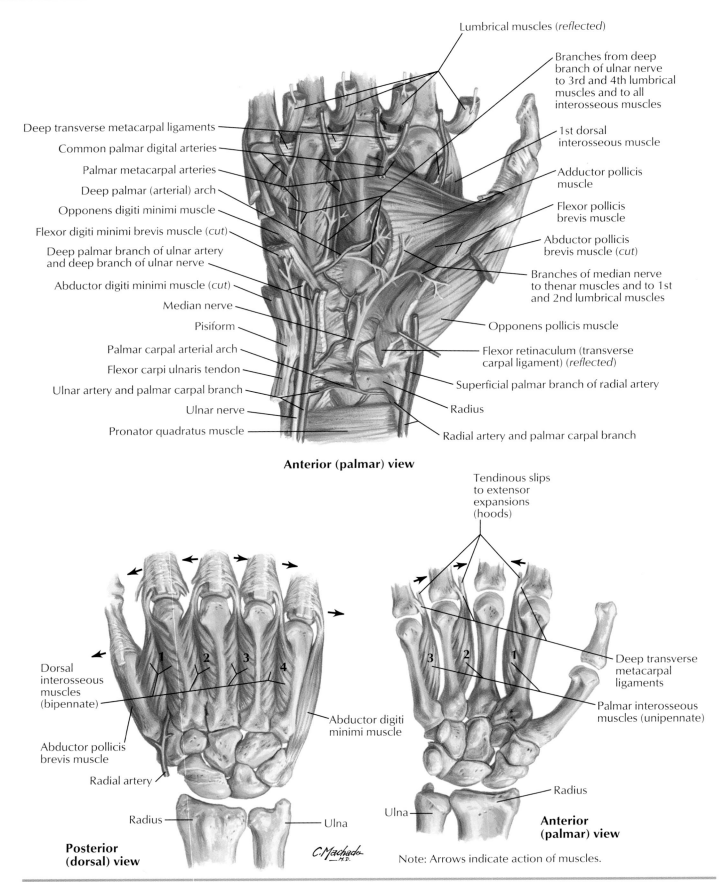

Lumbrical muscles (*reflected*)

Branches from deep branch of ulnar nerve to 3rd and 4th lumbrical muscles and to all interosseous muscles

1st dorsal interosseous muscle

Adductor pollicis muscle

Flexor pollicis brevis muscle

Abductor pollicis brevis muscle (*cut*)

Branches of median nerve to thenar muscles and to 1st and 2nd lumbrical muscles

Opponens pollicis muscle

Flexor retinaculum (transverse carpal ligament) (*reflected*)

Superficial palmar branch of radial artery

Radius

Radial artery and palmar carpal branch

Deep transverse metacarpal ligaments

Common palmar digital arteries

Palmar metacarpal arteries

Deep palmar (arterial) arch

Opponens digiti minimi muscle

Flexor digiti minimi brevis muscle (*cut*)

Deep palmar branch of ulnar artery and deep branch of ulnar nerve

Abductor digiti minimi muscle (*cut*)

Median nerve

Pisiform

Palmar carpal arterial arch

Flexor carpi ulnaris tendon

Ulnar artery and palmar carpal branch

Ulnar nerve

Pronator quadratus muscle

Anterior (palmar) view

Tendinous slips to extensor expansions (hoods)

Deep transverse metacarpal ligaments

Palmar interosseous muscles (unipennate)

Dorsal interosseous muscles (bipennate)

Abductor pollicis brevis muscle

Radial artery

Abductor digiti minimi muscle

Radius

Ulna

Posterior (dorsal) view

Ulna

Radius

Anterior (palmar) view

Note: Arrows indicate action of muscles.

C. Machado M.D.

Plate 453   **Wrist and Hand**

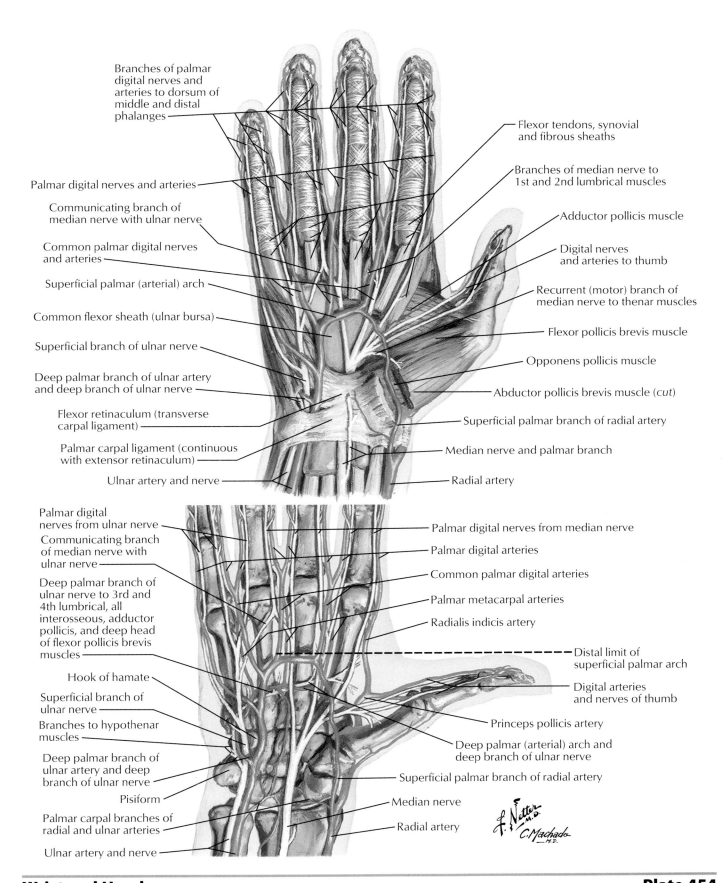

Branches of palmar digital nerves and arteries to dorsum of middle and distal phalanges

Palmar digital nerves and arteries

Communicating branch of median nerve with ulnar nerve

Common palmar digital nerves and arteries

Superficial palmar (arterial) arch

Common flexor sheath (ulnar bursa)

Superficial branch of ulnar nerve

Deep palmar branch of ulnar artery and deep branch of ulnar nerve

Flexor retinaculum (transverse carpal ligament)

Palmar carpal ligament (continuous with extensor retinaculum)

Ulnar artery and nerve

Flexor tendons, synovial and fibrous sheaths

Branches of median nerve to 1st and 2nd lumbrical muscles

Adductor pollicis muscle

Digital nerves and arteries to thumb

Recurrent (motor) branch of median nerve to thenar muscles

Flexor pollicis brevis muscle

Opponens pollicis muscle

Abductor pollicis brevis muscle (*cut*)

Superficial palmar branch of radial artery

Median nerve and palmar branch

Radial artery

Palmar digital nerves from ulnar nerve

Communicating branch of median nerve with ulnar nerve

Deep palmar branch of ulnar nerve to 3rd and 4th lumbrical, all interosseous, adductor pollicis, and deep head of flexor pollicis brevis muscles

Hook of hamate

Superficial branch of ulnar nerve

Branches to hypothenar muscles

Deep palmar branch of ulnar artery and deep branch of ulnar nerve

Pisiform

Palmar carpal branches of radial and ulnar arteries

Ulnar artery and nerve

Palmar digital nerves from median nerve

Palmar digital arteries

Common palmar digital arteries

Palmar metacarpal arteries

Radialis indicis artery

Distal limit of superficial palmar arch

Digital arteries and nerves of thumb

Princeps pollicis artery

Deep palmar (arterial) arch and deep branch of ulnar nerve

Superficial palmar branch of radial artery

Median nerve

Radial artery

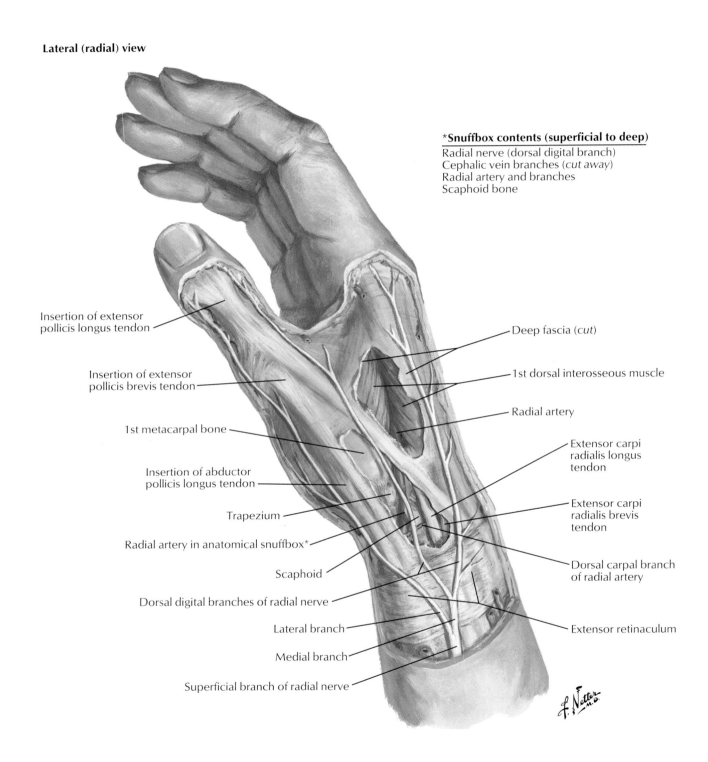

Lateral (radial) view

*Snuffbox contents (superficial to deep)
Radial nerve (dorsal digital branch)
Cephalic vein branches (*cut away*)
Radial artery and branches
Scaphoid bone

Insertion of extensor
pollicis longus tendon

Insertion of extensor
pollicis brevis tendon

1st metacarpal bone

Insertion of abductor
pollicis longus tendon

Trapezium

Radial artery in anatomical snuffbox*

Scaphoid

Dorsal digital branches of radial nerve

Lateral branch

Medial branch

Superficial branch of radial nerve

Deep fascia (*cut*)

1st dorsal interosseous muscle

Radial artery

Extensor carpi
radialis longus
tendon

Extensor carpi
radialis brevis
tendon

Dorsal carpal branch
of radial artery

Extensor retinaculum

Plate 455

Wrist and Hand

Posterior (dorsal) view

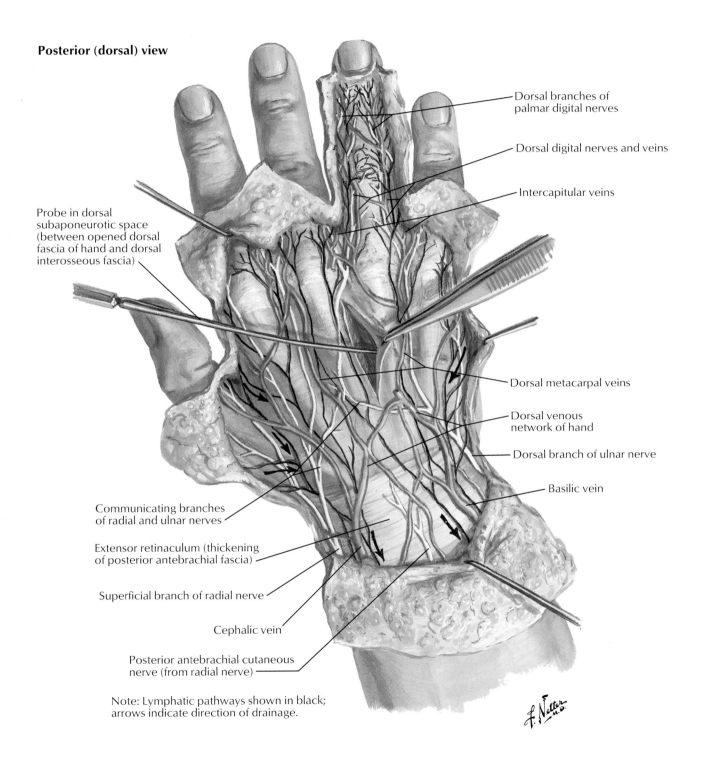

Dorsal branches of
palmar digital nerves

Dorsal digital nerves and veins

Intercapitular veins

Probe in dorsal
subaponeurotic space
(between opened dorsal
fascia of hand and dorsal
interosseous fascia)

Dorsal metacarpal veins

Dorsal venous
network of hand

Dorsal branch of ulnar nerve

Basilic vein

Communicating branches
of radial and ulnar nerves

Extensor retinaculum (thickening
of posterior antebrachial fascia)

Superficial branch of radial nerve

Cephalic vein

Posterior antebrachial cutaneous
nerve (from radial nerve)

Note: Lymphatic pathways shown in black;
arrows indicate direction of drainage.

f. Netter M.D.

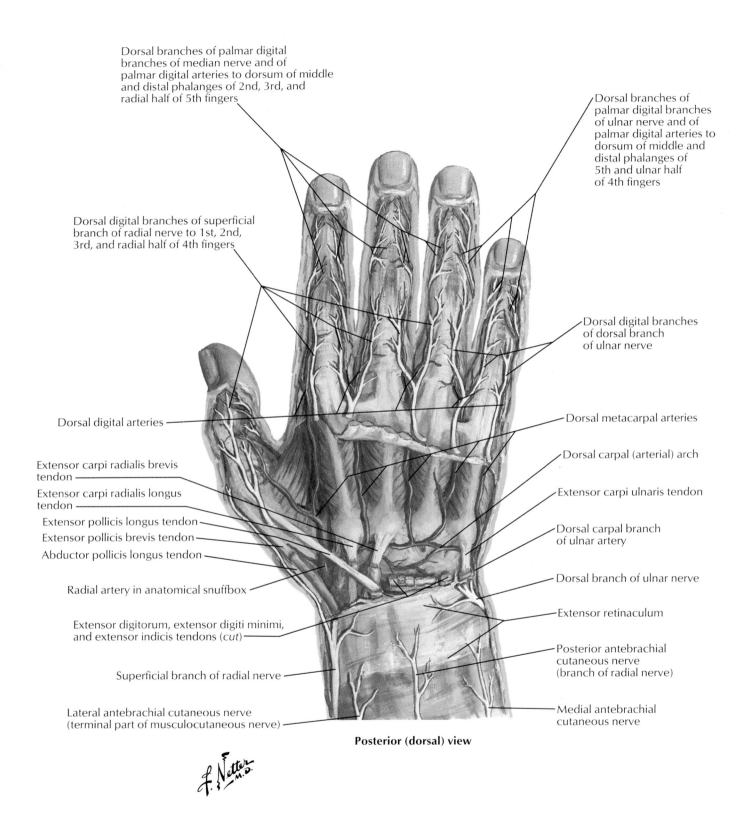

Dorsal branches of palmar digital branches of median nerve and of palmar digital arteries to dorsum of middle and distal phalanges of 2nd, 3rd, and radial half of 5th fingers

Dorsal branches of palmar digital branches of ulnar nerve and of palmar digital arteries to dorsum of middle and distal phalanges of 5th and ulnar half of 4th fingers

Dorsal digital branches of superficial branch of radial nerve to 1st, 2nd, 3rd, and radial half of 4th fingers

Dorsal digital branches of dorsal branch of ulnar nerve

Dorsal digital arteries

Dorsal metacarpal arteries

Extensor carpi radialis brevis tendon

Dorsal carpal (arterial) arch

Extensor carpi radialis longus tendon

Extensor carpi ulnaris tendon

Extensor pollicis longus tendon

Dorsal carpal branch of ulnar artery

Extensor pollicis brevis tendon

Abductor pollicis longus tendon

Radial artery in anatomical snuffbox

Dorsal branch of ulnar nerve

Extensor retinaculum

Extensor digitorum, extensor digiti minimi, and extensor indicis tendons (*cut*)

Posterior antebrachial cutaneous nerve (branch of radial nerve)

Superficial branch of radial nerve

Lateral antebrachial cutaneous nerve (terminal part of musculocutaneous nerve)

Medial antebrachial cutaneous nerve

Posterior (dorsal) view

Plate 457 **Wrist and Hand**

Posterior (dorsal) view

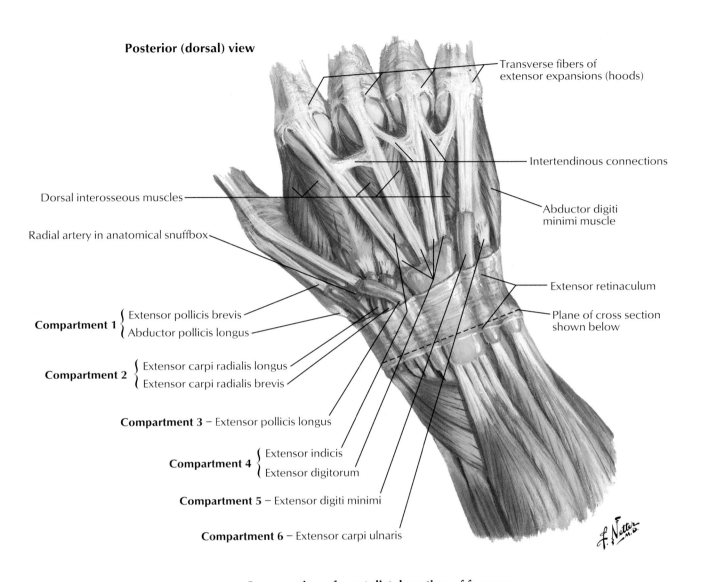

Transverse fibers of
extensor expansions (hoods)

Intertendinous connections

Dorsal interosseous muscles

Abductor digiti
minimi muscle

Radial artery in anatomical snuffbox

Extensor retinaculum

Plane of cross section
shown below

Compartment 1 { Extensor pollicis brevis
Abductor pollicis longus

Compartment 2 { Extensor carpi radialis longus
Extensor carpi radialis brevis

Compartment 3 – Extensor pollicis longus

Compartment 4 { Extensor indicis
Extensor digitorum

Compartment 5 – Extensor digiti minimi

Compartment 6 – Extensor carpi ulnaris

Cross section of most distal portion of forearm

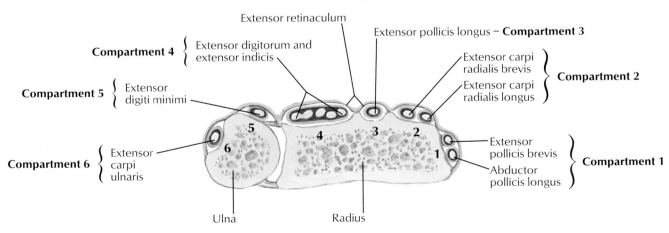

Extensor retinaculum

Extensor pollicis longus – **Compartment 3**

Compartment 4 { Extensor digitorum and
extensor indicis

Extensor carpi
radialis brevis

Extensor carpi
radialis longus

Compartment 2

Compartment 5 { Extensor
digiti minimi

Extensor
pollicis brevis

Compartment 6 { Extensor
carpi
ulnaris

Abductor
pollicis longus

Compartment 1

Ulna

Radius

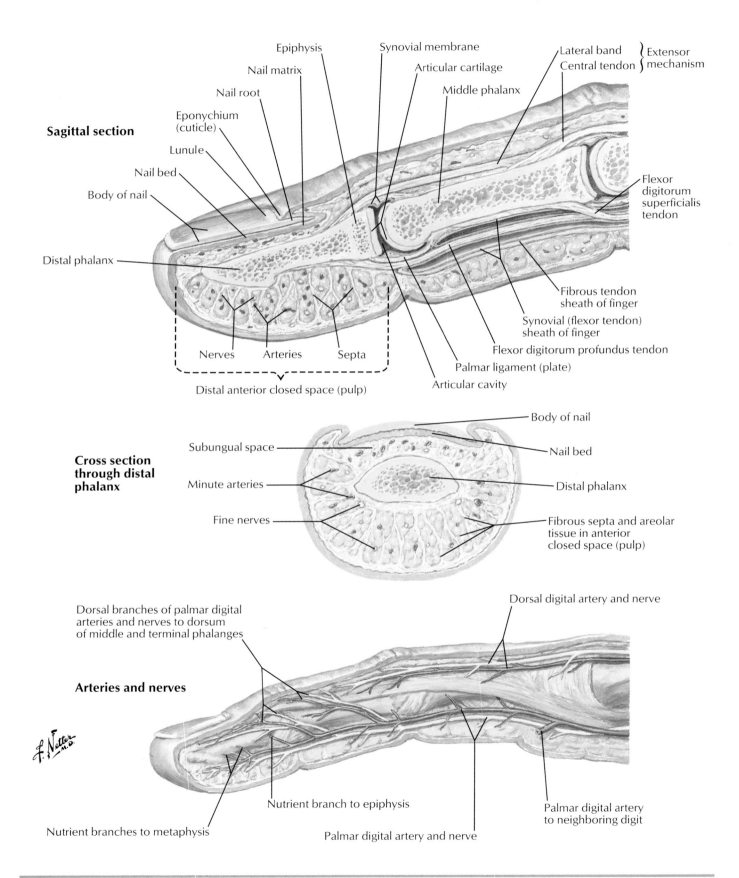

Sagittal section

Epiphysis

Nail matrix

Nail root

Eponychium (cuticle)

Lunule

Nail bed

Body of nail

Distal phalanx

Synovial membrane

Articular cartilage

Middle phalanx

Lateral band ⎫ Extensor
Central tendon ⎬ mechanism

Flexor digitorum superficialis tendon

Fibrous tendon sheath of finger

Synovial (flexor tendon) sheath of finger

Flexor digitorum profundus tendon

Palmar ligament (plate)

Articular cavity

Nerves   Arteries   Septa

Distal anterior closed space (pulp)

Cross section through distal phalanx

Subungual space

Minute arteries

Fine nerves

Body of nail

Nail bed

Distal phalanx

Fibrous septa and areolar tissue in anterior closed space (pulp)

Arteries and nerves

Dorsal branches of palmar digital arteries and nerves to dorsum of middle and terminal phalanges

Dorsal digital artery and nerve

Nutrient branches to metaphysis

Nutrient branch to epiphysis

Palmar digital artery and nerve

Palmar digital artery to neighboring digit

Plate 459   **Wrist and Hand**

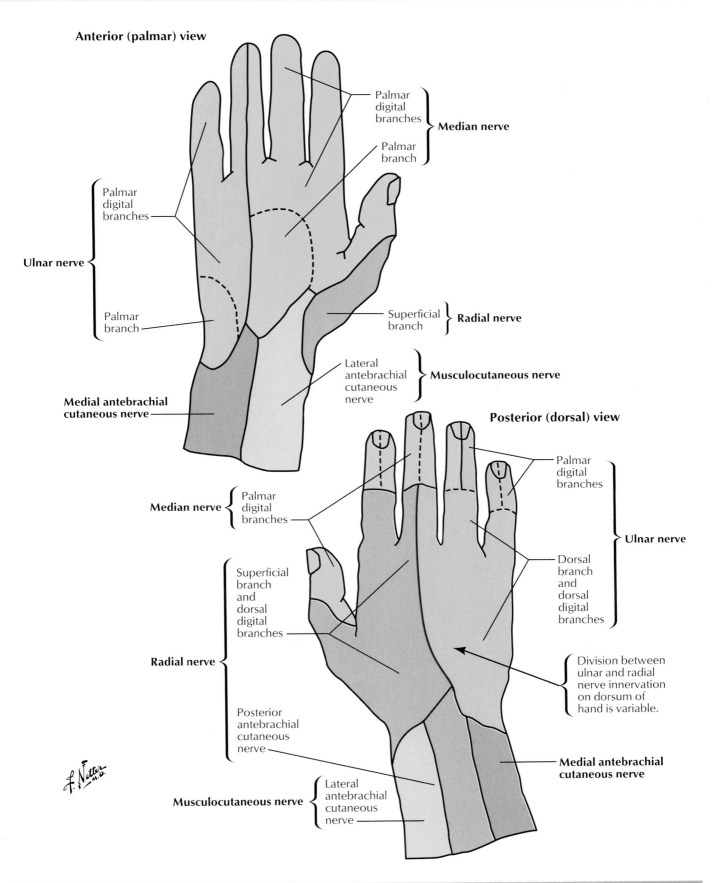

Anterior (palmar) view

Palmar
digital
branches

Median nerve

Palmar
branch

Palmar
digital
branches

Ulnar nerve

Palmar
branch

Superficial
branch

Radial nerve

Lateral
antebrachial
cutaneous
nerve

Musculocutaneous nerve

Medial antebrachial
cutaneous nerve

Posterior (dorsal) view

Median nerve

Palmar
digital
branches

Palmar
digital
branches

Ulnar nerve

Superficial
branch
and
dorsal
digital
branches

Dorsal
branch
and
dorsal
digital
branches

Radial nerve

Division between
ulnar and radial
nerve innervation
on dorsum of
hand is variable.

Posterior
antebrachial
cutaneous
nerve

Medial antebrachial
cutaneous nerve

Lateral
antebrachial
cutaneous
nerve

Musculocutaneous nerve

Anterior view

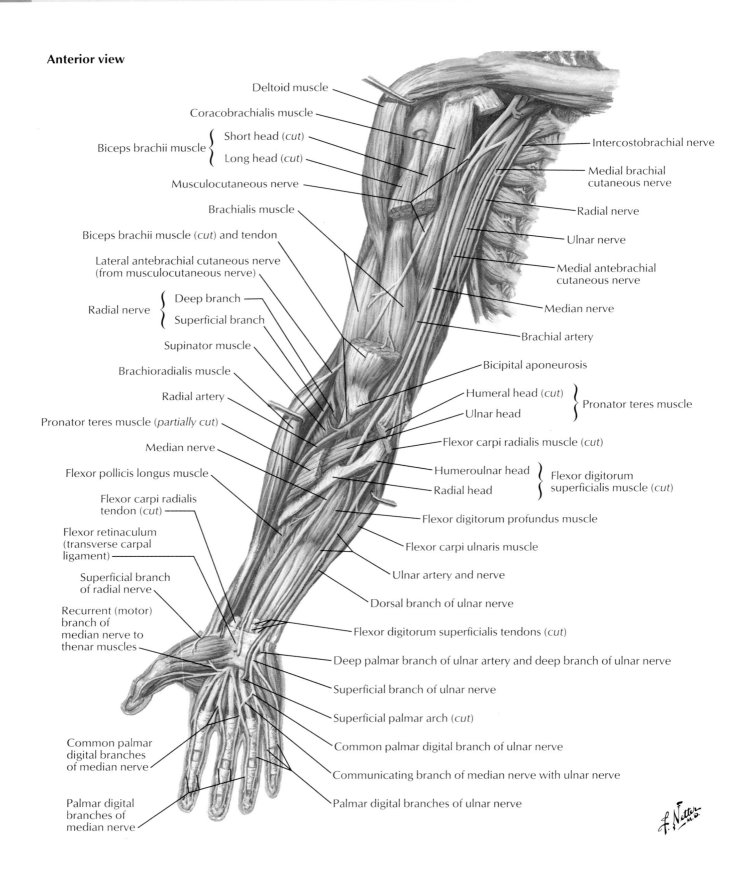

Deltoid muscle

Coracobrachialis muscle

Biceps brachii muscle {
Short head (*cut*)
Long head (*cut*)

Musculocutaneous nerve

Brachialis muscle

Biceps brachii muscle (*cut*) and tendon

Lateral antebrachial cutaneous nerve (from musculocutaneous nerve)

Radial nerve {
Deep branch
Superficial branch

Supinator muscle

Brachioradialis muscle

Radial artery

Pronator teres muscle (*partially cut*)

Median nerve

Flexor pollicis longus muscle

Flexor carpi radialis tendon (*cut*)

Flexor retinaculum (transverse carpal ligament)

Superficial branch of radial nerve

Recurrent (motor) branch of median nerve to thenar muscles

Common palmar digital branches of median nerve

Palmar digital branches of median nerve

Intercostobrachial nerve

Medial brachial cutaneous nerve

Radial nerve

Ulnar nerve

Medial antebrachial cutaneous nerve

Median nerve

Brachial artery

Bicipital aponeurosis

Humeral head (*cut*)
Ulnar head } Pronator teres muscle

Flexor carpi radialis muscle (*cut*)

Humeroulnar head
Radial head } Flexor digitorum superficialis muscle (*cut*)

Flexor digitorum profundus muscle

Flexor carpi ulnaris muscle

Ulnar artery and nerve

Dorsal branch of ulnar nerve

Flexor digitorum superficialis tendons (*cut*)

Deep palmar branch of ulnar artery and deep branch of ulnar nerve

Superficial branch of ulnar nerve

Superficial palmar arch (*cut*)

Common palmar digital branch of ulnar nerve

Communicating branch of median nerve with ulnar nerve

Palmar digital branches of ulnar nerve

Plate 461

Neurovasculature

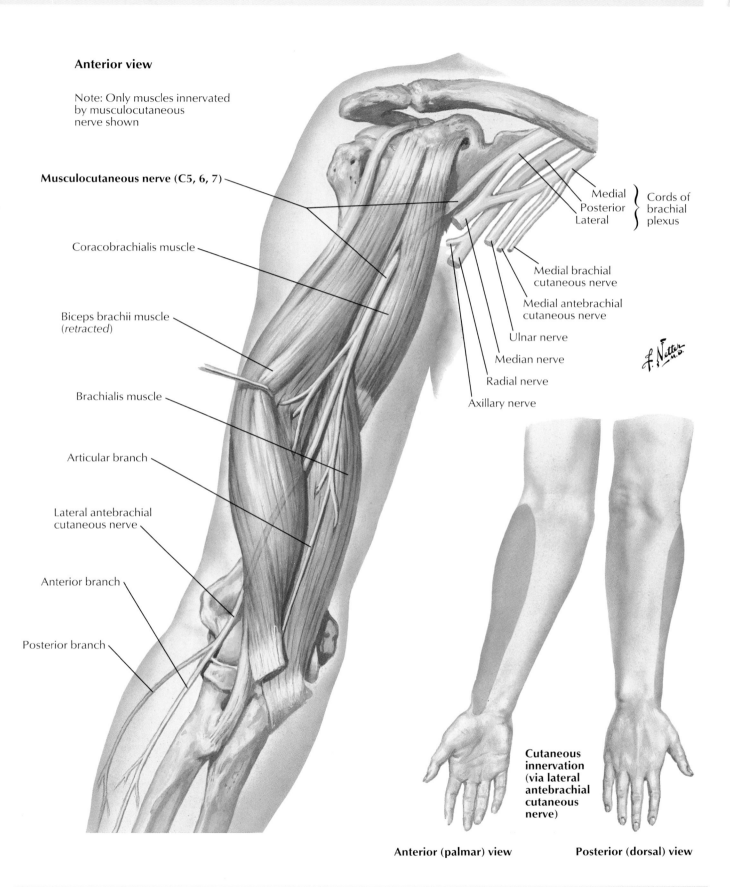

Anterior view

Note: Only muscles innervated by musculocutaneous nerve shown

Musculocutaneous nerve (C5, 6, 7)

Coracobrachialis muscle

Biceps brachii muscle (*retracted*)

Brachialis muscle

Articular branch

Lateral antebrachial cutaneous nerve

Anterior branch

Posterior branch

Medial
Posterior } Cords of brachial plexus
Lateral

Medial brachial cutaneous nerve

Medial antebrachial cutaneous nerve

Ulnar nerve

Median nerve

Radial nerve

Axillary nerve

Cutaneous innervation (via lateral antebrachial cutaneous nerve)

Anterior (palmar) view

Posterior (dorsal) view

Anterior view

Note: Only muscles innervated by median nerve shown

Musculocutaneous nerve

Median nerve (C5, 6, 7, 8, T1)
Inconstant contribution

Medial
Posterior
Lateral

Cords of
brachial
plexus

Medial brachial
cutaneous nerve

Pronator teres muscle (humeral head)

Articular branch

Medial antebrachial
cutaneous nerve

Flexor carpi radialis muscle

Palmaris longus muscle

Axillary nerve

Pronator teres muscle (ulnar head)

Radial nerve

Flexor digitorum superficialis muscle
(*turned up*)

Ulnar nerve

Flexor digitorum profundus muscle
(lateral part supplied by median
[anterior interosseous] nerve; medial
part supplied by ulnar nerve)

Anterior interosseous nerve

Flexor pollicis longus muscle

Pronator quadratus muscle

Palmar branch of median nerve

Abductor pollicis brevis

Opponens pollicis

Thenar
muscles

Superficial head of
flexor pollicis brevis
(deep head
supplied by
ulnar nerve)

Communicating branch
of median nerve with
ulnar nerve

1st and 2nd
lumbrical muscles

Common palmar
digital nerves

Palmar
digital nerves

Dorsal branches to
dorsum of middle and
distal phalanges

**Cutaneous
innervation**

Palmar view

Posterior (dorsal) view

Plate 463   **Neurovasculature**

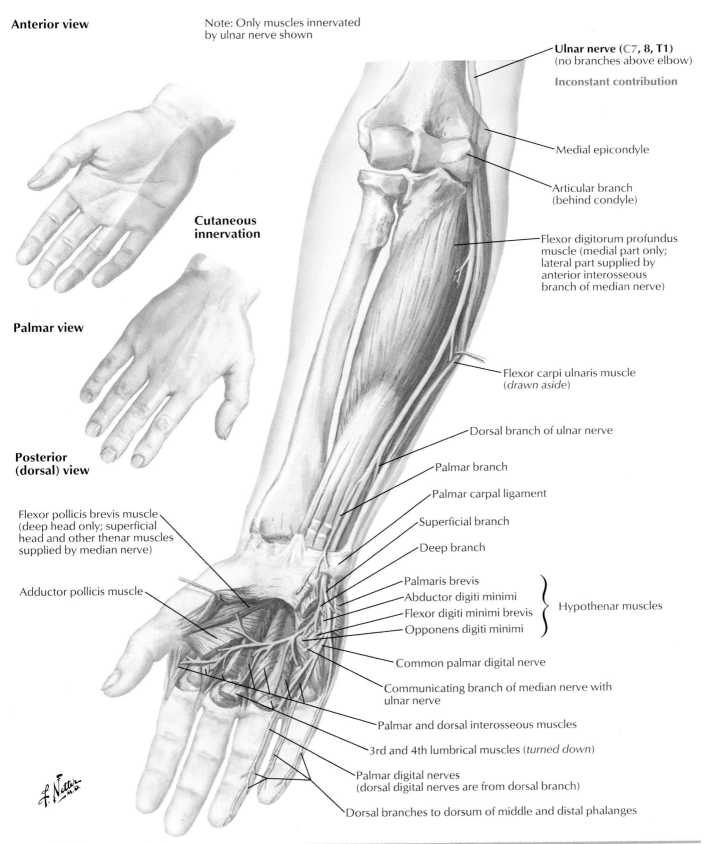

Anterior view

Note: Only muscles innervated by ulnar nerve shown

Ulnar nerve (C7, 8, T1)
(no branches above elbow)

Inconstant contribution

Medial epicondyle

Articular branch
(behind condyle)

Flexor digitorum profundus
muscle (medial part only;
lateral part supplied by
anterior interosseous
branch of median nerve)

**Cutaneous
innervation**

Palmar view

Flexor carpi ulnaris muscle
(*drawn aside*)

**Posterior
(dorsal) view**

Dorsal branch of ulnar nerve

Palmar branch

Palmar carpal ligament

Superficial branch

Deep branch

Flexor pollicis brevis muscle
(deep head only; superficial
head and other thenar muscles
supplied by median nerve)

Adductor pollicis muscle

Palmaris brevis
Abductor digiti minimi
Flexor digiti minimi brevis
Opponens digiti minimi

} Hypothenar muscles

Common palmar digital nerve

Communicating branch of median nerve with
ulnar nerve

Palmar and dorsal interosseous muscles

3rd and 4th lumbrical muscles (*turned down*)

Palmar digital nerves
(dorsal digital nerves are from dorsal branch)

Dorsal branches to dorsum of middle and distal phalanges

f. Netter.

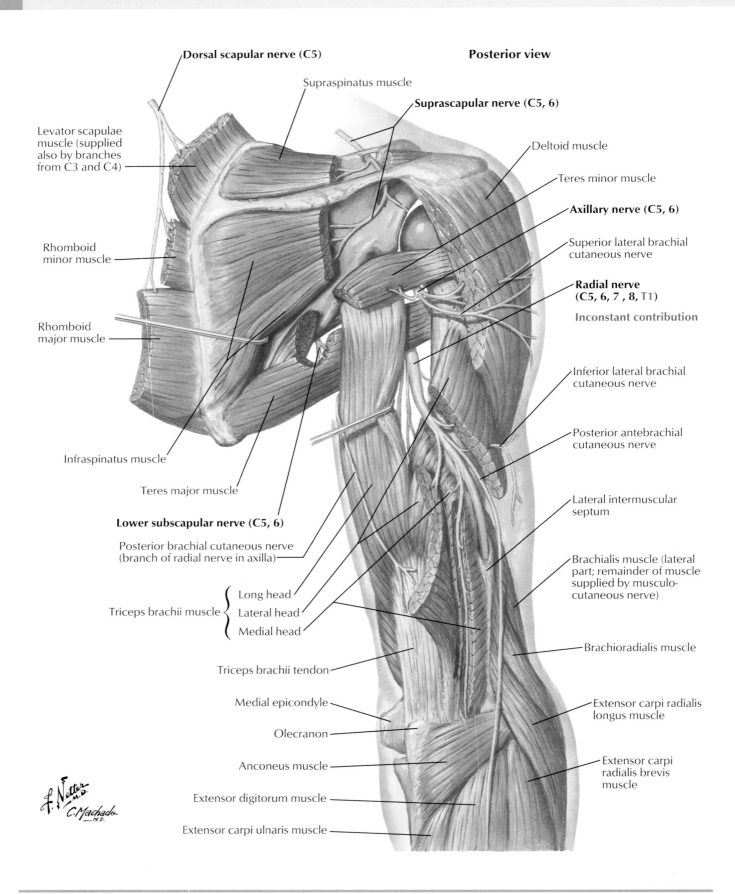

Dorsal scapular nerve (C5)

Posterior view

Supraspinatus muscle

Suprascapular nerve (C5, 6)

Levator scapulae muscle (supplied also by branches from C3 and C4)

Deltoid muscle

Teres minor muscle

Axillary nerve (C5, 6)

Superior lateral brachial cutaneous nerve

Rhomboid minor muscle

Radial nerve (C5, 6, 7 , 8, T1)

Inconstant contribution

Rhomboid major muscle

Inferior lateral brachial cutaneous nerve

Posterior antebrachial cutaneous nerve

Infraspinatus muscle

Teres major muscle

Lateral intermuscular septum

Lower subscapular nerve (C5, 6)

Brachialis muscle (lateral part; remainder of muscle supplied by musculo-cutaneous nerve)

Posterior brachial cutaneous nerve (branch of radial nerve in axilla)

Triceps brachii muscle
{
Long head
Lateral head
Medial head

Brachioradialis muscle

Triceps brachii tendon

Medial epicondyle

Extensor carpi radialis longus muscle

Olecranon

Anconeus muscle

Extensor carpi radialis brevis muscle

Extensor digitorum muscle

Extensor carpi ulnaris muscle

Plate 465

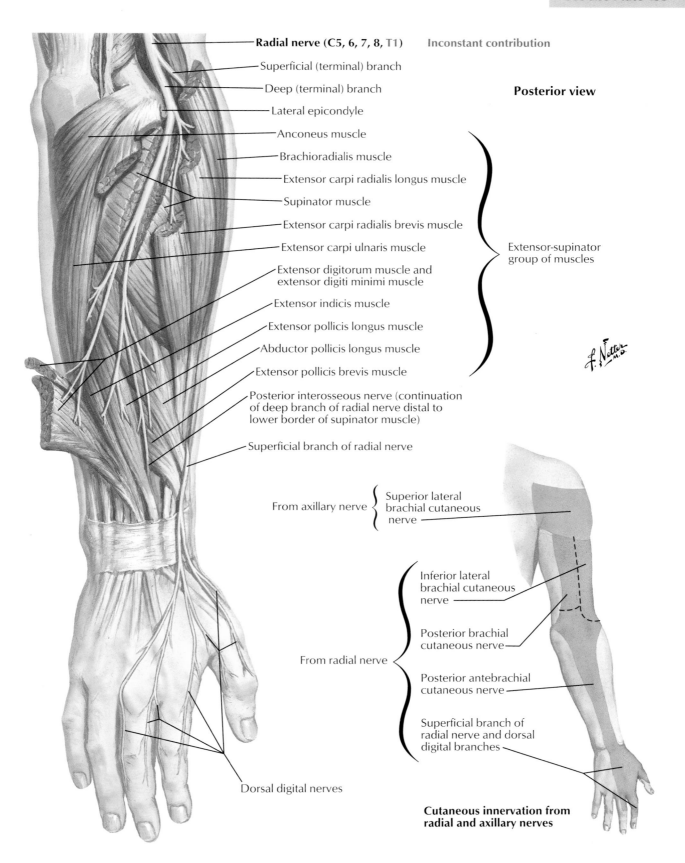

Radial nerve (C5, 6, 7, 8, T1)   Inconstant contribution

Superficial (terminal) branch

Deep (terminal) branch

Lateral epicondyle

Anconeus muscle

Brachioradialis muscle

Extensor carpi radialis longus muscle

Supinator muscle

Extensor carpi radialis brevis muscle

Extensor carpi ulnaris muscle

Extensor digitorum muscle and extensor digiti minimi muscle

Extensor indicis muscle

Extensor pollicis longus muscle

Abductor pollicis longus muscle

Extensor pollicis brevis muscle

Posterior interosseous nerve (continuation of deep branch of radial nerve distal to lower border of supinator muscle)

Superficial branch of radial nerve

Dorsal digital nerves

Posterior view

Extensor-supinator group of muscles

F. Netter M.D.

From axillary nerve {
Superior lateral brachial cutaneous nerve

Inferior lateral brachial cutaneous nerve

Posterior brachial cutaneous nerve

From radial nerve {
Posterior antebrachial cutaneous nerve

Superficial branch of radial nerve and dorsal digital branches

Cutaneous innervation from radial and axillary nerves

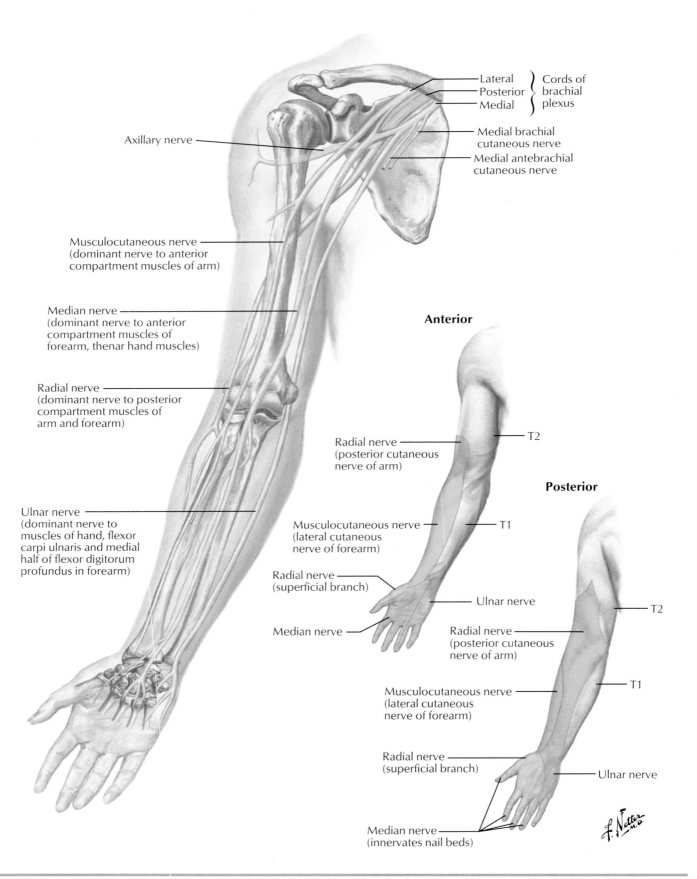

Lateral ⎫
Posterior ⎬ Cords of brachial plexus
Medial ⎭

Axillary nerve

Medial brachial cutaneous nerve

Medial antebrachial cutaneous nerve

Musculocutaneous nerve (dominant nerve to anterior compartment muscles of arm)

Median nerve (dominant nerve to anterior compartment muscles of forearm, thenar hand muscles)

Radial nerve (dominant nerve to posterior compartment muscles of arm and forearm)

Ulnar nerve (dominant nerve to muscles of hand, flexor carpi ulnaris and medial half of flexor digitorum profundus in forearm)

Anterior

Radial nerve (posterior cutaneous nerve of arm)

T2

Musculocutaneous nerve (lateral cutaneous nerve of forearm)

T1

Radial nerve (superficial branch)

Ulnar nerve

Median nerve

Posterior

Radial nerve (posterior cutaneous nerve of arm)

T2

Musculocutaneous nerve (lateral cutaneous nerve of forearm)

T1

Radial nerve (superficial branch)

Ulnar nerve

Median nerve (innervates nail beds)

Plate 467   **Neurovasculature**

Arthrogram: glenohumeral joint

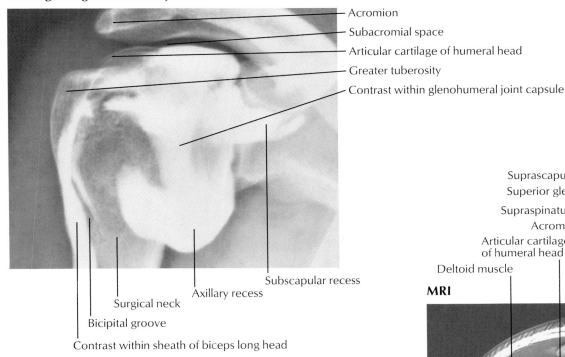

Acromion

Subacromial space

Articular cartilage of humeral head

Greater tuberosity

Contrast within glenohumeral joint capsule

Subscapular recess

Axillary recess

Surgical neck

Bicipital groove

Contrast within sheath of biceps long head

Suprascapular nerve, artery, vein

Superior glenoid labrum

Supraspinatus muscle

Acromion

Articular cartilage of humeral head

Deltoid muscle

MRI

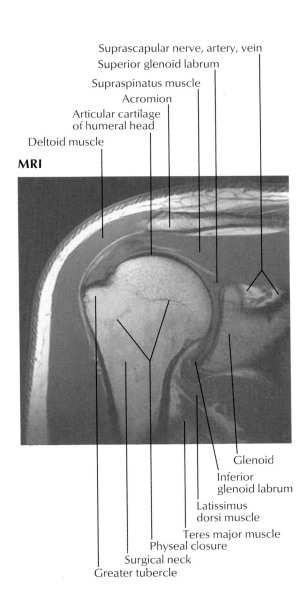

Glenoid

Inferior glenoid labrum

Latissimus dorsi muscle

Teres major muscle

Physeal closure

Surgical neck

Greater tubercle

Deltoid muscle

Humeral head

Glenoid

CT

Sternal end of clavicle

1st rib

2nd rib

Bicipital groove with long head of biceps tendon

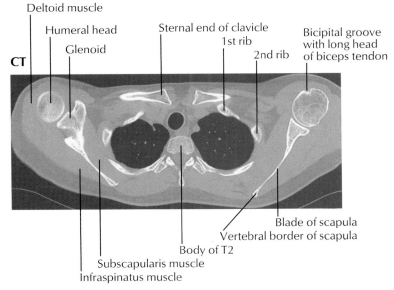

Blade of scapula

Vertebral border of scapula

Body of T2

Subscapularis muscle

Infraspinatus muscle

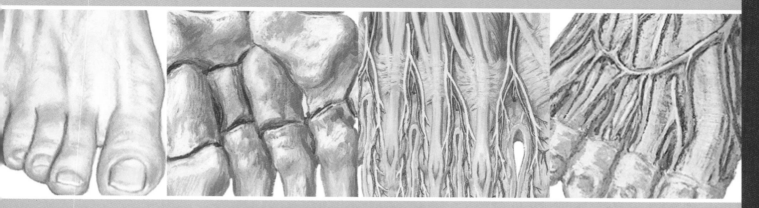

Section 7 **LOWER LIMB**

Topographic Anatomy
Plate 469

469 Lower Limb

Cutaneous Anatomy
Plates 470-473

470 Dermatomes of Lower Limb

471 Superficial Nerves and Veins of Lower Limb: Anterior View

472 Superficial Nerves and Veins of Lower Limb: Posterior View

473 Lymph Vessels and Nodes of Lower Limb

Hip and Thigh
Plates 474-493

474 Hip (Coxal) Bone

475 Hip Joint

476 Hip Joint: Anteroposterior Radiograph

477 Femur

478 Bony Attachments of Muscles of Hip and Thigh: Anterior View

479 Bony Attachments of Muscles of Hip and Thigh: Posterior View

480 Muscles of Thigh: Anterior Views

481 Muscles of Thigh: Anterior Views (continued)

482 Muscles of Hip and Thigh: Lateral View

483 Muscles of Hip and Thigh: Posterior Views

484 Psoas and Iliacus Muscles

485 Lumbosacral and Coccygeal Plexuses

486 Lumbar Plexus

487 Sacral and Coccygeal Plexuses

488 Arteries and Nerves of Thigh: Anterior Views

489 Arteries and Nerves of Thigh: Anterior Views (continued)

490 Arteries and Nerves of Thigh: Posterior View

491 Nerves of Hip and Buttock

492 Arteries of Femoral Head and Neck

493 Thigh: Serial Cross Sections

Knee
Plates 494-500

494 Knee: Medial and Lateral Views

495 Knee: Anterior Views

496 Knee: Interior

497 Knee: Cruciate and Collateral Ligaments

498 Knee: Anteroposterior Radiograph

499 Knee: Posterior and Sagittal Views

500 Arteries of Thigh and Knee: Schema

Leg
Plates 501-510

501 Tibia and Fibula

502 Tibia and Fibula (continued)

503 Attachments of Muscles of Leg

504 Muscles of Leg (Superficial Dissection): Posterior View

505 Muscles of Leg (Intermediate Dissection): Posterior View

506 Muscles of Leg (Deep Dissection): Posterior View

507 Muscles of Leg (Superficial Dissection): Anterior View

508 Muscles of Leg (Deep Dissection): Anterior View

509 Muscles of Leg: Lateral View

510 Leg: Cross Sections and Fascial Compartments

Ankle and Foot
Plates 511-525

511 Bones of Foot

512 Bones of Foot (continued)

513 Calcaneus

514 Ankle: Radiographs

515 Ligaments and Tendons of Ankle

516 Ligaments and Tendons of Foot: Plantar View

517 Tendon Sheaths of Ankle

518 Muscles of Dorsum of Foot: Superficial Dissection

519 Dorsum of Foot: Deep Dissection

520 Sole of Foot: Superficial Dissection

521 Muscles of Sole of Foot: First Layer

522 Muscles of Sole of Foot: Second Layer

523 Muscles of Sole of Foot: Third Layer

524 Interosseous Muscles and Deep Arteries of Foot

525 Interosseous Muscles of Foot

Neurovasculature
Plates 526-530

526 Femoral Nerve and Lateral Cutaneous Nerve of Thigh

527 Obturator Nerve

528 Sciatic Nerve and Posterior Cutaneous Nerve of Thigh

529 Tibial Nerve

530 Common Fibular (Peroneal) Nerve

Regional Scans
Plate 531

531 Hip Radiograph, Arthrogram, and MR

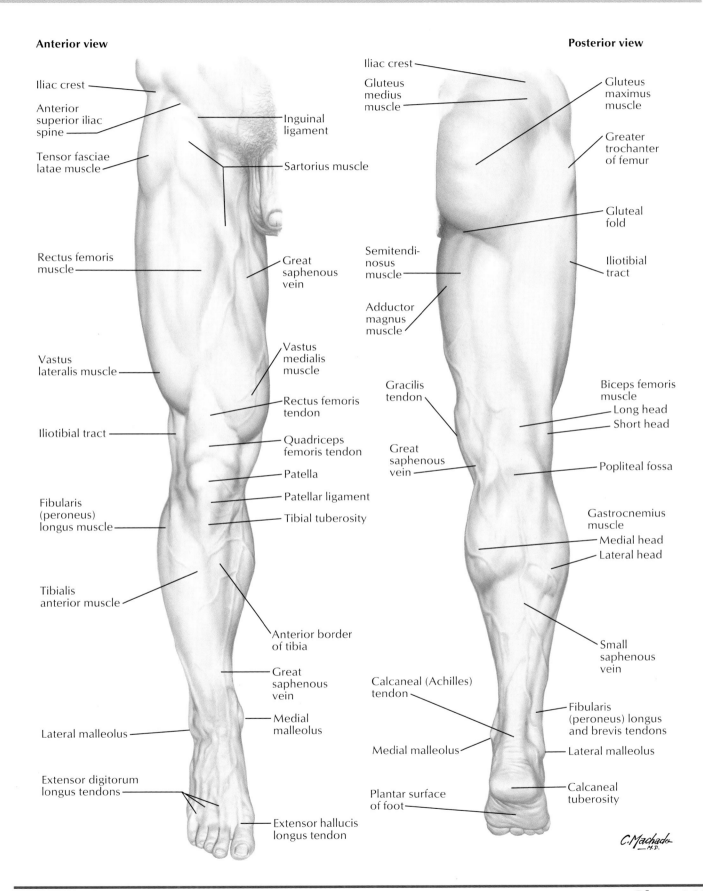

Anterior view

Iliac crest

Anterior superior iliac spine

Tensor fasciae latae muscle

Inguinal ligament

Sartorius muscle

Rectus femoris muscle

Great saphenous vein

Vastus medialis muscle

Vastus lateralis muscle

Rectus femoris tendon

Iliotibial tract

Quadriceps femoris tendon

Patella

Fibularis (peroneus) longus muscle

Patellar ligament

Tibial tuberosity

Tibialis anterior muscle

Anterior border of tibia

Great saphenous vein

Medial malleolus

Lateral malleolus

Extensor digitorum longus tendons

Extensor hallucis longus tendon

Posterior view

Iliac crest

Gluteus medius muscle

Gluteus maximus muscle

Greater trochanter of femur

Gluteal fold

Iliotibial tract

Semitendinosus muscle

Adductor magnus muscle

Gracilis tendon

Biceps femoris muscle

Long head

Short head

Great saphenous vein

Popliteal fossa

Gastrocnemius muscle

Medial head

Lateral head

Small saphenous vein

Calcaneal (Achilles) tendon

Fibularis (peroneus) longus and brevis tendons

Medial malleolus

Lateral malleolus

Plantar surface of foot

Calcaneal tuberosity

C. Machado
—M.D.

Schematic demarcation of dermatomes (according to Keegan and Garrett) shown as distinct segments. There is actually considerable overlap between any two adjacent dermatomes. An alternative dermatome map is online.

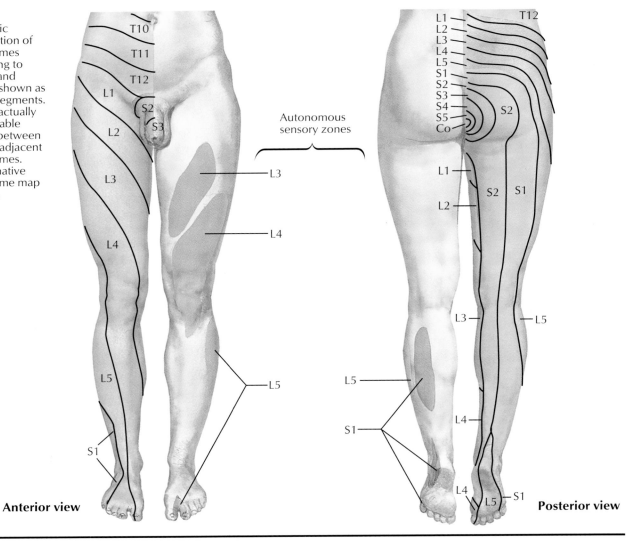

Anterior view

Posterior view

Autonomous sensory zones

Segmental innervation of lower limb movements

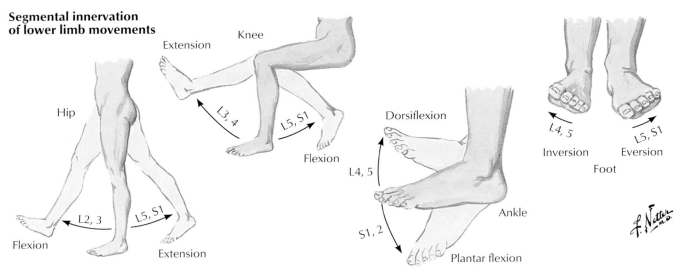

Hip

Flexion

L2, 3

L5, S1

Extension

Knee

Extension

L3, 4

L5, S1

Flexion

Dorsiflexion

L4, 5

S1, 2

Plantar flexion

Ankle

Inversion

L4, 5

Eversion

L5, S1

Foot

Plate 470   **Cutaneous Anatomy**

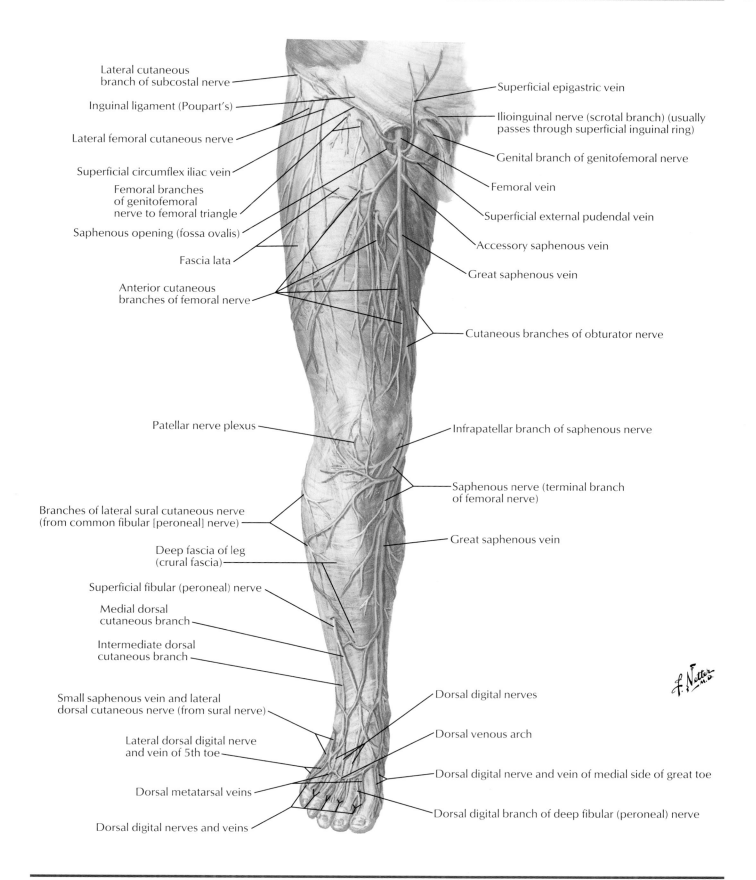

Lateral cutaneous branch of subcostal nerve

Inguinal ligament (Poupart's)

Lateral femoral cutaneous nerve

Superficial circumflex iliac vein

Femoral branches of genitofemoral nerve to femoral triangle

Saphenous opening (fossa ovalis)

Fascia lata

Anterior cutaneous branches of femoral nerve

Patellar nerve plexus

Branches of lateral sural cutaneous nerve (from common fibular [peroneal] nerve)

Deep fascia of leg (crural fascia)

Superficial fibular (peroneal) nerve

Medial dorsal cutaneous branch

Intermediate dorsal cutaneous branch

Small saphenous vein and lateral dorsal cutaneous nerve (from sural nerve)

Lateral dorsal digital nerve and vein of 5th toe

Dorsal metatarsal veins

Dorsal digital nerves and veins

Superficial epigastric vein

Ilioinguinal nerve (scrotal branch) (usually passes through superficial inguinal ring)

Genital branch of genitofemoral nerve

Femoral vein

Superficial external pudendal vein

Accessory saphenous vein

Great saphenous vein

Cutaneous branches of obturator nerve

Infrapatellar branch of saphenous nerve

Saphenous nerve (terminal branch of femoral nerve)

Great saphenous vein

Dorsal digital nerves

Dorsal venous arch

Dorsal digital nerve and vein of medial side of great toe

Dorsal digital branch of deep fibular (peroneal) nerve

f. Netter m.d.

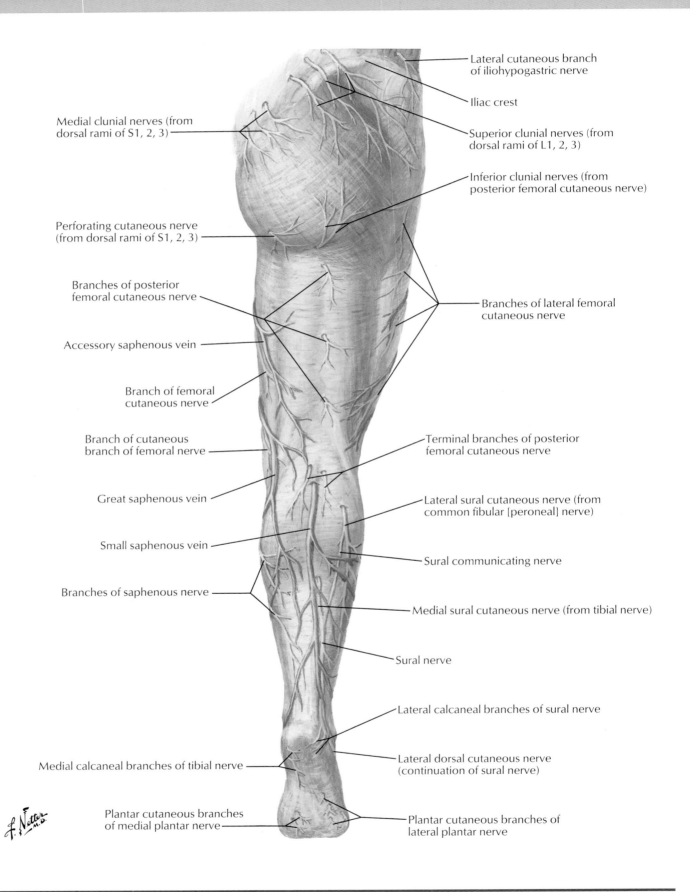

Lateral cutaneous branch of iliohypogastric nerve

Iliac crest

Superior clunial nerves (from dorsal rami of L1, 2, 3)

Medial clunial nerves (from dorsal rami of S1, 2, 3)

Inferior clunial nerves (from posterior femoral cutaneous nerve)

Perforating cutaneous nerve (from dorsal rami of S1, 2, 3)

Branches of lateral femoral cutaneous nerve

Branches of posterior femoral cutaneous nerve

Accessory saphenous vein

Branch of femoral cutaneous nerve

Branch of cutaneous branch of femoral nerve

Terminal branches of posterior femoral cutaneous nerve

Great saphenous vein

Lateral sural cutaneous nerve (from common fibular [peroneal] nerve)

Small saphenous vein

Sural communicating nerve

Branches of saphenous nerve

Medial sural cutaneous nerve (from tibial nerve)

Sural nerve

Lateral calcaneal branches of sural nerve

Medial calcaneal branches of tibial nerve

Lateral dorsal cutaneous nerve (continuation of sural nerve)

Plantar cutaneous branches of medial plantar nerve

Plantar cutaneous branches of lateral plantar nerve

Plate 472 **Cutaneous Anatomy**

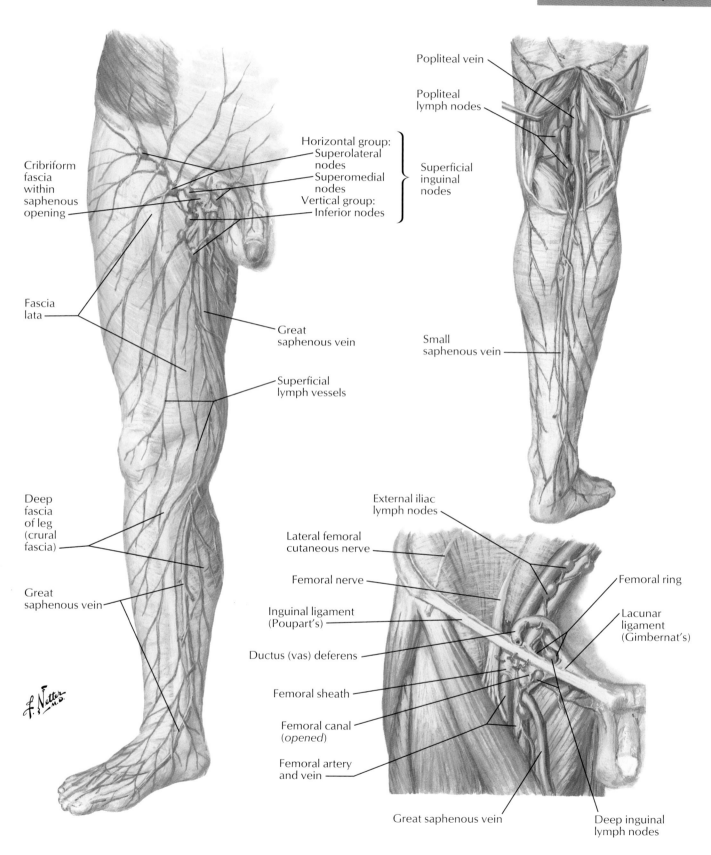

Cribriform fascia within saphenous opening

Horizontal group:
Superolateral nodes
Superomedial nodes
Vertical group:
Inferior nodes

Fascia lata

Great saphenous vein

Superficial lymph vessels

Deep fascia of leg (crural fascia)

Great saphenous vein

Popliteal vein

Popliteal lymph nodes

Superficial inguinal nodes

Small saphenous vein

External iliac lymph nodes

Lateral femoral cutaneous nerve

Femoral nerve

Inguinal ligament (Poupart's)

Ductus (vas) deferens

Femoral sheath

Femoral canal (opened)

Femoral artery and vein

Femoral ring

Lacunar ligament (Gimbernat's)

Great saphenous vein

Deep inguinal lymph nodes

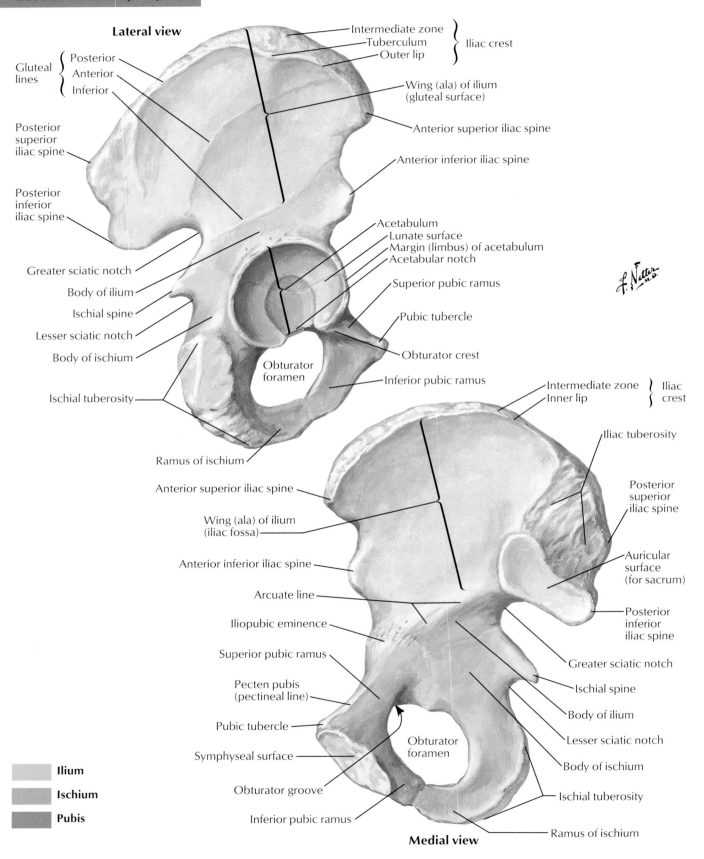

Lateral view

Gluteal lines { Posterior / Anterior / Inferior

Intermediate zone
Tuberculum } Iliac crest
Outer lip

Posterior superior iliac spine

Posterior inferior iliac spine

Wing (ala) of ilium (gluteal surface)

Anterior superior iliac spine

Anterior inferior iliac spine

Acetabulum
Lunate surface
Margin (limbus) of acetabulum
Acetabular notch

Greater sciatic notch

Body of ilium

Ischial spine

Lesser sciatic notch

Body of ischium

Superior pubic ramus

Pubic tubercle

Obturator crest

Obturator foramen

Inferior pubic ramus

Ischial tuberosity

Ramus of ischium

Anterior superior iliac spine

Wing (ala) of ilium (iliac fossa)

Anterior inferior iliac spine

Arcuate line

Iliopubic eminence

Superior pubic ramus

Pecten pubis (pectineal line)

Pubic tubercle

Symphyseal surface

Obturator groove

Inferior pubic ramus

Intermediate zone
Inner lip } Iliac crest

Iliac tuberosity

Posterior superior iliac spine

Auricular surface (for sacrum)

Posterior inferior iliac spine

Greater sciatic notch

Ischial spine

Body of ilium

Lesser sciatic notch

Body of ischium

Ischial tuberosity

Ramus of ischium

Obturator foramen

Medial view

Ilium

Ischium

Pubis

Plate 474 | **Hip and Thigh**

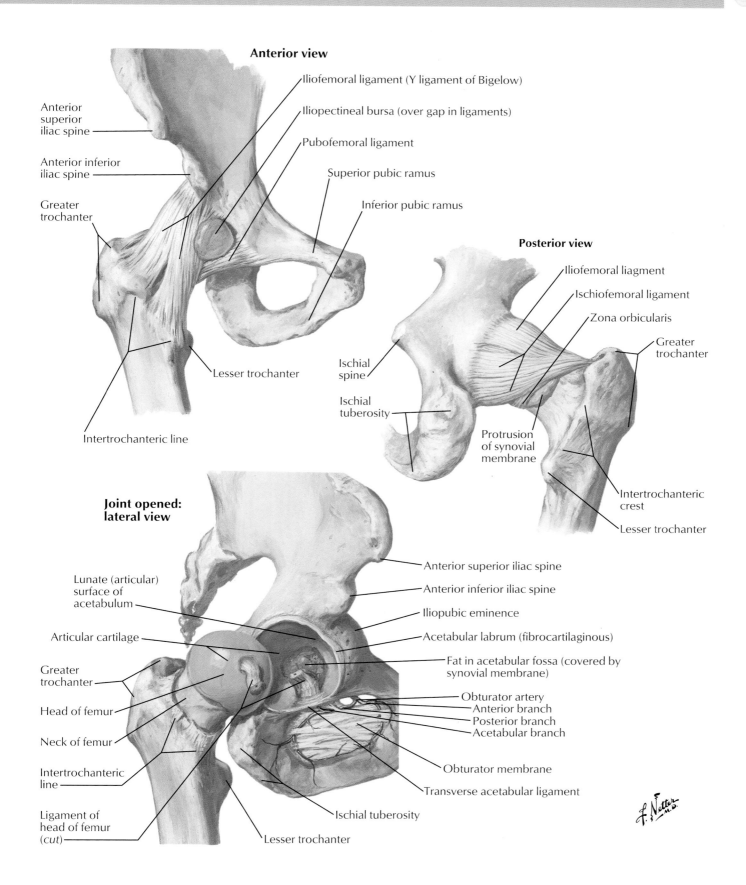

Anterior view

Iliofemoral ligament (Y ligament of Bigelow)

Iliopectineal bursa (over gap in ligaments)

Pubofemoral ligament

Superior pubic ramus

Inferior pubic ramus

Anterior superior iliac spine

Anterior inferior iliac spine

Greater trochanter

Lesser trochanter

Intertrochanteric line

Posterior view

Iliofemoral liagment

Ischiofemoral ligament

Zona orbicularis

Greater trochanter

Ischial spine

Ischial tuberosity

Protrusion of synovial membrane

Intertrochanteric crest

Lesser trochanter

Joint opened: lateral view

Lunate (articular) surface of acetabulum

Articular cartilage

Greater trochanter

Head of femur

Neck of femur

Intertrochanteric line

Ligament of head of femur (cut)

Lesser trochanter

Ischial tuberosity

Anterior superior iliac spine

Anterior inferior iliac spine

Iliopubic eminence

Acetabular labrum (fibrocartilaginous)

Fat in acetabular fossa (covered by synovial membrane)

Obturator artery

Anterior branch

Posterior branch

Acetabular branch

Obturator membrane

Transverse acetabular ligament

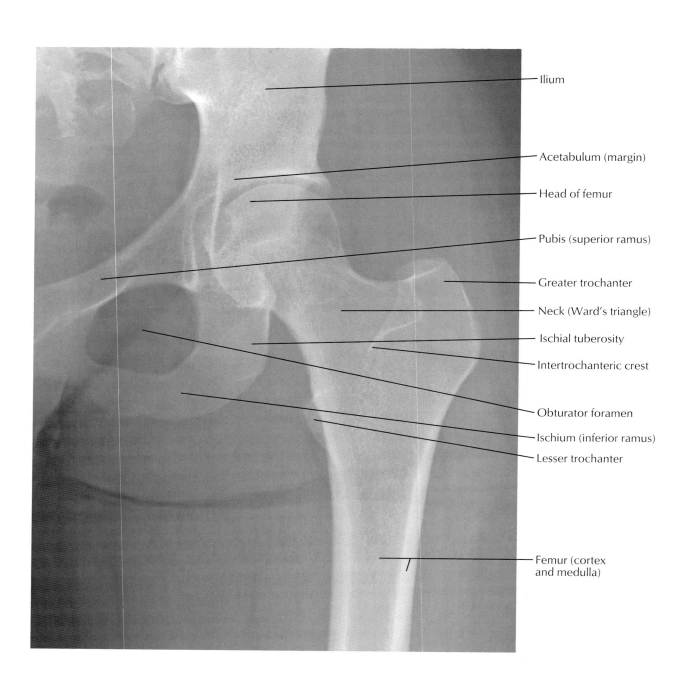

Ilium

Acetabulum (margin)

Head of femur

Pubis (superior ramus)

Greater trochanter

Neck (Ward's triangle)

Ischial tuberosity

Intertrochanteric crest

Obturator foramen

Ischium (inferior ramus)

Lesser trochanter

Femur (cortex and medulla)

Plate 476

Hip and Thigh

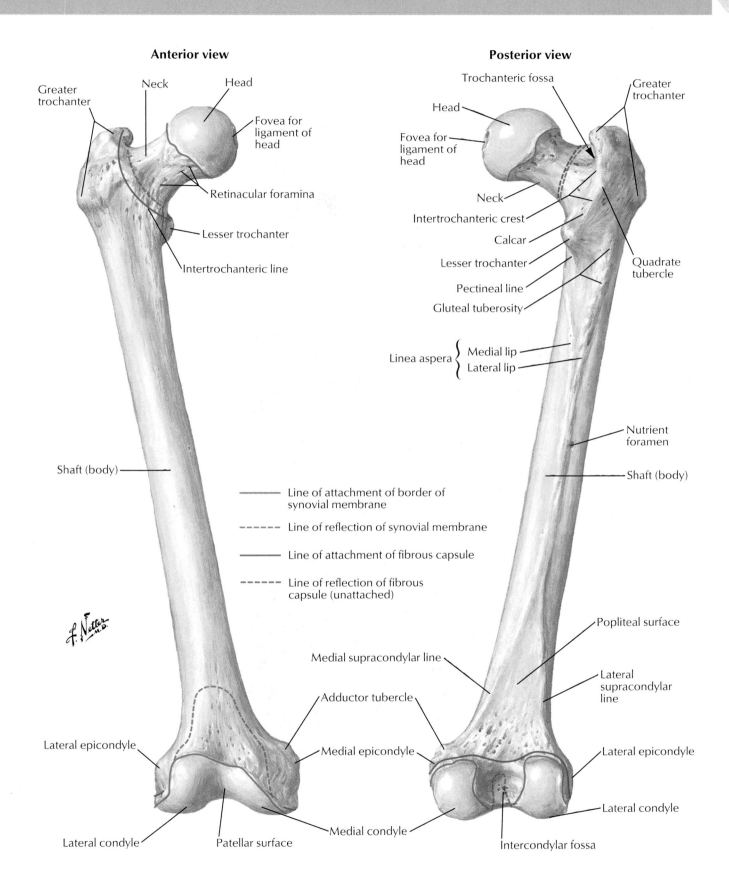

Anterior view

Greater trochanter

Neck

Head

Fovea for ligament of head

Retinacular foramina

Lesser trochanter

Intertrochanteric line

Shaft (body)

Line of attachment of border of synovial membrane

Line of reflection of synovial membrane

Line of attachment of fibrous capsule

Line of reflection of fibrous capsule (unattached)

Adductor tubercle

Lateral epicondyle

Medial epicondyle

Lateral condyle

Patellar surface

Medial condyle

Posterior view

Trochanteric fossa

Greater trochanter

Head

Fovea for ligament of head

Neck

Intertrochanteric crest

Calcar

Lesser trochanter

Pectineal line

Gluteal tuberosity

Quadrate tubercle

Linea aspera { Medial lip / Lateral lip }

Nutrient foramen

Shaft (body)

Popliteal surface

Medial supracondylar line

Lateral supracondylar line

Lateral epicondyle

Lateral condyle

Intercondylar fossa

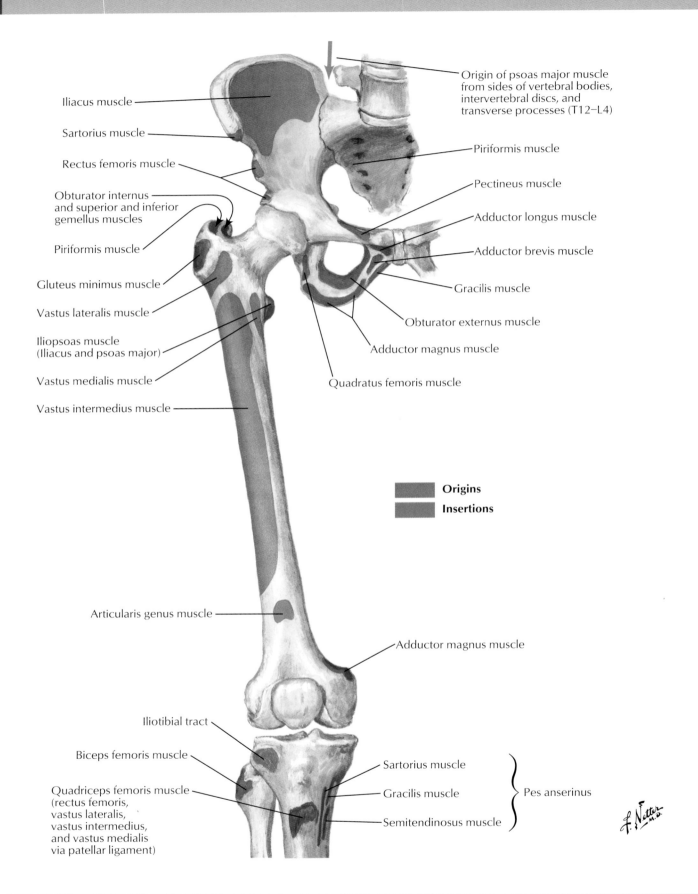

Iliacus muscle

Sartorius muscle

Rectus femoris muscle

Obturator internus
and superior and inferior
gemellus muscles

Piriformis muscle

Gluteus minimus muscle

Vastus lateralis muscle

Iliopsoas muscle
(Iliacus and psoas major)

Vastus medialis muscle

Vastus intermedius muscle

Articularis genus muscle

Iliotibial tract

Biceps femoris muscle

Quadriceps femoris muscle
(rectus femoris,
vastus lateralis,
vastus intermedius,
and vastus medialis
via patellar ligament)

Origin of psoas major muscle
from sides of vertebral bodies,
intervertebral discs, and
transverse processes (T12–L4)

Piriformis muscle

Pectineus muscle

Adductor longus muscle

Adductor brevis muscle

Gracilis muscle

Obturator externus muscle

Adductor magnus muscle

Quadratus femoris muscle

Adductor magnus muscle

Sartorius muscle

Gracilis muscle

Semitendinosus muscle

Pes anserinus

Origins

Insertions

Plate 478 **Hip and Thigh**

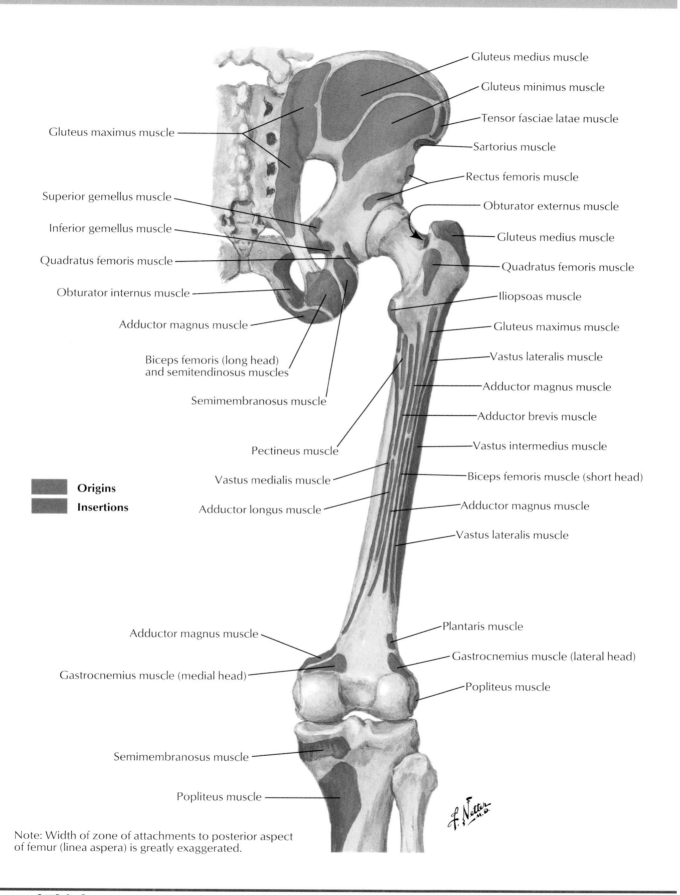

Gluteus medius muscle

Gluteus minimus muscle

Tensor fasciae latae muscle

Gluteus maximus muscle

Sartorius muscle

Rectus femoris muscle

Superior gemellus muscle

Obturator externus muscle

Inferior gemellus muscle

Gluteus medius muscle

Quadratus femoris muscle

Quadratus femoris muscle

Obturator internus muscle

Iliopsoas muscle

Adductor magnus muscle

Gluteus maximus muscle

Vastus lateralis muscle

Biceps femoris (long head)
and semitendinosus muscles

Adductor magnus muscle

Adductor brevis muscle

Semimembranosus muscle

Vastus intermedius muscle

Pectineus muscle

Biceps femoris muscle (short head)

Vastus medialis muscle

Adductor magnus muscle

Adductor longus muscle

Vastus lateralis muscle

Origins

Insertions

Adductor magnus muscle

Plantaris muscle

Gastrocnemius muscle (lateral head)

Gastrocnemius muscle (medial head)

Popliteus muscle

Semimembranosus muscle

Popliteus muscle

Note: Width of zone of attachments to posterior aspect
of femur (linea aspera) is greatly exaggerated.

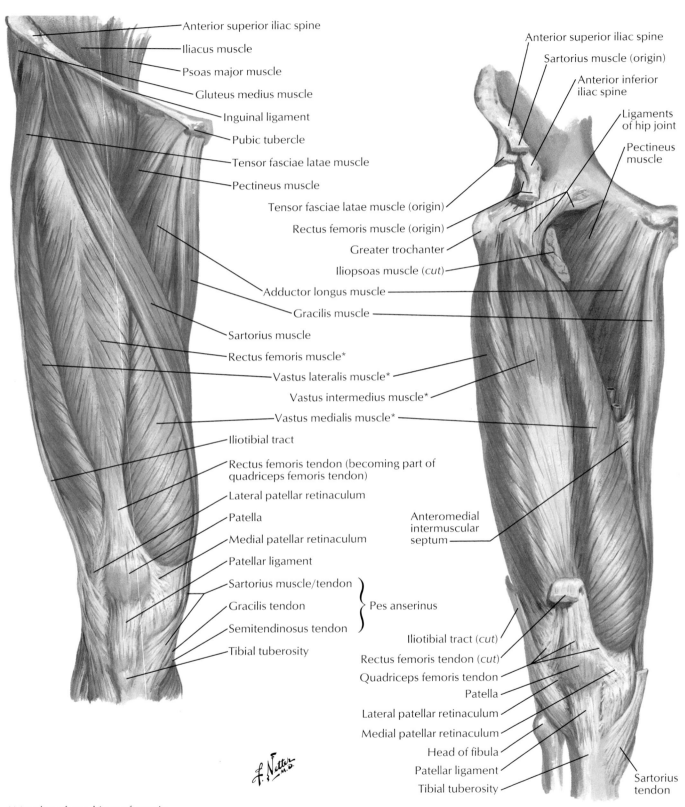

Anterior superior iliac spine

Iliacus muscle

Psoas major muscle

Gluteus medius muscle

Inguinal ligament

Pubic tubercle

Tensor fasciae latae muscle

Pectineus muscle

Tensor fasciae latae muscle (origin)

Rectus femoris muscle (origin)

Greater trochanter

Iliopsoas muscle (cut)

Adductor longus muscle

Gracilis muscle

Sartorius muscle

Rectus femoris muscle*

Vastus lateralis muscle*

Vastus intermedius muscle*

Vastus medialis muscle*

Iliotibial tract

Rectus femoris tendon (becoming part of quadriceps femoris tendon)

Lateral patellar retinaculum

Patella

Medial patellar retinaculum

Patellar ligament

Sartorius muscle/tendon

Gracilis tendon

Semitendinosus tendon

Tibial tuberosity

Pes anserinus

Anterior superior iliac spine

Sartorius muscle (origin)

Anterior inferior iliac spine

Ligaments of hip joint

Pectineus muscle

Anteromedial intermuscular septum

Iliotibial tract (cut)

Rectus femoris tendon (cut)

Quadriceps femoris tendon

Patella

Lateral patellar retinaculum

Medial patellar retinaculum

Head of fibula

Patellar ligament

Tibial tuberosity

Sartorius tendon

*Muscles of quadriceps femoris

Plate 480 **Hip and Thigh**

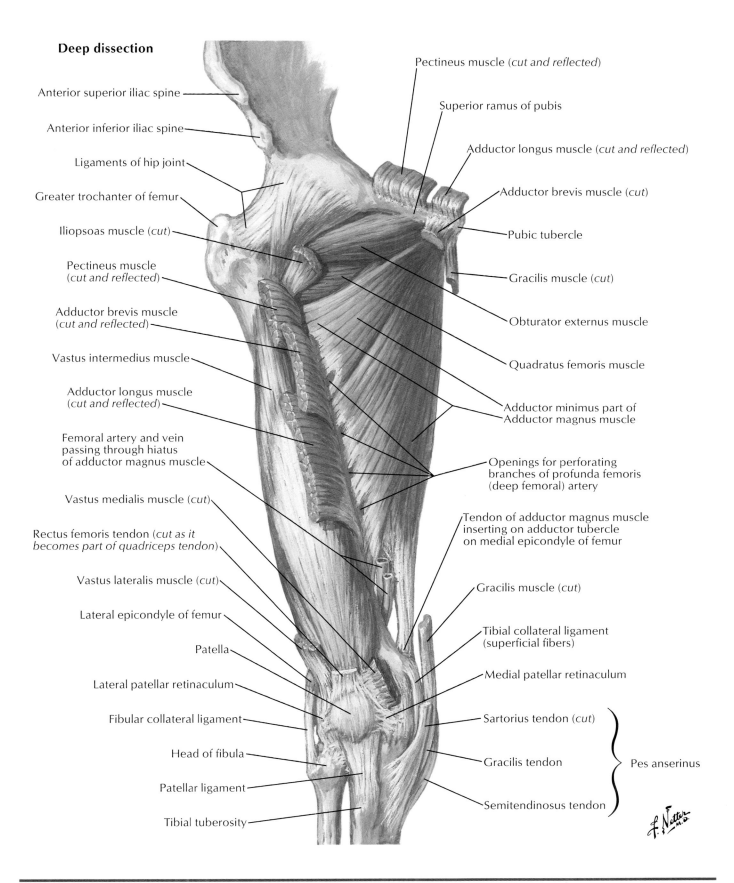

Deep dissection

Anterior superior iliac spine

Anterior inferior iliac spine

Ligaments of hip joint

Greater trochanter of femur

Iliopsoas muscle (*cut*)

Pectineus muscle (*cut and reflected*)

Adductor brevis muscle (*cut and reflected*)

Vastus intermedius muscle

Adductor longus muscle (*cut and reflected*)

Femoral artery and vein passing through hiatus of adductor magnus muscle

Vastus medialis muscle (*cut*)

Rectus femoris tendon (*cut as it becomes part of quadriceps tendon*)

Vastus lateralis muscle (*cut*)

Lateral epicondyle of femur

Patella

Lateral patellar retinaculum

Fibular collateral ligament

Head of fibula

Patellar ligament

Tibial tuberosity

Pectineus muscle (*cut and reflected*)

Superior ramus of pubis

Adductor longus muscle (*cut and reflected*)

Adductor brevis muscle (*cut*)

Pubic tubercle

Gracilis muscle (*cut*)

Obturator externus muscle

Quadratus femoris muscle

Adductor minimus part of Adductor magnus muscle

Openings for perforating branches of profunda femoris (deep femoral) artery

Tendon of adductor magnus muscle inserting on adductor tubercle on medial epicondyle of femur

Gracilis muscle (*cut*)

Tibial collateral ligament (superficial fibers)

Medial patellar retinaculum

Sartorius tendon (*cut*)

Gracilis tendon

Semitendinosus tendon

Pes anserinus

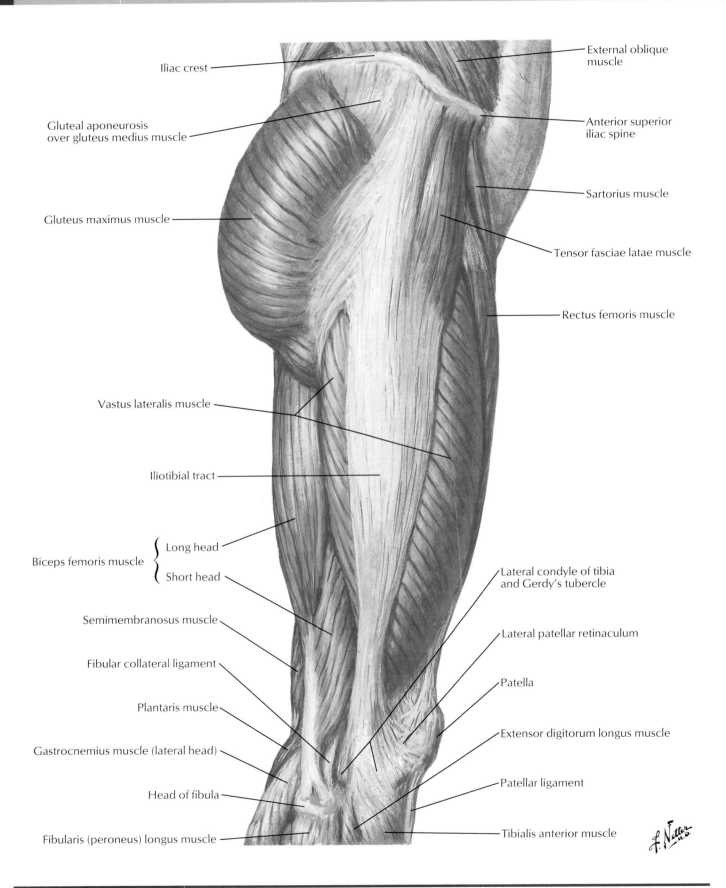

Iliac crest

External oblique muscle

Gluteal aponeurosis over gluteus medius muscle

Anterior superior iliac spine

Gluteus maximus muscle

Sartorius muscle

Tensor fasciae latae muscle

Rectus femoris muscle

Vastus lateralis muscle

Iliotibial tract

Biceps femoris muscle { Long head

Short head

Lateral condyle of tibia and Gerdy's tubercle

Semimembranosus muscle

Lateral patellar retinaculum

Fibular collateral ligament

Patella

Plantaris muscle

Extensor digitorum longus muscle

Gastrocnemius muscle (lateral head)

Patellar ligament

Head of fibula

Fibularis (peroneus) longus muscle

Tibialis anterior muscle

Plate 482

Hip and Thigh

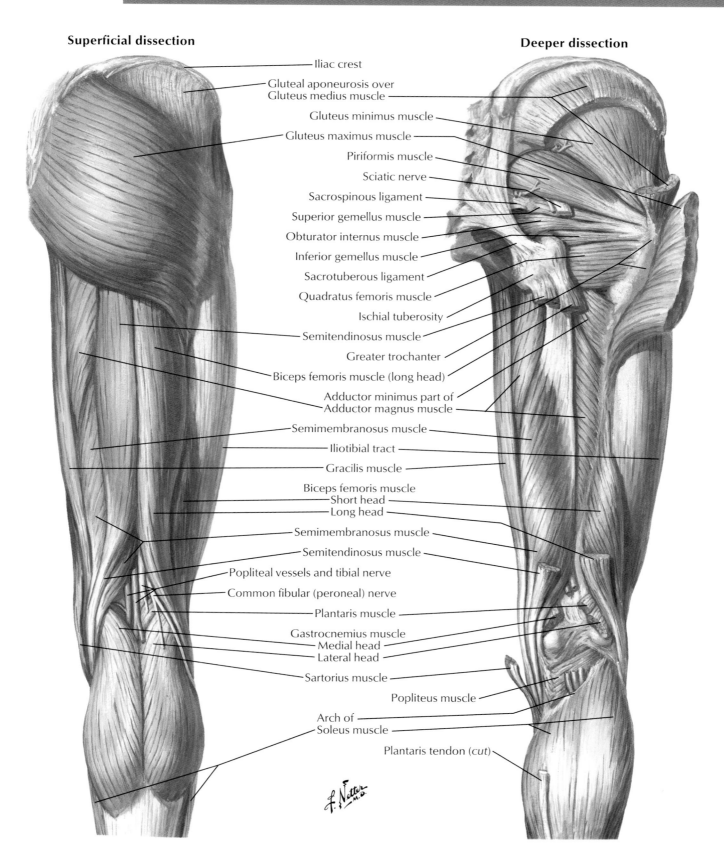

Superficial dissection

Deeper dissection

Iliac crest

Gluteal aponeurosis over
Gluteus medius muscle

Gluteus minimus muscle

Gluteus maximus muscle

Piriformis muscle

Sciatic nerve

Sacrospinous ligament

Superior gemellus muscle

Obturator internus muscle

Inferior gemellus muscle

Sacrotuberous ligament

Quadratus femoris muscle

Ischial tuberosity

Semitendinosus muscle

Greater trochanter

Biceps femoris muscle (long head)

Adductor minimus part of
Adductor magnus muscle

Semimembranosus muscle

Iliotibial tract

Gracilis muscle

Biceps femoris muscle
Short head
Long head

Semimembranosus muscle

Semitendinosus muscle

Popliteal vessels and tibial nerve

Common fibular (peroneal) nerve

Plantaris muscle

Gastrocnemius muscle
Medial head
Lateral head

Sartorius muscle

Popliteus muscle

Arch of
Soleus muscle

Plantaris tendon (*cut*)

Hip and Thigh

Plate 483

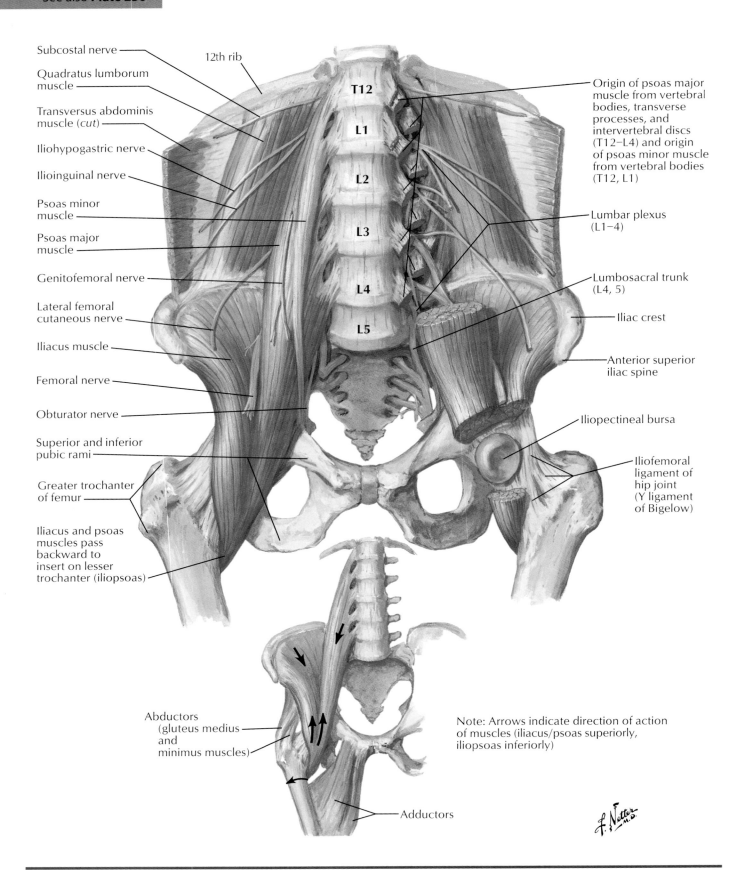

Subcostal nerve

12th rib

Quadratus lumborum muscle

Transversus abdominis muscle (*cut*)

Iliohypogastric nerve

Ilioinguinal nerve

Psoas minor muscle

Psoas major muscle

Genitofemoral nerve

Lateral femoral cutaneous nerve

Iliacus muscle

Femoral nerve

Obturator nerve

Superior and inferior pubic rami

Greater trochanter of femur

Iliacus and psoas muscles pass backward to insert on lesser trochanter (iliopsoas)

T12

L1

L2

L3

L4

L5

Origin of psoas major muscle from vertebral bodies, transverse processes, and intervertebral discs (T12–L4) and origin of psoas minor muscle from vertebral bodies (T12, L1)

Lumbar plexus (L1–4)

Lumbosacral trunk (L4, 5)

Iliac crest

Anterior superior iliac spine

Iliopectineal bursa

Iliofemoral ligament of hip joint (Y ligament of Bigelow)

Abductors (gluteus medius and minimus muscles)

Note: Arrows indicate direction of action of muscles (iliacus/psoas superiorly, iliopsoas inferiorly)

Adductors

Plate 484

Hip and Thigh

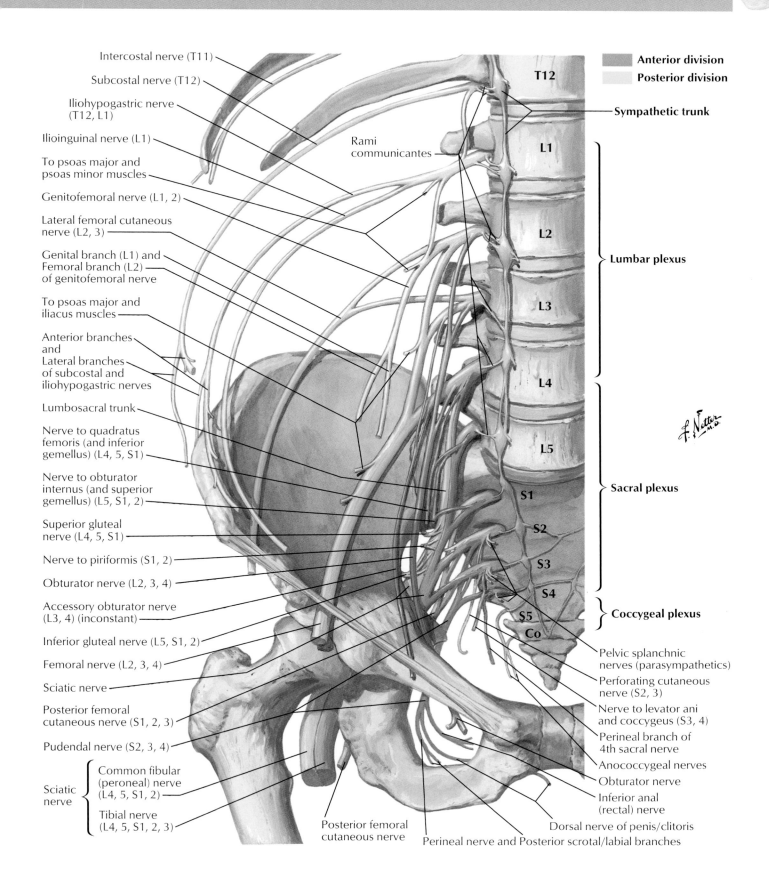

Intercostal nerve (T11)

Subcostal nerve (T12)

Iliohypogastric nerve (T12, L1)

Ilioinguinal nerve (L1)

To psoas major and psoas minor muscles

Genitofemoral nerve (L1, 2)

Lateral femoral cutaneous nerve (L2, 3)

Genital branch (L1) and Femoral branch (L2) of genitofemoral nerve

To psoas major and iliacus muscles

Anterior branches and Lateral branches of subcostal and iliohypogastric nerves

Lumbosacral trunk

Nerve to quadratus femoris (and inferior gemellus) (L4, 5, S1)

Nerve to obturator internus (and superior gemellus) (L5, S1, 2)

Superior gluteal nerve (L4, 5, S1)

Nerve to piriformis (S1, 2)

Obturator nerve (L2, 3, 4)

Accessory obturator nerve (L3, 4) (inconstant)

Inferior gluteal nerve (L5, S1, 2)

Femoral nerve (L2, 3, 4)

Sciatic nerve

Posterior femoral cutaneous nerve (S1, 2, 3)

Pudendal nerve (S2, 3, 4)

Sciatic nerve {
Common fibular (peroneal) nerve (L4, 5, S1, 2)
Tibial nerve (L4, 5, S1, 2, 3)
}

Rami communicantes

T12

L1

L2

L3

L4

L5

S1

S2

S3

S4

S5

Co

Anterior division
Posterior division

Sympathetic trunk

Lumbar plexus

Sacral plexus

Coccygeal plexus

Pelvic splanchnic nerves (parasympathetics)

Perforating cutaneous nerve (S2, 3)

Nerve to levator ani and coccygeus (S3, 4)

Perineal branch of 4th sacral nerve

Anococcygeal nerves

Obturator nerve

Inferior anal (rectal) nerve

Dorsal nerve of penis/clitoris

Posterior femoral cutaneous nerve

Perineal nerve and Posterior scrotal/labial branches

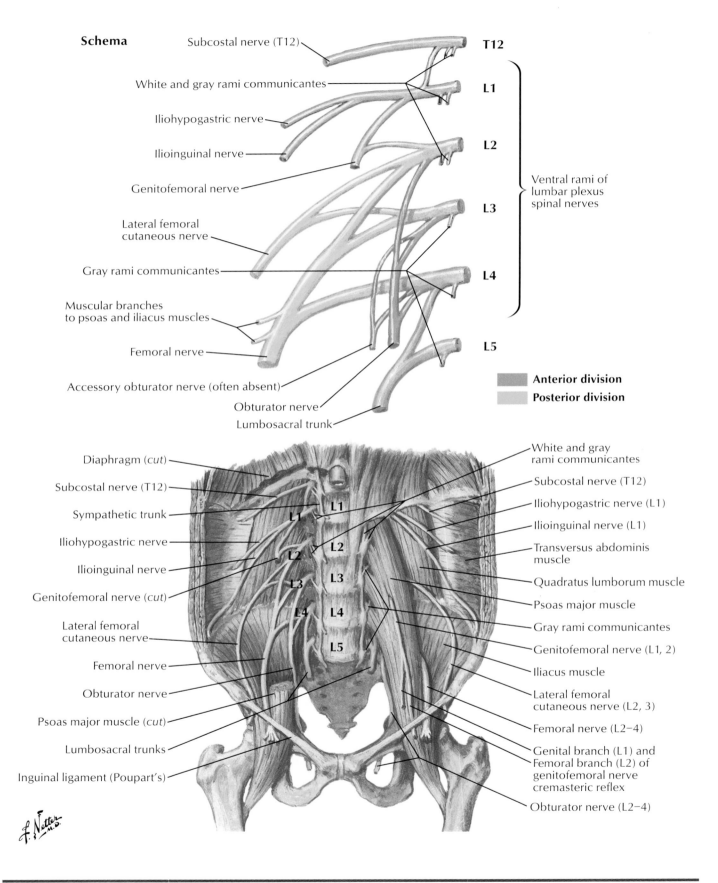

Schema

Subcostal nerve (T12)

White and gray rami communicantes

Iliohypogastric nerve

Ilioinguinal nerve

Genitofemoral nerve

Lateral femoral cutaneous nerve

Gray rami communicantes

Muscular branches to psoas and iliacus muscles

Femoral nerve

Accessory obturator nerve (often absent)

Obturator nerve

Lumbosacral trunk

T12
L1
L2
L3
L4
L5

Ventral rami of lumbar plexus spinal nerves

■ **Anterior division**
□ **Posterior division**

Diaphragm (cut)

Subcostal nerve (T12)

Sympathetic trunk

Iliohypogastric nerve

Ilioinguinal nerve

Genitofemoral nerve (cut)

Lateral femoral cutaneous nerve

Femoral nerve

Obturator nerve

Psoas major muscle (cut)

Lumbosacral trunks

Inguinal ligament (Poupart's)

White and gray rami communicantes

Subcostal nerve (T12)

Iliohypogastric nerve (L1)

Ilioinguinal nerve (L1)

Transversus abdominis muscle

Quadratus lumborum muscle

Psoas major muscle

Gray rami communicantes

Genitofemoral nerve (L1, 2)

Iliacus muscle

Lateral femoral cutaneous nerve (L2, 3)

Femoral nerve (L2–4)

Genital branch (L1) and Femoral branch (L2) of genitofemoral nerve cremasteric reflex

Obturator nerve (L2–4)

Plate 486

Hip and Thigh

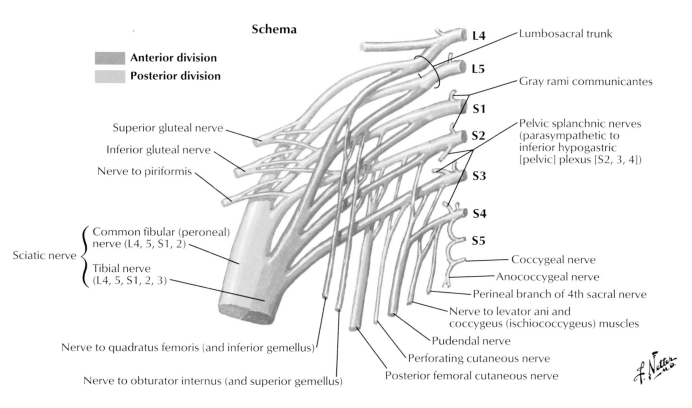

Schema

Anterior division
Posterior division

Superior gluteal nerve

Inferior gluteal nerve

Nerve to piriformis

Sciatic nerve
{ Common fibular (peroneal) nerve (L4, 5, S1, 2)
Tibial nerve (L4, 5, S1, 2, 3) }

Nerve to quadratus femoris (and inferior gemellus)

Nerve to obturator internus (and superior gemellus)

L4 — Lumbosacral trunk

L5 — Gray rami communicantes

S1

S2 — Pelvic splanchnic nerves (parasympathetic to inferior hypogastric [pelvic] plexus [S2, 3, 4])

S3

S4

S5

Coccygeal nerve

Anococcygeal nerve

Perineal branch of 4th sacral nerve

Nerve to levator ani and coccygeus (ischiococcygeus) muscles

Pudendal nerve

Perforating cutaneous nerve

Posterior femoral cutaneous nerve

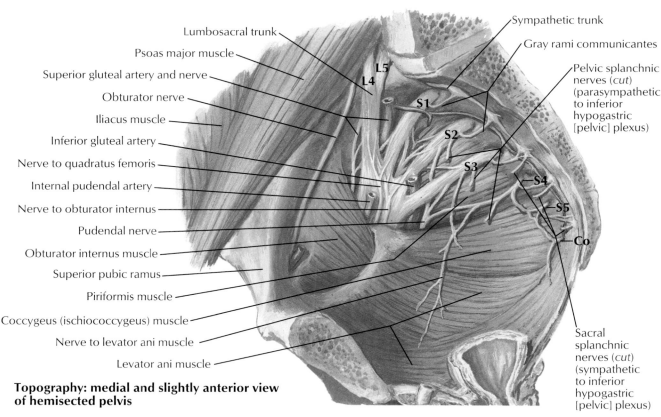

Lumbosacral trunk

Psoas major muscle

Superior gluteal artery and nerve

Obturator nerve

Iliacus muscle

Inferior gluteal artery

Nerve to quadratus femoris

Internal pudendal artery

Nerve to obturator internus

Pudendal nerve

Obturator internus muscle

Superior pubic ramus

Piriformis muscle

Coccygeus (ischiococcygeus) muscle

Nerve to levator ani muscle

Levator ani muscle

Topography: medial and slightly anterior view of hemisected pelvis

Sympathetic trunk

Gray rami communicantes

Pelvic splanchnic nerves (cut) (parasympathetic to inferior hypogastric [pelvic] plexus)

L5
L4

S1

S2

S3

S4

S5

Co

Sacral splanchnic nerves (cut) (sympathetic to inferior hypogastric [pelvic] plexus)

Superficial dissections

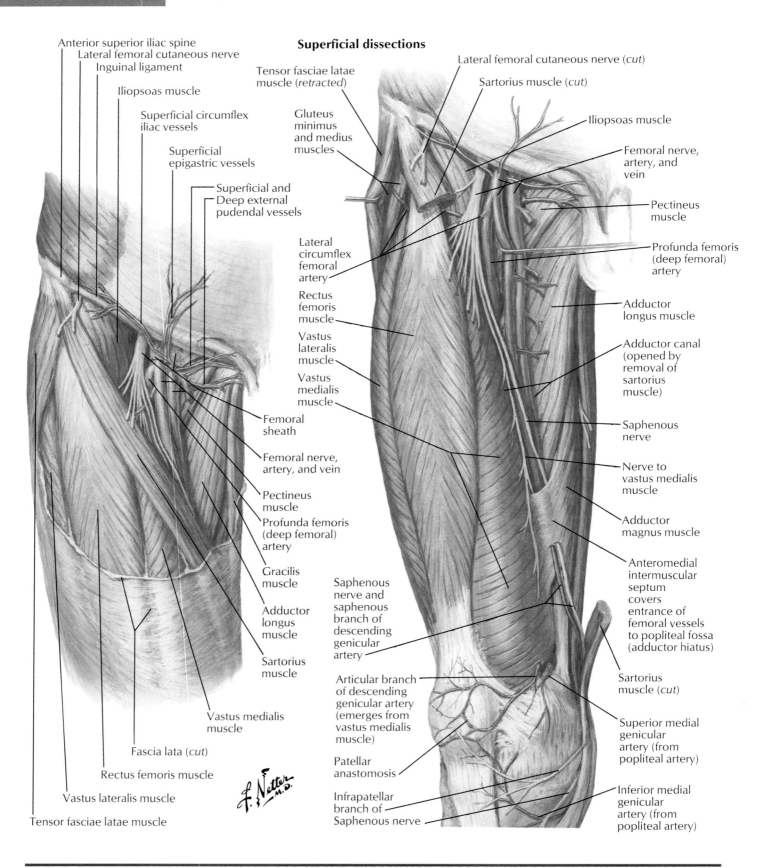

Anterior superior iliac spine
Lateral femoral cutaneous nerve
Inguinal ligament

Iliopsoas muscle

Superficial circumflex iliac vessels

Superficial epigastric vessels

Superficial and Deep external pudendal vessels

Tensor fasciae latae muscle (*retracted*)

Gluteus minimus and medius muscles

Lateral circumflex femoral artery

Rectus femoris muscle

Vastus lateralis muscle

Vastus medialis muscle

Femoral sheath

Femoral nerve, artery, and vein

Pectineus muscle

Profunda femoris (deep femoral) artery

Gracilis muscle

Adductor longus muscle

Sartorius muscle

Vastus medialis muscle

Fascia lata (*cut*)

Rectus femoris muscle

Vastus lateralis muscle

Tensor fasciae latae muscle

Lateral femoral cutaneous nerve (*cut*)

Sartorius muscle (*cut*)

Iliopsoas muscle

Femoral nerve, artery, and vein

Pectineus muscle

Profunda femoris (deep femoral) artery

Adductor longus muscle

Adductor canal (opened by removal of sartorius muscle)

Saphenous nerve

Nerve to vastus medialis muscle

Adductor magnus muscle

Anteromedial intermuscular septum covers entrance of femoral vessels to popliteal fossa (adductor hiatus)

Sartorius muscle (*cut*)

Superior medial genicular artery (from popliteal artery)

Inferior medial genicular artery (from popliteal artery)

Saphenous nerve and saphenous branch of descending genicular artery

Articular branch of descending genicular artery (emerges from vastus medialis muscle)

Patellar anastomosis

Infrapatellar branch of Saphenous nerve

F. Netter, M.D.

Plate 488

Hip and Thigh

Deep dissection

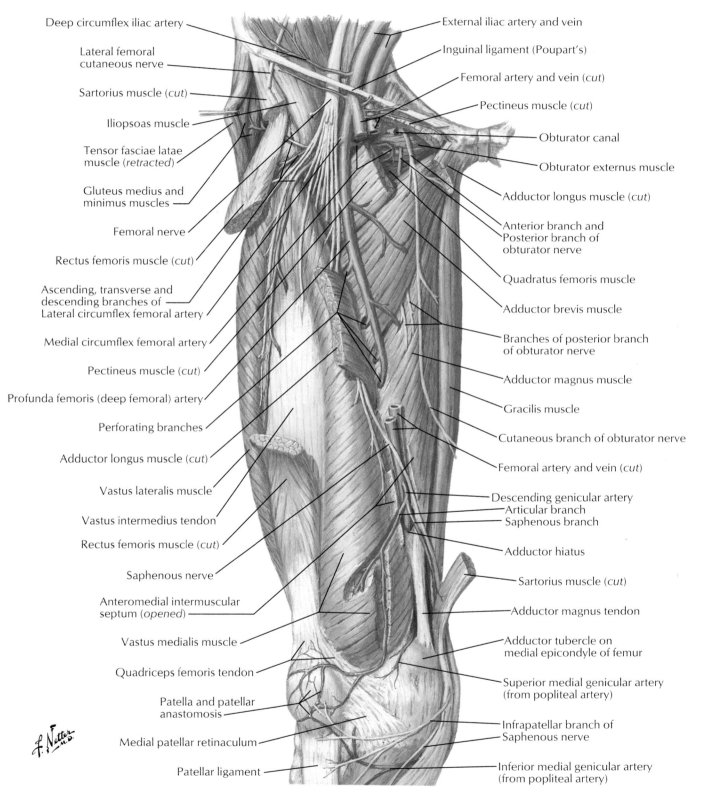

Deep circumflex iliac artery

Lateral femoral cutaneous nerve

Sartorius muscle (*cut*)

Iliopsoas muscle

Tensor fasciae latae muscle (*retracted*)

Gluteus medius and minimus muscles

Femoral nerve

Rectus femoris muscle (*cut*)

Ascending, transverse and descending branches of Lateral circumflex femoral artery

Medial circumflex femoral artery

Pectineus muscle (*cut*)

Profunda femoris (deep femoral) artery

Perforating branches

Adductor longus muscle (*cut*)

Vastus lateralis muscle

Vastus intermedius tendon

Rectus femoris muscle (*cut*)

Saphenous nerve

Anteromedial intermuscular septum (*opened*)

Vastus medialis muscle

Quadriceps femoris tendon

Patella and patellar anastomosis

Medial patellar retinaculum

Patellar ligament

External iliac artery and vein

Inguinal ligament (Poupart's)

Femoral artery and vein (*cut*)

Pectineus muscle (*cut*)

Obturator canal

Obturator externus muscle

Adductor longus muscle (*cut*)

Anterior branch and Posterior branch of obturator nerve

Quadratus femoris muscle

Adductor brevis muscle

Branches of posterior branch of obturator nerve

Adductor magnus muscle

Gracilis muscle

Cutaneous branch of obturator nerve

Femoral artery and vein (*cut*)

Descending genicular artery
Articular branch
Saphenous branch

Adductor hiatus

Sartorius muscle (*cut*)

Adductor magnus tendon

Adductor tubercle on medial epicondyle of femur

Superior medial genicular artery (from popliteal artery)

Infrapatellar branch of Saphenous nerve

Inferior medial genicular artery (from popliteal artery)

Deep dissection

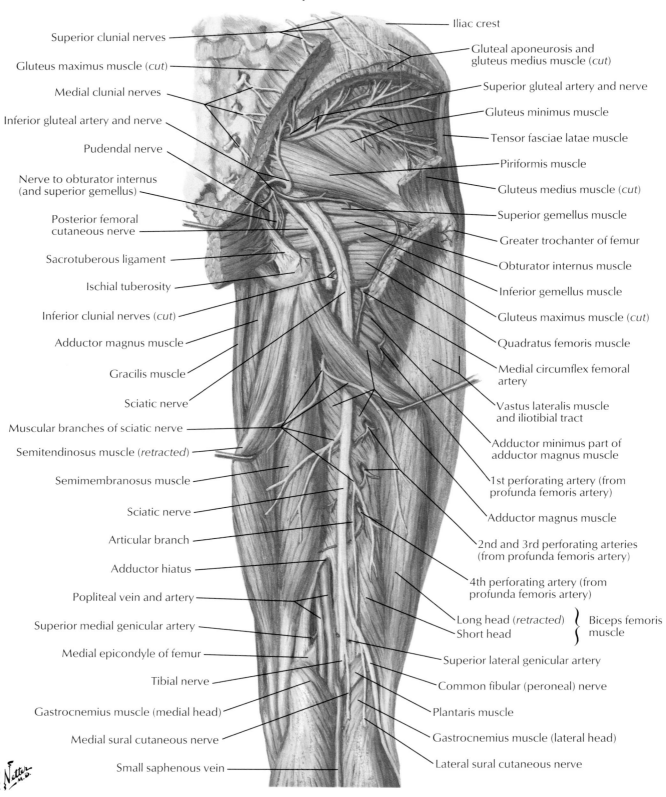

Superior clunial nerves

Gluteus maximus muscle (*cut*)

Medial clunial nerves

Inferior gluteal artery and nerve

Pudendal nerve

Nerve to obturator internus
(and superior gemellus)

Posterior femoral
cutaneous nerve

Sacrotuberous ligament

Ischial tuberosity

Inferior clunial nerves (*cut*)

Adductor magnus muscle

Gracilis muscle

Sciatic nerve

Muscular branches of sciatic nerve

Semitendinosus muscle (*retracted*)

Semimembranosus muscle

Sciatic nerve

Articular branch

Adductor hiatus

Popliteal vein and artery

Superior medial genicular artery

Medial epicondyle of femur

Tibial nerve

Gastrocnemius muscle (medial head)

Medial sural cutaneous nerve

Small saphenous vein

Iliac crest

Gluteal aponeurosis and
gluteus medius muscle (*cut*)

Superior gluteal artery and nerve

Gluteus minimus muscle

Tensor fasciae latae muscle

Piriformis muscle

Gluteus medius muscle (*cut*)

Superior gemellus muscle

Greater trochanter of femur

Obturator internus muscle

Inferior gemellus muscle

Gluteus maximus muscle (*cut*)

Quadratus femoris muscle

Medial circumflex femoral
artery

Vastus lateralis muscle
and iliotibial tract

Adductor minimus part of
adductor magnus muscle

1st perforating artery (from
profunda femoris artery)

Adductor magnus muscle

2nd and 3rd perforating arteries
(from profunda femoris artery)

4th perforating artery (from
profunda femoris artery)

Long head (*retracted*) ⎱ Biceps femoris
Short head ⎰ muscle

Superior lateral genicular artery

Common fibular (peroneal) nerve

Plantaris muscle

Gastrocnemius muscle (lateral head)

Lateral sural cutaneous nerve

Plate 490 **Hip and Thigh**

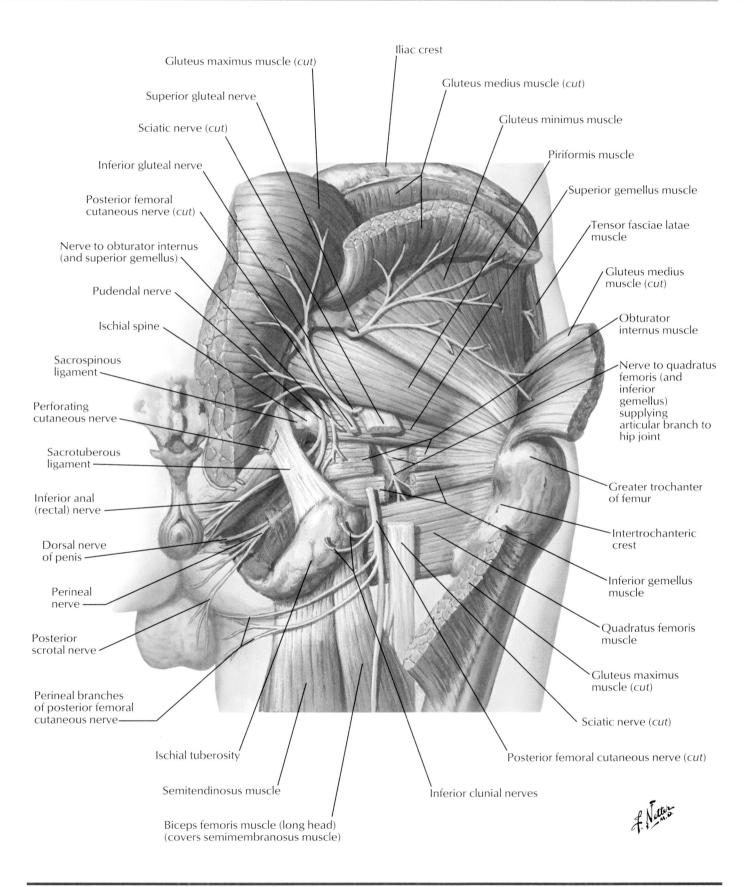

Gluteus maximus muscle (*cut*)

Superior gluteal nerve

Sciatic nerve (*cut*)

Inferior gluteal nerve

Posterior femoral cutaneous nerve (*cut*)

Nerve to obturator internus (and superior gemellus)

Pudendal nerve

Ischial spine

Sacrospinous ligament

Perforating cutaneous nerve

Sacrotuberous ligament

Inferior anal (rectal) nerve

Dorsal nerve of penis

Perineal nerve

Posterior scrotal nerve

Perineal branches of posterior femoral cutaneous nerve

Ischial tuberosity

Semitendinosus muscle

Biceps femoris muscle (long head) (covers semimembranosus muscle)

Iliac crest

Gluteus medius muscle (*cut*)

Gluteus minimus muscle

Piriformis muscle

Superior gemellus muscle

Tensor fasciae latae muscle

Gluteus medius muscle (*cut*)

Obturator internus muscle

Nerve to quadratus femoris (and inferior gemellus) supplying articular branch to hip joint

Greater trochanter of femur

Intertrochanteric crest

Inferior gemellus muscle

Quadratus femoris muscle

Gluteus maximus muscle (*cut*)

Sciatic nerve (*cut*)

Posterior femoral cutaneous nerve (*cut*)

Inferior clunial nerves

f. Netter

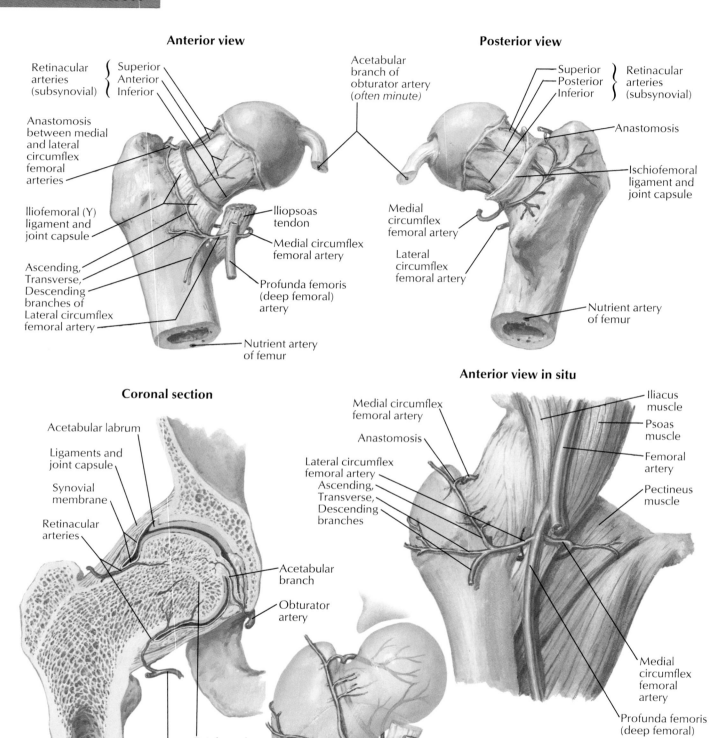

Anterior view

Retinacular arteries (subsynovial) { Superior / Anterior / Inferior

Anastomosis between medial and lateral circumflex femoral arteries

Iliofemoral (Y) ligament and joint capsule

Ascending, Transverse, Descending branches of Lateral circumflex femoral artery

Iliopsoas tendon

Medial circumflex femoral artery

Profunda femoris (deep femoral) artery

Nutrient artery of femur

Posterior view

Acetabular branch of obturator artery (often minute)

Retinacular arteries (subsynovial) { Superior / Posterior / Inferior

Anastomosis

Ischiofemoral ligament and joint capsule

Medial circumflex femoral artery

Lateral circumflex femoral artery

Nutrient artery of femur

Coronal section

Acetabular labrum

Ligaments and joint capsule

Synovial membrane

Retinacular arteries

Acetabular branch

Obturator artery

Epiphyseal plate

Medial circumflex femoral artery

Anterior view in situ

Medial circumflex femoral artery

Anastomosis

Lateral circumflex femoral artery

Ascending, Transverse, Descending branches

Iliacus muscle

Psoas muscle

Femoral artery

Pectineus muscle

Medial circumflex femoral artery

Profunda femoris (deep femoral) artery

Medial circumflex femoral artery

Iliopsoas tendon

Lateral circumflex femoral artery

Femur of child: anterior view

Plate 492

Hip and Thigh

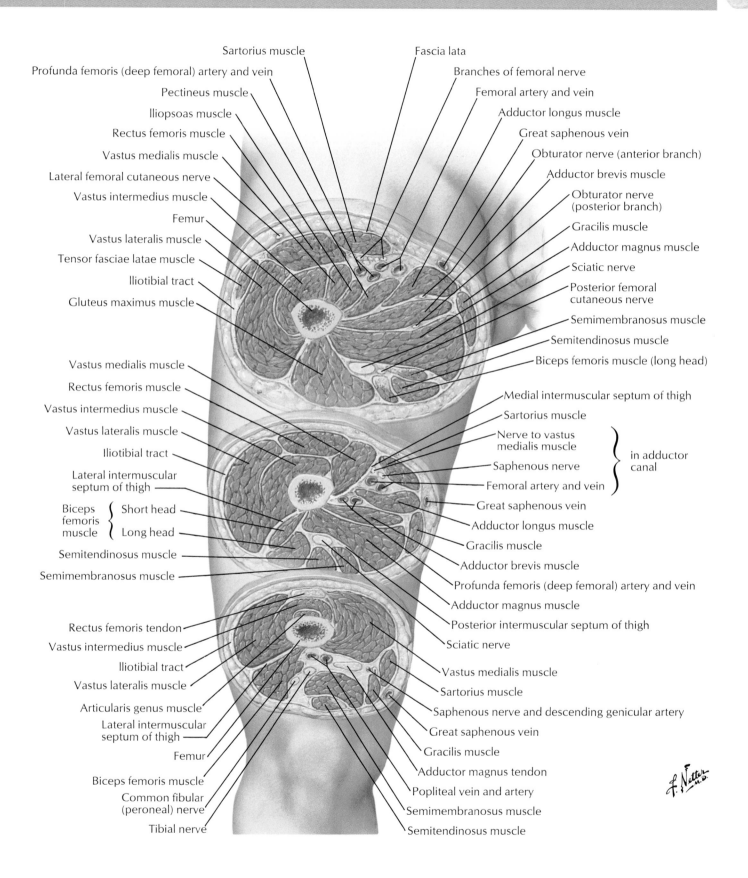

Sartorius muscle

Profunda femoris (deep femoral) artery and vein

Pectineus muscle

Iliopsoas muscle

Rectus femoris muscle

Vastus medialis muscle

Lateral femoral cutaneous nerve

Vastus intermedius muscle

Femur

Vastus lateralis muscle

Tensor fasciae latae muscle

Iliotibial tract

Gluteus maximus muscle

Fascia lata

Branches of femoral nerve

Femoral artery and vein

Adductor longus muscle

Great saphenous vein

Obturator nerve (anterior branch)

Adductor brevis muscle

Obturator nerve (posterior branch)

Gracilis muscle

Adductor magnus muscle

Sciatic nerve

Posterior femoral cutaneous nerve

Semimembranosus muscle

Semitendinosus muscle

Biceps femoris muscle (long head)

Vastus medialis muscle

Rectus femoris muscle

Vastus intermedius muscle

Vastus lateralis muscle

Iliotibial tract

Lateral intermuscular septum of thigh

Biceps femoris muscle { Short head / Long head }

Semitendinosus muscle

Semimembranosus muscle

Medial intermuscular septum of thigh

Sartorius muscle

Nerve to vastus medialis muscle

Saphenous nerve

Femoral artery and vein

} in adductor canal

Great saphenous vein

Adductor longus muscle

Gracilis muscle

Adductor brevis muscle

Profunda femoris (deep femoral) artery and vein

Adductor magnus muscle

Posterior intermuscular septum of thigh

Sciatic nerve

Rectus femoris tendon

Vastus intermedius muscle

Iliotibial tract

Vastus lateralis muscle

Articularis genus muscle

Lateral intermuscular septum of thigh

Femur

Biceps femoris muscle

Common fibular (peroneal) nerve

Tibial nerve

Vastus medialis muscle

Sartorius muscle

Saphenous nerve and descending genicular artery

Great saphenous vein

Gracilis muscle

Adductor magnus tendon

Popliteal vein and artery

Semimembranosus muscle

Semitendinosus muscle

Medial view

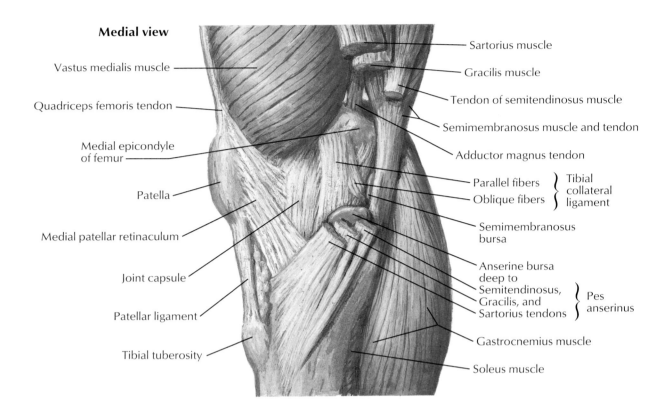

Vastus medialis muscle

Quadriceps femoris tendon

Medial epicondyle of femur

Patella

Medial patellar retinaculum

Joint capsule

Patellar ligament

Tibial tuberosity

Sartorius muscle

Gracilis muscle

Tendon of semitendinosus muscle

Semimembranosus muscle and tendon

Adductor magnus tendon

Parallel fibers } Tibial
Oblique fibers } collateral ligament

Semimembranosus bursa

Anserine bursa deep to
Semitendinosus,
Gracilis, and } Pes anserinus
Sartorius tendons }

Gastrocnemius muscle

Soleus muscle

Lateral view

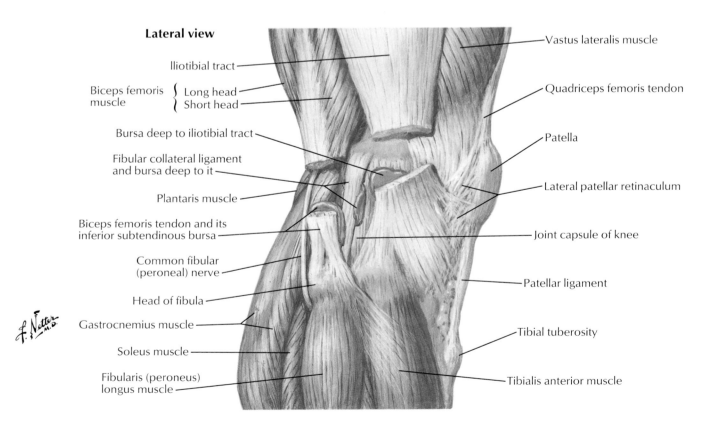

Iliotibial tract

Biceps femoris { Long head
muscle { Short head

Bursa deep to iliotibial tract

Fibular collateral ligament and bursa deep to it

Plantaris muscle

Biceps femoris tendon and its inferior subtendinous bursa

Common fibular (peroneal) nerve

Head of fibula

Gastrocnemius muscle

Soleus muscle

Fibularis (peroneus) longus muscle

Vastus lateralis muscle

Quadriceps femoris tendon

Patella

Lateral patellar retinaculum

Joint capsule of knee

Patellar ligament

Tibial tuberosity

Tibialis anterior muscle

Plate 494 **Knee**

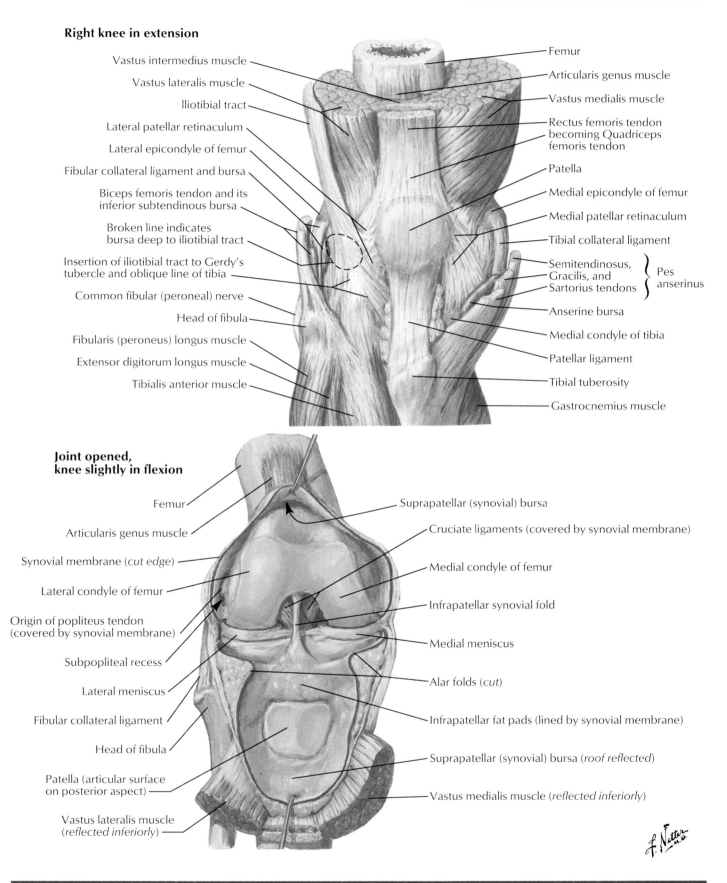

Right knee in extension

Vastus intermedius muscle

Vastus lateralis muscle

Iliotibial tract

Lateral patellar retinaculum

Lateral epicondyle of femur

Fibular collateral ligament and bursa

Biceps femoris tendon and its inferior subtendinous bursa

Broken line indicates bursa deep to iliotibial tract

Insertion of iliotibial tract to Gerdy's tubercle and oblique line of tibia

Common fibular (peroneal) nerve

Head of fibula

Fibularis (peroneus) longus muscle

Extensor digitorum longus muscle

Tibialis anterior muscle

Femur

Articularis genus muscle

Vastus medialis muscle

Rectus femoris tendon becoming Quadriceps femoris tendon

Patella

Medial epicondyle of femur

Medial patellar retinaculum

Tibial collateral ligament

Semitendinosus, Gracilis, and Sartorius tendons } Pes anserinus

Anserine bursa

Medial condyle of tibia

Patellar ligament

Tibial tuberosity

Gastrocnemius muscle

Joint opened, knee slightly in flexion

Femur

Articularis genus muscle

Synovial membrane (*cut edge*)

Lateral condyle of femur

Origin of popliteus tendon (covered by synovial membrane)

Subpopliteal recess

Lateral meniscus

Fibular collateral ligament

Head of fibula

Patella (articular surface on posterior aspect)

Vastus lateralis muscle (*reflected inferiorly*)

Suprapatellar (synovial) bursa

Cruciate ligaments (covered by synovial membrane)

Medial condyle of femur

Infrapatellar synovial fold

Medial meniscus

Alar folds (*cut*)

Infrapatellar fat pads (lined by synovial membrane)

Suprapatellar (synovial) bursa (*roof reflected*)

Vastus medialis muscle (*reflected inferiorly*)

Inferior view

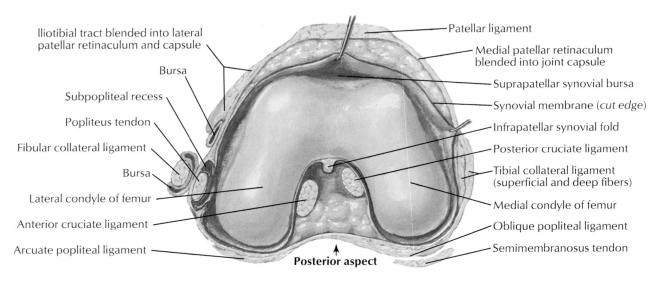

Iliotibial tract blended into lateral patellar retinaculum and capsule

Bursa

Subpopliteal recess

Popliteus tendon

Fibular collateral ligament

Bursa

Lateral condyle of femur

Anterior cruciate ligament

Arcuate popliteal ligament

Patellar ligament

Medial patellar retinaculum blended into joint capsule

Suprapatellar synovial bursa

Synovial membrane (*cut edge*)

Infrapatellar synovial fold

Posterior cruciate ligament

Tibial collateral ligament (superficial and deep fibers)

Medial condyle of femur

Oblique popliteal ligament

Semimembranosus tendon

Posterior aspect

Superior view

Posterior meniscofemoral ligament

Arcuate popliteal ligament

Fibular collateral ligament

Bursa

Popliteus tendon

Subpopliteal recess

Lateral meniscus

Superior articular surface of tibia (lateral facet)

Iliotibial tract blended into capsule

Infrapatellar fat pad

Semimembranosus tendon

Oblique popliteal ligament

Posterior cruciate ligament

Tibial collateral ligament (deep fibers bound to medial meniscus)

Medial meniscus

Synovial membrane

Superior articular surface of tibia (medial facet)

Joint capsule

Anterior cruciate ligament

Patellar ligament

Anterior aspect ↑

Superior view: ligaments and cartilage removed

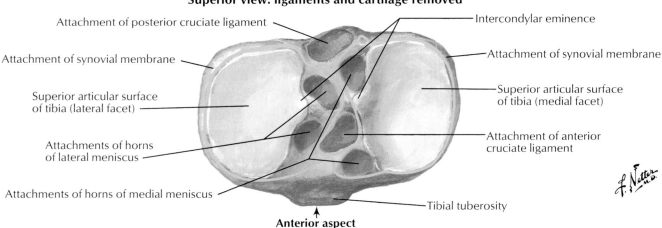

Attachment of posterior cruciate ligament

Attachment of synovial membrane

Superior articular surface of tibia (lateral facet)

Attachments of horns of lateral meniscus

Attachments of horns of medial meniscus

Intercondylar eminence

Attachment of synovial membrane

Superior articular surface of tibia (medial facet)

Attachment of anterior cruciate ligament

Tibial tuberosity

Anterior aspect ↑

Plate 496   **Knee**

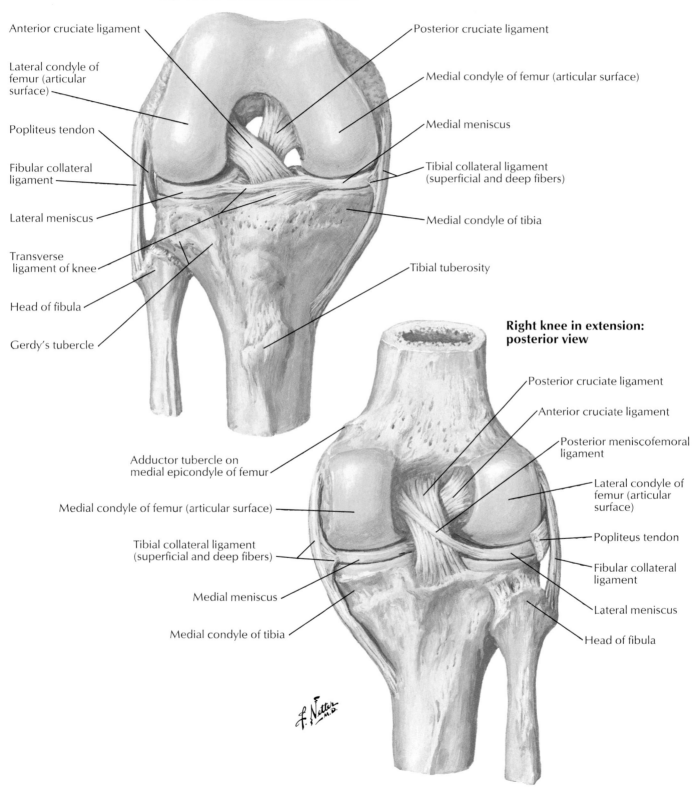

Right knee in flexion: anterior view

Anterior cruciate ligament

Lateral condyle of femur (articular surface)

Popliteus tendon

Fibular collateral ligament

Lateral meniscus

Transverse ligament of knee

Head of fibula

Gerdy's tubercle

Posterior cruciate ligament

Medial condyle of femur (articular surface)

Medial meniscus

Tibial collateral ligament (superficial and deep fibers)

Medial condyle of tibia

Tibial tuberosity

Right knee in extension: posterior view

Adductor tubercle on medial epicondyle of femur

Medial condyle of femur (articular surface)

Tibial collateral ligament (superficial and deep fibers)

Medial meniscus

Medial condyle of tibia

Posterior cruciate ligament

Anterior cruciate ligament

Posterior meniscofemoral ligament

Lateral condyle of femur (articular surface)

Popliteus tendon

Fibular collateral ligament

Lateral meniscus

Head of fibula

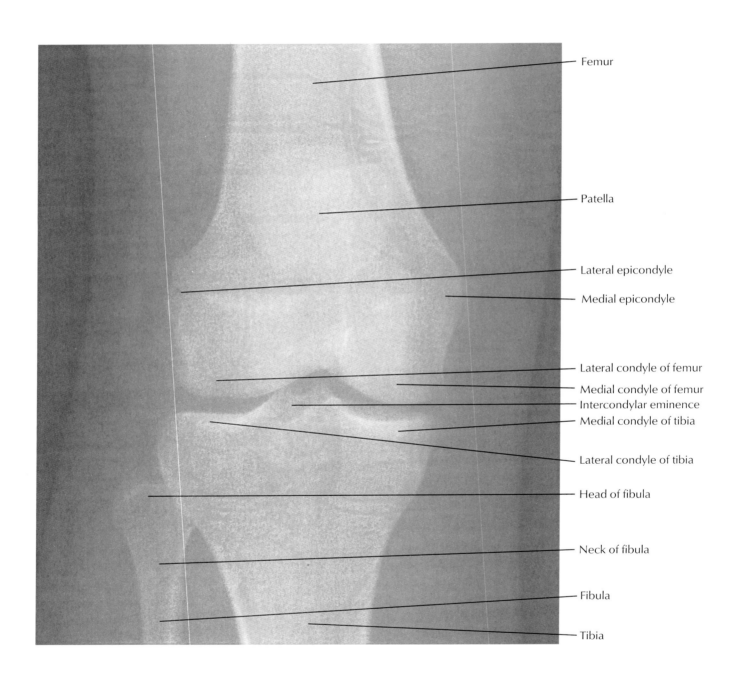

Femur

Patella

Lateral epicondyle

Medial epicondyle

Lateral condyle of femur

Medial condyle of femur

Intercondylar eminence

Medial condyle of tibia

Lateral condyle of tibia

Head of fibula

Neck of fibula

Fibula

Tibia

Plate 498 Anteroposterior Radiograph **Knee**

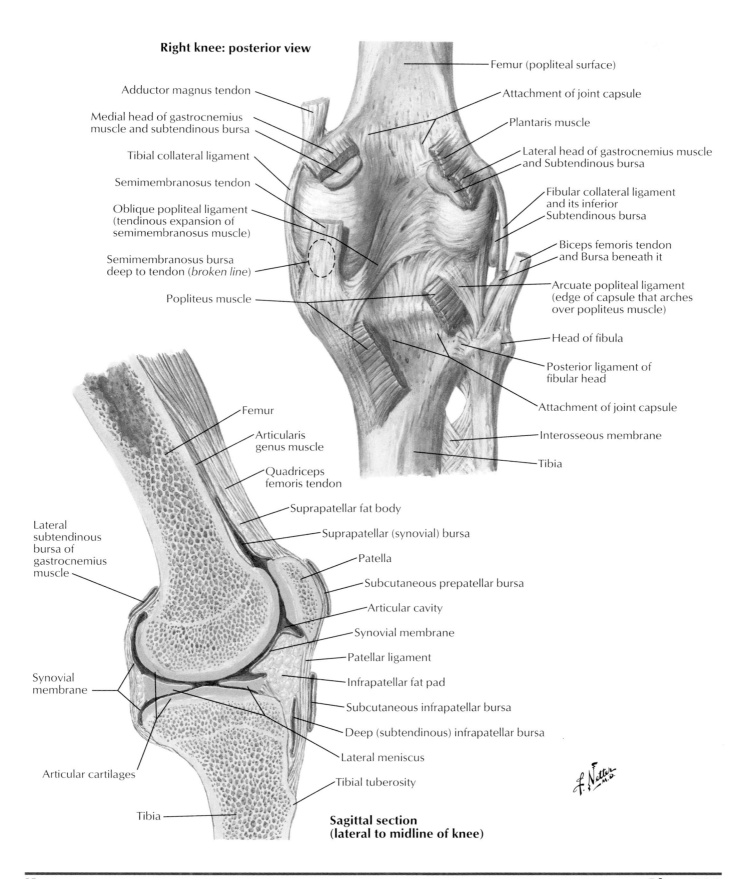

Right knee: posterior view

Adductor magnus tendon

Medial head of gastrocnemius muscle and subtendinous bursa

Tibial collateral ligament

Semimembranosus tendon

Oblique popliteal ligament (tendinous expansion of semimembranosus muscle)

Semimembranosus bursa deep to tendon (*broken line*)

Popliteus muscle

Femur (popliteal surface)

Attachment of joint capsule

Plantaris muscle

Lateral head of gastrocnemius muscle and Subtendinous bursa

Fibular collateral ligament and its inferior Subtendinous bursa

Biceps femoris tendon and Bursa beneath it

Arcuate popliteal ligament (edge of capsule that arches over popliteus muscle)

Head of fibula

Posterior ligament of fibular head

Attachment of joint capsule

Interosseous membrane

Tibia

Femur

Articularis genus muscle

Quadriceps femoris tendon

Suprapatellar fat body

Suprapatellar (synovial) bursa

Patella

Subcutaneous prepatellar bursa

Articular cavity

Synovial membrane

Patellar ligament

Infrapatellar fat pad

Subcutaneous infrapatellar bursa

Deep (subtendinous) infrapatellar bursa

Lateral meniscus

Tibial tuberosity

Lateral subtendinous bursa of gastrocnemius muscle

Synovial membrane

Articular cartilages

Tibia

Sagittal section (lateral to midline of knee)

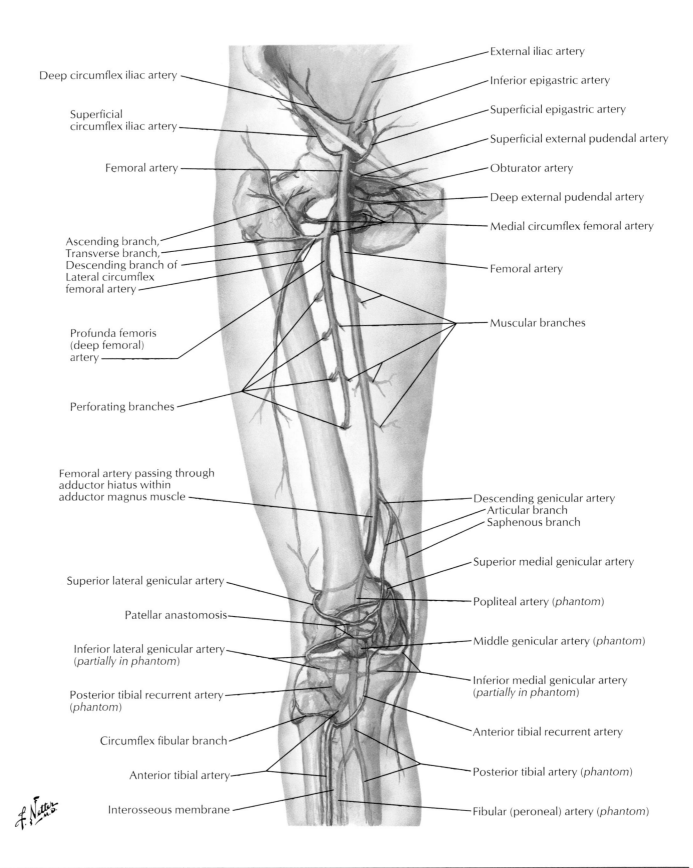

Deep circumflex iliac artery

Superficial circumflex iliac artery

Femoral artery

Ascending branch,
Transverse branch,
Descending branch of
Lateral circumflex
femoral artery

Profunda femoris
(deep femoral)
artery

Perforating branches

Femoral artery passing through
adductor hiatus within
adductor magnus muscle

Superior lateral genicular artery

Patellar anastomosis

Inferior lateral genicular artery
(*partially in phantom*)

Posterior tibial recurrent artery
(*phantom*)

Circumflex fibular branch

Anterior tibial artery

Interosseous membrane

External iliac artery

Inferior epigastric artery

Superficial epigastric artery

Superficial external pudendal artery

Obturator artery

Deep external pudendal artery

Medial circumflex femoral artery

Femoral artery

Muscular branches

Descending genicular artery
Articular branch
Saphenous branch

Superior medial genicular artery

Popliteal artery (*phantom*)

Middle genicular artery (*phantom*)

Inferior medial genicular artery
(*partially in phantom*)

Anterior tibial recurrent artery

Posterior tibial artery (*phantom*)

Fibular (peroneal) artery (*phantom*)

Plate 500 **Knee**

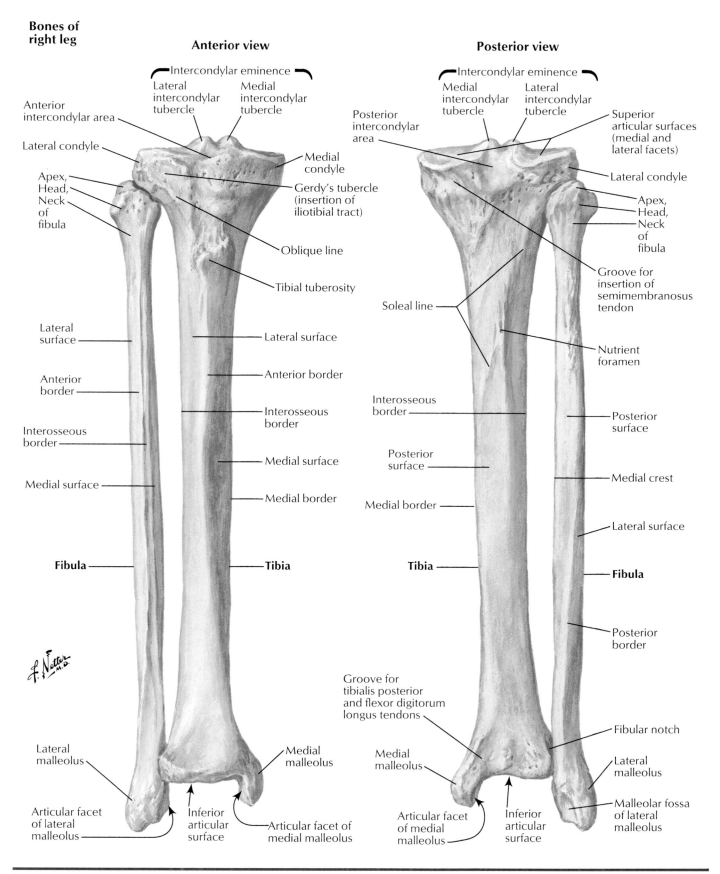

Bones of right leg

Anterior view

Intercondylar eminence

Lateral intercondylar tubercle

Medial intercondylar tubercle

Anterior intercondylar area

Lateral condyle

Medial condyle

Apex, Head, Neck of fibula

Gerdy's tubercle (insertion of iliotibial tract)

Oblique line

Tibial tuberosity

Lateral surface

Lateral surface

Anterior border

Anterior border

Interosseous border

Interosseous border

Medial surface

Medial surface

Medial border

Fibula

Tibia

Lateral malleolus

Medial malleolus

Articular facet of lateral malleolus

Inferior articular surface

Articular facet of medial malleolus

Posterior view

Intercondylar eminence

Medial intercondylar tubercle

Lateral intercondylar tubercle

Posterior intercondylar area

Superior articular surfaces (medial and lateral facets)

Lateral condyle

Apex, Head, Neck of fibula

Groove for insertion of semimembranosus tendon

Soleal line

Nutrient foramen

Interosseous border

Posterior surface

Posterior surface

Medial crest

Medial border

Lateral surface

Tibia

Fibula

Posterior border

Groove for tibialis posterior and flexor digitorum longus tendons

Medial malleolus

Fibular notch

Lateral malleolus

Articular facet of medial malleolus

Inferior articular surface

Malleolar fossa of lateral malleolus

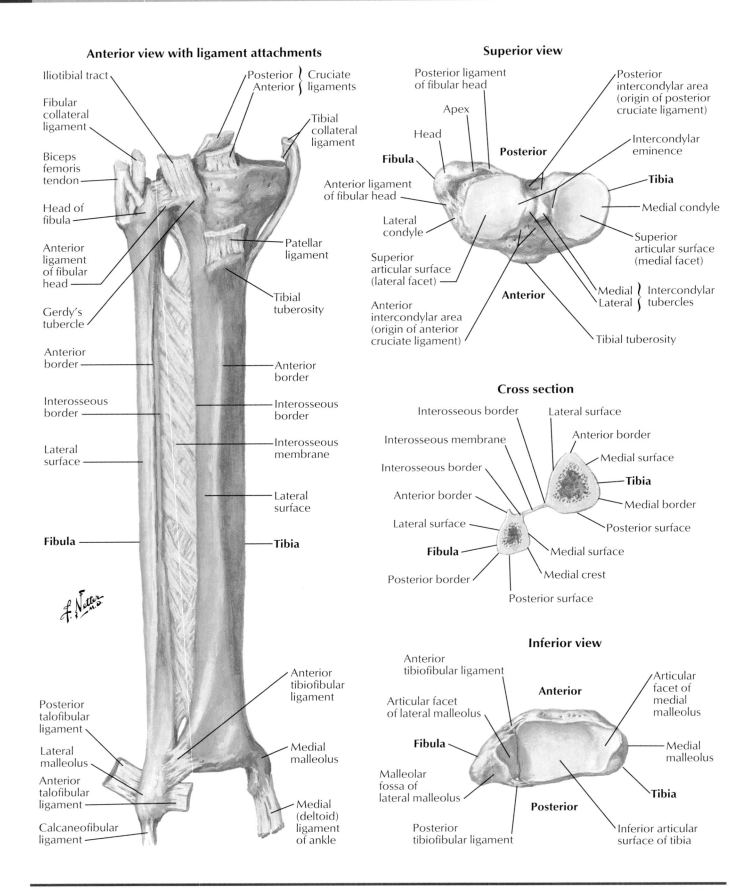

Anterior view with ligament attachments

Iliotibial tract

Fibular collateral ligament

Biceps femoris tendon

Head of fibula

Anterior ligament of fibular head

Gerdy's tubercle

Anterior border

Interosseous border

Lateral surface

Fibula

Posterior talofibular ligament

Lateral malleolus

Anterior talofibular ligament

Calcaneofibular ligament

Posterior } Cruciate
Anterior } ligaments

Tibial collateral ligament

Patellar ligament

Tibial tuberosity

Anterior border

Interosseous border

Interosseous membrane

Lateral surface

Tibia

Anterior tibiofibular ligament

Medial malleolus

Medial (deltoid) ligament of ankle

Superior view

Posterior ligament of fibular head

Apex

Head

Fibula

Anterior ligament of fibular head

Lateral condyle

Superior articular surface (lateral facet)

Anterior intercondylar area (origin of anterior cruciate ligament)

Posterior intercondylar area (origin of posterior cruciate ligament)

Intercondylar eminence

Posterior

Tibia

Medial condyle

Superior articular surface (medial facet)

Medial } Intercondylar
Lateral } tubercles

Tibial tuberosity

Anterior

Cross section

Interosseous border

Interosseous membrane

Interosseous border

Anterior border

Lateral surface

Fibula

Posterior border

Posterior surface

Lateral surface

Anterior border

Medial surface

Tibia

Medial border

Posterior surface

Medial surface

Medial crest

Inferior view

Anterior tibiofibular ligament

Articular facet of lateral malleolus

Fibula

Malleolar fossa of lateral malleolus

Posterior tibiofibular ligament

Anterior

Articular facet of medial malleolus

Medial malleolus

Tibia

Inferior articular surface of tibia

Posterior

Plate 502 **Leg**

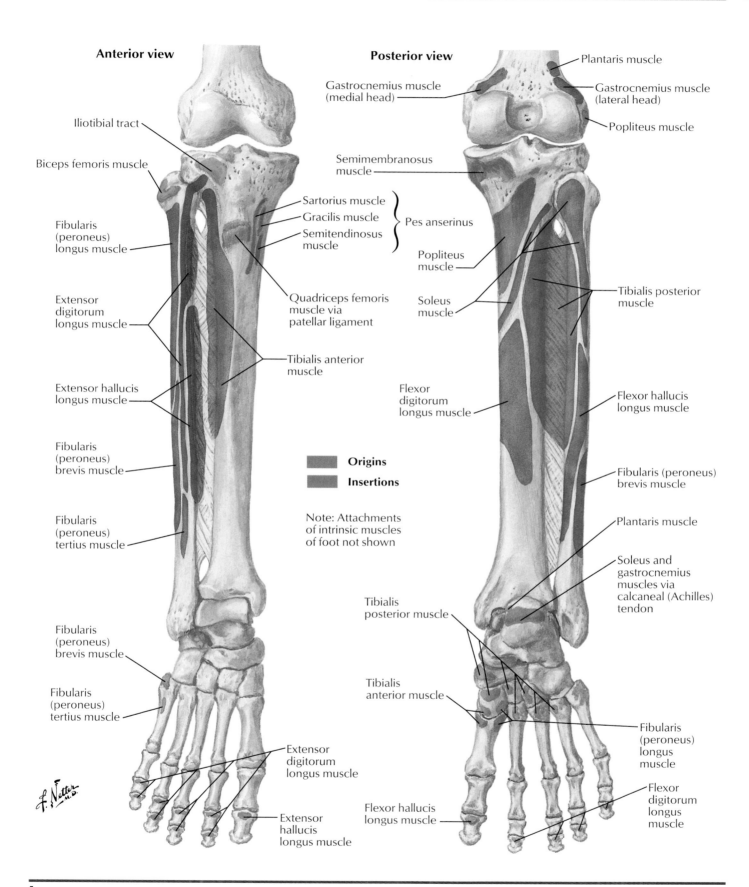

Anterior view

Iliotibial tract

Biceps femoris muscle

Fibularis (peroneus) longus muscle

Extensor digitorum longus muscle

Extensor hallucis longus muscle

Fibularis (peroneus) brevis muscle

Fibularis (peroneus) tertius muscle

Fibularis (peroneus) brevis muscle

Fibularis (peroneus) tertius muscle

Extensor digitorum longus muscle

Extensor hallucis longus muscle

Sartorius muscle
Gracilis muscle
Semitendinosus muscle

} Pes anserinus

Quadriceps femoris muscle via patellar ligament

Tibialis anterior muscle

Posterior view

Plantaris muscle

Gastrocnemius muscle (medial head)

Gastrocnemius muscle (lateral head)

Popliteus muscle

Semimembranosus muscle

Popliteus muscle

Soleus muscle

Tibialis posterior muscle

Flexor digitorum longus muscle

Flexor hallucis longus muscle

Fibularis (peroneus) brevis muscle

Plantaris muscle

Soleus and gastrocnemius muscles via calcaneal (Achilles) tendon

Tibialis posterior muscle

Tibialis anterior muscle

Fibularis (peroneus) longus muscle

Flexor hallucis longus muscle

Flexor digitorum longus muscle

Origins

Insertions

Note: Attachments of intrinsic muscles of foot not shown

F. Netter M.D.

Muscles of Leg (Superficial Dissection): Posterior View

See also **Plate 529**

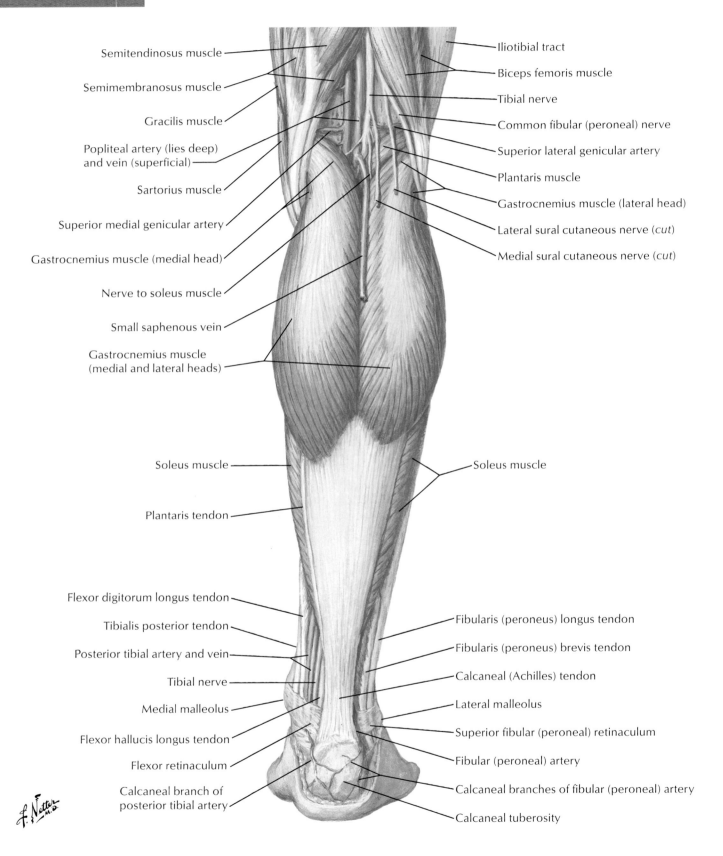

Semitendinosus muscle

Semimembranosus muscle

Gracilis muscle

Popliteal artery (lies deep) and vein (superficial)

Sartorius muscle

Superior medial genicular artery

Gastrocnemius muscle (medial head)

Nerve to soleus muscle

Small saphenous vein

Gastrocnemius muscle (medial and lateral heads)

Soleus muscle

Plantaris tendon

Flexor digitorum longus tendon

Tibialis posterior tendon

Posterior tibial artery and vein

Tibial nerve

Medial malleolus

Flexor hallucis longus tendon

Flexor retinaculum

Calcaneal branch of posterior tibial artery

Iliotibial tract

Biceps femoris muscle

Tibial nerve

Common fibular (peroneal) nerve

Superior lateral genicular artery

Plantaris muscle

Gastrocnemius muscle (lateral head)

Lateral sural cutaneous nerve (*cut*)

Medial sural cutaneous nerve (*cut*)

Soleus muscle

Fibularis (peroneus) longus tendon

Fibularis (peroneus) brevis tendon

Calcaneal (Achilles) tendon

Lateral malleolus

Superior fibular (peroneal) retinaculum

Fibular (peroneal) artery

Calcaneal branches of fibular (peroneal) artery

Calcaneal tuberosity

Plate 504   **Leg**

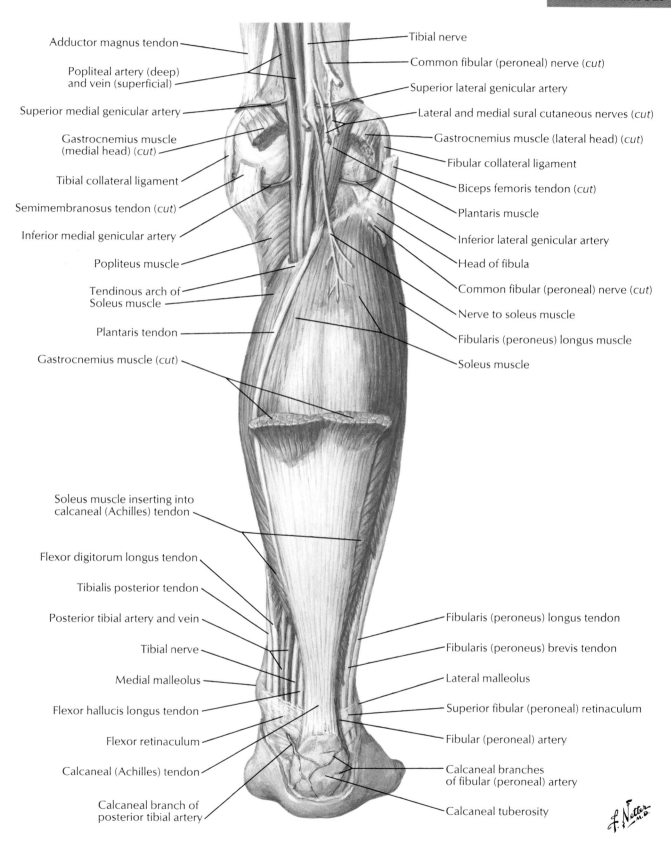

Adductor magnus tendon

Popliteal artery (deep) and vein (superficial)

Superior medial genicular artery

Gastrocnemius muscle (medial head) (*cut*)

Tibial collateral ligament

Semimembranosus tendon (*cut*)

Inferior medial genicular artery

Popliteus muscle

Tendinous arch of Soleus muscle

Plantaris tendon

Gastrocnemius muscle (*cut*)

Soleus muscle inserting into calcaneal (Achilles) tendon

Flexor digitorum longus tendon

Tibialis posterior tendon

Posterior tibial artery and vein

Tibial nerve

Medial malleolus

Flexor hallucis longus tendon

Flexor retinaculum

Calcaneal (Achilles) tendon

Calcaneal branch of posterior tibial artery

Tibial nerve

Common fibular (peroneal) nerve (*cut*)

Superior lateral genicular artery

Lateral and medial sural cutaneous nerves (*cut*)

Gastrocnemius muscle (lateral head) (*cut*)

Fibular collateral ligament

Biceps femoris tendon (*cut*)

Plantaris muscle

Inferior lateral genicular artery

Head of fibula

Common fibular (peroneal) nerve (*cut*)

Nerve to soleus muscle

Fibularis (peroneus) longus muscle

Soleus muscle

Fibularis (peroneus) longus tendon

Fibularis (peroneus) brevis tendon

Lateral malleolus

Superior fibular (peroneal) retinaculum

Fibular (peroneal) artery

Calcaneal branches of fibular (peroneal) artery

Calcaneal tuberosity

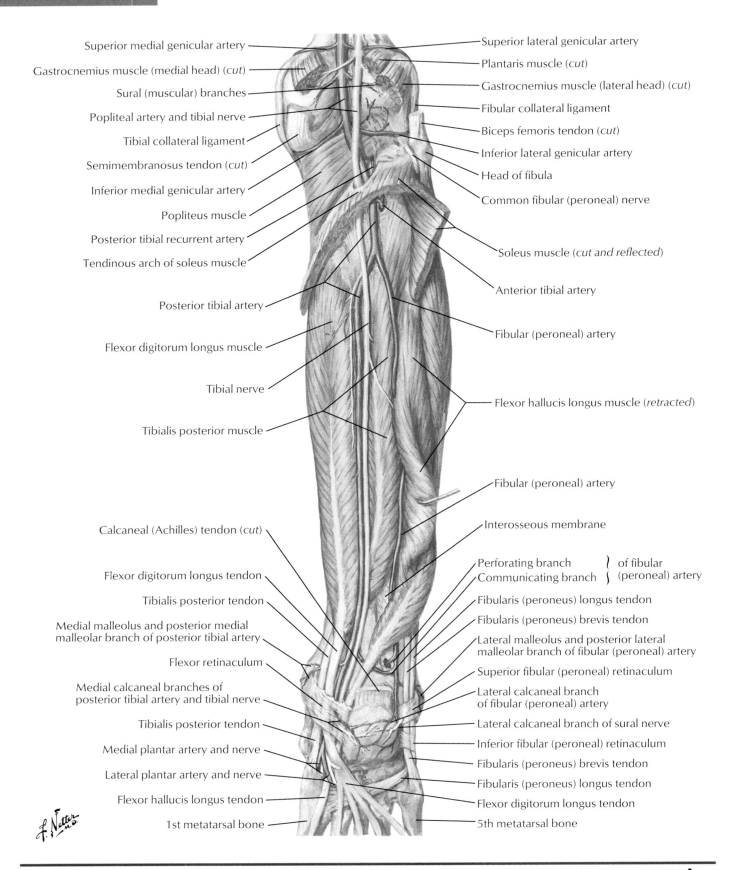

Superior medial genicular artery

Gastrocnemius muscle (medial head) *(cut)*

Sural (muscular) branches

Popliteal artery and tibial nerve

Tibial collateral ligament

Semimembranosus tendon *(cut)*

Inferior medial genicular artery

Popliteus muscle

Posterior tibial recurrent artery

Tendinous arch of soleus muscle

Posterior tibial artery

Flexor digitorum longus muscle

Tibial nerve

Tibialis posterior muscle

Calcaneal (Achilles) tendon *(cut)*

Flexor digitorum longus tendon

Tibialis posterior tendon

Medial malleolus and posterior medial
malleolar branch of posterior tibial artery

Flexor retinaculum

Medial calcaneal branches of
posterior tibial artery and tibial nerve

Tibialis posterior tendon

Medial plantar artery and nerve

Lateral plantar artery and nerve

Flexor hallucis longus tendon

1st metatarsal bone

Superior lateral genicular artery

Plantaris muscle *(cut)*

Gastrocnemius muscle (lateral head) *(cut)*

Fibular collateral ligament

Biceps femoris tendon *(cut)*

Inferior lateral genicular artery

Head of fibula

Common fibular (peroneal) nerve

Soleus muscle *(cut and reflected)*

Anterior tibial artery

Fibular (peroneal) artery

Flexor hallucis longus muscle *(retracted)*

Fibular (peroneal) artery

Interosseous membrane

Perforating branch } of fibular
Communicating branch } (peroneal) artery

Fibularis (peroneus) longus tendon

Fibularis (peroneus) brevis tendon

Lateral malleolus and posterior lateral
malleolar branch of fibular (peroneal) artery

Superior fibular (peroneal) retinaculum

Lateral calcaneal branch
of fibular (peroneal) artery

Lateral calcaneal branch of sural nerve

Inferior fibular (peroneal) retinaculum

Fibularis (peroneus) brevis tendon

Fibularis (peroneus) longus tendon

Flexor digitorum longus tendon

5th metatarsal bone

Plate 506

Leg

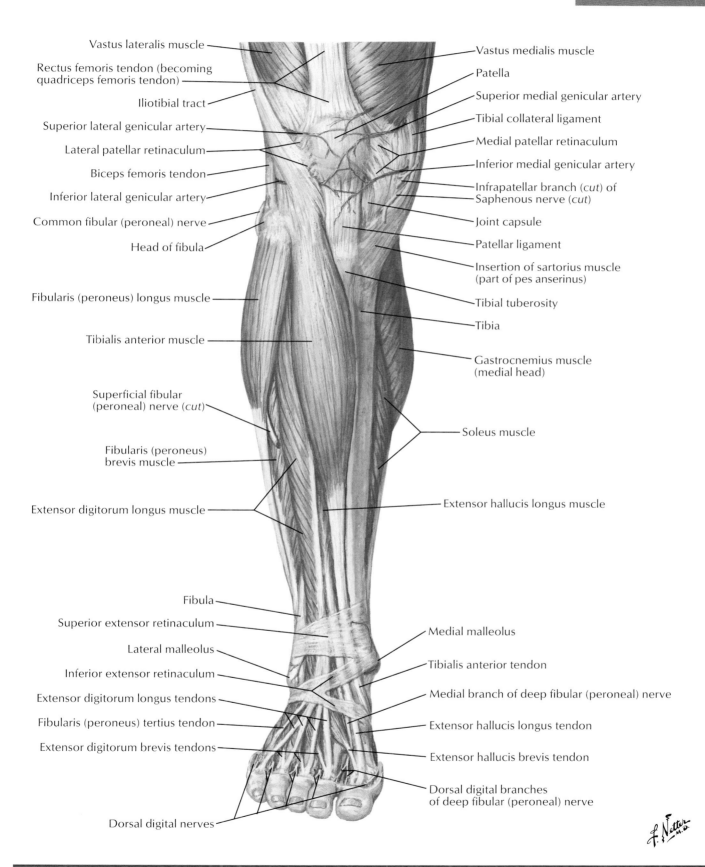

Vastus lateralis muscle

Rectus femoris tendon (becoming quadriceps femoris tendon)

Iliotibial tract

Superior lateral genicular artery

Lateral patellar retinaculum

Biceps femoris tendon

Inferior lateral genicular artery

Common fibular (peroneal) nerve

Head of fibula

Fibularis (peroneus) longus muscle

Tibialis anterior muscle

Superficial fibular (peroneal) nerve (*cut*)

Fibularis (peroneus) brevis muscle

Extensor digitorum longus muscle

Fibula

Superior extensor retinaculum

Lateral malleolus

Inferior extensor retinaculum

Extensor digitorum longus tendons

Fibularis (peroneus) tertius tendon

Extensor digitorum brevis tendons

Dorsal digital nerves

Vastus medialis muscle

Patella

Superior medial genicular artery

Tibial collateral ligament

Medial patellar retinaculum

Inferior medial genicular artery

Infrapatellar branch (*cut*) of Saphenous nerve (*cut*)

Joint capsule

Patellar ligament

Insertion of sartorius muscle (part of pes anserinus)

Tibial tuberosity

Tibia

Gastrocnemius muscle (medial head)

Soleus muscle

Extensor hallucis longus muscle

Medial malleolus

Tibialis anterior tendon

Medial branch of deep fibular (peroneal) nerve

Extensor hallucis longus tendon

Extensor hallucis brevis tendon

Dorsal digital branches of deep fibular (peroneal) nerve

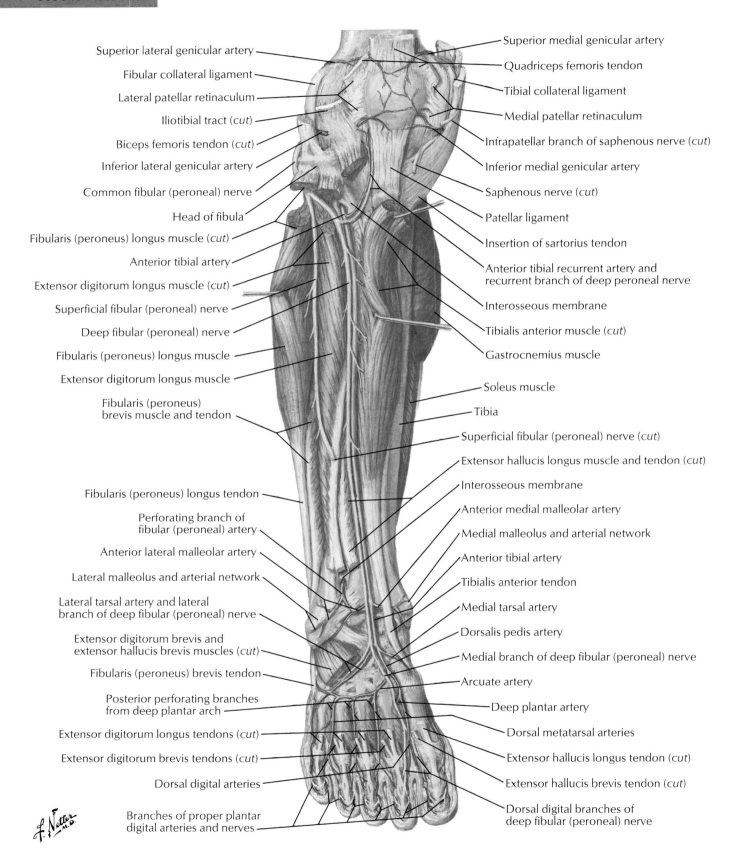

Superior lateral genicular artery

Fibular collateral ligament

Lateral patellar retinaculum

Iliotibial tract (*cut*)

Biceps femoris tendon (*cut*)

Inferior lateral genicular artery

Common fibular (peroneal) nerve

Head of fibula

Fibularis (peroneus) longus muscle (*cut*)

Anterior tibial artery

Extensor digitorum longus muscle (*cut*)

Superficial fibular (peroneal) nerve

Deep fibular (peroneal) nerve

Fibularis (peroneus) longus muscle

Extensor digitorum longus muscle

Fibularis (peroneus) brevis muscle and tendon

Fibularis (peroneus) longus tendon

Perforating branch of fibular (peroneal) artery

Anterior lateral malleolar artery

Lateral malleolus and arterial network

Lateral tarsal artery and lateral branch of deep fibular (peroneal) nerve

Extensor digitorum brevis and extensor hallucis brevis muscles (*cut*)

Fibularis (peroneus) brevis tendon

Posterior perforating branches from deep plantar arch

Extensor digitorum longus tendons (*cut*)

Extensor digitorum brevis tendons (*cut*)

Dorsal digital arteries

Branches of proper plantar digital arteries and nerves

Superior medial genicular artery

Quadriceps femoris tendon

Tibial collateral ligament

Medial patellar retinaculum

Infrapatellar branch of saphenous nerve (*cut*)

Inferior medial genicular artery

Saphenous nerve (*cut*)

Patellar ligament

Insertion of sartorius tendon

Anterior tibial recurrent artery and recurrent branch of deep peroneal nerve

Interosseous membrane

Tibialis anterior muscle (*cut*)

Gastrocnemius muscle

Soleus muscle

Tibia

Superficial fibular (peroneal) nerve (*cut*)

Extensor hallucis longus muscle and tendon (*cut*)

Interosseous membrane

Anterior medial malleolar artery

Medial malleolus and arterial network

Anterior tibial artery

Tibialis anterior tendon

Medial tarsal artery

Dorsalis pedis artery

Medial branch of deep fibular (peroneal) nerve

Arcuate artery

Deep plantar artery

Dorsal metatarsal arteries

Extensor hallucis longus tendon (*cut*)

Extensor hallucis brevis tendon (*cut*)

Dorsal digital branches of deep fibular (peroneal) nerve

Plate 508

Leg

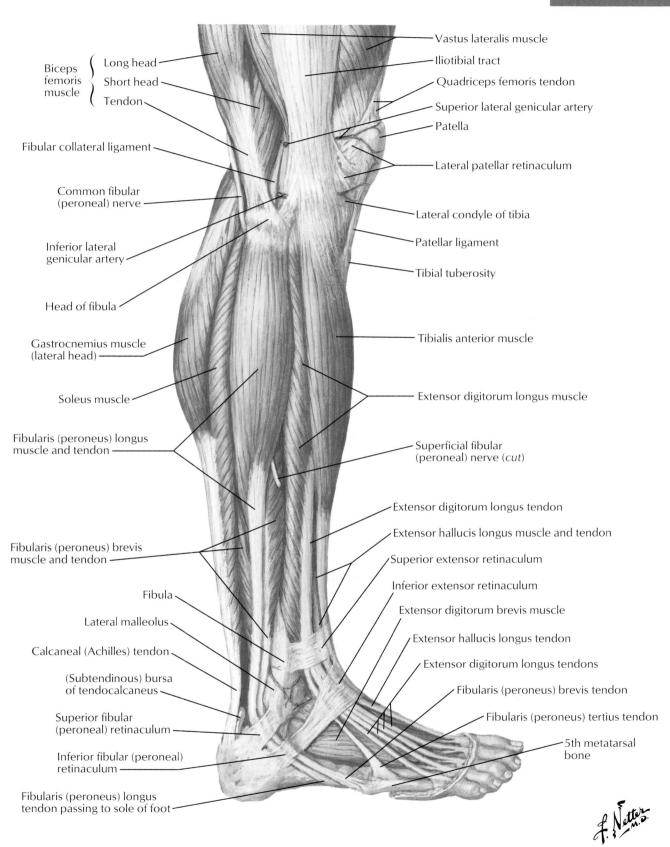

Biceps femoris muscle
{ Long head
Short head
Tendon

Fibular collateral ligament

Common fibular (peroneal) nerve

Inferior lateral genicular artery

Head of fibula

Gastrocnemius muscle (lateral head)

Soleus muscle

Fibularis (peroneus) longus muscle and tendon

Fibularis (peroneus) brevis muscle and tendon

Fibula

Lateral malleolus

Calcaneal (Achilles) tendon

(Subtendinous) bursa of tendocalcaneus

Superior fibular (peroneal) retinaculum

Inferior fibular (peroneal) retinaculum

Fibularis (peroneus) longus tendon passing to sole of foot

Vastus lateralis muscle

Iliotibial tract

Quadriceps femoris tendon

Superior lateral genicular artery

Patella

Lateral patellar retinaculum

Lateral condyle of tibia

Patellar ligament

Tibial tuberosity

Tibialis anterior muscle

Extensor digitorum longus muscle

Superficial fibular (peroneal) nerve (*cut*)

Extensor digitorum longus tendon

Extensor hallucis longus muscle and tendon

Superior extensor retinaculum

Inferior extensor retinaculum

Extensor digitorum brevis muscle

Extensor hallucis longus tendon

Extensor digitorum longus tendons

Fibularis (peroneus) brevis tendon

Fibularis (peroneus) tertius tendon

5th metatarsal bone

F. Netter M.D.

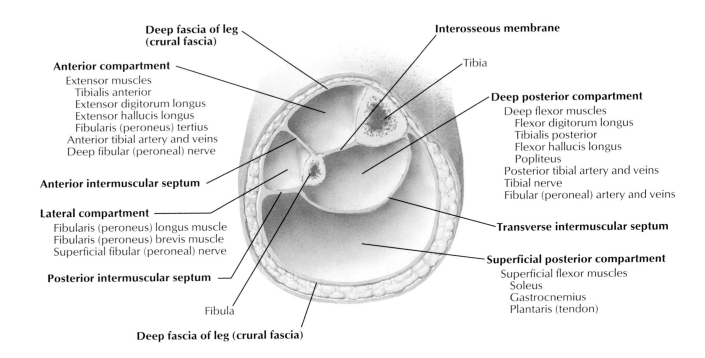

Cross section just above middle of leg

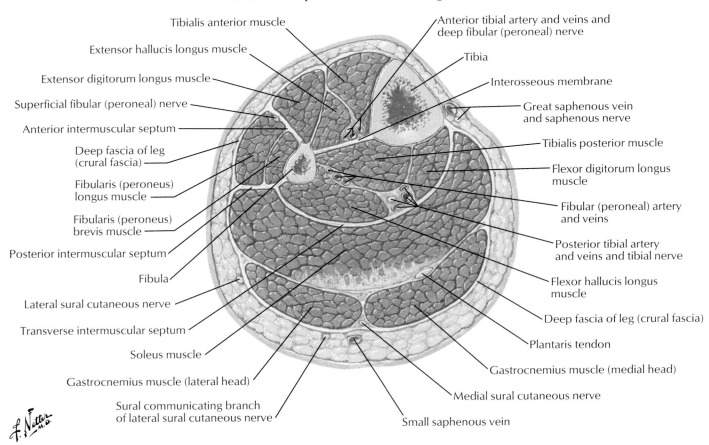

Plate 510

Leg

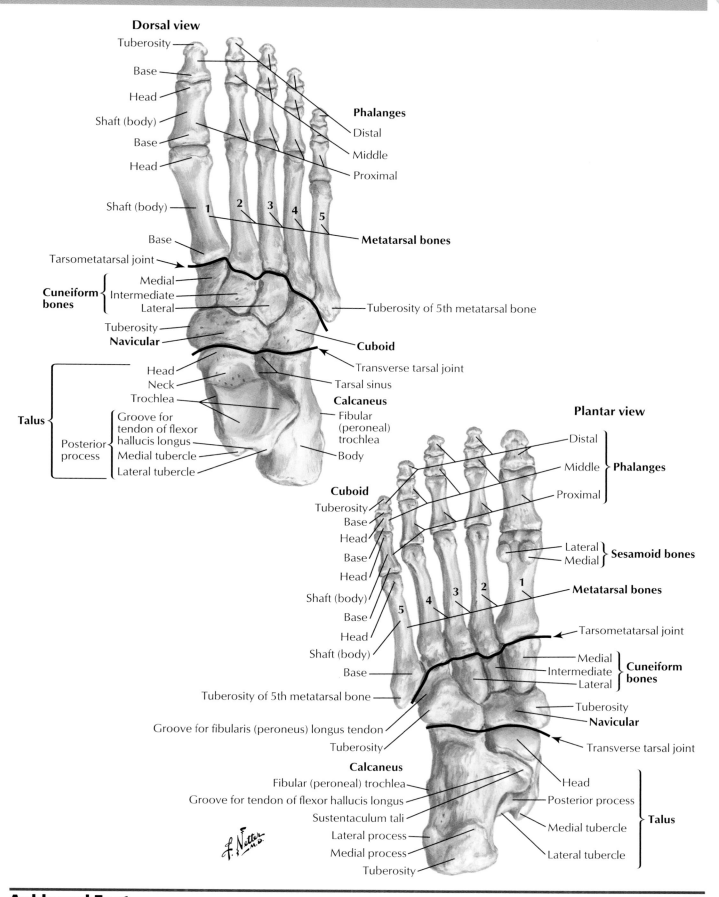

Dorsal view

Tuberosity

Base

Head

Shaft (body)

Base

Head

Shaft (body)

Phalanges

Distal

Middle

Proximal

1 2 3 4 5

Metatarsal bones

Base

Tarsometatarsal joint

Cuneiform bones

Medial
Intermediate
Lateral

Tuberosity of 5th metatarsal bone

Tuberosity

Navicular

Cuboid

Transverse tarsal joint

Head

Neck

Trochlea

Tarsal sinus

Calcaneus

Talus

Posterior process

Groove for tendon of flexor hallucis longus

Medial tubercle

Lateral tubercle

Fibular (peroneal) trochlea

Body

Plantar view

Distal

Middle

Proximal

Phalanges

Lateral

Medial

Sesamoid bones

Metatarsal bones

1 2 3 4 5

Tarsometatarsal joint

Medial
Intermediate
Lateral

Cuneiform bones

Tuberosity

Navicular

Transverse tarsal joint

Head

Posterior process

Medial tubercle

Lateral tubercle

Talus

Cuboid

Tuberosity

Base

Head

Base

Head

Shaft (body)

Base

Head

Shaft (body)

Base

Tuberosity of 5th metatarsal bone

Groove for fibularis (peroneus) longus tendon

Tuberosity

Calcaneus

Fibular (peroneal) trochlea

Groove for tendon of flexor hallucis longus

Sustentaculum tali

Lateral process

Medial process

Tuberosity

F. Netter M.D.

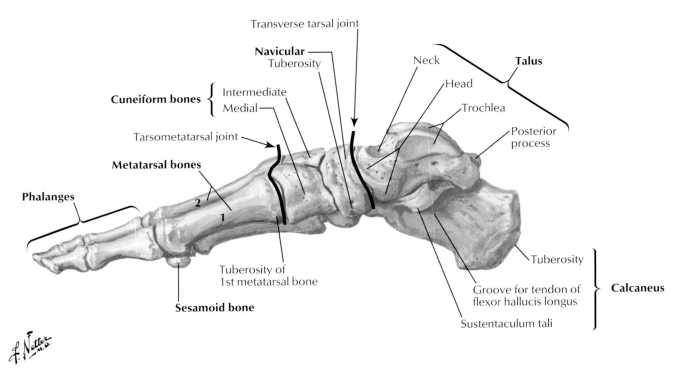

Lateral view

Talus
- Head
- Neck
- Trochlea
- Lateral process
- Posterior process

Transverse tarsal joint

Navicular

Intermediate
Lateral } **Cuneiform bones**

Tarsometatarsal joint

Metatarsal bones

Phalanges

Tarsal sinus

Calcaneus
- Body
- Fibular (peroneal) trochlea
- Tuberosity
- Groove for fibularis (peroneus) longus tendon

Cuboid

Tuberosity

Groove for fibularis (peroneus) longus tendon

Tuberosity of 5th metatarsal bone

2
3
4
5

Medial view

Transverse tarsal joint

Navicular
Tuberosity

Neck

Talus

Head

Trochlea

Posterior process

Cuneiform bones {
Intermediate
Medial

Tarsometatarsal joint

Metatarsal bones

Phalanges

2
1

Tuberosity of 1st metatarsal bone

Sesamoid bone

Tuberosity

Groove for tendon of flexor hallucis longus

Sustentaculum tali

} **Calcaneus**

Plate 512

Ankle and Foot

Right foot

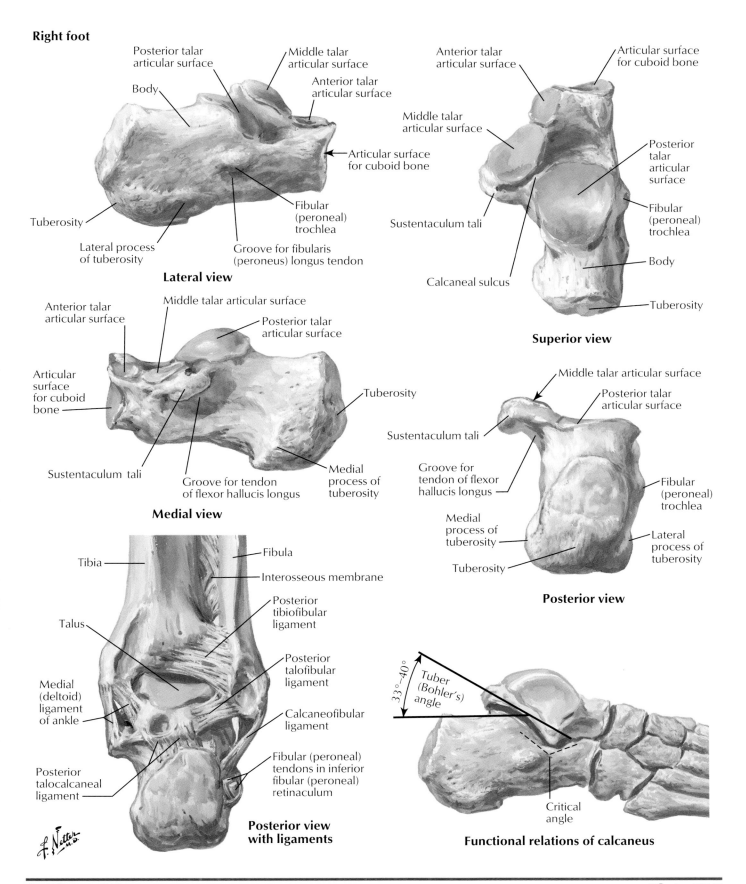

Posterior talar articular surface

Body

Middle talar articular surface

Anterior talar articular surface

Articular surface for cuboid bone

Tuberosity

Lateral process of tuberosity

Fibular (peroneal) trochlea

Groove for fibularis (peroneus) longus tendon

Lateral view

Anterior talar articular surface

Middle talar articular surface

Articular surface for cuboid bone

Posterior talar articular surface

Tuberosity

Sustentaculum tali

Groove for tendon of flexor hallucis longus

Medial process of tuberosity

Medial view

Anterior talar articular surface

Articular surface for cuboid bone

Middle talar articular surface

Sustentaculum tali

Posterior talar articular surface

Fibular (peroneal) trochlea

Body

Calcaneal sulcus

Tuberosity

Superior view

Middle talar articular surface

Posterior talar articular surface

Sustentaculum tali

Groove for tendon of flexor hallucis longus

Medial process of tuberosity

Tuberosity

Fibular (peroneal) trochlea

Lateral process of tuberosity

Posterior view

Tibia

Talus

Medial (deltoid) ligament of ankle

Posterior talocalcaneal ligament

Fibula

Interosseous membrane

Posterior tibiofibular ligament

Posterior talofibular ligament

Calcaneofibular ligament

Fibular (peroneal) tendons in inferior fibular (peroneal) retinaculum

Posterior view with ligaments

33°–40°

Tuber (Bohler's) angle

Critical angle

Functional relations of calcaneus

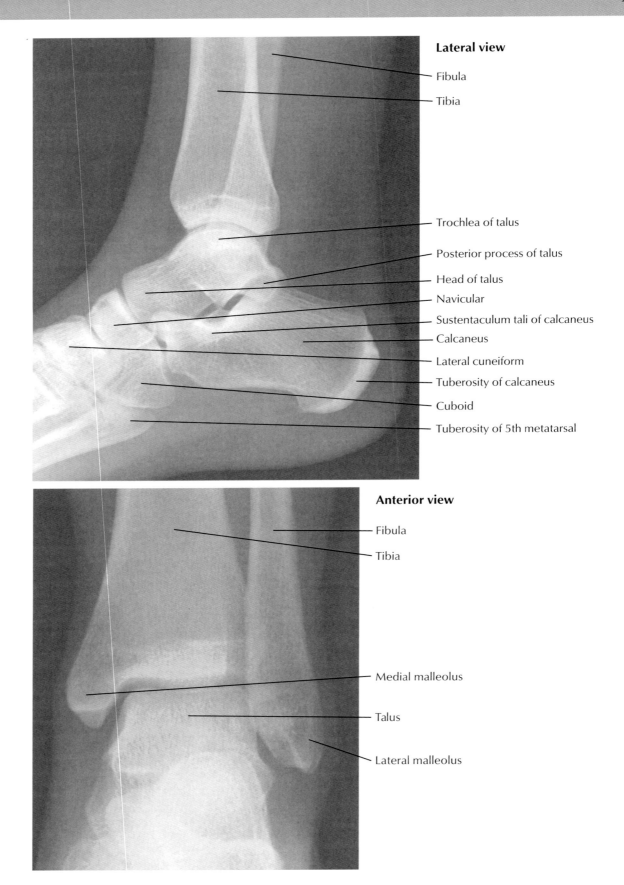

Lateral view

Fibula

Tibia

Trochlea of talus

Posterior process of talus

Head of talus

Navicular

Sustentaculum tali of calcaneus

Calcaneus

Lateral cuneiform

Tuberosity of calcaneus

Cuboid

Tuberosity of 5th metatarsal

Anterior view

Fibula

Tibia

Medial malleolus

Talus

Lateral malleolus

Plate 514　　　　　　　　　　　　　　　　　　**Ankle and Foot**

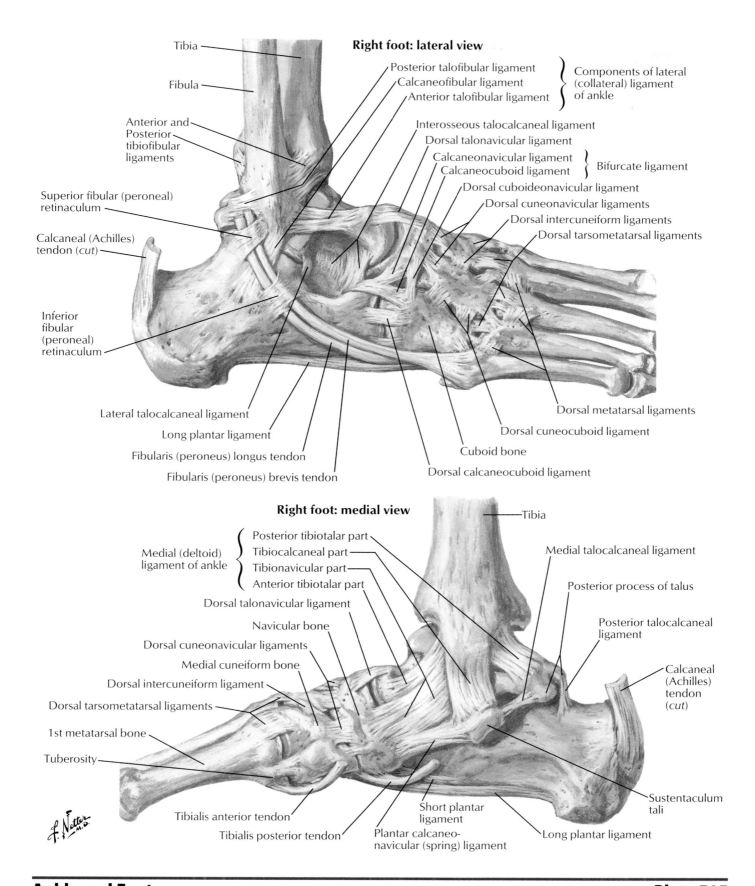

Right foot: lateral view

Tibia

Fibula

Posterior talofibular ligament
Calcaneofibular ligament
Anterior talofibular ligament
} Components of lateral (collateral) ligament of ankle

Anterior and Posterior tibiofibular ligaments

Interosseous talocalcaneal ligament
Dorsal talonavicular ligament
Calcaneonavicular ligament
Calcaneocuboid ligament
} Bifurcate ligament
Dorsal cuboideonavicular ligament
Dorsal cuneonavicular ligaments
Dorsal intercuneiform ligaments
Dorsal tarsometatarsal ligaments

Superior fibular (peroneal) retinaculum

Calcaneal (Achilles) tendon (cut)

Inferior fibular (peroneal) retinaculum

Lateral talocalcaneal ligament

Long plantar ligament

Fibularis (peroneus) longus tendon

Fibularis (peroneus) brevis tendon

Dorsal metatarsal ligaments

Dorsal cuneocuboid ligament

Cuboid bone

Dorsal calcaneocuboid ligament

Right foot: medial view

Tibia

Medial (deltoid) ligament of ankle
{ Posterior tibiotalar part
Tibiocalcaneal part
Tibionavicular part
Anterior tibiotalar part

Medial talocalcaneal ligament

Posterior process of talus

Posterior talocalcaneal ligament

Calcaneal (Achilles) tendon (cut)

Dorsal talonavicular ligament

Navicular bone

Dorsal cuneonavicular ligaments

Medial cuneiform bone

Dorsal intercuneiform ligament

Dorsal tarsometatarsal ligaments

1st metatarsal bone

Tuberosity

Tibialis anterior tendon

Tibialis posterior tendon

Short plantar ligament

Plantar calcaneonavicular (spring) ligament

Long plantar ligament

Sustentaculum tali

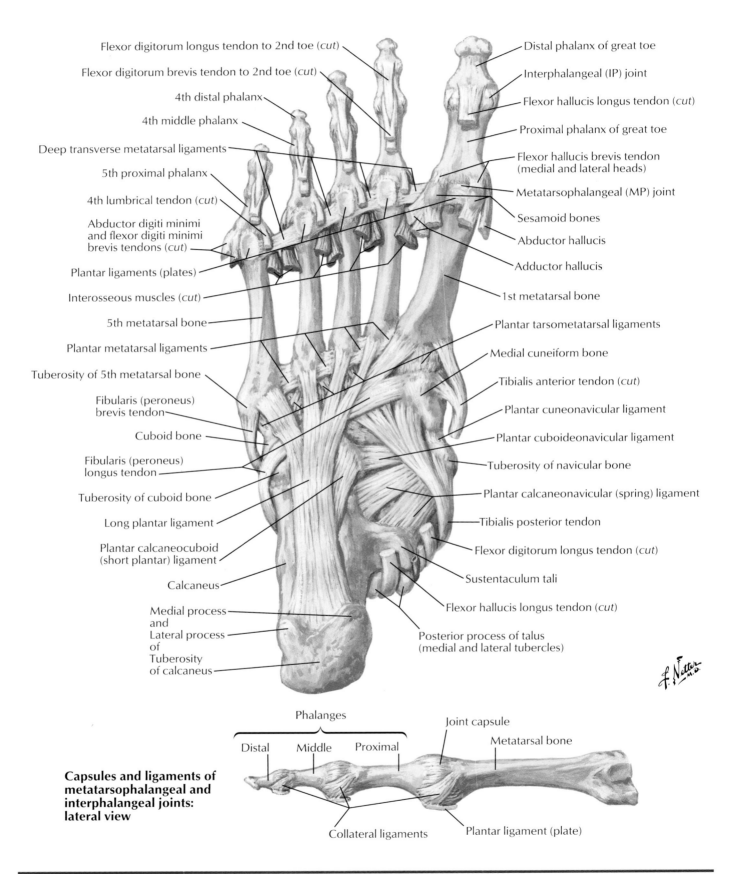

Flexor digitorum longus tendon to 2nd toe (*cut*)

Flexor digitorum brevis tendon to 2nd toe (*cut*)

4th distal phalanx

4th middle phalanx

Deep transverse metatarsal ligaments

5th proximal phalanx

4th lumbrical tendon (*cut*)

Abductor digiti minimi and flexor digiti minimi brevis tendons (*cut*)

Plantar ligaments (plates)

Interosseous muscles (*cut*)

5th metatarsal bone

Plantar metatarsal ligaments

Tuberosity of 5th metatarsal bone

Fibularis (peroneus) brevis tendon

Cuboid bone

Fibularis (peroneus) longus tendon

Tuberosity of cuboid bone

Long plantar ligament

Plantar calcaneocuboid (short plantar) ligament

Calcaneus

Medial process and Lateral process of Tuberosity of calcaneus

Distal phalanx of great toe

Interphalangeal (IP) joint

Flexor hallucis longus tendon (*cut*)

Proximal phalanx of great toe

Flexor hallucis brevis tendon (medial and lateral heads)

Metatarsophalangeal (MP) joint

Sesamoid bones

Abductor hallucis

Adductor hallucis

1st metatarsal bone

Plantar tarsometatarsal ligaments

Medial cuneiform bone

Tibialis anterior tendon (*cut*)

Plantar cuneonavicular ligament

Plantar cuboideonavicular ligament

Tuberosity of navicular bone

Plantar calcaneonavicular (spring) ligament

Tibialis posterior tendon

Flexor digitorum longus tendon (*cut*)

Sustentaculum tali

Flexor hallucis longus tendon (*cut*)

Posterior process of talus (medial and lateral tubercles)

Phalanges

Distal   Middle   Proximal

Joint capsule

Metatarsal bone

Capsules and ligaments of metatarsophalangeal and interphalangeal joints: lateral view

Collateral ligaments

Plantar ligament (plate)

Plate 516

Ankle and Foot

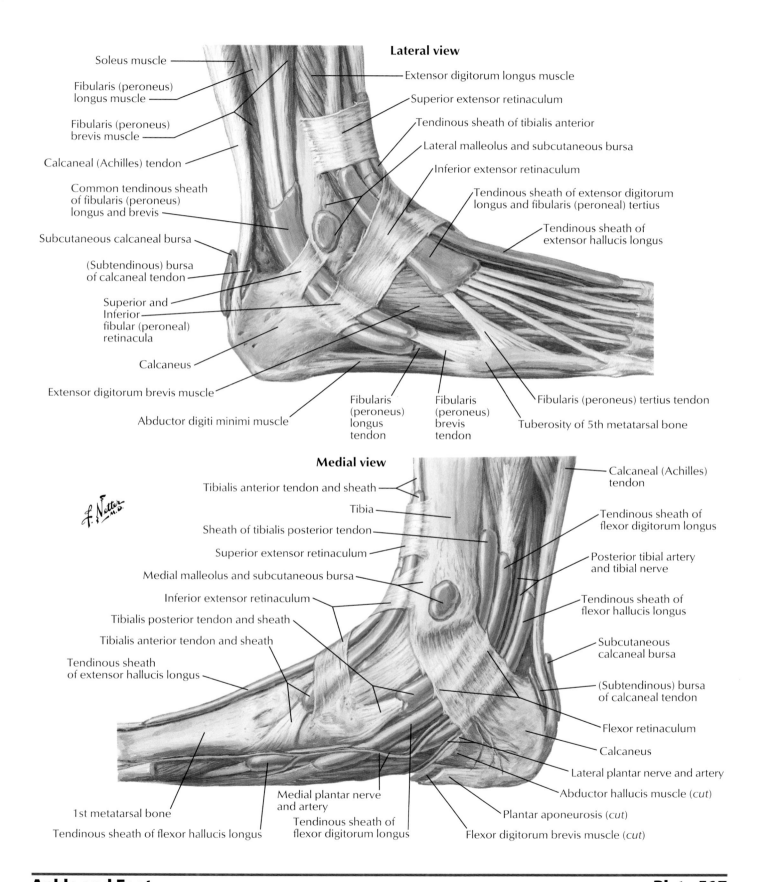

Lateral view

Soleus muscle

Fibularis (peroneus) longus muscle

Fibularis (peroneus) brevis muscle

Calcaneal (Achilles) tendon

Common tendinous sheath of fibularis (peroneus) longus and brevis

Subcutaneous calcaneal bursa

(Subtendinous) bursa of calcaneal tendon

Superior and Inferior fibular (peroneal) retinacula

Calcaneus

Extensor digitorum brevis muscle

Abductor digiti minimi muscle

Extensor digitorum longus muscle

Superior extensor retinaculum

Tendinous sheath of tibialis anterior

Lateral malleolus and subcutaneous bursa

Inferior extensor retinaculum

Tendinous sheath of extensor digitorum longus and fibularis (peroneal) tertius

Tendinous sheath of extensor hallucis longus

Fibularis (peroneus) longus tendon

Fibularis (peroneus) brevis tendon

Fibularis (peroneus) tertius tendon

Tuberosity of 5th metatarsal bone

Medial view

Tibialis anterior tendon and sheath

Tibia

Sheath of tibialis posterior tendon

Superior extensor retinaculum

Medial malleolus and subcutaneous bursa

Inferior extensor retinaculum

Tibialis posterior tendon and sheath

Tibialis anterior tendon and sheath

Tendinous sheath of extensor hallucis longus

1st metatarsal bone

Tendinous sheath of flexor hallucis longus

Medial plantar nerve and artery

Tendinous sheath of flexor digitorum longus

Calcaneal (Achilles) tendon

Tendinous sheath of flexor digitorum longus

Posterior tibial artery and tibial nerve

Tendinous sheath of flexor hallucis longus

Subcutaneous calcaneal bursa

(Subtendinous) bursa of calcaneal tendon

Flexor retinaculum

Calcaneus

Lateral plantar nerve and artery

Abductor hallucis muscle (*cut*)

Plantar aponeurosis (*cut*)

Flexor digitorum brevis muscle (*cut*)

f. Netter M.D.

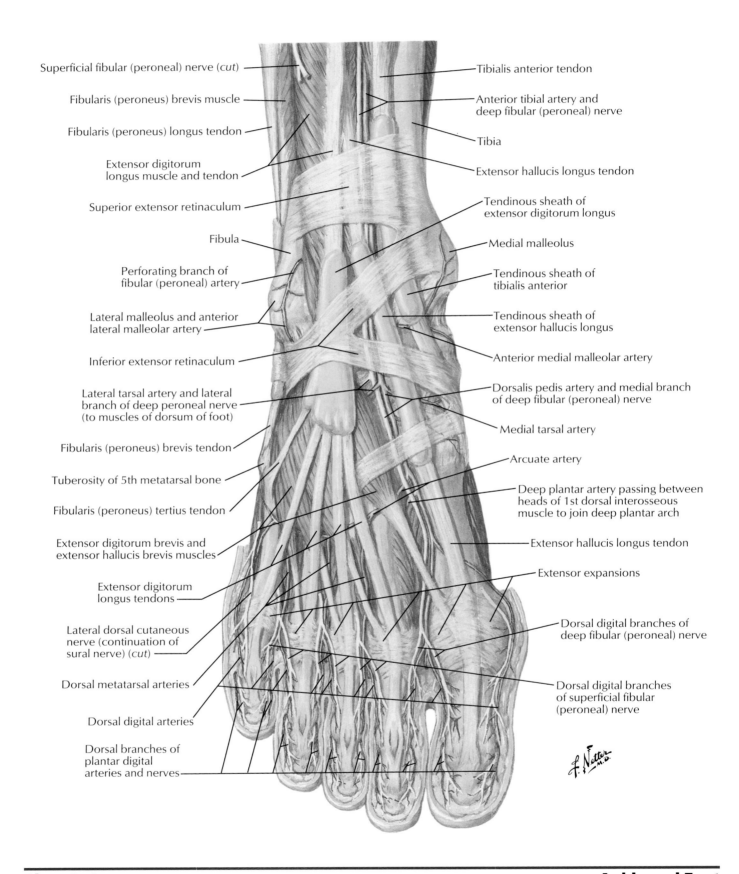

Superficial fibular (peroneal) nerve (*cut*)

Fibularis (peroneus) brevis muscle

Fibularis (peroneus) longus tendon

Extensor digitorum longus muscle and tendon

Superior extensor retinaculum

Fibula

Perforating branch of fibular (peroneal) artery

Lateral malleolus and anterior lateral malleolar artery

Inferior extensor retinaculum

Lateral tarsal artery and lateral branch of deep peroneal nerve (to muscles of dorsum of foot)

Fibularis (peroneus) brevis tendon

Tuberosity of 5th metatarsal bone

Fibularis (peroneus) tertius tendon

Extensor digitorum brevis and extensor hallucis brevis muscles

Extensor digitorum longus tendons

Lateral dorsal cutaneous nerve (continuation of sural nerve) (*cut*)

Dorsal metatarsal arteries

Dorsal digital arteries

Dorsal branches of plantar digital arteries and nerves

Tibialis anterior tendon

Anterior tibial artery and deep fibular (peroneal) nerve

Tibia

Extensor hallucis longus tendon

Tendinous sheath of extensor digitorum longus

Medial malleolus

Tendinous sheath of tibialis anterior

Tendinous sheath of extensor hallucis longus

Anterior medial malleolar artery

Dorsalis pedis artery and medial branch of deep fibular (peroneal) nerve

Medial tarsal artery

Arcuate artery

Deep plantar artery passing between heads of 1st dorsal interosseous muscle to join deep plantar arch

Extensor hallucis longus tendon

Extensor expansions

Dorsal digital branches of deep fibular (peroneal) nerve

Dorsal digital branches of superficial fibular (peroneal) nerve

Plate 518

Ankle and Foot

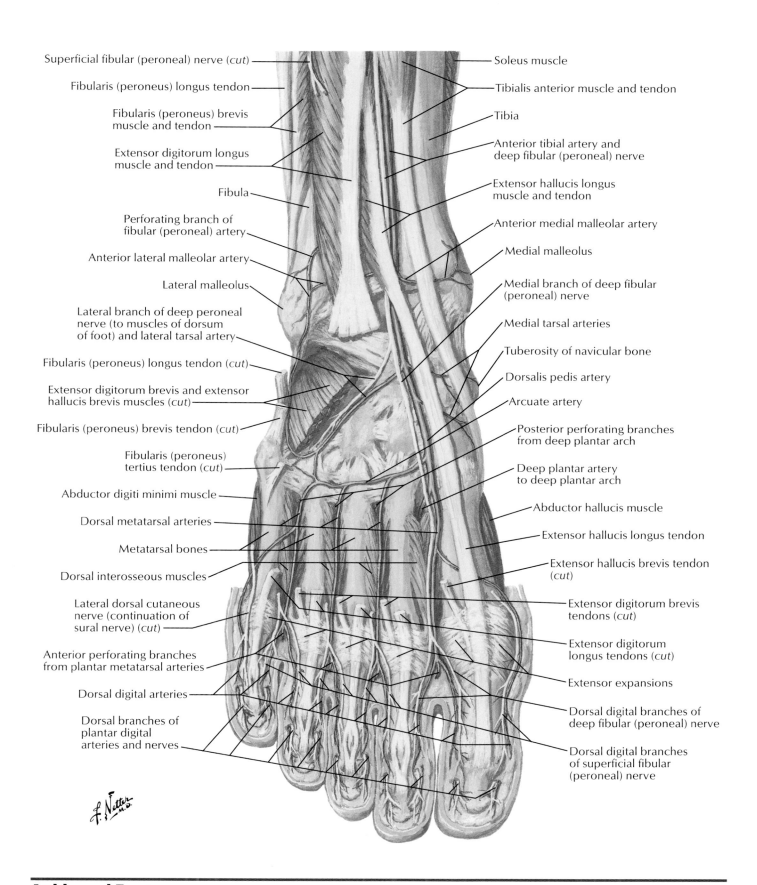

Superficial fibular (peroneal) nerve (*cut*)

Fibularis (peroneus) longus tendon

Fibularis (peroneus) brevis
muscle and tendon

Extensor digitorum longus
muscle and tendon

Fibula

Perforating branch of
fibular (peroneal) artery

Anterior lateral malleolar artery

Lateral malleolus

Lateral branch of deep peroneal
nerve (to muscles of dorsum
of foot) and lateral tarsal artery

Fibularis (peroneus) longus tendon (*cut*)

Extensor digitorum brevis and extensor
hallucis brevis muscles (*cut*)

Fibularis (peroneus) brevis tendon (*cut*)

Fibularis (peroneus)
tertius tendon (*cut*)

Abductor digiti minimi muscle

Dorsal metatarsal arteries

Metatarsal bones

Dorsal interosseous muscles

Lateral dorsal cutaneous
nerve (continuation of
sural nerve) (*cut*)

Anterior perforating branches
from plantar metatarsal arteries

Dorsal digital arteries

Dorsal branches of
plantar digital
arteries and nerves

Soleus muscle

Tibialis anterior muscle and tendon

Tibia

Anterior tibial artery and
deep fibular (peroneal) nerve

Extensor hallucis longus
muscle and tendon

Anterior medial malleolar artery

Medial malleolus

Medial branch of deep fibular
(peroneal) nerve

Medial tarsal arteries

Tuberosity of navicular bone

Dorsalis pedis artery

Arcuate artery

Posterior perforating branches
from deep plantar arch

Deep plantar artery
to deep plantar arch

Abductor hallucis muscle

Extensor hallucis longus tendon

Extensor hallucis brevis tendon
(*cut*)

Extensor digitorum brevis
tendons (*cut*)

Extensor digitorum
longus tendons (*cut*)

Extensor expansions

Dorsal digital branches of
deep fibular (peroneal) nerve

Dorsal digital branches
of superficial fibular
(peroneal) nerve

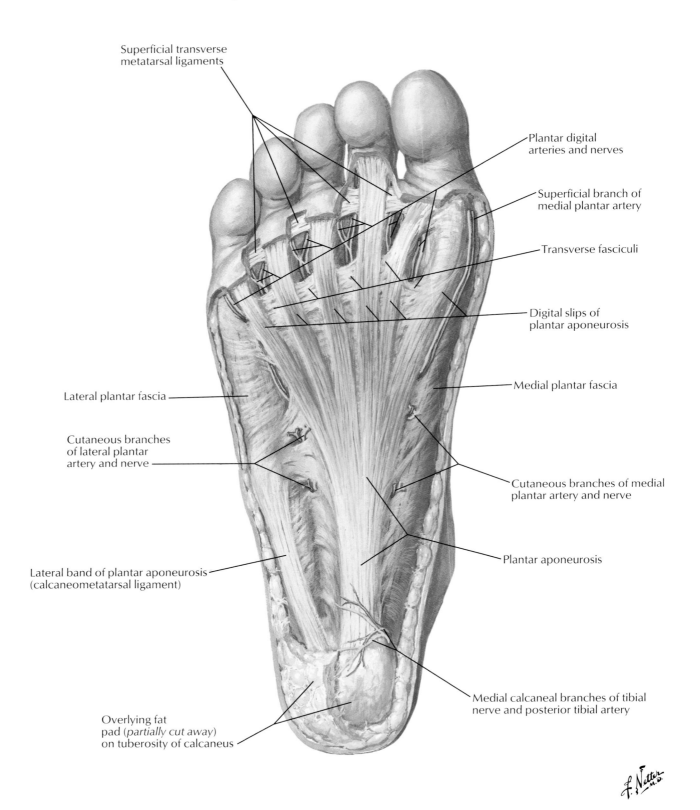

Superficial transverse
metatarsal ligaments

Plantar digital
arteries and nerves

Superficial branch of
medial plantar artery

Transverse fasciculi

Digital slips of
plantar aponeurosis

Medial plantar fascia

Cutaneous branches of medial
plantar artery and nerve

Plantar aponeurosis

Medial calcaneal branches of tibial
nerve and posterior tibial artery

Lateral plantar fascia

Cutaneous branches
of lateral plantar
artery and nerve

Lateral band of plantar aponeurosis
(calcaneometatarsal ligament)

Overlying fat
pad (*partially cut away*)
on tuberosity of calcaneus

Plate 520   **Ankle and Foot**

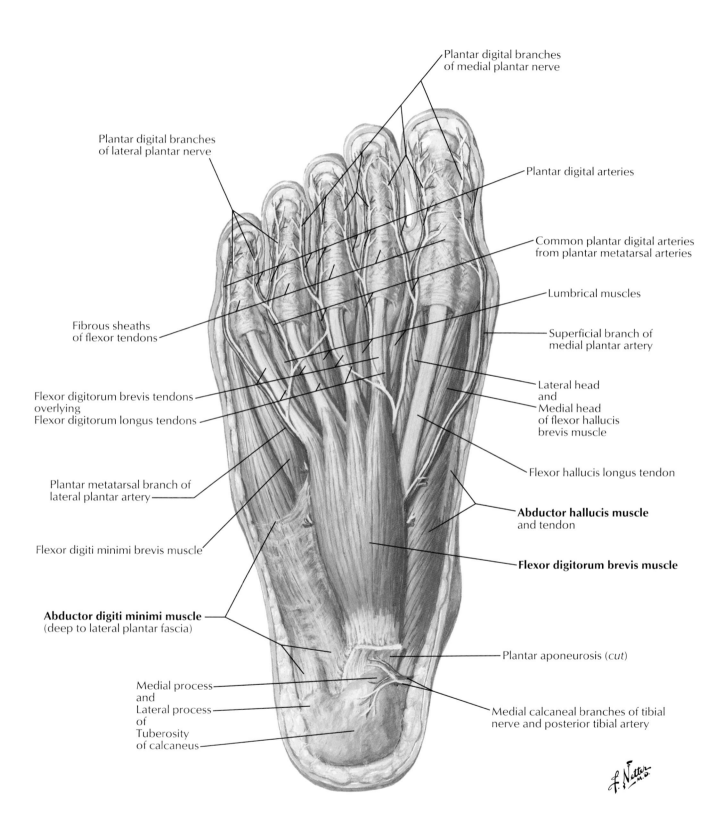

Plantar digital branches of medial plantar nerve

Plantar digital branches of lateral plantar nerve

Plantar digital arteries

Common plantar digital arteries from plantar metatarsal arteries

Lumbrical muscles

Fibrous sheaths of flexor tendons

Superficial branch of medial plantar artery

Flexor digitorum brevis tendons overlying
Flexor digitorum longus tendons

Lateral head and
Medial head of flexor hallucis brevis muscle

Flexor hallucis longus tendon

Plantar metatarsal branch of lateral plantar artery

Abductor hallucis muscle and tendon

Flexor digiti minimi brevis muscle

Flexor digitorum brevis muscle

Abductor digiti minimi muscle (deep to lateral plantar fascia)

Plantar aponeurosis (cut)

Medial process and
Lateral process of
Tuberosity of calcaneus

Medial calcaneal branches of tibial nerve and posterior tibial artery

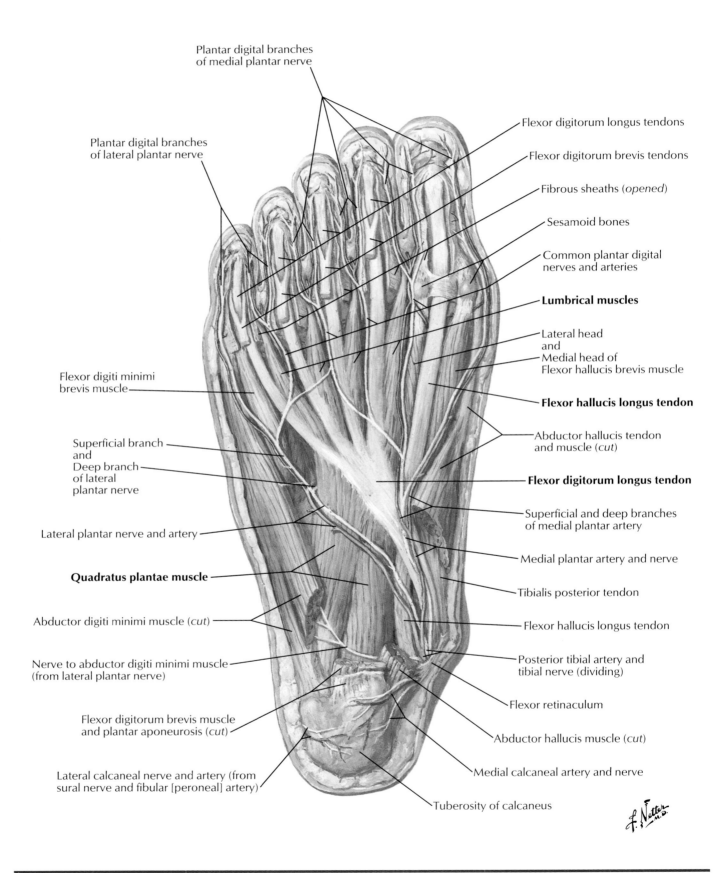

Plantar digital branches
of medial plantar nerve

Plantar digital branches
of lateral plantar nerve

Flexor digiti minimi
brevis muscle

Superficial branch
and
Deep branch
of lateral
plantar nerve

Lateral plantar nerve and artery

Quadratus plantae muscle

Abductor digiti minimi muscle (cut)

Nerve to abductor digiti minimi muscle
(from lateral plantar nerve)

Flexor digitorum brevis muscle
and plantar aponeurosis (cut)

Lateral calcaneal nerve and artery (from
sural nerve and fibular [peroneal] artery)

Flexor digitorum longus tendons

Flexor digitorum brevis tendons

Fibrous sheaths (opened)

Sesamoid bones

Common plantar digital
nerves and arteries

Lumbrical muscles

Lateral head
and
Medial head of
Flexor hallucis brevis muscle

Flexor hallucis longus tendon

Abductor hallucis tendon
and muscle (cut)

Flexor digitorum longus tendon

Superficial and deep branches
of medial plantar artery

Medial plantar artery and nerve

Tibialis posterior tendon

Flexor hallucis longus tendon

Posterior tibial artery and
tibial nerve (dividing)

Flexor retinaculum

Abductor hallucis muscle (cut)

Medial calcaneal artery and nerve

Tuberosity of calcaneus

f. Netter M.D.

Plate 522

Ankle and Foot

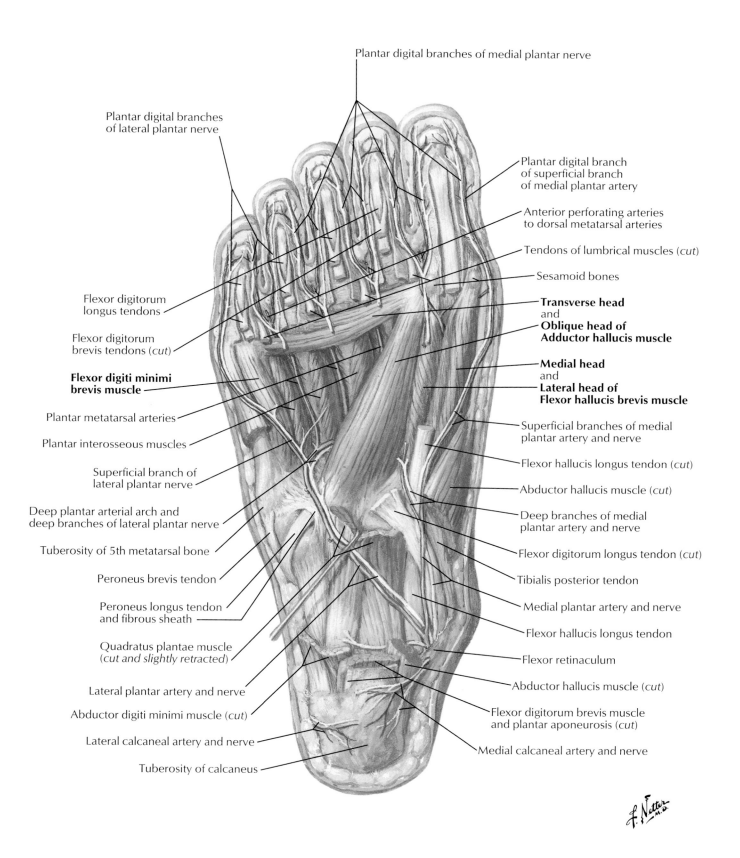

Plantar digital branches of medial plantar nerve

Plantar digital branches of lateral plantar nerve

Plantar digital branch of superficial branch of medial plantar artery

Anterior perforating arteries to dorsal metatarsal arteries

Tendons of lumbrical muscles (*cut*)

Sesamoid bones

Flexor digitorum longus tendons

Flexor digitorum brevis tendons (*cut*)

Transverse head and **Oblique head of Adductor hallucis muscle**

Flexor digiti minimi brevis muscle

Medial head and **Lateral head of Flexor hallucis brevis muscle**

Plantar metatarsal arteries

Superficial branches of medial plantar artery and nerve

Plantar interosseous muscles

Flexor hallucis longus tendon (*cut*)

Superficial branch of lateral plantar nerve

Abductor hallucis muscle (*cut*)

Deep plantar arterial arch and deep branches of lateral plantar nerve

Deep branches of medial plantar artery and nerve

Tuberosity of 5th metatarsal bone

Flexor digitorum longus tendon (*cut*)

Peroneus brevis tendon

Tibialis posterior tendon

Peroneus longus tendon and fibrous sheath

Medial plantar artery and nerve

Flexor hallucis longus tendon

Quadratus plantae muscle (*cut and slightly retracted*)

Flexor retinaculum

Lateral plantar artery and nerve

Abductor hallucis muscle (*cut*)

Abductor digiti minimi muscle (*cut*)

Flexor digitorum brevis muscle and plantar aponeurosis (*cut*)

Lateral calcaneal artery and nerve

Medial calcaneal artery and nerve

Tuberosity of calcaneus

Dorsal view

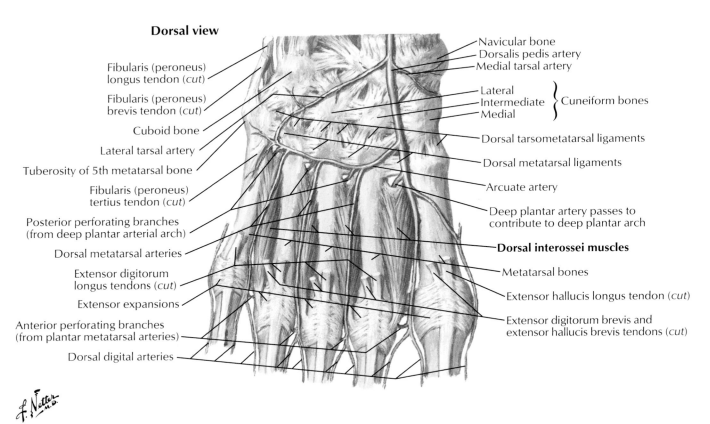

Fibularis (peroneus) longus tendon (*cut*)

Fibularis (peroneus) brevis tendon (*cut*)

Cuboid bone

Lateral tarsal artery

Tuberosity of 5th metatarsal bone

Fibularis (peroneus) tertius tendon (*cut*)

Posterior perforating branches (from deep plantar arterial arch)

Dorsal metatarsal arteries

Extensor digitorum longus tendons (*cut*)

Extensor expansions

Anterior perforating branches (from plantar metatarsal arteries)

Dorsal digital arteries

Navicular bone
Dorsalis pedis artery
Medial tarsal artery

Lateral
Intermediate } Cuneiform bones
Medial

Dorsal tarsometatarsal ligaments

Dorsal metatarsal ligaments

Arcuate artery

Deep plantar artery passes to contribute to deep plantar arch

Dorsal interossei muscles

Metatarsal bones

Extensor hallucis longus tendon (*cut*)

Extensor digitorum brevis and extensor hallucis brevis tendons (*cut*)

Plantar view

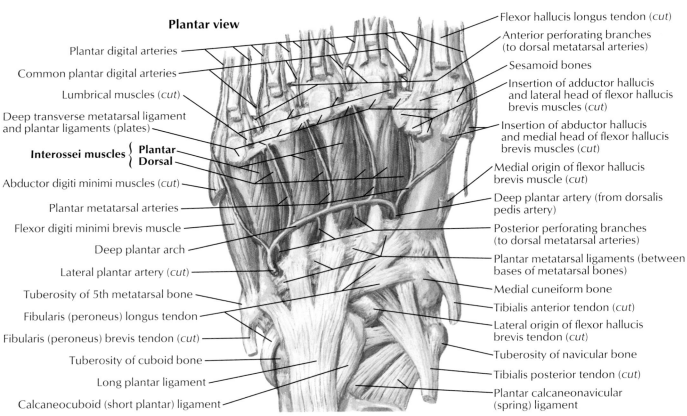

Plantar digital arteries

Common plantar digital arteries

Lumbrical muscles (*cut*)

Deep transverse metatarsal ligament and plantar ligaments (plates)

Interossei muscles { **Plantar** **Dorsal**

Abductor digiti minimi muscles (*cut*)

Plantar metatarsal arteries

Flexor digiti minimi brevis muscle

Deep plantar arch

Lateral plantar artery (*cut*)

Tuberosity of 5th metatarsal bone

Fibularis (peroneus) longus tendon

Fibularis (peroneus) brevis tendon (*cut*)

Tuberosity of cuboid bone

Long plantar ligament

Calcaneocuboid (short plantar) ligament

Flexor hallucis longus tendon (*cut*)

Anterior perforating branches (to dorsal metatarsal arteries)

Sesamoid bones

Insertion of adductor hallucis and lateral head of flexor hallucis brevis muscles (*cut*)

Insertion of abductor hallucis and medial head of flexor hallucis brevis muscles (*cut*)

Medial origin of flexor hallucis brevis muscle (*cut*)

Deep plantar artery (from dorsalis pedis artery)

Posterior perforating branches (to dorsal metatarsal arteries)

Plantar metatarsal ligaments (between bases of metatarsal bones)

Medial cuneiform bone

Tibialis anterior tendon (*cut*)

Lateral origin of flexor hallucis brevis tendon (*cut*)

Tuberosity of navicular bone

Tibialis posterior tendon (*cut*)

Plantar calcaneonavicular (spring) ligament

Plate 524   **Ankle and Foot**

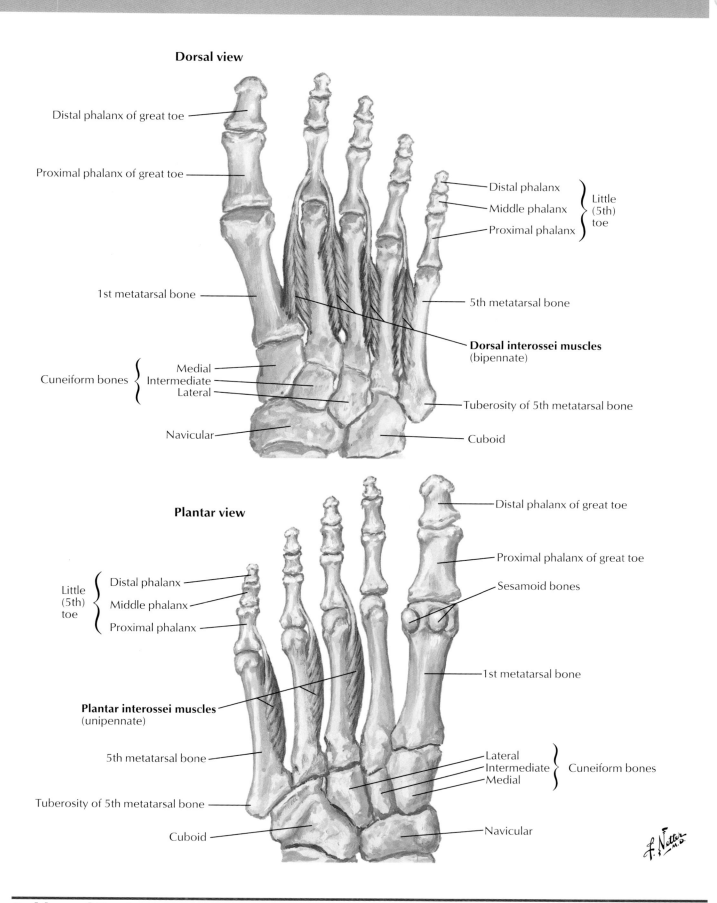

Dorsal view

Distal phalanx of great toe

Proximal phalanx of great toe

Distal phalanx
Middle phalanx } Little (5th) toe
Proximal phalanx }

1st metatarsal bone

5th metatarsal bone

Dorsal interossei muscles (bipennate)

Cuneiform bones {
Medial
Intermediate
Lateral

Tuberosity of 5th metatarsal bone

Navicular

Cuboid

Plantar view

Distal phalanx of great toe

Proximal phalanx of great toe

Sesamoid bones

Little (5th) toe {
Distal phalanx
Middle phalanx
Proximal phalanx

1st metatarsal bone

Plantar interossei muscles (unipennate)

5th metatarsal bone

Lateral
Intermediate } Cuneiform bones
Medial

Tuberosity of 5th metatarsal bone

Cuboid

Navicular

f. Netter m.d.

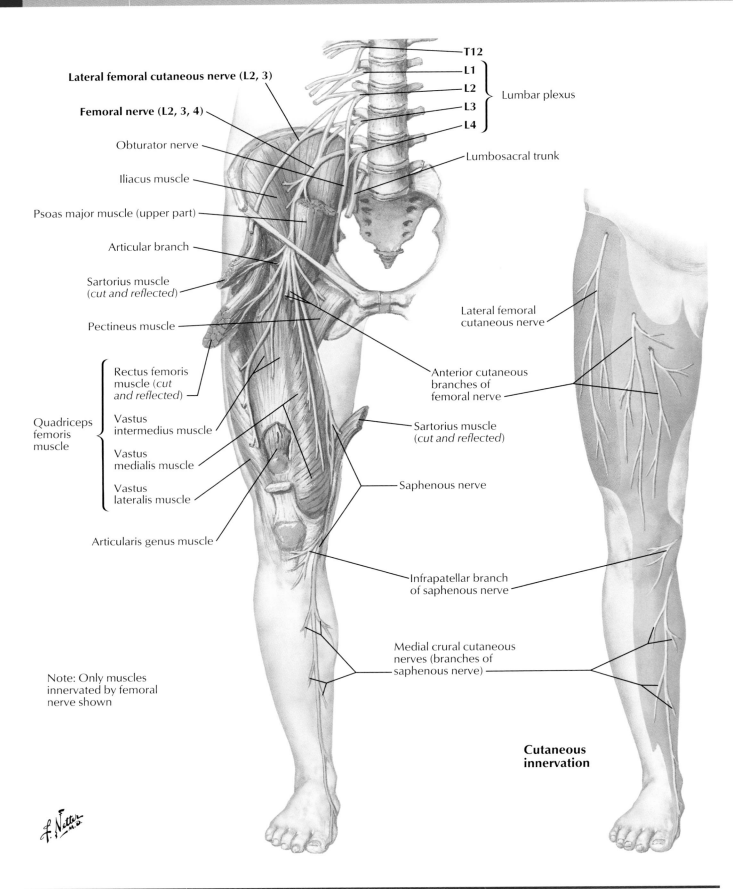

Lateral femoral cutaneous nerve (L2, 3)

Femoral nerve (L2, 3, 4)

Obturator nerve

Iliacus muscle

Psoas major muscle (upper part)

Articular branch

Sartorius muscle
(*cut and reflected*)

Pectineus muscle

Rectus femoris
muscle (*cut
and reflected*)

Quadriceps
femoris
muscle

Vastus
intermedius muscle

Vastus
medialis muscle

Vastus
lateralis muscle

Articularis genus muscle

Note: Only muscles
innervated by femoral
nerve shown

T12
L1
L2
L3
L4

Lumbar plexus

Lumbosacral trunk

Lateral femoral
cutaneous nerve

Anterior cutaneous
branches of
femoral nerve

Sartorius muscle
(*cut and reflected*)

Saphenous nerve

Infrapatellar branch
of saphenous nerve

Medial crural cutaneous
nerves (branches of
saphenous nerve)

**Cutaneous
innervation**

Plate 526   **Neurovasculature**

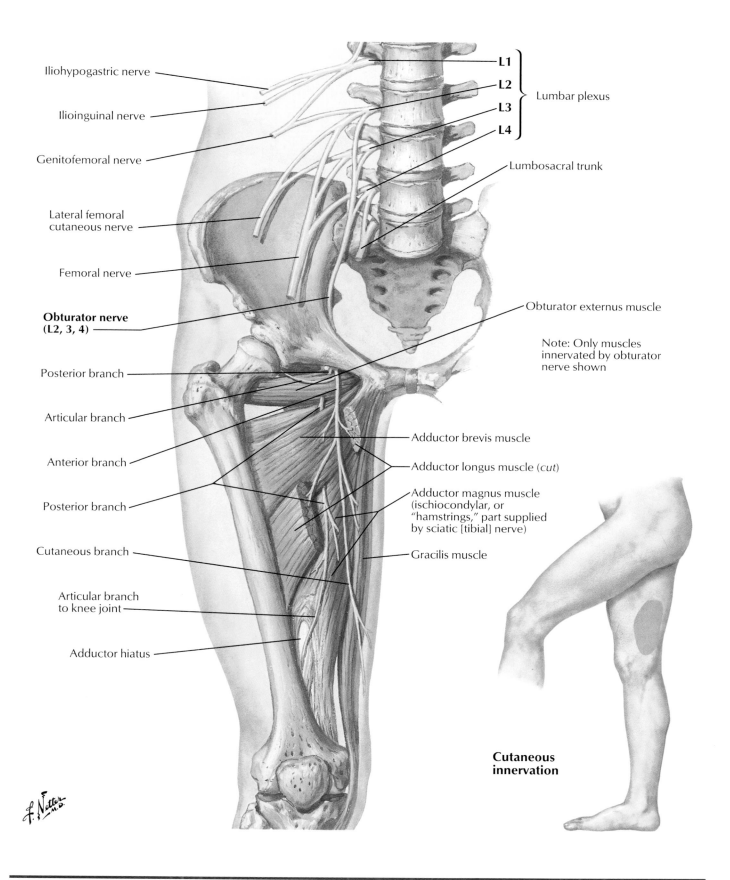

Iliohypogastric nerve

Ilioinguinal nerve

Genitofemoral nerve

Lateral femoral
cutaneous nerve

Femoral nerve

**Obturator nerve
(L2, 3, 4)**

Posterior branch

Articular branch

Anterior branch

Posterior branch

Cutaneous branch

Articular branch
to knee joint

Adductor hiatus

L1
L2
L3
L4
} Lumbar plexus

Lumbosacral trunk

Obturator externus muscle

Note: Only muscles
innervated by obturator
nerve shown

Adductor brevis muscle

Adductor longus muscle (*cut*)

Adductor magnus muscle
(ischiocondylar, or
"hamstrings," part supplied
by sciatic [tibial] nerve)

Gracilis muscle

**Cutaneous
innervation**

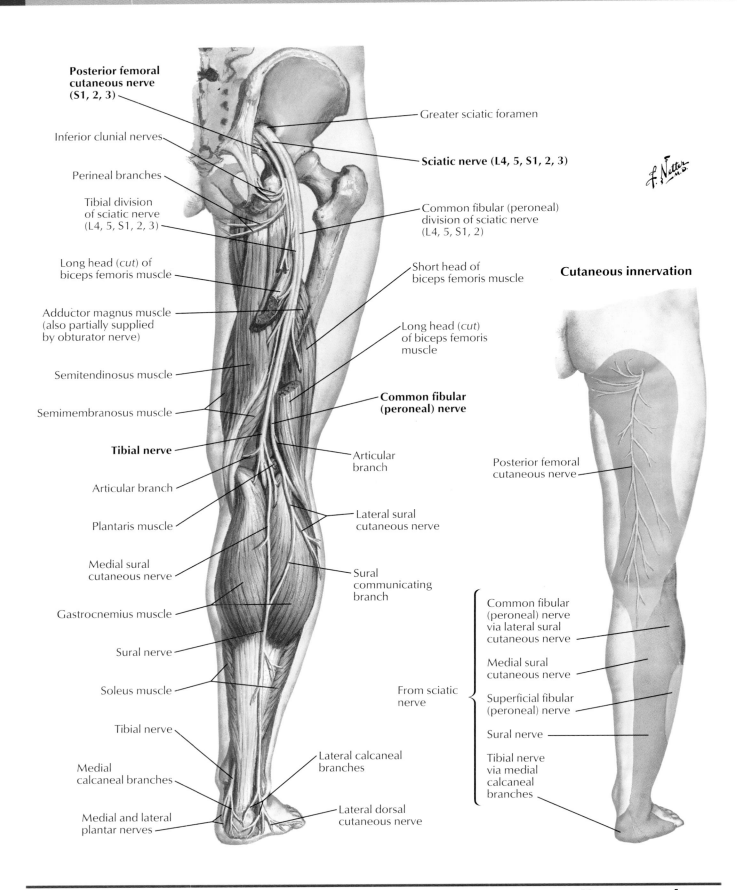

Posterior femoral cutaneous nerve (S1, 2, 3)

Inferior clunial nerves

Perineal branches

Tibial division of sciatic nerve (L4, 5, S1, 2, 3)

Long head (*cut*) of biceps femoris muscle

Adductor magnus muscle (also partially supplied by obturator nerve)

Semitendinosus muscle

Semimembranosus muscle

Tibial nerve

Articular branch

Plantaris muscle

Medial sural cutaneous nerve

Gastrocnemius muscle

Sural nerve

Soleus muscle

Tibial nerve

Medial calcaneal branches

Medial and lateral plantar nerves

Greater sciatic foramen

Sciatic nerve (L4, 5, S1, 2, 3)

Common fibular (peroneal) division of sciatic nerve (L4, 5, S1, 2)

Short head of biceps femoris muscle

Long head (*cut*) of biceps femoris muscle

Common fibular (peroneal) nerve

Articular branch

Lateral sural cutaneous nerve

Sural communicating branch

Lateral calcaneal branches

Lateral dorsal cutaneous nerve

F. Netter M.D.

Cutaneous innervation

Posterior femoral cutaneous nerve

Common fibular (peroneal) nerve via lateral sural cutaneous nerve

Medial sural cutaneous nerve

Superficial fibular (peroneal) nerve

Sural nerve

Tibial nerve via medial calcaneal branches

From sciatic nerve

Plate 528

Neurovasculature

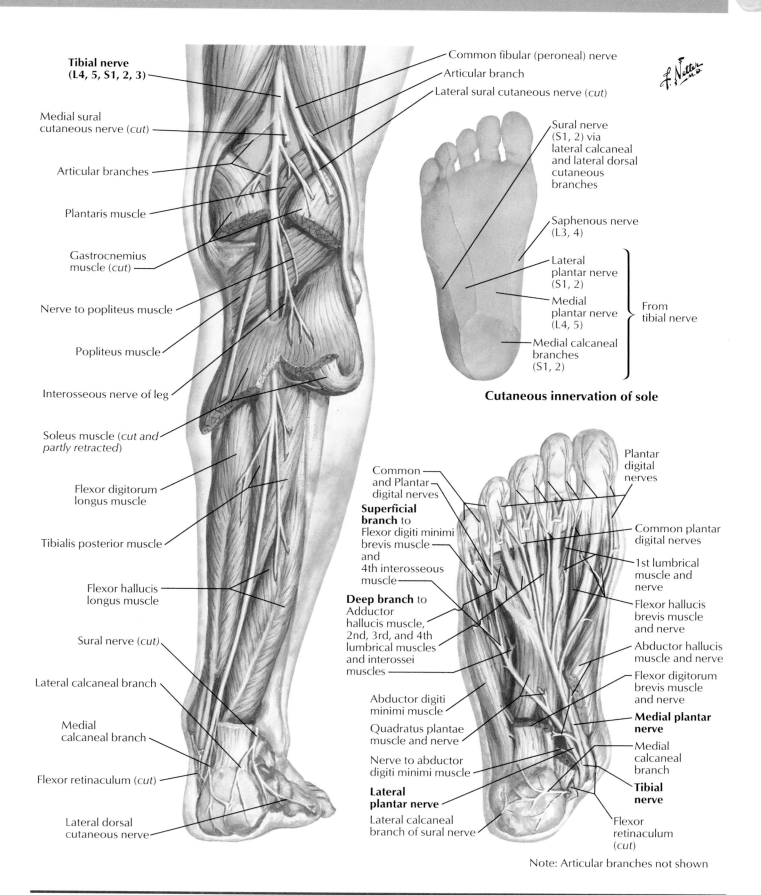

Tibial nerve
(L4, 5, S1, 2, 3)

Medial sural
cutaneous nerve (*cut*)

Articular branches

Plantaris muscle

Gastrocnemius
muscle (*cut*)

Nerve to popliteus muscle

Popliteus muscle

Interosseous nerve of leg

Soleus muscle (*cut and
partly retracted*)

Flexor digitorum
longus muscle

Tibialis posterior muscle

Flexor hallucis
longus muscle

Sural nerve (*cut*)

Lateral calcaneal branch

Medial
calcaneal branch

Flexor retinaculum (*cut*)

Lateral dorsal
cutaneous nerve

Common fibular (peroneal) nerve

Articular branch

Lateral sural cutaneous nerve (*cut*)

F. Netter

Sural nerve
(S1, 2) via
lateral calcaneal
and lateral dorsal
cutaneous
branches

Saphenous nerve
(L3, 4)

Lateral
plantar nerve
(S1, 2)

Medial
plantar nerve
(L4, 5)

Medial calcaneal
branches
(S1, 2)

From
tibial nerve

Cutaneous innervation of sole

Common
and Plantar
digital nerves

**Superficial
branch** to
Flexor digiti minimi
brevis muscle
and
4th interosseous
muscle

Deep branch to
Adductor
hallucis muscle,
2nd, 3rd, and 4th
lumbrical muscles
and interossei
muscles

Abductor digiti
minimi muscle

Quadratus plantae
muscle and nerve

Nerve to abductor
digiti minimi muscle

**Lateral
plantar nerve**

Lateral calcaneal
branch of sural nerve

Plantar
digital
nerves

Common plantar
digital nerves

1st lumbrical
muscle and
nerve

Flexor hallucis
brevis muscle
and nerve

Abductor hallucis
muscle and nerve

Flexor digitorum
brevis muscle
and nerve

**Medial plantar
nerve**

Medial
calcaneal
branch

**Tibial
nerve**

Flexor
retinaculum
(*cut*)

Note: Articular branches not shown

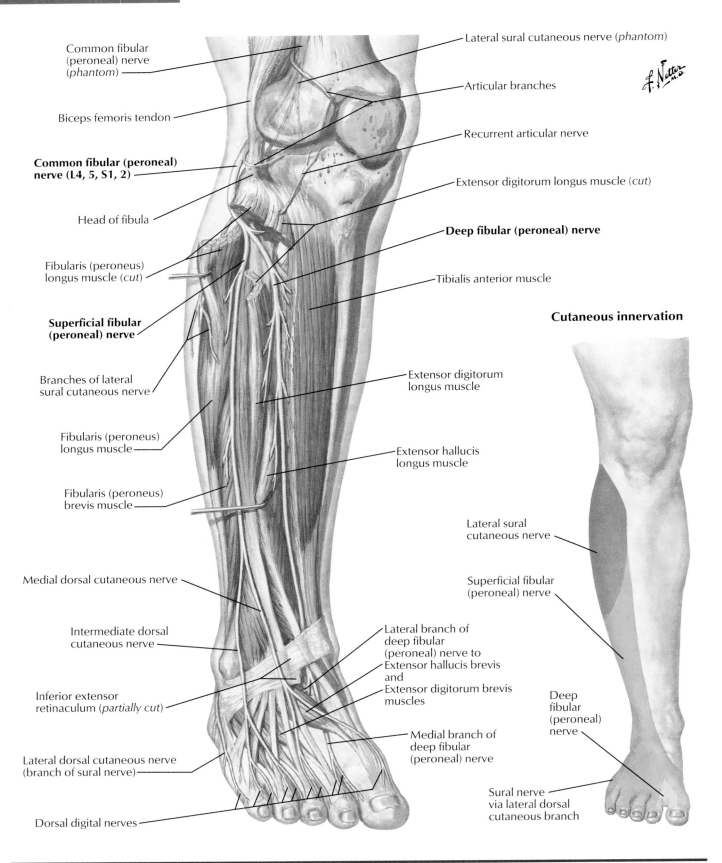

Common fibular (peroneal) nerve (*phantom*)

Biceps femoris tendon

Common fibular (peroneal) nerve (L4, 5, S1, 2)

Head of fibula

Fibularis (peroneus) longus muscle (*cut*)

Superficial fibular (peroneal) nerve

Branches of lateral sural cutaneous nerve

Fibularis (peroneus) longus muscle

Fibularis (peroneus) brevis muscle

Medial dorsal cutaneous nerve

Intermediate dorsal cutaneous nerve

Inferior extensor retinaculum (*partially cut*)

Lateral dorsal cutaneous nerve (branch of sural nerve)

Dorsal digital nerves

Lateral sural cutaneous nerve (*phantom*)

Articular branches

Recurrent articular nerve

Extensor digitorum longus muscle (*cut*)

Deep fibular (peroneal) nerve

Tibialis anterior muscle

Extensor digitorum longus muscle

Extensor hallucis longus muscle

Lateral branch of deep fibular (peroneal) nerve to Extensor hallucis brevis and Extensor digitorum brevis muscles

Medial branch of deep fibular (peroneal) nerve

Cutaneous innervation

Lateral sural cutaneous nerve

Superficial fibular (peroneal) nerve

Deep fibular (peroneal) nerve

Sural nerve via lateral dorsal cutaneous branch

Plate 530

Neurovasculature

Radiograph

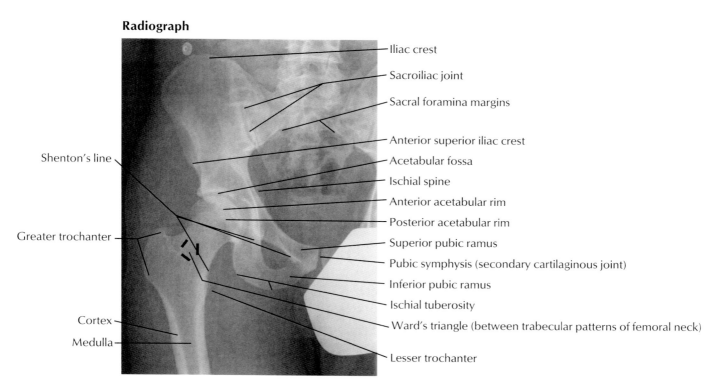

- Iliac crest
- Sacroiliac joint
- Sacral foramina margins
- Anterior superior iliac crest
- Acetabular fossa
- Ischial spine
- Anterior acetabular rim
- Posterior acetabular rim
- Superior pubic ramus
- Pubic symphysis (secondary cartilaginous joint)
- Inferior pubic ramus
- Ischial tuberosity
- Ward's triangle (between trabecular patterns of femoral neck)
- Lesser trochanter

- Shenton's line
- Greater trochanter
- Cortex
- Medulla

Arthrogram of hip

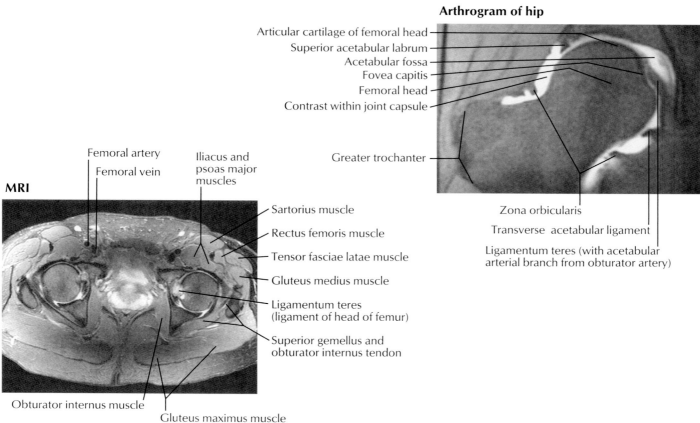

- Articular cartilage of femoral head
- Superior acetabular labrum
- Acetabular fossa
- Fovea capitis
- Femoral head
- Contrast within joint capsule
- Greater trochanter
- Zona orbicularis
- Transverse acetabular ligament
- Ligamentum teres (with acetabular arterial branch from obturator artery)

MRI

- Femoral artery
- Femoral vein
- Iliacus and psoas major muscles
- Sartorius muscle
- Rectus femoris muscle
- Tensor fasciae latae muscle
- Gluteus medius muscle
- Ligamentum teres (ligament of head of femur)
- Superior gemellus and obturator internus tendon
- Obturator internus muscle
- Gluteus maximus muscle

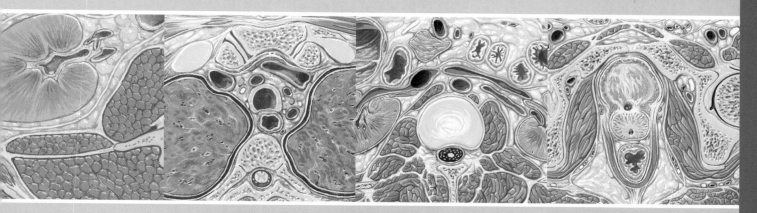

Section 8 CROSS-SECTIONAL ANATOMY

Cross-sectional Anatomy
Plate 532

532 Key Figures for Cross Sections

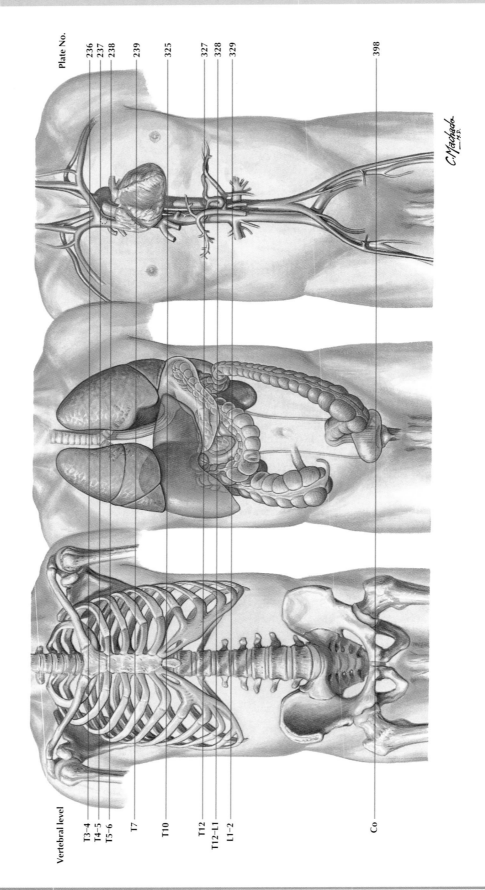

Plate No.

236
237
238

239

325

327
328
329

398

Vertebral level

T3–4
T4–5
T5–6

T7

T10

T12
T12–L1
L1–2

Co

C. Machado —M.D.

Plate 532   **Cross-sectional Anatomy**

References

Plates 8, 36-38, 48-50
Lang J. Clinical Anatomy of the Nose, Nasal Cavity and Paranasal Sinuses. New York, Thieme Medical Publishers, Inc., 1989.

Plate 23
Tubbs RS, Kelly DR, Humphrey ER, Chua GD, et al. The tectorial membrane: anatomical, biomechanical, and histological analysis. Clin Anat 2007; 20(4):382-386.

Plates 25-28, 53-55, 67-68
Noden DM, Francis-West P. The differentiation and morphogenesis of craniofacial muscles. Dev Dyn 2006; 235(5):1194-1218.

Plates 31, 33, 124-130
Tubbs RS, Salter EG, Oakes WJ. Anatomic landmarks for nerves of the neck: a vade mecum for neurosurgeons. Neurosurgery 2005; 56 (2 Suppl):256-260; discussion 256-260.

Plates 65, 93, 94
Kierner AC, Mayer R, v Kirschhofer K. Do the tensor tympani and tensor veli palatini muscles of man form a functional unit? A histochemical investigation of their putative connections. Hear Res 2002; 165(1-2):48-52.

Plates 78-80
Ludlow CL. Central nervous system control of the laryngeal muscles in humans. Respir Physiol Neurobiol 2005; 147(2-3):205-222.

Plates 100-114
Rhoton AL. Cranial Anatomy and Surgical Approaches. Schaumburg, Ill, The Congress of Neurological Surgeons, 2003.

Plates 103, 138
Tubbs RS, Hansasuta A, Loukas M, et al. Branches of the petrous and cavernous segments of the internal carotid artery. Clin Anat 2007; 20(6):596-601.

Plates 115-117, 123
Schrott-Fischer A, Kammen-Jolly K, Scholtz AW, et al. Patterns of GABA-like immunoreactivity in efferent fibers of the human cochlea. Hear Res 2002; 174(1-2):75-85.

Plate 157, 172
Tubbs RS, Loukas M, Slappy JB, et al. Clinical anatomy of the CI doral root, ganglion, and ramus: a review and anatomical study. Clin Anat 2007; 20:624-627.

Plate 159
Lee MWL, McPhee RW, Stringer MD. An evidence-based approach to human dermatomes. Clin Anat 2008; 21:363-373.

Plates 159, 401, 513, 470
Forester O. The dermatomes in man. Brain 1933; 56:1.

Garrett FD. The segmental distribution of the cutaneous nerves in the limbs of man. Anat Rec 1948; 102:409.

Keegan JJ. Dermatome hypalgesia with posterolateral herniation of lower cervical intervertebral disc. J Neurosurg 1947; 4:115.

Plate 165
Turnball IM. Bloody supply of the spinal cord. In Vinken PJ, Bruyn GW (eds). Handbook of Clinical Neurology, XII. Amsterdam, North-Holland, 1972, pp 478–491.

Plates 194, 195
Jackson CL, Huber JF. Correlated applied anatomy of the bronchial tree and lungs with a system of nomenclature. Dis Chest 1943; 9:319.

Plate 197
Ikeda S, Ono Y, Miyazawa S, et al. Flexible broncho-fiberscope. Otolaryngology (Tokyo) 1970; 42:855.

Plate 211
Angelini P, Velasco JA, Flamm S. Coronary anomalies: incidence, pathophysiology and clinical relevance. Circulation 2002; 105:2449-2454.

Plate 219
James TN. The internodal pathways of the human heart. Prog Cardiovas Dis 2001; 43:495.

Plate 234
Ang H-J, Gill Y-C, Lee W-J, et al. Anatomy of thoracic splanchnic nerves for surgical resection. Clin Anat 2008; 21:171-177.

Plate 279
Elias H. Morphology of the Liver. New York, Academic Press, 1969.

Robinson PJ. MRI of the Liver: A Practical Guide. New York, Taylor & Francis, 2006.

MacSween RNM, Anthony PP, Scheuer PJ, et al (eds). Pathology of the Liver. London, Churchill Livingstone, 2002.

Plates 283, 284
Odze RD. Surgical Pathology of the GI Tract, Liver, Biliary Tract, and Pancreas. Philadelphia, Saunders, 2004.

Plate 305
Thomas MD. In The Ciba Collection of Medical Illustrations, Vol 3, Part II. Summit NJ, CIBA, p 78.

Plates 323, 346, 364, 376, 394
Stormont TJ, Cahill DR, King BF, Myers RP. Fascias of the male external genitalia and perineum. Clin Anat 1994; 7:115.

Plates 337, 342, 348, 352, 357, 358
Oelrich TM. The striated urogenital sphincter muscle in the female. Anat Rec 1983; 205:223.

References

Plates 341, 346

Myers RP, Goellner JR, Cahill DR. Prostate shape, external striated urethral sphincter and radical prostatectomy: the apical dissection. J Urol 1987; 138:543.

Plates 341, 346, 363, 364

Oelrich TM. The urethral sphincter muscle in the male. Am J Anat 1980; 158:229.

Plate 383

Flocks RH, Kerr HD, Elkins HB, et al. Treatment of carcinoma of the prostate by interstitial radiation with radio-active gold (Au 198): a preliminary report. J Urol 1952; 68(2):510.

Plate 401

Keegan JJ, Garrett FD. The segmental distribution of the cutaneous nerves in the limbs of man. Anat Rec 1948; 102:409.

Plate 470

Keegan JJ. Neurological interpretation of dermatome hypalgesia with herniation of the lumbar intervertebral disc. J Bone Joint Surg 1944; 26:238.

Last RJ. Innervation of the limbs. J Bone Joint Surg (Br) 1949; 31:452.

References are to plate numbers. In most cases, structures are listed under singular nouns.

A

Abdomen
autonomic nerves and ganglia of, 297
axial CT images of, 324
bony framework of, 241
cross sections of
at L3, L4 level, 330
at L1-L2 level, 329
at middle T12 level, 327
at T12-L1 level, 328
left lower quadrant of, 242
left upper quadrant of, 242
regions and planes of, 242
right lower quadrant of, 242
right upper quadrant of, 242
subcutaneous tissue of, 243
surface anatomy of, 240
transverse section of, at T12, 326
viscera of, 261
Abdominal aortic plexus. See Intermesenteric plexus
Abdominal cavity, contrast medium in, 354
Abdominal muscles, 343, 347
Abdominal wall
anterior, 257, 258
arteries of, 249
deep dissection of, 245
intermediate dissection of, 244
internal view of, 247
nerves of, 251
parietal peritoneum of, 323
superficial dissection of, 243
veins of, 250
paramedian (parasagittal) section of, 323
posterior
arteries of, 257
internal view of, 256
lymph vessels and nodes of, 259
nerves of, 260
peritoneum of, 266
veins of, 258
posterolateral, 248, 330
Abdominis aponeurosis, transverse, 249, 330
Abdominis muscle
rectus, 175, 182, 183, 185, 240, 244, 245, 246, 247, 252, 253, 254, 323, 327, 330, 343, 345, 357
axial CT image of, 324
MR sagittal images of, 377
transverse section of, 325
tendon of origin of, 169, 170, 173
transversus, 169, 170, 173, 183, 184, 245, 246, 247, 249, 251, 252, 253, 254, 256, 260, 308, 309, 330, 343, 347, 484, 486
aponeurosis of, 246, 309
area for aponeurosis, 309
tendon of origin of, 248, 330
Abducent nerve (VI), 13, 83, 84, 86, 103, 113, 116, 120
distribution of, 117
schema of, 120
Abducent nucleus, 115, 116, 120
Abductor digiti minimi muscle, 453, 458, 464, 517, 523, 524
deep to lateral plantar fascia of, 521
nerve to, 522, 529
Abductor hallucis muscle, 516, 521, 522, 523, 529
Abductor hallucis nerve, 529
Abductor hallucis tendon, 516, 521, 522
Abductor muscle, 484
Abductor pollicis brevis muscle, 449, 453, 463
Abductor pollicis longus muscle, 429, 431, 433, 437, 466
area for, 427
insertion of, 438, 439

Abductor pollicis longus tendon, 436, 458
insertion of, 455
Aberrant ductule, 370
Abscess, perineal, 376
Accessory collateral ligament, 446
Accessory hemiazygos vein, 201
Accessory nerve (XI), 13, 31, 32, 33, 46, 47, 71, 72, 73, 103, 113, 115, 116, 128, 171, 414
cranial root of, 125, 126
distribution of, 117
in jugular fossa, 12
schema of, 126
spinal roots of, 13, 126
in foramen magnum, 12
Accessory nucleus, 115, 116
Accessory oculomotor nucleus, 131
Accessory pancreatic duct (of Santorini), 281
Accessory process, lumbar, 152
Acetabular fossa, 398
arthrogram of, 531
fat in, 475
radiograph of, 531
Acetabular labrum, 336, 475
superior, 531
arthrogram of, 531
Acetabular ligament, transverse, 336, 475, 531
arthrogram of, 531
Acetabular margin, 335, 340
Acetabular notch, 474
Acetabular rim
anterior, 531
radiograph of, 531
posterior, 531
radiograph of, 531
radiograph of, 531
Acetabulum, 336, 474
lunate (articular) surface of, 333, 475
margin (limbus) of, 333
radiograph of, 333, 476
Achilles tendon. See Calcaneal (Achilles) tendon
Acinus, 198
Acoustic artery, internal. See Labyrinthine artery
Acoustic meatus
external, 6, 10, 15, 92, 96
coronal oblique section of, 93
internal, 8, 13, 92, 122, 123
Acoustic opening, internal, 97
Acromial anastomosis, 415
Acromial angle, 407
Acromial facet, of clavicle, 406
Acromioclavicular joint, 413
capsule of, 410
Acromioclavicular ligament, 410
Acromion, 26, 179, 182, 400, 407, 410, 411, 413, 414, 415, 416, 419
arthrogram of, 468
magnetic resonance imaging of, 468
radiograph of, 409
Adamkiewicz, artery of, 164
Adductor brevis muscle, 481, 493, 527
insertion of, 479
origin of, 478
Adductor canal, 488, 493
Adductor hallucis muscle
insertion of, 524
oblique head of, 523
transverse head of, 523
Adductor hallucis tendon, 516
Adductor hiatus, 488, 490, 527
femoral artery passing through, 500
Adductor longus muscle, 480, 481, 488, 489, 493, 527
insertion of, 479
origin of, 478
Adductor magnus muscle, 469, 489, 490, 493, 500, 527
adductor minimus part of, 483, 490
insertion of, 478, 479
ischiocondylar part of, 527
origin of, 479

Adductor magnus tendon, 481, 488, 489, 493, 494, 505
Adductor muscles, 484
Adductor pollicis brevis muscle, 454
Adductor pollicis muscle, 450, 453, 454, 464
fascia over, 448, 450
Adductor tubercle, 489
Adenohypophysis, 138, 145, 146
Aditus (laryngeal inlet), 62
Afferent fibers, 120, 131
of brainstem, 116
of stomach and duodenum, 300
of tracheobronchial tree, 204
vestibular, 123
Afferent nerves, of nose and sinuses, 204
Agger nasi, 36, 37
Air cells
ethmoidal, 5, 48, 49, 83
anterior, 36, 37, 50
middle, openings of, 36, 37, 50
posterior, openings of, 36, 37, 50
mastoid, 7, 47
Airway
intrapulmonary, schema of, 198
to nasal meatus, 36
Airway reflexes, nerves initiating, 204
Ala, 1, 10, 241, 332, 336, 340, 474
gluteal surface of, 474
of sacrum, radiograph of, 333
wing of, 154
Alar fibrofatty tissue, 35, 37
Alar fold, 495
Alar ligament, 23
Albini's nodule, 217
Alcock's canal. See Pudendal (Alcock's) canal
Alveolar artery
inferior, 39, 53, 60, 69, 70
lingual branch of, 69
mental branch of, 39, 69
mylohyoid branch of, 18, 69
posterior superior, 39
superior
anterior, 39
middle, 39
posterior, 39, 69
Alveolar duct, 198
opening of, 198
Alveolar foramina, 6
Alveolar nerve, 39, 60
anterior superior, 44, 71
nasal branch of, 41
inferior, 18, 45, 53, 55, 60, 71, 121, 130, 133
entering mandibular foramen, 45
middle superior, 44, 71
posterior superior, 43, 44, 71
nasal branch of, 43
superior, 62
Alveolar periosteum, 57
Alveolar pores (of Kohn), 198
Alveolar process, 8
Alveolar sac, 198
Alveolar vein
inferior, 60, 70
posterior superior, 70
Alveolar wall
capillary bed within, 199
capillary plexus within, 199
Alveolus, 198
Alveus, of hippocampus, 111
Amacrine cells, 119
Ampulla
of ductus deferens, 364
of duodenum, 268
of ear, 92, 95, 96
anterior, 95
lateral, 95
posterior, 95
hepatopancreatic (of Vater), 280

Ampulla *(Continued)*
  of rectum, 348
  sphincter of, 280
  of uterine tube, 354
Amygdaloid body, 109, 111, 118, 134
Anal canal, 373
  anatomical, 373
  arteries of, 378
  beginning of, 398
  conjoined longitudinal muscle of, 340, 341
  MR sagittal images of, 377
  muscularis mucosae of, 373, 374
  surgical, 373
  veins of, 379
Anal columns (Morgagni's), 373
Anal crypt, 373
Anal glands, 373
Anal nerve, inferior, 303, 359, 390, 391, 393, 394, 485, 491
Anal pit, 368
Anal sinus, 373
Anal sphincter muscles, 368
  deep, 371
  external, 275, 303, 337, 342, 348, 358, 362, 363, 372, 375
    deep, 323, 374, 375, 376
    female, 375
    male, 346, 375
    perineal views of, 375
    subcutaneous, 323, 346, 374, 375, 376
    superficial, 323, 346, 374, 375, 376
  internal, 358, 372
    deep part of, 374
  subcutaneous, 371
  superficial, 371
Anal triangle, 360
Anal tubercle, 368
Anal valve, 373
Anal verge, 373
Anastomoses
  acromial, 415
  around elbow, 422
  around scapula, 415
  carotid-vertebral, 136
  in incisive canal, 39
  internal carotid–external carotid, 136
  with lower intercostal artery, 249
  with lumbar arteries, 249
  paravertebral, 165
  patellar, 488, 500
  portocaval, 292
  prevertebral, 165
  right-left, 136
  between septal sphenopalatine artery and greater palatine artery, 40
  subclavian-carotid, 136
  subclavian-vertebral, 136
  with subcostal artery, 249
Anastomotic loop
  of small intestine, 287
  to spinal arteries, 164
Anastomotic vein
  inferior (of Labbé), 101, 143
  superior (of Trolard), 101
Anatomical snuffbox, 400, 432
  contents of, 455
  radial artery in, 455, 457, 458
Anconeus muscle, 420, 432, 433, 437, 465, 466
  as extensor of elbow, 429
  insertion of, 439
  nerve to, 420
Anersine bursa, 495
Angular artery, 3, 35, 39, 69, 85, 136
Angular gyrus, 104
Angular vein, 3, 70, 85
Ankle
  dorsiflexion and plantar flexion of, 470
  ligaments of, 515
  radiograph of, 514
  tendon sheaths of, 517
  tendons of, 515

Annular ligament, 196, 426
Annular pulleys, 450
Anococcygeal body (ligament), 339, 357, 358, 362, 375, 376
Anococcygeal nerve, 391, 393, 485, 487
Anocutaneous line, 372, 373, 374
Anoderm, 373
Anorectal hiatus, 340
Anorectal junction
  circular muscle layer of, 341
  conjoined longitudinal muscle of, 341
Anorectal line, 373
Anorectal muscle, 374
Ansa cervicalis, 30, 127, 128
  inferior root of, 31, 32, 33, 71, 74, 127, 128
  superior root of, 31, 32, 33, 71, 74, 127
Ansa of Galen, 80
Ansa pectoralis, 417
Ansa subclavia, 129, 203, 220, 234
Anseriform semilunar fissure, 112
Anserine bursa, 494
Antebrachial vein, median, 437
Anterior chamber, 81, 87, 89, 90
  endothelium of, 88
Anterior nares, 1
Anterolateral central artery, 138, 141
Anteromedial intermuscular septum, 488
Antihelix, 1
  crura of, 93
Antitragus, 93
Anulus fibrosus, 21, 152
Anus, 339, 342, 356, 360, 362, 375
  fetal, 368
Aorta, 34, 201, 214, 306
  abdominal, 189, 226, 257, 262, 266, 270, 283, 284, 308, 310, 316, 317, 323, 327, 328, 329, 330, 343, 344, 378, 380, 381, 382, 383, 392
    cross section of, 173, 265
  arch of, 74, 75, 136, 190, 200, 204, 206, 208, 209, 215, 219, 225, 226, 227, 231, 237
    groove for, 193
    radiograph of, 207
  ascending, 136, 209, 214, 217, 218, 219, 238
    CT axial image of, 235
  axial CT image of, 324
  descending, 136, 238, 239
    axial CT image of, 235
    groove for, 193
  prenatal, 223
  thoracic
    descending, 165, 185, 188, 210, 225, 226, 231
    esophageal branches of, 231
    transverse section of, 326
Aortic arch. *See* Aorta, arch of
Aortic hiatus, 189
Aortic lymph node
  lateral, 259, 318, 386
  of ligamentum arteriosum, 202
Aorticorenal ganglion, 160, 260, 299, 300, 301, 303, 319, 320, 321, 390, 394, 395
  left, 297, 299, 302, 396
  right, 297, 299, 302
Aortic plexus, 203, 300, 330, 392, 396
Aortic sinus (of Valsalva), 217
Aortic valve, 207, 217
  left semilunar cusp of, 215, 216, 217, 218, 219
  posterior semilunar cusp of, 215, 216, 217, 218, 219
  right semilunar cusp of, 215, 216, 217, 218, 219
Aortobronchial constriction, 227
Apical axillary (subclavian) lymph nodes, 178
Apical collecting vessels, 73
Apical ligament of dens, 23
Aponeurosis
  abdominis, 330
    transverse, 330
  bicipital, 404, 419, 421, 434, 461
  epicranial, 3, 25, 172
  external oblique, 255
  of external oblique muscle, 243, 244, 245, 246, 253, 254, 367

Aponeurosis *(Continued)*
  galea, 3, 101
  gluteal, over gluteus medius muscle, 309, 482, 483
  of internal oblique muscle, 246
  oblique
    external, 330
    internal, 330
  palatine, 52
  palmar, 430, 434, 442, 447, 448, 450
    septa from, 448
  pharyngeal, 65, 67
  plantar, 517, 522, 523
    digital slips of, 520
  of transverse abdominis muscle, 246
  triangular, 452
Appendicular artery, 273, 287, 288, 302
  in mesoappendix, 301
Appendicular lymph nodes, 296
Appendicular nerve plexus, 301, 302
Appendicular vein, 291, 292
Appendix, 125
  of epididymis, 367
  omental (epiploic), 263, 276, 330
  of testis, 367
  vermiform, 263, 273, 274, 275, 276
    barium radiograph of, 275
    fixed retrocecal, 275
    orifice of, 274
    variations in position of, 275
  vesicular, 355, 369
Arachnoid, 99, 108
Arachnoid-dura interface, 101
Arachnoid granulation, 99, 100, 101, 108
  granular foveolae for, 9, 99
Arachnoid mater, 163
  lumbar, 163
  spinal, 162
  thoracic, 163
Arantius, body of, 217
Arcades, of small intestine, 287
Arcuate artery, 312, 314, 518, 524
  lymph vessels along, 318
Arcuate eminence, 11, 92
Arcuate ligament, 340, 348, 363
  inferior, 338, 341, 345, 357
  lateral, 189, 256
  medial, 189, 256
  median, 256
Arcuate line, 241, 245, 247, 249, 253, 332, 335, 336, 337, 338, 340, 474
Arcuate popliteal ligament, 496, 499
Arcuate vein, 314
Arcus tendinous fasciae pelvis, 353
Areola, 176
Areolar gland, 176
Areolar tissue, 173, 459
  loose, 101
Areolar venous plexus, 250
Arm. *See also* Forearm
  anterior view of, 403
  cutaneous nerves of, 403
  muscles of
    anterior view of, 419
    deep layer of, 419
    posterior view of, 420
    superficial layer of, 419
  posterior view of, 403
  radial nerve in, 465
  serial cross section of, 423
  superficial veins of, 403
Arrector pili muscle, innervation to, 160
Arteriae rectae, 287, 288, 305
Arteriogram
  celiac, 285
  of coronary arteries, 212
Arteriole
  glomerular, afferent and efferent, 313, 314
  inferior macular, 90
  inferior nasal retinal, 90

Arteriole (Continued)
inferior temporal retinal, 90
intralobular, 279
periportal, 279
superior macular, 90
superior nasal retinal, 90
superior temporal retinal, 90
Artery(ies). See also specific arteries
of abdominal wall, 257
of anal canal, 378
of brain, 135
frontal view of, 139
inferior views of, 137
lateral and medial views of, 140
schema of, 136
section of, 139
bronchial, 201
of cranial fossa, 141
of duodenum, 284, 286
of esophagus, 231
of eye, 90
of eyelid, 85
of face, 3
of female pelvic organs, 380
of femoral head and neck, 492
of fingers, 459
of foot, 524
of hand, 454
of hypothalamus and hypophysis, 146
of kidney, 314
of knee, 500
of large intestine, 288
of liver, 283, 284
of mammary gland, 177
of meninges, 135
of nasal cavity, 40
of oral and pharyngeal region, 69
of orbit, 85
of pancreas, 284, 286
of pelvis, 383
female, 382
male, 383
perineal, 384
of perineum
female, 384
male, 385
of pterygoid canal, 39
of rectum, 378
of scalp, 3
of small intestine, 287
of spinal cord
intrinsic distribution of, 165
schema, 164
of spleen, 283, 284
of stomach, 283
of suprarenal glands, 322
of testis, 381
of thigh
anterior view of, 489
anterior views of, 488
posterior view of, 490
schema of, 500
of upper limb, 461
of ureters, 316
of urinary bladder, 316
of uterus, 384
of wrist, 449
Artery of Adamkiewicz, 164
Arthrogram
of hip, 531
of shoulder, 468
Articular cavity, 180, 499
Articular disc, 18, 442
coronal section: dorsal view of, 443
cross section of, 236
region of, posterior view of, 443
sagittal section through, 441
Articular facet
inferior, 156
for sacrum, 152

Articular facet (Continued)
superior, 151
of rib head, 181
thoracic, superior, 151
of vertebral body, 180
Articularis genus muscle, 495, 499, 526
origin of, 478
Articular nerve, recurrent, 528, 530
Articular process
cervical
inferior, 20, 21
superior, 20, 21
inferior, 156
lumbar
inferior, 152, 153, 155
superior, 152, 153, 154, 155
transverse, 156
thoracic
inferior, 151
superior, 151
Articular tubercle, 6, 10, 18, 55
Aryepiglottic fold, 66, 67, 78
Aryepiglottic muscle, 78, 80
Arytenoid muscle
oblique, 67, 78, 80, 229
action of, 79
transverse, 63, 67, 78, 80, 229
action of, 79
Ascending fibers, 320
Asterion, 6
Atlantoaxial joint
lateral, 21, 22
capsule of, 22, 23
median, superior view of, 23
Atlantoaxial membrane, 23
Atlantooccipital joint capsule, 22, 23
Atlantooccipital joint complex, median, articular
cartilage for, 21
Atlantooccipital ligament, anterior, 23
Atlantooccipital membrane
anterior, 22, 63, 65
posterior, 22
Atlas (C1), 15, 21, 22, 23
anterior arch of, 7, 19, 21, 63, 167
anterior tubercle of, 19, 21, 23
anterior view of, 19, 150
dens of, 19
articular facet for, 19
groove for vertebral artery, 19
inferior view of, 19
lateral mass of, 19
left lateral view of, 150
posterior arch of, 19, 148, 172
posterior left lateral view of, 150
posterior tubercle of, 19, 169, 170
posterior view of, 150
posterosuperior view of, 19
superior articular surface of lateral mass of occipital condyle, 19
superior view of, 19
transverse foramen of, 19
transverse process of, 19, 22, 29, 170
tubercle for transverse ligament of atlas, 19
vertebral foramen of, 19
Atrial appendage, 218
Atrioventricular bundle (of His), 219
left, 219
right, 219
Atrioventricular node
left. See Mitral valve
right. See Tricuspid valve
Atrium, 218
left, 208, 209, 210, 215, 218, 239
oblique vein (of Marshall) of, 208, 209, 211, 215
right, 206, 208, 209, 210, 214, 217, 218, 239
opened, 214
radiograph of, 207
Auditory (pharyngotympanic, eustachian) tube,
92, 93, 94, 125
cartilage of, 47

Auditory (pharyngotympanic, eustachian) tube
(Continued)
cartilaginous part of, 52, 55, 64, 65, 67, 98
lateral lamina of, 98
medial lamina of, 98
groove for, 10
opening of, 36
pharyngeal opening of, 63, 64, 66, 124
Auerbach's plexus, 305
Auricle, 92, 97
concha of, 93
left, 206, 208, 209, 211, 215, 218, 219
lobule of, 93
right, 93, 206, 208, 214, 218
Auricular artery
anterior, 3
posterior, 3, 33, 39, 69, 100, 135, 136, 172
Auricularis muscle, 117
Auricularis posterior muscle, 25
Auricular muscle, facial nerve branches to, 122
Auricular nerve
anterior, 121
branches to auricular muscle, 122
great, 2, 30, 31, 32, 128, 171
greater, 172
posterior, 24, 45, 122
occipital branch of, 122
Auricular tubercle (of Darwin), 93
Auricular vein, posterior, 3, 31, 70
Auriculotemporal nerve, 2, 18, 39, 45, 55, 61, 69, 71,
121, 124, 133
meningeal branch of, 121
parotid branches of, 121
Auscultation
precordial areas of, 207
triangle of, 149, 239, 248
Autonomic nerves
of biliary tract, 306
of duodenum, 298, 299, 300
of head, 130
of kidneys, 319
of large intestine, 302, 303
of liver, 306
of neck, 129
of pancreas, 307
of small intestine, 301, 303
of stomach, 298, 299, 300
in thorax, 203
of ureters, 319
of urinary bladder, 319
Autonomic plexus, intrinsic, of intestines, 305
Autonomic reflex pathways, schema of, 304
Autonomic sensory zones, of lower limb, 470
Axilla, 175
dissection of, anterior view of, 417
oblique parasagittal section of, 416
suspensory ligament of, 416
Axillary artery, 177, 183, 192, 249, 415, 417, 421,
422
Axillary fold
anterior, 175
posterior, 175
Axillary fossa, 236, 237, 238
Axillary lymph nodes
anterior (pectoral), 178
apical, 178
central, 178, 416
lateral, 178, 405
pectoral, 416
posterior (subscapular), 178
Axillary nerve, 402, 412, 413, 414, 417, 418, 420, 462,
463, 465, 467
cutaneous innervation from, 466
in quadrangular space, 414
superior cutaneous, 403
superior lateral brachial cutaneous nerve from,
171, 412, 466
Axillary recess, 410
arthrogram of, 468
Axillary tail (of Spence), 177

Axillary vein, 183, 192, 250
    intercostal tributaries to, 250
    lateral axillary lymph nodes along, 405
Axis (C2), 21, 23
    anterior view of, 19, 150
    body of, 19, 22
    dens of, 7, 15, 19, 21, 22, 23, 63
    inferior articular facet of, 19
    interarticular part of, 19
    left lateral view of, 150
    pedicle of, 19
    posterior articular facet of, 19
    posterior view of, 150
    posterosuperior view of, 19
    spinous process of, 19
    superior articular facet of, 19
    transverse process of, 19
        posterior tubercle of, 29
Azygos vein, 186, 188, 200, 201, 203, 210, 224, 232, 238, 239, 327
    arch of, 224, 226, 237
    axial CT images of, 235
    groove for, 193
    junction with accessory hemiazygos vein, 232
    transverse section of, 325

B

Back
    lumbar region, cross-section of, 173
    muscles of
        deep, axial CT image of, 324
        deep layers of, 170
        intermediate layers of, 169
        superficial layers of, 168
    nerves of, 171
    surface anatomy of, 149
Bartholin's gland, 358, 359, 384
    opening of, 356
Basal collecting vessels, 73
Basal nucleus, organization of, 109
Basal vein (of Rosenthal), 142, 143, 144, 417
Basilar artery, 135, 136, 137, 138, 139, 141, 164
    computed tomography of, 147
    imaging of, 148
Basilar membrane, 96
Basilar venous plexus, 102, 103
Basilic vein, 400, 403, 404, 405, 423, 437, 456
    median, 404
Basivertebral vein, 166, 167
Batson, internal vertebral venous plexus of, 102, 163, 166
Bertin, renal column of, 311, 314
Biceps brachii muscle, 175, 400, 417, 421, 423, 434, 435, 462
    fascia over, 416
    insertion of, 438, 439
    long head of, 238, 407, 411, 412, 414, 416, 419, 423, 461
        tendon of, 237, 238
    short head of, 237, 407, 411, 412, 414, 416, 419, 423, 461
    tendon of, 461
Biceps brachii tendon, 419, 421, 426, 435, 436
    long head of, 410, 413, 414, 419
    short head of, 414, 419
Biceps femoris muscle, 493, 504
    insertion of, 503
    long head of, 482, 483, 490, 491, 493, 509
        origin of, 479
        tendon of, 335
    short head of, 482, 483, 490, 509
        origin of, 479
    tendon of, 495, 509
        bursa of, 495
Biceps femoris tendon, 494, 495, 499, 505, 506, 507, 528, 529
    bursa beneath, 499
Bicipital aponeurosis, 404, 419, 421, 434, 461

Bicipital groove
    arthrogram of, 468
    computed tomography of, 468
Bifid spinous process, cervical, 20
Bifurcate ligament, 515
Bigelow, Y ligament of, 475, 484
Bile canaliculi, 279
Bile duct, 125, 161, 279
    common, 265, 266, 270, 271, 277, 278, 281, 283, 286, 326
        sphincter of, 280
    extrahepatic, 280
    innervation of, 160
    periportal, 279
Biliary disease, common areas of referred pain in, 306
Biliary tract, innervation of, 306
Bipolar cell, 119
Bladder-prostate junction, 398
Blood circulation
    intrapulmonary, schema of, 199
    postnatal, 223
    prenatal, 223
Bloodless fold of Treves, 273
Blood vessels. *See also specific arteries and veins*
    innervation of, 222
Bones. *See also names of specific bones*
    of elbow, 424
    of foot, 511, 512
        lateral view of, 512
        medal view of, 512
    of forearm, 427
    of hand, 444
    of pelvis, 332, 335, 336
    of wrist, 444
Bony labyrinth. *See* Labyrinth, bony
Bowman's capsule, 313
Brachial artery, 177, 415, 417, 419, 421, 422, 423, 434, 435, 436, 461
    acromial branch of, 422
    clavicular branch of, 422
    deep, 417, 420, 421, 422, 423
        middle collateral branch of, 433
        in triangular interval, 414
    deltoid branch of, 422
    inferior ulnar collateral branch of, 433
    in situ, 421
    muscular branch of, 421
    pectoral branch of, 422
    posterior branch of, 433
    superior ulnar collateral branch of, 433
Brachial cutaneous nerve
    inferior lateral, 402, 403, 420
    medial, 403, 417, 418, 421, 423
    posterior, 402, 403, 420
    superior lateral, 402, 403, 414, 420
Brachialis muscle, 407, 417, 419, 421, 423, 434, 435, 436, 461, 462
    innervation of, 465
    insertion of, 426, 438
    origin of, 438
Brachial plexus, 1, 26, 29, 30, 31, 71, 157, 177, 183, 187, 192, 200, 205, 224, 225, 226, 414, 417
    anterior divisions of, 418
    communication to, 128
    cords of, 418
        lateral, 416, 421, 462, 463, 467
        medial, 416, 421, 462, 463, 467
        posterior, 416, 462, 463, 467
    inferior, 418
    middle, 418
    posterior divisions of, 418
    roots of, 418
    schema of, 418
    superior, 418
    terminal branches of, 418
    trunks of, 412, 418
Brachial vein, 423
Brachiocephalic trunk, 32, 74, 75, 76, 135, 136, 184, 187, 200, 205, 206, 208, 226, 231, 236

Brachiocephalic vein, 74, 184, 202
    left, 70, 75, 76, 167, 186, 200, 205, 206, 224, 225, 226, 232
    groove for, 193
Brachiocephalic vein *(Continued)*
    right, 75, 167, 186, 200, 205, 206, 224
        cross section of, 236
Brachioradialis muscle, 400, 407, 419, 420, 421, 423, 432, 433, 434, 435, 437, 461, 465, 466
    as flexor of elbow, 430
    insertion of, 438, 439
Brachioradialis tendon, 436, 437
Brain
    arteries of, 135
        frontal view of, 139
        inferior views of, 137
        lateral and medial views of, 140
        schema of, 136
        section of, 139
    coronal section of, 48, 99, 107
    deep veins of, 143
    horizontal section of, 48
    inferior view of, 143
    sagittal section of, in situ, 105
    subependymal veins of, 144
    superior view of, 143
    ventricles of, 107
Brainstem
    anterior view of, 113
    cranial nerve in, 115
    posterolateral view of, 113
    sectioned, 106
Bregma, 9
Bridging vein, 99, 101, 102, 108
    computed tomography of, 147
    inferior, 99
Broad ligament, 342, 343, 344, 352, 369
    laminae of
        anterior, 354
        posterior, 354
    mesometrium of, 355
    mesosalpinx of, 344
    subdivisions and contents of, 354
Bronchial artery, 199, 201, 224, 225
    esophageal branches of, 201, 231
    inferior left, 201
    left, 193
        esophageal branch of, 231
        inferior, 231
        superior, 231
    right, 193, 201, 231
        esophageal branch of, 231
    superior left, 201
Bronchial vein, 201
    left, 201
    right, 201
Bronchiole
    respiratory, 198, 199
    terminal, 198, 199
Bronchomediastinal lymphatic trunk, 202
Bronchopulmonary (hilar) lymph nodes, 193, 202, 224, 225
Bronchopulmonary segments, 194, 195
    anterior view of, 194
    lateral view of, 195
    medial view of, 195
    nomenclature of: schema, 197
    posterior view of, 194
Bronchus, 161
    anterior basal, 197
    anteromedial basal, 197
    apical, 197
    apicoposterior, 197
    inferior lobar, 196
    innervation of, 160
    intermediate, 196
    intermediate right, 193
    lateral basal, 197
    left main, 193, 200, 201, 225, 226, 227, 228, 238
        axial CT image of, 235

Bronchus, left main *(Continued)*
  branches of, 196, 210
  lingular, 196
  major, 196
    cross section of, 196
  middle lobar, 196, 197
  nomenclature of: schema, 197
  posterior, 197
  right intermediate, 200
  right main, 201, 224, 226
    axial CT image of, 235
    branches of, 196, 210
    cross-section of, 238
  right superior lobar, 193, 200
  superior lingular, 197
  superior lobar, 196, 197
Brunner's glands, 271
Buccal artery, 39, 69
Buccal nerve, 2, 39, 45, 71, 121
Buccinator lymph node, 72
Buccinator muscle, 25, 45, 48, 52, 54, 55, 60, 61, 65, 68, 69, 122
Buccopharyngeal fascia, 34, 60
Bulbar conjunctiva, 81, 87, 88, 90
Bulbocavenous muscle, 384
Bulb of vestibule, 384
  artery to, 384
Bulb of vorticose (choroid) vein, 91
Bulbospongiosus muscle, 323, 350, 357, 358, 359, 363, 375, 376, 385
  fascia of, 363
Bulbourethral (Cowper's) gland, 247, 323, 346, 350, 363, 384
  duct of, 363
  opening of, 369
  primordium of, 369
Bulging septum, 36
Burns, suprasternal space of, 27, 34, 63
Bursae
  of fingers, 451
  omental, cross section of, 265
  subdeltoid, 410, 419
Buttock, nerves of, 491

C

Calcaneal (Achilles) tendon, 469, 504, 505, 506, 509, 515, 517
Calcaneal artery
  lateral, 522, 523
  medial, 522, 523
Calcaneal bursa, subcutaneous, 517
Calcaneal nerve
  lateral, 522, 523
  medial, 522, 523
Calcaneal tendon, subtendinous bursa of, 517
Calcaneocuboid ligament, 515, 524
  dorsal, 515
Calcaneofibular ligament, 515
Calcaneonavicular ligament, 515
  plantar, 515, 524
Calcaneus, 511, 513
  body of, 512
  fibular (peroneal) trochlea of, 511, 512
  functional relationships of, 513
  groove for fibularis longus tendon, 512
  lateral process of, 511
  lateral view of, 514
  medial process of, 511
  radiograph of, 514
  sustentaculum tali of, 511
    radiograph of, 514
  tuberosity of, 469, 504, 505, 511, 512, 522, 523
    fat pad overlying, 520
    lateral process of, 516, 521
    medial process of, 516, 521
    radiograph of, 514
Calcar, 477

Calcar avis, 110, 111
Calcarine artery, 140, 141
Calcarine sulcus, 104, 105, 106, 110, 119
Callosomarginal artery, 139, 140
Calot, cystic lymph node of, 294
Calot's (cystohepatic) triangle, 280, 284
Calvaria, 101
  inferior view of, 9
  superior view of, 9
Calyx, major, 329
Camper chiasm, 451
Camper's layer, 243, 323, 346, 357, 360
Canal of Schlemm, 87, 88, 90, 91
  veins draining, 91
Canine teeth, 56
Capillary, subpleural, 199
Capillary bed, within alveolar wall, 199
Capillary plexus
  within alveolar wall, 199
  medullary, 314
Capitate, 442, 449
  anterior (palmar) view of, 440, 441, 444
  coronal section: dorsal view of, 443
  posterior (dorsal) view of, 440, 443, 444
  radiograph of, 445
  sagittal section through, 441
Capitate ligament, radiate, 442
Capitotriquetral ligament, 442
Capitulum, 407, 424
  radiograph of, 425
Capsular ligament, 410
Capsular tissue, superficial, 443
Capsular vein, 314
Capsule
  external, 109
  internal, 109, 139
    cleft for, 109
    retrolenticular part of, 109
Cardia
  hepatic plexus branch to, 299
  lymph nodes around, 293
Cardiac nerve
  cervical, sympathetic and vagal, 129, 130, 203
  thoracic, 129, 187
  vagal, 129
Cardiac notch, 190, 192, 230, 267
Cardiac plexus, 125, 203, 220, 234
Cardiac vein, 211
  anterior, 211
  great, 211
  middle, 211
  small, 211
Cardinal (Mackenrodt's) ligament, 344, 345, 352, 353, 355
Caroticotympanic nerve, 122
  from internal carotid plexus, 124
Carotid artery, 33
  common, 3, 30, 32, 33, 34, 46, 69, 70, 71, 74, 75, 76, 124, 127, 129, 130, 132, 133, 135, 136, 184, 192, 204, 226, 231
    left, 167, 187, 205, 206, 208, 236
    right, 29, 167, 187, 200
  external, 3, 27, 28, 30, 33, 39, 40, 46, 59, 60, 61, 69, 70, 71, 74, 75, 76, 100, 124, 129, 130, 132, 133, 135, 136
    schema of, 33
  internal, 3, 33, 43, 46, 47, 55, 60, 69, 71, 74, 75, 76, 85, 86, 94, 103, 120, 122, 127, 129, 130, 131, 132, 133, 135, 136, 137, 138, 139
    in carotid canal, 12, 13, 98
    carotid groove for, 11
    computed tomography of, 147
    left, 140, 141
    meningohypophyseal trunk of, 100
    right, 140
Carotid autonomic plexus, 12
Carotid body, 33, 71, 124, 129, 135, 204
Carotid canal, 12, 13
  external opening of, 10
Carotid groove, for internal carotid artery, 11

Carotid nerve
  external, 160
  internal, 46, 129, 130, 132
Carotid plexus
  common, 129, 130
  external, 129, 130, 132, 160
  internal, 13, 43, 86, 120, 122, 130, 131, 160
    caroticotympanic nerve from, 124
Carotid sheath, 27, 34, 60
Carotid sinus, 124, 129, 130, 135, 204
Carotid sinus nerve (of Hering), 33, 71, 124, 129, 130
Carotid tubercle of Chassaignac, 21, 22
Carpal arterial arch, palmar, 453
Carpal bones. *See also specific carpal bones*
  in abduction, 441
  anterior (palmar) view of, 440, 441, 444
  posterior (dorsal) view of, 440, 444
Carpal ligament
  palmar, 448
    continuous with extensor retinaculum, 404, 434, 447
  transverse, 435, 442, 449, 450, 453, 461
Carpal tunnel, palmar view of, 442
Carpometacarpal joint
  articular capsule of, 442
  coronal section: dorsal view of, 443
  in extension, 441
  first, capsule of, 443
  in flexion, 441
  sagittal section through, 441
Carpometacarpal ligament
  dorsal, posterior view of, 443
  palmar, 442
Cartilage
  of airway, 198
  alar
    lateral and medial crus of, 35
    major, 35, 37, 38, 47
    minor, 35
  articular, 410, 475, 499
    of dens, 21
    of elbow, 426
    of femoral head, 521, 531
  arytenoid, 65, 77
    muscular process of, 77, 78
    vocal process of, 77, 78
  of auditory tube, 47
  auricular, 47
  corniculate, 65, 77
  costal, 180, 190, 241, 406
    cross-section of, 236
    fifth, 188
    fifth left, 210
    second, 238
    seventh, 192, 327
    sixth, 411
    transverse section of, 325
  cricoid, 15, 27, 28, 63, 65, 68, 74, 77, 78, 190, 196, 200, 227, 228, 229
    arch of, 77
    arytenoid surface of, 77
    lamina of, 77, 78
    prominence over lamina of, 66
  of larynx, 77
  nasal accessory, 35
  nasal septal, 35, 47
    lateral process of, 35, 37, 38
  prevertebral, 60
  septal, 35
  thyroid, 1, 15, 28, 63, 65, 68, 74, 78, 80, 190, 196, 200, 227, 228, 229
    lamina of, 78
    oblique line of, 28
    superior horn of, 66, 67, 68, 77
  tracheal, 196
  triticeal, 77
Caruncle
  hymenal, 356
  lacrimal, 82
  sublingual, 51, 61

Cauda equina, 157, 158, 163, 329
  cross section of, 174
Cauda equina artery, 164
Caudal mesonephric tubule, 370
Caudate nucleus, 109, 139
  anterior vein of, 143, 144
  body of, 107, 109
  head of, 109, 110, 141, 143, 148
  posterior terminal vein of, 144
  posterior vein of, 143
  tail of, 107, 111
  transverse veins of, 143, 144
Caudate process, 277
Caval opening, 189, 256
Caval tributaries, 292
Cave of Retzius, 323
Cavernous nerve, 390, 396
Cavernous plexus, 120
Cavernous sinus, 85, 100, 103, 135
Cavum septum pellucidum, 99
Cecal artery, 302
  anterior, 273, 287, 288
  posterior, 273, 287, 288
Cecal folds, 273, 343, 347
Cecal plexus, 302
Cecal vein
  anterior, 291, 292
  posterior, 291, 292
Cecum, 125, 261, 263, 275, 276, 343, 347
  vascular fold of, 273
Celiac ganglion, 125, 160, 161, 234, 260, 297, 298,
  299, 300, 301, 302, 303, 306, 307, 319, 320, 327,
  389, 390, 394, 395, 396
Celiac lymph node, 233, 259, 293, 294, 295
Celiac plexus, 125, 234, 298, 299, 301, 302, 319, 320,
  390, 395
  vagal branch to, 125, 234
Celiac trunk, 226, 231, 257, 262, 266, 270, 281, 283, 284,
  286, 287, 300, 303, 307, 308, 310, 323, 328, 390
  arteriogram of, 285
  bifurcation of, 326
  prenatal, 223
Central artery
  anterolateral, 137, 138, 139
  posteromedial, 138
Central band, 452
Central canal, 116
Central collecting vessels, 73
Central retinal artery, 87
Central retinal vein, 87
Central sulcus of Rolando, 104, 105
Central tendon
  middle leaflet of, 188
  right leaflet of, 199
Central vein, 278, 279
Cephalic vein, 175, 182, 183, 250, 400, 403, 404, 405,
  411, 416, 417, 423, 437, 456
  accessory, 403, 404
  median, 404
Cerebellar artery
  anterior inferior, 135, 136, 137, 138, 139, 164
  posterior inferior, 135, 136, 137, 164
  superior, 135, 137, 138, 139, 164
Cerebellar hemispheric vein, inferior, 142
Cerebellar notch
  anterior, 112
  posterior, 112
Cerebellar nucleus
  dentate, 111
  emboliform, 111
  fastigial, 111
  globose, 111
Cerebellar peduncle
  inferior, 112, 114, 142
  middle, 112, 113, 114, 142
  superior, 112, 113, 114, 142
    decussation of, 112
Cerebellar vein
  precentral, 142
  superior (inconstant), 142

Cerebellomedullary cistern, 108
  vein of, 142
Cerebellum, 97, 105, 110, 144
  anterior lobe of, 112
Cerebellum (Continued)
  biventer lobule of, 112
  central lobule of, 142
  culmen of, 142
  declive of, 142
  dentate nucleus of, 114
  flocculonodular lobe of, 112
  flocculus of, 113
  folium of, 142
  horizontal fissure of, 112
  imaging of, 148
  inferior semilunar lobule of, 112
  inferior surface of, 112
  lingula of, 142
  median sagittal section of, 114
  nodule of, 142
  parts of, 142
  posterior lobe of, 112
  posterior view of, 114
  posterolateral (dorsolateral) fissure of, 112
  postlunate fissure of, 112
  primary fissure of, 112
  pyramid of, 142
  quadrangular lobule of, 112
  retrotonsillar fissure of, 112
  secondary (postpyramidal) fissure of, 112
  simple lobule of, 112
  superior semilunar lobule of, 112
  superior surface of, 112
  surface in plane of superior cerebellar peduncle,
    112
  tonsil of, 112, 142
  tuber of, 142
  uvula of, 142
  vermis of
    central lobule, 114
    culmen, 114
    declive, 114
    folium, 114
    lingula, 114
    nodulus, 114
    pyramid, 114
    tuber, 114
    uvula, 114
  wing of central lobule of, 112
Cerebral aqueduct, 105, 106, 107, 108, 114, 116, 144,
  145
  imaging of, 148
Cerebral arterial circle of Willis, 137, 138
  inferior view of, 138
  vessels dissected out, 138
  vessels in situ, 138
Cerebral artery, 101
  anterior, 135, 136, 137, 139, 141, 143, 144
    A₂ section of, 138
    branches of, 139
    computed tomography of, 147
    imaging of, 148
    left, 140
    right, 140
    temporal branches of, 140
  anterior inferior, 141
  calcarine branch of, 140, 141
  deep, 99
  dorsal branch to corpus callosum, 140
  inferior, 138
  middle, 135, 136, 137, 138, 139, 141
    computed tomography of, 147
    left, 140
    temporal branches of, 139
  parietooccipital branch of, 140, 141
  posterior, 135, 136, 137, 138, 139, 141, 164
    anterior temporal branch of, 140
    computed tomography of, 147
    inferior temporal branch of, 140
    inferior terminal branch of, 140

Cerebral artery, posterior (Continued)
    middle temporal branch of, 140
    occipitotemporal branches of, 140
    P₁ segment of, 138
    P₂ segment of, 138
    right, 140
    superior temporal branch of, 140
    superior terminal branch of, 140
    temporal branches of, 141
    terminal branches of, 140
  posterior inferior, 139, 141
    cerebellar tonsillar branch of, 141
  superior, 99, 141
Cerebral crus, 106, 113, 143
Cerebral fissure, longitudinal, 106, 141, 143
Cerebral hemisphere, 101
  medial surface of, 105
Cerebral peduncle, 105, 114
Cerebral vein
  anterior, 142, 143
  deep middle, 142, 143, 144
  great (of Galen), 103, 114, 142, 143, 144
  inferior, 103, 143
    beneath arachnoid, 101
  internal, 99, 107, 110, 142, 143
    computed tomography of, 147
    left, 144
    right, 144
  penetrating subdural space, 99
  superficial, 101
    middle, 101, 103, 143
  superior, 101
    beneath arachnoid, 101
    opening of, 100
    penetrating arachnoid and dura mater,
      101
Cerebrospinal fluid, circulation of, 108
Cerebrum
  frontal lobe of, 104
  frontal pole of, 104, 106
  gyri of, 104
  horizontal section through, 109
  inferior margin of, 106
  inferior view of, 106
  lateral view of, 104
  medial view of, 105
  occipital lobe of, 104
  occipital pole of, 104, 106
  parietal lobe of, 104
  sulci of, 104
  temporal lobe of, 104
  temporal pole of, 104, 106
Cervical artery
  ascending, 32, 69, 71, 74, 75, 76, 136, 164,
    415
  deep, 135, 136, 164
  superficial, 74, 75, 136
  transverse, 31, 32, 76, 171, 415
Cervical canal, with palmate folds, 355
Cervical cardiac nerve
  inferior, 69, 220
  middle, 220
  superior, 69, 220
  sympathetic and vagal, 203, 234
Cervical curvature, 150
Cervical ganglion
  middle, 71, 127
  superior, 43, 46, 160
Cervical ligament, transverse, 344
Cervical lymph nodes
  anterior superficial, 72
  deep lateral (internal jugular), 73
  inferior deep (internal jugular), 233
  inferior deep lateral, 72
  inferior deep (scalene), 202
  posterior lateral superficial, 72
  superior deep lateral, 72
  superior lateral superficial, 72
  transverse chain of, 72
Cervical muscles, deep, 34

Cervical nerves. *See also* Cervical spinal nerves
transverse, 2, 30, 32, 128
ventral ramus of, 31
Cervical plexus, 172
ansa cervicalis of, 127
branches from, 2
schema of, 32, 128
Cervical spinal nerves
C1, 126, 157
dorsal ramus of, 22, 127
relation to cervical vertebrae, 158
schema of, 160
ventral ramus of, 71, 127
C2, 126
dorsal ramus of, 172
relation to cervical vertebrae, 158
schema of, 160
ventral ramus of, 31, 71, 127, 171
C3, 126
dorsal ramus of, 171, 172
intervertebral foramen for, 21
relation to cervical vertebrae, 158
schema of, 160
ventral ramus of, 127, 171
C4, 126
dorsal ramus of, 2, 171, 172
groove for, 20, 21
relation to cervical vertebrae, 158
schema of, 160
ventral ramus of, 71
C5
dorsal ramus of, 2, 155, 172
relation to cervical vertebrae, 158
schema of, 160
ventral ramus of, 31
C6
dorsal ramus of, 2, 172
relation to cervical vertebrae, 158
schema of, 160
C7
groove for, 20
relation to cervical vertebrae, 158
schema of, 160
C8, 157
relation to cervical vertebrae, 158
schema of, 160
dorsal rami of, medial branches of, 2
Cervical sympathetic cardiac nerves
inferior, 129
middle, 129
sympathetic, 130
Cervical sympathetic ganglion
middle, 32, 220
superior, 127, 131, 204, 220
Cervical triangle, posterior, 34
Cervical vein
deep, 167
left, 167
right, 167
transverse, 171
Cervical vertebrae
anterior view of, 21
C1, 7, 157
C2, 7
axis of, 157
spinous process of, 168, 170
C3, 15, 19
inferior view of, 20
transverse process of, 29
tubercles of, 29
venous communications of, 167
C4, 19
anterior view of, 20
area for articulation of left uncinate process
of, 20
body of, 20
spinous process of, 20
superior view of, 20
transverse process of, 20

Cervical vertebrae *(Continued)*
C6
anterior tubercle of, 22
transverse process of, 135
C7, 15, 34, 157
anterior view of, 20, 150
left lateral view of, 150
posterior tubercle of, 29
posterior view of, 150
spinous process of, 22, 149, 169, 170, 411
superior view of, 20
transverse process of, 29
facets of, 20, 21
inferior aspect of, 20
posterior view of, 150
uncovertebral articulations of, 20
uncovertebral joints of, 21
upper, 19
ventral rami of, 187
Cervicofacial division, 24
Cervicothoracic (stellate) ganglion, 129, 203, 220,
234
Cervix, 342, 345, 352, 353, 355
Chassaignac, carotid tubercle of, 21
Cheek ligament, 83
Chest
axial CT images of, 235
radiograph of, 207
Chest. *See also* Thorax
Chiasmatic cistern, 108
Choana, 10, 16, 36, 38, 52, 55, 66, 67, 98
posterior, 16
Chordae tendineae, 214, 215, 217
Chorda tympani nerve, 12, 45, 46, 71, 93, 94, 121,
122, 123, 130, 132, 133
Choroid, 87, 89, 90, 119
vascular arrangements within, 91
Choroidal artery
anterior, 137, 138, 141
posterior, 85
posterior lateral, 137, 141
posterior medial, 137, 141
Choroidal vein, 99
Choroid plexus, 111, 114
of lateral ventricle, 108
Choroid vein, superior, 143, 144
Ciliary artery
anterior, 90, 91
recurrent branch of, 91
long posterior, 90, 91
short posterior, 90, 91
Ciliary body, 87, 88, 90
blood vessels of, 90
orbiculus ciliaris of, 89
Ciliary ganglion, 44, 46, 86, 120, 121, 130, 131,
161
nasociliary root of, 131
oculomotor root of, 131
parasympathetic root of, 86, 120, 130
schema of, 131
sensory root of, 86, 120, 130
sympathetic root of, 86, 120, 130, 131
Ciliary muscle, 87, 117, 120, 131
circular fibers of, 88
meridional fibers of, 88
Ciliary nerve
long, 44, 86, 120, 121, 130, 131
short, 44, 86, 120, 121, 131
Ciliary process, 87, 88, 89
Ciliary vein, anterior, 88, 90, 91
Cingulate gyrus, 105
isthmus of, 105
Cingulate sulcus, 105
Circle of Willis
inferior view of, 138
vessels dissected out, 138
vessels in situ, 138
Circular folds (valves of Kerckring), 271, 272
Circular intramuscular plexus, 305

Circular muscle, 305
of duodenum, 271, 280
of esophagus, 228, 229
rectal, 373, 374
Circumflex humeral vein, 403
Cisterna chyli, 259, 295, 297
gastric lymph drainage to, 293
lumbar lymph nodes to, 318
Claustrum, 109
Clavicle, 25, 26, 27, 28, 30, 79, 175, 176, 180, 182, 183,
184, 190, 191, 192, 224, 225, 400, 406, 410, 411,
412, 413, 415, 416, 417
acromial end of, 406
acromial facet of, 406
anterior view of, 407
coronoid tubercle of, 406
cross-section of, 236
glenoid cavity of, 407
impression for costoclavicular ligament, 406
inferior angle of, 407
inferior surface of, 406
infraglenoid fossa of, 407
lateral border of, 407
ligament insertion sites on, 406
medial border of, 407
muscle origin and insertion sites on, 406
neck of, 407
radiograph of, 207, 409
right, 406
shaft of, 406
sternal end of, 406
computed tomography of, 468
sternal facet of, 406
subclavian groove of, 406
subscapular fossa of, 407
superior angle of, 407
superior border of, 407
superior surface of, 406
suprascapular notch of, 407
trapezoid line of, 406
Clavicular head, 175
Clavipectoral fascia, 416
Cleft of Luschka, 21
Clinoid process
anterior, 8, 11
posterior, 11
Clitoral artery, 359, 384
Clitoris, 358, 359, 375
body of, 342, 368
crus of, 342, 350, 352, 358, 359
deep artery of, 359, 384
deep dorsal vein of, 338, 339, 342, 345, 348, 359
dorsal artery of, 359, 384
dorsal nerve of, 359, 393, 394, 485
passing superior to perineal membrane, 393
frenulum of, 356
glans of, 356, 368
prepuce of, 356
suspensory ligament of, 357, 358, 359
Clivus, 11, 23
Cloquet's lymph node, 255, 388
Clunial nerves
inferior, 171, 391, 393, 472, 490, 491
medial, 171, 472, 490
superior, 171, 248, 472, 490
Coccygeal cornu, 154
Coccygeal ligament, 157, 158
Coccygeal nerve, 157, 158, 487
Coccygeal plexus, 485, 487
Coccygeus muscle, 256, 337, 338, 341, 378, 382, 390,
391, 392, 487
nerve to, 485, 487
Coccyx, 157, 158, 332, 335, 336, 337, 338, 339, 371,
398
anterior view of, 150
left lateral view of, 150, 155
pelvic surface of, 154
posterior view of, 150
tip of, 334, 339, 341, 360, 362, 375
transverse process of, 154

Cochlea, 46, 95, 97
helicotrema of, 92, 96
modiolus of, 96
osseous, 96
scala tympani of, 92
scala vestibuli of, 92
turn of, section through, 96
Cochlear aqueduct, 96
Cochlear capsule, 95
Cochlear duct, 92, 96, 97
basal turn of, 95
Cochlear ganglion, 123
Cochlear nerve, 92, 95, 96, 97, 123
Cochlear nucleus
anterior, 116, 123
posterior, 116, 123
Cochlear recess, 95
Cochlear (round) window, 92
fossa of, 93, 94
Colic artery
ascending branch of, 288
descending branch of, 288
left, 257, 288, 297, 302, 378
ascending branch of, 378
descending branch of, 378
middle, 281, 284, 287, 288, 301, 302, 323
right, 287, 288, 301, 302, 315
Colic (hepatic) flexure
left, 261, 262, 263, 264, 267, 270, 276, 278, 281, 322
right, 261, 263, 264, 267, 270, 276, 278, 281, 317, 328
transverse section of, 326
Colic impression, 282
Colic lymph node
left, 296
middle, 296
right, 296
Colic plexus
left, 297, 302
middle, 301, 302
right, 301, 302
Colic vein
left, 292
middle, 281, 290, 291, 292
right, 290, 291, 292
Collar of Helvetius, 230
Collateral artery
middle, 420, 422, 423
radial, 420, 422, 423
ulnar, 421
inferior, 421, 422, 433
superior, 422, 432, 433
Collateral eminence, 110
Collateral ligament, 446, 452, 497, 516
accessory, 446
fibular, 495, 497, 505, 509
inferior subtendinous bursa of, 499
radial, 426, 442, 446
posterior (dorsal) view of, 443
tibial, 495, 497, 499, 505, 507
superficial and deep fibers of, 496
ulnar, 426, 446
posterior (dorsal) view of, 443
Collateral sulcus, 105, 106
Collateral trigone, 110
Collecting duct, 314
Collecting tubule, 314
schema of, 313
Collecting vessels
apical, 73
basal, 73
central, 73
marginal, 73
Colles' (perineal) fascia, 359
Colliculus
facial, 114
inferior, 105, 110, 113, 114
brachium of, 110, 113
left
inferior, 142
superior, 142

Colliculus (Continued)
seminal, 350, 364
superior, 105, 110, 113, 114, 115, 131, 141
brachium of, 110, 113
of corporal quadrigemina, 106
Colli muscle, nerves to, 132
Colon
air in, radiograph of, 333
area for, 308
ascending, 125, 261, 263, 266, 270, 276, 309, 328, 329, 330, 343, 347
axial CT image of, 324
circular muscle of, 274
descending, 161, 263, 270, 276, 317, 328, 329, 330, 343
area for, 308
innervation of, 160
site of, 266
transverse section of, 326
right colic flexure of
transverse section of, 326
sigmoid, 161, 261, 263, 276, 343, 344, 347, 371, 372, 373, 374, 392
innervation of, 160
reflected, 263
transverse, 261, 262, 263, 265, 270, 276, 280, 281, 282, 290, 328, 329, 330
axial CT image of, 324
transverse section of, 326
tributary from, 291
Commissure
anterior, 105, 114, 139, 144, 145, 356
habenular, 105, 110, 114
of labia majora, 356
posterior, 105, 110, 114, 139, 356, 368
of semilunar valve cusps, 217
Common tendinous ring (of Zinn), 84, 86, 120
Communicating artery
anterior, 135, 136, 137, 138, 139, 140
computed tomography of, 147
posterior, 103, 135, 136, 137, 138, 140, 141
Communicating vein, 30, 167
Compressor urethrae muscle, 349, 359
Computed tomography (CT)
abdominal, 324
of chest, 235
of shoulder, 468
Concha
of auricle, 93
inferior, 16
nasal. See Nasal concha
Condylar canal, 13
Condylar process, 17
Condyle
lateral, 424
radiograph of, 498
medial, 424, 501
radiograph of, 498
occipital, 10, 16
Cone of light, 93
Cones, retinal, 119
Conjoined longitudinal muscle, 372, 374
Conjoined tendon, 244, 245, 247, 253, 254
Conjunctiva, 81, 91
bulbar, 81, 83
palpebral, 83
inferior, 81
superior, 81
Conjunctival artery, posterior, 91
Conjunctival fornix
inferior, 81
superior, 81
Conjunctival vein, posterior, 91
Conjunctival vessels, 90
Connective tissue
of liver, 279
of skull, 101
subserous, 306
Connective tissue sheath, 196
Conoid ligament, 410, 413
attachment of, 406

Conoid tubercle, of clavicle, 406
Conus arteriosus, 206, 214, 215, 216
Conus elasticus, 78, 80
Conus medullaris, 157, 158, 329
Convoluted tubule
distal, 313
proximal, 313
Cooper's ligament, 88, 176, 244, 245, 247, 253, 255, 256
Corabrachialis muscle, 407, 412, 414
Corabrachialis tendon, 414
Coracoacromial ligament, 410, 413, 414, 419
Coracobrachialis muscle, 237, 238, 417, 419, 421, 423, 461, 462
fascia over, 416
Coracoclavicular ligament, 410, 413
attachment of, 406
Coracohumeral ligament, 410
Coracoid process, 179, 182, 183, 407, 410, 412, 413, 414, 415, 416, 417, 419, 421
radiograph of, 409
Cornea, 81, 83, 87, 88, 90, 91
Corneal limbus, 81
Corneoscleral junction, 81
Corniculate tubercle, 66
Cornuate tubercle, 67
Coronal sulcus, 368
Coronal suture, 4, 7, 8, 9, 14
Coronary artery
left, 211, 213
anterior interventricular branch of, 206, 211, 213
arteriographic view of, 213
circumflex branch of, 211, 213, 216
left anterior oblique view of, 213
left (obtuse) marginal branch of, 213
(perforating) interventricular septal branches of, 213
posterolateral branches of, 213
right anterior oblique view of, 213
opening of, 217, 218
right, 206, 211, 212, 216
arteriographic view of, 213
atrial branch of, 211
atrioventricular nodal branch of, 212, 216
conus (arteriosus) branch of, 212
diaphragmatic surface of, 211
interventricular septal branches of, 211
left anterior oblique view of, 212
left marginal branch of, 211
opening of, 217
posterior interventricular branch of, 208, 211, 212, 216
posterior left ventricular branch of, 211
posterior ventricular branch of, 212
right (acute) marginal branch of, 211, 212
right anterior oblique view of, 212
right posterolateral branches of, 212
sinuatrial nodal branch of, 211, 212
sternocostal surface of, 211
Coronary ligament, 277
enclosing bare area of liver, 323
hepatorenal portion of, 277
of liver, 266
Coronary sinus, 208, 209, 211, 215, 239
opening of, 214, 217
valve (thebesian) of, 214
Coronary sulcus, 206
Coronary vein
diaphragmatic surface of, 211
sternocostal surface of, 211
Coronoid fossa, 424
Coronoid process, 7, 17, 424, 431
radiograph of, 207, 425
Corpora cavernosa, 362
Corpora quadrigemina, superior colliculus of, 106
Corpus albicans, 355

Corpus callosum, 105, 107, 110, 139, 141
  cistern of, 108
  dorsal vein of, 142, 144
  genu of, 105, 106, 109, 111, 144
    imaging of, 148
  imaging of, 148
  right dorsal branch of pericallosal artery to,
    141
  rostrum of, 105, 139, 143
  splenium of, 105, 106, 109, 111, 114, 141, 143,
    144
    imaging of, 148
  sulcus of, 105
  trunk of, 105, 139
Corpus cavernosum, 346, 363, 365
  MR sagittal images of, 377
Corpus luteum, 355
Corpus spongiosum, 346, 350, 362, 363, 365
  MR sagittal images of, 377
Corpus striatum, 109, 139
Corrugator cutis ani muscle, 373, 374
Corrugator supercilii muscle, 25, 35, 122
Corti, spiral organ of, 92, 96
Cortical capillary plexus, 314
Cortical glomerulus, 314
Cortical radiate artery, 312, 314
  cortical lymph vessels along, 318
Cortical radiate vein, 314
Corticomedullary glomerulus, 314
Costal facet
  inferior, 151, 181
  superior, 151, 181
  transverse, 151
Costal impression, 277
Costal lamella, 20
Costal pleura, 225, 226
Costocervical trunk, 32, 135, 136, 167
Costochondral joint, 180
Costoclavicular ligament, 180, 406, 416
  impression for, 406
Costocoracoid ligament, 416
Costocoracoid membrane, 416
Costodiaphragmatic recess, 190, 191, 192, 224, 225,
  309, 317, 327
Costomediastinal recess, 190
  left, 188
  right, 188
Costomediastinal space, 192
Costotransverse joint, 236
Costotransverse ligament, 181
  lateral, 181
  superior, 181
Costovertebral joint, 181
  left lateral view of, 181
  right posterolateral view of, 181
  transverse section: superior view of, 181
Costoxiphoid ligament, 180
Cough receptors, 204
Cowper's gland, 247, 323, 346, 350, 363, 384
  duct of, 363
  opening of, 369
  primordium of, 369
Coxal bone. *See* Hip bone
Cranial base
  blood vessels of, orientation of, 46
  foramina and canals of
    inferior view of, 12
    superior view of, 13
  inferior view of, 10
  nerves of, orientation of, 46
  superior view of, 11
Cranial fossa
  anterior, 11
  middle, 11
  posterior, 11
    arteries of, 141
    veins of, 142
Cranial imaging, 148
Cranial mesonephric duct, 369

Cranial mesonephric tubule, 369
Cranial nerve
  motor and sensory distribution of, 117
  nuclei of, in brainstem, 115, 116
Craniocervical ligaments
  external
    anterior view of, 22
    posterior view of, 22
    right lateral view of, 22
  internal, 23
Cremaster fascia, 244, 245
Cremaster muscle, 244, 245, 251, 254, 367
  lateral origin of, 244, 253
  medial origin of, 244, 253
Cremasteric artery, 249, 255
Cremasteric reflex, 486
Cremasteric vessels, 254, 381
Cribriform plate, 8, 37, 38, 42, 118
  foramina of, 13
Cricoarytenoid muscle
  action of, 79
  lateral, 78, 80
    action of, 79
  posterior, 67, 78, 80, 229
    action of, 79
Cricoesophageal tendon, 229
Cricopharyngeal muscle, 67
Cricopharyngeus muscle, 65, 67, 68, 75, 76, 80, 227,
  228, 229
  inferior, 80
Cricothyroid artery, 69, 74
Cricothyroid joint, 77
  pivot point of, 79
Cricothyroid ligament, 74
  median, 28, 65, 68, 77, 196
Cricothyroid muscle, 28, 68, 74, 78, 80, 125
  action of, 79
  oblique part of, 78
  posterior, action of, 79
  straight part of, 78
Crista galli, 5, 8, 38
Crista terminalis, 219
Cross section
  of abdomen
    at L1-L2 level, 329
    at L3-L4 level, 330
    at middle T12 level, 327
    at T10 levels, 325
    at T12-L1 level, 328
  of forearm, 437, 458
    serial, 437
  of leg, 510
  of omental bursa, 265
  of prostate gland, 364
  of rectus sheath, 246
  of spleen, 282
  of thorax, 236
    at T7 level, 239
  of trachea, 196
Cruciate ligament, 497
  anterior, 496, 497, 502
    attachment of, 496
    origin of, 496
  covered by synovial membrane, 495
  inferior longitudinal band of, 23
  posterior, 496, 497, 502
    attachment of, 496
  superior longitudinal band of, 23
  transverse ligament of atlas of, 23
Cubital fossa, 400
Cubital lymph nodes, 405
Cubital vein, median, 400, 403, 405
  as tributary to basilic vein, 404
Cuboid bone, 511, 515, 524, 525
  base of, 511
  head of, 511
  lateral view of, 514
  radiograph of, 514
  shaft (body) of, 511
  tuberosity of, 511, 512, 516, 524

Cuboideonavicular ligament, dorsal, 515
Culmen, 112, 142
Cuneate fasciculus, 114
Cuneate tubercle, 113, 114
Cuneiform bone, 511
  intermediate, 511, 524, 525
  lateral, 511, 524, 525
    lateral view of, 514
    radiograph of, 514
  medial, 511, 515, 516, 524, 525
Cuneiform tubercle, 66
Cuneocuboid ligament, dorsal, 515
Cuneonavicular ligament, dorsal, 515
Cuneus, 105
  apex of, 106
Cutaneous muscle, dorsal
  intermediate, 528
  lateral, 528
Cutaneous nerves
  antebrachial
    intermediate, 403
    lateral, 402, 403, 404, 419, 423, 435, 436, 437,
      457, 460, 461, 462
    lateral, anterior branch of, 462
    lateral, posterior branch of, 462
    lateral branches of, 403, 404
    medial, 417, 418, 421, 423, 457, 460, 461, 462,
      463
    medial, posterior branches of, 404
    medial branches of, 403
    median, 404
    posterior, 402, 403, 404, 420, 423, 456, 460, 465,
      466
  brachial
    inferior lateral, 402, 403, 420, 465, 466
    medial, 251, 403, 461, 462, 463
    posterior, 402, 403, 465, 466
    superior lateral, 171, 402, 403, 414, 465,
      466
  dorsal
    intermediate, 530
    lateral, 518, 529, 530
    medial, 530
  femoral
    cutaneous branch of, 472
    lateral, 255, 260, 308, 389, 471, 473, 484, 485,
      486, 488, 489, 526, 527
    lateral, branches of, 472
    posterior, 157, 391, 485, 487, 490,
      491
      branches of, 472
        perineal, 393, 491
  of forearm, 404
  of hand, 460
  of head and neck, 2
  inferior lateral, 402
  intermediate, 530
  lateral, of forearm, 434
  lateral dorsal, 471, 529, 530
  medial crural, 526
  medial dorsal, 530
  of neck, 30
  perforating, 391, 393, 491
  sural
    lateral, 471, 504, 510, 528, 529, 530
    medial, 472, 490, 504, 529
      branches of, 529
  of upper limb, 402
  of wrist, 460
Cuticle, 459
Cystic artery, 280, 283, 284
Cystic duct, 277, 283, 327
  smooth part of, 280
  spiral fold of, 280
Cystic lymph node (of Calot), 294
Cystohepatic (Calor's) triangle, 280, 284
Cystourethrogram, voiding
  female, 351
  male, 351

D

Darwin, auricular tubercle of, 93
Declive, 112, 142
Deep (Buck's) fascia, 243, 244, 245, 323, 346, 360,
    362, 363, 375, 376, 381, 383
    intercavernous septum of, 362
Deep facial vein, 3
Deltoid ligament, medial, 515
Deltoid muscle, 26, 27, 149, 160, 171, 236, 238, 240,
    400, 407, 410, 411, 412, 414, 416, 417, 420, 421,
    423, 461, 465
    computed tomography of, 468
    magnetic resonance imaging of, 468
    origin of, 406
    reflected, 419
Deltoid tuberosity, 407
Deltopectoral groove, 400
Deltopectoral lymph node, 405
Deltopectoral triangle, 240, 411
Denonvillier's fascia, 323, 341, 346, 371, 376
Dens, 19, 21, 167
    apical ligament of, 23, 63, 65
    articular cartilage on, 21
    of axis, 7
Dental plexus
    inferior, 121
    superior, 44
Dental pulp, 57
Dentate gyrus, 105, 107, 110, 111, 118
Dentate line, 373
Dentate nucleus, 114
Denticulate ligament, 162, 163
Dentinal tubule, 57
Dentine, 57
Depressor anguli oris muscle, 25, 54, 122
Depressor labii inferioris muscle, 25
Depressor septi nasi muscle, 25, 35, 122
Dermatomes
    levels of, 159
    of lower limb, 470
    schematic demarcation of, 159
    of upper limb, anterior and posterior views of,
        401
Descemet's membrane, 88
Descending pathway, 131
Diaphragm, 184, 192, 200, 203, 205, 226, 227, 230,
    231, 232, 247, 256, 258, 264, 267, 277, 282, 306,
    308, 309, 317, 327, 390, 486
    abdominal surface of, 189
    area for, 309
    central tendon of, 189, 256, 323
    costal part of, 189
    covered by parietal pleura, 224, 225
    cross section of, 265
    crus of, 173, 317
        left, 189, 226, 256, 262, 325, 326, 328, 329
        right, 189, 226, 256, 262, 325, 326, 327, 328, 329
    dome of
        left, 190, 191
        radiograph of, 207
        right, 190, 191
    lumbar part of, 189
    pelvic, 342
        fascia of, 344, 348, 357, 358, 362, 372, 374, 376,
          385
        female, 337, 338, 339
        male, 340, 341
Diaphragmatic constriction, 227
Diaphragmatic ligament, 366, 369
Digastric fossa, 17
Digastric muscle
    anterior belly of, 26, 27, 28, 30, 33, 45, 48, 53, 61,
        68, 117
    intermediate tendon of, 59
    mastoid notch of, 10
    phantom, 33
    posterior belly of, 26, 28, 33, 39, 45, 53, 59, 60, 61,
        67, 68, 73, 117, 122
        nerve to, 24

Digastric tendon, intermediate, 60
    fibrous loop for, 27, 28, 53, 59
Digital artery
    dorsal, 518, 524
    palmar, 447, 448, 454
        common, 448, 450, 453, 454
    plantar, 459, 520, 521, 524
        common, 524
        dorsal branches of, 518
        to neighboring digit, 459
Digital fibrous sheath, 446
Digital nerve
    dorsal, 404, 456, 466, 471, 528, 530
    of fourth and fifth digits, 447
    palmar, 404, 447, 448, 454
        branches to phalanges, 454
        common, 450
        dorsal branches of, 456
        to fourth and fifth fingers, 448
        from superficial branch of ulnar nerve, 447
        of thumb, 448
    plantar, 520
        dorsal branches of, 518
Digital vein
    dorsal, 404, 456, 471
    palmar, 404
Dilator pupillae muscle, 88, 120, 131
Diploë, 9
Diploic vein, 99, 101
    occipital, 99
    temporal
        anterior, 99
        posterior, 99
Direct vein, lateral, 143, 144
Distal interphalangeal (DIP) joint
    in extension: medial view of, 446
    site of, 400
Distal medial striate artery (recurrent artery of
    Heubner), 137, 138, 139, 140
Distributing vein, 279
Dorsalis pedis artery, 518, 524
Dorsal ramus, spinal, 252, 418
Dorsal root ganglion, 131, 174, 252, 300, 303, 304,
    306, 307, 320
Dorsal tubercle of radius (Lister's), 427
    posterior (dorsal) view of, 440
Dorsal venous network, 404
Dorsiflexion, of lower limb, 470
Dorsum sellae, 11
Douglas, retrouterine pouch of, 342, 344
Ductus arteriosus
    obliterated, 223
    prenatal, 223
Ductus choledochus. *See* Bile duct. common
Ductus (vas) deferens, 247, 253, 254, 255, 257, 346,
    350, 364, 366, 367, 370, 371, 383, 389, 390, 396,
    473
    ampulla of, 364
    artery to, 249, 257, 367, 378, 381, 383
    covered by peritoneum, 254
    in peritoneal fold, 347
Ductus plexus, 389, 390, 396
Ductus reuniens, 96
Ductus venosus
    obliterated, 223
    prenatal, 223
Duodenal cap, 268
Duodenal flexure
    inferior, 271
    superior, 271
Duodenal fold
    circular, 271
    inferior, 262, 270
    superior, 262
Duodenal fossa
    inferior, 262, 270
    superior, 262
Duodenal glands, 271
Duodenal impression, 277

Duodenal papillae
    major, 271
    minor (inconstant), 271
Duodenal wall, layers of, 271
Duodenojejunal flexure, 262, 270, 281, 317, 322
Duodenojejunal junction, 173
Duodenum, 125, 265, 266, 267, 277, 278, 280, 281,
    315, 317, 322
    arteries of, 284, 286
    ascending (4th) part of, 262, 270, 271
    autonomic innervation of, 298, 299
        schema of, 300
    circular folds of, 280
    circular muscle layer of, 269, 271
    descending (2nd) part of, 262, 270, 271, 328
        cross section of, 173
        minor papilla of, 280
    inferior (horizontal or 3rd) part of, 270, 271, 323
    in situ, 270
    junction of second and third parts of, 329
    longitudinal fold of, 280
    longitudinal muscle layer of, 269, 271
    minor papilla of, 280
    mucosa of, 271
    muscles of, 271, 280
    posterior view of, 286
    reflected to left, 286
    superior (1st) part of, 268, 270, 280
        transverse section of, 326
    suspensory muscle of, 262
    veins of, 289
Dural sac
    MR sagittal images of, 377
    termination of, 157, 158
Dural venous sinuses
    coronal section through, 103
    sagittal section of, 102
Dura mater, 38, 93, 96, 100, 101, 108, 118
    lumbar, 163
    meningeal layer of, 99
    periosteal layer of, 99
    spinal, 157, 162
    thoracic, 163
    of vertebral column, 167
Dura-skull interface, 99, 101

E

Ear
    bony and membranous labyrinths of, 95
    external
        coronal oblique section of, 93
        lateral view of, 93
    middle, coronal oblique section of, 93
    tympanic cavity of, 94
Edinger-Westphal nucleus, 115, 116, 120, 131
Efferent ductule, 369, 370
Efferent fibers, 120
    of brainstem, 116
Ejaculatory duct, 398
    beginning of, 364
    opening of, 364, 369
Elastic fibers, of airway, 198
Elbow
    anastomosis around, 422
    bones of, 424
    in extension
        lateral view of, 424
        medial view of, 424
    fat pads of, 426
    joint capsule of, 426
    ligaments of, 426
    in 90° flexion, 424, 426
    opened
        anterior view of, 426
        posterior view of, 426
    radiographs of, 425
        anteroposterior, 425
        lateral, 425

Elbow *(Continued)*
  right
    anterior view of, 426
    in extension: anterior view of, 424
Elliptical recess, 95
Emissary vein, 13, 99, 101
  communicating with cavernous sinus, 70
  condylar, 167
  mastoid, 3, 99, 167
    in mastoid foramen, 12
  occipital, 99
  parietal, 3, 99
  parietal foramen of, 9
  of the skull, 99
  to superior sagittal sinus, 13
Enamel, of teeth, 57
Endolymphatic duct, 13, 95, 96
  in vestibular aqueduct, 96
Endolymphatic sac, 96
Endometrium, 355
Endopelvic fascia, 345
Endothelium, of anterior chamber, 88
Enteric plexus, of gut, 304
Ependyma, 107
Epicolic lymph node, 296
Epicondyle
  lateral, 419, 426, 428, 430, 431, 436
    radiograph of, 425, 498
  medial, 407, 419, 428, 429, 430, 431, 432, 435, 464,
    465
    radiograph of, 425, 498
Epicranial aponeurosis, 3, 25, 172
Epicranius muscle
  frontal belly (frontalis) of, 25
  occipital belly (occipitalis) of, 25
Epididymal duct, 370
Epididymis, 366, 367, 369, 396
  appendix of, 367, 369
  body of, 370
  head of, 370
  sinus of, 370
  tail of, 370
Epidural hematoma, 99, 101
Epidural space, fat in, 163, 167
Epigastric artery
  inferior, 245, 249, 257, 316, 345, 378, 380, 500
    cremasteric branch of, 245, 247, 257
    pubic branch of, 245, 247, 257, 345
  superficial, 245, 249, 257
  superior, 182, 183, 184, 185, 205, 249, 500
Epigastric lymph nodes, inferior, 259
Epigastric region, 242
Epigastric vein
  inferior, 245, 250, 258, 380
  superficial, 240, 250, 331, 471
  superior, 183, 184, 186, 250
Epigastric vessels
  inferior, 245, 247, 253, 254, 255, 343, 383
    branches of, 330
    pubic branches of, 253
    within umbilical fold, 247, 266
  superficial, 243, 488
  superior, 245, 327
Epiglottis, 15, 58, 63, 66, 67, 76, 77, 78, 80, 134, 227,
  229
Epiphysis, 459
Epiploic (omental) appendices, 263, 276, 330
Epiploic (omental) foramen (of Winslow), 265, 267,
  278, 327
Epiploic vein, 232
Episcleral artery, 90
Episcleral space, 83, 87
Episcleral vein, 90
  anastomosis with vorticose veins, 91
  drainage of, 91
Epithelial tag, 368
Epithelium, gingival, 57
Epitympanic recess, 92, 93, 94
Eponychium, 459
Epoophoron, 355, 369

Erector spinae muscle, 149, 168, 169, 170, 173, 174,
  185, 236, 252, 309, 327, 330
  transverse section of, 325
Esophageal artery, 201
Esophageal hiatus, 189
Esophageal impression, 277
Esophageal muscle, 63, 196
  circular, 65, 67, 230
  longitudinal, 65, 67, 75, 230
    cricoid attachment of, 65, 67
Esophageal plexus, 125, 200, 203, 210, 224, 225,
  226, 300
  anterior portion of, 234
  sympathetic branches to, 234
Esophageal portocaval anastomosis, 292
Esophageal prominence, 209
Esophageal tributary, 289
Esophageal veins, plexus of, 232
Esophagogastric junction, 230, 325
Esophagus, 34, 63, 68, 76, 78, 125, 188, 200, 210, 224,
  225, 239, 256, 258, 262, 266, 302, 308, 310, 323
  abdominal part of, 226, 227, 231, 267
  anterior view of, 234
  area for, 193
  arteries of, 231
  average length of, 227
  bare area on ventral surface of, 228
  cervical part of, 226, 231
  circular muscle layer of, 228
  constrictions of, 227
  cross-section of, 236, 237, 238
  fibroelastic membranes of, 228
  groove for, 193
  in situ, 226
  longitudinal muscle layer of, 228, 269
  lymph nodes and vessels of, 233
  mucosa of, 230
    junction with gastric mucosa, 268
  muscles of, 63, 228
  nerves of, anterior and posterior views of, 234
  nerve to, 189
  opened posterior view of, 66
  posterior view of, 234
  submucosa of, 230
  surface anatomy of, 227
  thoracic part of, 226, 231
  veins of, 232
  zone of sparse muscle fibers of, 228
Ethmoidal artery
  anterior, 13, 85
    anterior meningeal branch of, 100
    external nasal branch of, 40
    lateral nasal branch of, 40
    septal branch of, 40
  posterior, 13, 85, 100
    septal and lateral nasal branches of, 40
Ethmoidal bone, 8
  anterior ethmoidal foramen of, 14
  cribriform plate of, 8, 11, 36, 37, 38, 118
  crista galli of, 8, 11, 38
  highest nasal concha of, 37
  middle nasal concha of, 4, 8, 37
  orbital plate of, 4, 6, 14
  perpendicular plate of, 4, 8, 38
  superior nasal concha of, 8, 37
  uncinate process of, 37, 50
Ethmoidal bulla, 36, 37
Ethmoidal cells, 5, 48, 83
  anterior
    openings of, 36, 37
    semilunar hiatus of, 50
  middle, openings of, 36, 37, 50
  posterior, openings of, 36, 37, 50
Ethmoidal foramen
  anterior, 4, 13, 14
  posterior, 4
Ethmoidal nerve
  anterior, 13, 44, 86, 120, 121
    external nasal branches of, 121
    external nasal branch of, 2, 42, 44

Ethmoidal nerve, anterior *(Continued)*
    internal nasal branches of, 121
    lateral internal nasal branch of, 42
    medial internal nasal branch of, 42
  posterior, 13, 44, 86, 120, 121
Ethmoidal vein
  anterior, 13
  posterior, 13
Eustachian tube. *See* Auditory (pharyngotympanic,
  eustachian) tube
Extension, of lower limb, 470
Extensor carpi radialis brevis muscle, 429, 432, 433,
  465, 466
  groove for, 427
  origin of, 438
Extensor carpi radialis brevis tendon, 437, 457,
  458
Extensor carpi radialis longus muscle, 400, 407,
  420, 423, 429, 432, 433, 465, 466
  groove for, 427
  insertion of, 438
  origin of, 438
Extensor carpi radialis longus tendon, 432, 437,
  455, 458
Extensor carpi ulnaris muscle, 400, 420, 429, 432,
  465, 466
  insertion of, 438
  origin of, 438
Extensor carpi ulnaris tendon, 432, 433, 458
Extensor digiti minimi muscle, 429, 432, 466
  insertion of, 438
  origin of, 438
Extensor digiti minimi tendon, 429, 432, 433, 458
Extensor digitorum brevis muscle, 509, 517, 518,
  519, 528, 530
Extensor digitorum brevis tendon, 524
Extensor digitorum hallucis muscle, 528
Extensor digitorum longus muscle, 482, 495, 509,
  510, 517, 518, 519, 528, 530
  origin of, 503
  tendinous sheath of, 518
Extensor digitorum longus tendon, 469, 509, 518,
  519, 524
Extensor digitorum muscle, 420, 429, 432, 437, 465, 466
  central bands of, insertions of, 439
  lateral bands of, insertions of, 439
  origin of, 438
Extensor digitorum tendon, 400, 429, 432, 433, 458
Extensor expansions, 452, 518, 524
  distal lumbrical tendon insertion into, 451
  tendinous slips to, 453
  transverse fibers (hoods) of, 458
Extensor hallucis brevis muscle, 518, 519, 528, 530
Extensor hallucis brevis tendon, 507, 524
Extensor hallucis longus muscle, 507, 509, 510, 530
Extensor hallucis longus tendon, 507, 509, 518, 524
Extensor hallucis longus tendon sheath, 517
Extensor indicis muscle, 429, 433, 437, 466
  insertion of, 439
  origin of, 438
Extensor indicis tendon, 400, 429, 432, 437, 458
Extensor pollicis brevis muscle, 429, 466
  area for, 427
  insertion of, 439
Extensor pollicis brevis tendon, 432, 436, 437, 458
  insertion of, 455
Extensor pollicis longus muscle, 429, 432, 433, 466
Extensor pollicis longus tendon, 400, 432, 437, 458
  insertion of, 455
Extensor retinaculum, 404, 432, 433, 455, 456, 458
  inferior, 509, 518, 528, 530
  superior, 509, 518, 528, 530
Extensor-supinator muscles, 466
Extensor tendon, 450
  common, 429, 432, 433
    origin of, 438
  in fingers, 452
  long, 452
  at wrist, 458
External occipital protuberance (inion), 6, 8, 16

Extrinsic eye muscle, 90
Extrinsic eye muscle, 90
Eye, 161
  anterior and posterior chambers of, 87, 88
  extrinsic muscles of, 84
    innervation of, 84
  innervation of, 160
  intrinsic arteries and veins of, 90
  muscles of, 117
  vascular supply of, 91
Eyeball, 87, 89
  fasciae of, 83
  fascial sheath (Tenon's capsule) of, 83, 87
  horizontal section of, 87
  transverse section of, 48
Eyelash (cilia), 81
Eyelid, 81
  arteries and veins of, 85
  tarsus of, 83

F

Face
  arterial supply sources of, 3
  muscles of, 117, 122
  sensory nerves of, 117
  superficial arteries and veins of, 3
  superficial view of, 24
Facet (zygapophyseal) joint, 239
Facets, 239
  articular
    inferior, 156
    of rib head, 181
    of sacrum, 152
    superior, 151
    thoracic, superior, 151
    of vertebral body, 180
  cervical, 20, 21
  costal
    inferior, 181
    superior, 181
Facial artery, 3, 30, 33, 35, 39, 47, 60, 61, 69, 70, 71,
      75, 85, 130, 132, 135, 136
  lateral nasal alar branch of, 40
  superior labial branch of, 40
  tonsillar branch of, 64
  transverse, 3, 33, 35, 61, 69, 85
Facial canal, 123
  prominence of, 93, 94
Facial colliculus, 114
Facial expression muscles, 25, 60
  lateral view of, 25
Facial lymph node, 72
Facial nerve (VII), 13, 33, 39, 43, 45, 46, 47, 60, 62, 92,
      94, 97, 103, 113, 115, 116, 121, 130, 132, 133, 134
  branches of, 24, 61, 161
  buccal branches of, 24
  cervical branch of, 24
  chorda tympani of, 12
  common, 70
  communication with glossopharyngeal nerve, 124
  deep, 70
  distribution of, 117
  emerging from stylomastoid foramen, 24
  geniculum (geniculate ganglion) of, 43, 45, 94, 97,
      123, 124, 130
  internal genu of, 116
  marginal mandibular branch of, 24, 30
  motor nucleus of, 122
  motor root of, 123
  schema of, 122
  in stylomastoid foramen, 12, 94
  temporal branches of, 24
  trunk of, 24
  zygomatic branches of, 24
Facial nucleus, 115, 116
Facial plexus, 130
Facial vein, 3, 30, 31, 45, 47, 59, 60, 61, 70, 85, 113
  common, 3, 31, 59, 61
  common trunk for, 59, 61

Facial vein (Continued)
  deep, 3
  transverse, 3, 70
Falciform ligament, 246, 247, 261, 266, 267, 277,
      292, 327
  nerve to, 249
Fallopian tube. See Uterine tube
False pelvis, 336
Falx cerebelli, 102
Falx cerebri, 38, 48, 101, 102, 103, 139, 142
Fascia
  alar, 34
  antebrachial, 437
    deep, thickening of, 442, 447
  axillary, 416
  brachial, 416, 423
  buccopharyngeal, 34, 60, 63
  Camper's, 243, 323, 357, 360
  cervical, 34
    investing (deep) layer of, 25, 27, 34, 63, 182, 411
    pretracheal layer of, 27
  clavicopectoral, 416
    investing layer of, 182
  cremasteric, 244, 245, 254, 367, 370
  cribriform, 250
    within saphenous opening, 473
  crural, 471, 473, 510
  dartos, 243, 346, 367, 370, 375
  deep, 455
    of leg, 510
  deep antebrachial, thickening of, 442, 447
  deep (Buck's), 243, 244, 245, 323, 360, 362, 363,
      375, 376, 381, 383
    intercavernous septum of, 362
  Denonvillier's, 323, 341, 346, 371, 376
  diaphragmatic, 230, 317
  endopelvic paravesical, 350
  extraperitoneal, 173, 245, 246, 254, 255, 392
  geniohyoid, 34
  of hand, 450
  iliac, 255, 345, 372
  infradiaphragmatic, 230
  infrahyoid, 27, 34
  infraspinatus, 168, 171
  interosseous
    dorsal, 450
    palmar, 450
  intraspinous, 248
  investing omohyoid muscle, 416
  investing subclavius muscle, 416
  of leg/lower limb, 473
    deep, 471, 473
  masseteric, 25
  medial plantar, 520
  obturator, 338, 340, 344, 345, 348, 352, 358, 372,
      382, 391
  of orbit and eyeball, 83
  over adductor pollicis muscle, 448
  paravesical endopelvic, 350
  parotid, 25
  pectineal, 245, 255
  pectoral, 176, 416
  of pectoralis major muscle, 416
  of pectoralis minor muscle, 416
  pelvic, 371
    of pelvic diaphragm, 348, 358, 372, 374, 385
    tendinous arch of, 345, 350
  penile, 243, 244, 245, 381
    deep (Buck's), 243, 244, 245, 346, 362, 363, 376,
      381, 383
  perianal, deep (investing or Gallaudet's), 346, 350,
      357, 362, 363, 371, 376, 385
  perineal
    of deep perineal muscles, 338
    deep transverse, 364
    superficial (Colles'), 346, 350, 357, 358, 360, 362,
      363, 367, 371, 375, 376, 384, 385, 391
  pharyngobasilar, 59, 65, 67, 68, 73
  plantar, 521
    lateral, 520

Fascia (Continued)
  posterior antebrachial, thickening of, 456
  presacral, 345, 376
  pretracheal, 34, 63, 196
  prevertebral, 63, 65
  psoas, 173, 317
  pubocervical
    distal (vertical) portion of, 353
    horizontal portion of, 353
  of quadratus lumborum muscle, 173
  rectal, 344, 345, 357, 364, 371, 372, 373, 374, 376
  renal, 329
    anterior layer of, 173, 317
    Gerota's, 317
    posterior layer of, 173, 317
    transverse section of, 317
  retrovesical or rectoprostatic (Denonvillier's), 323,
      341, 346, 371, 376
  scrotal, 243, 244
    superficial (dartos), 346, 370, 375, 385
  serratus anterior, 416
  Sibson's, 225
  slips of costal origin of, 184
  spermatic, 254
    external, 243, 244, 245, 253, 346, 360, 367, 370, 385
      investing spermatic cord, 251, 362
    internal, 245, 255, 367, 370
      origin of, 254
  subclavius, 416
  supradiaphragmatic, 230
  temporal, 25, 45, 54
    deep layer of, 54
    superficial layer of, 54
  thoracolumbar, 168, 171, 248
    anterior layer of, 173
    combined layer of, 330
    middle layer of, 173, 330
    posterior layer of, 169, 170, 173, 309, 330
  transversalis, 173, 230, 245, 246, 247, 253, 254, 255,
      257, 317, 323, 327, 343, 346, 347, 348, 357
    continuation of, 317
    deep inguinal ring in, 253
    transverse section of, 325
  ulna, 437
  umbilical prevesical, 247, 254, 345, 346, 348
  uterine, 345, 353
  uterovaginal, 344, 357
  vaginorectal, 345
  vesical, 344, 345, 346, 350, 357, 371, 376
Fascia lata, 243, 244, 352, 357, 387, 471, 473, 488,
      493
Fascial compartments, of leg, 510
Fascial sheath
  of eyeball (Tenon's capsule), 83, 87
  of lumbrical muscles, 450, 451
Fasciculus
  cuneate, 114
  gracile, 114
  longitudinal
    dorsal, 114
    medial, 112, 145
  mammillothalamic, 105
  transverse, 520
Fat
  in acetabular fossa, 475
  epidural, 163, 167
  of mammary gland, 176
  orbital, 48
  pararenal, 317
  perirenal, 173, 317, 329
    interlobar artery and vein in, 314
  in posterior cervical triangle, 34
  in renal sinus, 311
  retrobulbar, 83
  in retropubic space, 245, 341
  transverse section of, 399
Fat body
  of ischioanal fossa, 357, 360, 372, 398
  orbital, 83
  suprapatellar, 499

Fat pad
of elbow, 426
infrapatellar, 495, 496, 499
mediastinal, 225
on tuberosity of calcaneus, 520
Fat ring, subhiatal, 230
Fauces, 64
Femoral artery, 249, 257, 398, 473, 488, 489, 493, 500
anastomosis between, 492
ascending branch of, 500
deep, 488, 489, 500
openings for, 481
descending branch of, 500
in femoral sheath, 245
lateral circumflex, 488, 500
ascending transverse branch of, 489, 492
descending transverse branch of, 489, 492
magnetic resonance imaging of, 531
medial circumflex, 489, 490, 500
muscular branches of, 500
passing through adductor hiatus, 500
perforating branches of, 489, 500
transverse section of, 399
Femoral canal, 473
Femoral nerve, 157, 247, 253, 260, 387, 389, 398, 473, 484, 485, 486, 488, 489, 527
anterior cutaneous branches of, 389, 471, 526
articular branch of, 526
braches of, 493
cutaneous
cutaneous branch of, 472
lateral, 255, 260, 308, 389, 471, 473, 484, 485, 486, 488, 489, 526, 527
lateral, branches of, 472
posterior, 157, 391, 485, 487, 490, 491, 493
posterior, branches of, 472
posterior, perineal branches of, 491
posterior, perineal branch of, 393
deep to iliopsoas fascia, 255
muscles innervated by, 526
terminal branches of, 471, 472
transverse section of, 399
Femoral ring, 253, 255, 343, 345, 347, 473
Femoral sheath, 245, 247, 255, 473, 488
anterior wall of, 255
Femoral triangle, 471
Femoral vein, 250, 258, 471, 473, 488, 489, 493
in femoral sheath, 244, 245
magnetic resonance imaging of, 531
MRI of, 531
transverse section of, 399
Femoral vessels, 254, 381, 387
in femoral sheath, 255
opening for, 256
Femur, 495, 499
adductor tubercle of, 477
anterior view of, 477
calcar of, 477
of child, 492
condyles of
lateral, 477, 495, 496, 498
medial, 477, 495, 496, 498
cortex of, 531
radiograph of, 476
epicondyles of
lateral, 477, 495
medial, 477, 490, 495, 497
medial, adductor tubercle on, 489, 497
fovea for ligament of head of, 477
gluteal tuberosity of, 477
head of, 398, 475, 477
arteries of, 492
arthrogram of, 531
cartilage of, 531
ligament of, 475, 531
MRI of, 531
radiograph of, 333, 476
intercondylar fossa of, 477
intertrochanteric crest of, 477

Femur *(Continued)*
lateral supracondylar line of, 477
linea aspera of, 477, 479
medulla of, 531
radiograph of, 476
neck of, 475, 477
arteries of, 492
radiograph of, 476
nutrient artery of, 492
nutrient foramen of, 477
patellar surface of, 477
pectineal line of, 477
popliteal surface of, 477, 499
posterior view of, 477
quadrate tubercle of, 477
radiograph of, 333, 476, 498
retinacular foramina of, 477
shaft (body) of, 477
trochanteric fossa of, 477
trochanter of
greater, 149, 241, 477
lesser, 241, 477
transverse sectcin of, 399
Fetus
blood circulation in, 223
external genitalia development in, 368
Fibrocartilaginous labrum, 475
Fibrofatty tissue, 372
Fibrous capsule, of spleen, 282
Fibrous (Albini's) nodule, 217
Fibrous ring, of tricuspid valve, 219
Fibrous septum, 372, 374
transverse, 373
Fibrous sheath
annular and cruciform parts of, 448
digital, 446
of fingers, 459
of sole of foot, 522
Fibrous trabecula, 145
Fibrous trigone
left, 216
right, 216
Fibula, 501, 507, 509, 510, 515, 518, 519
anterior border of, 501
anterior intercondylar area of, 501
anterior view of, 501, 502, 524
with ligament attachments, 502
apex of, 501
head of, 480, 481, 482, 495, 499, 501, 502, 505, 506, 509, 528, 529
anterior ligament of, 502
fibular ligament of, 499
posterior ligament of, 499
radiograph of, 498
inferior view of, 502
interosseous border of, 501, 502
lateral surface of, 501, 502
lateral view of, 514
ligaments of, 502
medial surface of, 501
neck of, 501
posterior view of, 501
radiograph of, 498, 514
superior view of, 502
Fibular artery, 500, 504, 505, 506
calcaneal branches of, 504, 505
communicating branch of, 506
lateral calcaneal branch of, 506
perforating branch of, 506, 518
posterior malleolar branch of, 506
Fibular collateral bursa, 495
Fibular collateral ligament, 482, 495, 496, 499, 505, 506, 509
inferior subtendinous bursa of, 499
Fibularis brevis muscle, 507, 509, 510, 517, 518, 528, 530
common tendinous sheath of, 517
origin of, 503
Fibularis brevis tendon, 469, 504, 506, 509, 515, 518, 524

Fibularis longus muscle, 469, 482, 495, 505, 509, 510, 517, 528, 530
common tendinous sheath of, 517
insertion of, 503
origin of, 503
Fibularis longus tendon, 469, 504, 505, 506, 509, 515, 518, 519, 524
groove for, 511, 512
Fibularis tertius tendon, 507, 509, 518, 519, 524
Fibular nerve, 506
common, 409, 471, 483, 485, 487, 490, 495, 504, 505, 506, 528, 529, 530
articular branch of, 529
muscles innervated by, 530
deep, 518, 528, 530
dorsal digital branches of, 471, 518
lateral branch of, 528, 530
medial branch of, 518, 528, 530
superficial, 471, 509, 510, 518, 519, 528, 530
dorsal digital branches of, 518
intermediate dorsal cutaneous branch of, 471
medial dorsal cutaneous branch of, 471
Fibular notch, 501
Fibular retinaculum
inferior, 506, 509, 515, 517
superior, 504, 506, 509, 515, 517
Filiform papillae, 58
Filum terminale externum, 157, 158
Filum terminale internum, 157, 158, 163
Fimbria, hippocampal, 118
Fimbriated fold, 51
Fine nerves, of fingers, 459
Finger(s), 400, 459
anterior closed space of, 459
arteries of, 459
bursae of, 451
common names of, 400
dorsum of, lymph vessels passing to, 405
in extension, 452
extensor muscles of, 429
extensor tendons of, 452, 459
fibrous and synovial sheaths of, 450
fibrous tendon sheath of, 459
fifth (little)
flexor tendons to, 450
palmar digital nerves to, 448
synovial tendinous sheath of, 448
fine nerves of, 459
in flexion, 452
flexor muscles of, 431
flexor tendons of, 452
fourth, 400
palmar digital nerves to, 448
index, 400
minute arteries of, 459
nerves of, 457, 459
fine, 459
ring, 400
distal phalanx of, radiograph of, 445
sagittal section of, 441, 459
septa of, 459
subungual space of, 459
synovial sheath of, 450
synovial sheaths of, 448
tendinous sheaths of, 451
third (middle)
middle phalanx of, radiograph of, 445
sagittal section through, 441
thumb, 400
carpometacarpal joint of, 442
digital arteries to, 454
digital nerves to, 454
metacarpal joint base of, radiograph of, 445
palmar digital nerves of, 448
Flank
left, 242
right, 242
Flexion, of lower limb, 470

Flexor carpi radialis muscle, 419, 421, 430, 434, 437, 461, 463
  innervation of, 464
  insertion of, 438
  origin of, 438
Flexor carpi radialis tendon, 400, 435, 436, 442, 448, 449, 461
Flexor carpi ulnaris muscle, 400, 420, 430, 432, 433, 434, 435, 461, 464
  humeral origin of, 438
  innervation of, 464
  origin of, 438
    humeral origin, 439
    ulnar origin, 439
Flexor carpi ulnaris tendon, 400, 442, 448, 449, 453
Flexor digiti minimi brevis muscle, 449, 453, 464, 521, 522, 523, 524, 529
Flexor digitorum brevis muscle, 521, 522, 523, 529
Flexor digitorum brevis nerve, 529
Flexor digitorum brevis tendon, 521, 523
Flexor digitorum longus muscle, 503, 506, 529
  insertion of, 503
  origin of, 503
Flexor digitorum longus tendon, 504, 505, 506, 521, 522, 523
  groove for insertion of, 501
Flexor digitorum longus tendon sheath, 517
Flexor digitorum profundus muscle, 436, 461, 463
  innervation of, 464
  insertion of, 438
  origin of, 438
Flexor digitorum profundus tendon, 442, 446, 449, 450, 451, 452
  insertion of, 448
Flexor digitorum superficialis muscle, 431, 434, 435, 437, 463
  humeroulnar head of, 435, 461
    origin of, 438
  insertion of, 438
    origin of, 439
  radial head of, 435, 436, 461
    insertion of, 438
Flexor digitorum superficialis tendon, 400, 431, 434, 442, 446, 449, 450, 451, 461
  insertion of, 448
Flexor hallucis brevis muscle, 529
  lateral head of, 521, 522, 523, 524
  medial head of, 521, 522, 523
  medial origin of, 524
Flexor hallucis brevis nerve, 529
Flexor hallucis brevis tendon
  lateral origin of, 524
Flexor hallucis longus muscle, 506, 522, 529
  insertion of, 503
  origin of, 503
Flexor hallucis longus tendon, 504, 505, 506, 521, 522, 523
  groove for, 511
Flexor hallucis longus tendon sheath, 517
Flexor muscles
  of digits, 431
  superficial, 434
  of wrist, 430
Flexor pollicis brevis muscle, 437, 453
  innervation of, 464
  superficial head of, 463
Flexor pollicis longus muscle, 431, 435, 436, 449, 454, 461, 463
  insertion of, 438
  origin of, 438
  tendinous sheath of, 448, 449, 450, 451
Flexor pollicis longus tendon, 436, 442, 449
  in tendon sheath, 449
Flexor retinaculum, 435, 442, 449, 450, 453, 461, 504, 505, 506, 522, 523, 529
Flexor sheath, common, 448, 449, 450, 451
Flexor tendons
  common, 430, 431, 434
    origin of, 438
  fibrous sheaths of, 454, 521

Flexor tendons *(Continued)*
  in fingers, 452
  profundus, 448
  profundus and superficialis, 450
  superficialis, 448
  synovial sheaths of, 454
  at wrist, 449
Flocculus, 112
Foliate papillae, 58, 134
Folium, 112, 142
Follicles, graafian, 355
Fontana, iridocorneal angle of, 88
Fontanelle
  anterior, 14
  mastoid, 14
  posterior, 14
  sphenoidal, 14
Foot
  arteries of, 524
  bones of, 511, 512
    lateral view of, 512
    medial view of, 512
  dorsal view of, 511, 524, 525
  dorsum of
    deep dissection of, 519
    muscles of: superficial dissection of, 518
  eversion of, 470
  innervation of, 530
  interosseous muscles of, 524, 525
  inversion of, 470
  ligaments of, plantar view of, 516
  plantar surface of, 469
  plantar view of, 511, 524, 525
  right
    lateral view of, 513, 515
    medial view of, 513, 515
    superior view of, 513
  sole of
    cutaneous innervation of, 529
    muscles of, 521, 522, 523
    superficial dissection of, 520
  tendons of, plantar view of, 516
Foramen
  apical, of the teeth, 57
  of the cranial base, 12
  interventricular (of Monro), 143
  nasolacrimal, 50
Foramen cecum, 11, 13, 58, 63
Foramen lacerum, 10, 12, 13, 98
Foramen magnum, 8, 10, 12, 13, 16, 98, 126
Foramen of Luschka, 107, 108
Foramen of Magendie, 108, 114, 116
Foramen ovale, 6, 12, 13, 16, 44, 45, 55, 98
  obliterated, 223
  prenatal, 223
  valve of, 215
Foramen rotundum, 13, 44
  maxillary nerve entering, 43
Foramen spinosum, 13, 16, 45, 98
Foramen transversarium, 20, 21
  bony spicule dividing, 20
  septated, 20
Forearm
  anterior view of, 404
  bones of, 427
  cross section of, 437
  cutaneous nerves of, 404
  most distal portion of, cross section of, 458
  muscles of, 428, 429, 430, 431
    attachments of: anterior view of, 438
    attachments of: posterior view of, 439
    deep layer: anterior view of, 436
    deep layer: posterior view of, 433
    intermediate layer: anterior view of, 435
    superficial layer: anterior view of, 434
    superficial layer of, 432
  posterior view of, 404, 466
  pronated position of, 428
  radial nerve in, 466

Forearm *(Continued)*
  right
    anterior view of, 428, 430, 431
    posterior view of, 429
  serial cross sections of, 437
  superficial veins of, 404
  supinated position of, 428
Fornix, 105
  body of, 105, 107, 111, 114
  columns of, 105, 107, 109, 111, 143
  commissure of, 111
  crura of, 109, 111, 141
  crus of, 105
  imaging of, 148
  schema of, 111
  vaginal, 355
    posterior, 342
Fossa ovalis, 214, 223, 471
  limbus of, 214
Fovea
  inferior, 114
  superior, 114
Fovea capitis, 531
  arthrogram of, 531
Fovea centralis, 87, 90
Free taenia, 263, 273, 274, 371, 374
Frenulum, 274, 362
  of clitoris, 356
  of labia minora, 356
  of tongue, 51, 61
  of upper lip, 51
Frontal artery, 3
  polar, 140
Frontal bone, 1, 4, 8, 9, 10, 35, 82
  foramen cecum of, 11
  frontal crest of, 11
  glabella of, 4, 6
  groove for anterior meningeal vessels of, 11
  groove for superior sagittal sinus of, 11
  lateral view of, 14
  nasal spine of, 37, 38
  of newborn, 14
  orbital surface of, 4
  sinus of, 37, 38
  squamous part of, 14, 37, 38
  superior surface of superior part of, 11
  superior view of, 14
  supraorbital notch of, 4, 6, 14
Frontal crest, 9, 11
Frontal gyrus
  inferior
    opercular part of, 104
    orbital part of, 104
    triangular part of, 104
  medial, 105
  middle, 104
  superior, 104
Frontalis muscle, 35
Frontal lobe, 104
Frontal nerve, 44, 83, 86, 120, 121, 130
Frontal operculum, 104
Frontal pole, 104
Frontal sinus, 5, 7, 8, 36, 37, 38, 48, 49, 63
  growth throughout life, 50
Frontal suture, 14
Frontobasal artery
  lateral, 137, 139, 140
  medial, 137, 139, 140
Frontonasal canal, 37
Frontonasal duct, opening of, 49
Fundiform ligament, 243, 253
Fundus, vagal branch to, 234
Fungiform papillae, 58, 134
Funiculus, lateral, 114

G

Galea aponeurosis, 3, 101
Galen
  ansa of, 80

Galen (Continued)
  great cerebral vein of, 102, 105, 108, 142, 147
Gallbladder, 125, 161, 190, 261, 264, 267, 278, 280, 284, 327
  body of, 280
  ducts of, 280
  fundus of, 277, 280
  innervation of, 160
  neck of, 280
  transverse section of, 326
Ganglion cells, retinal, 119
Gartner's duct, 369
Gasserian ganglion, 103, 115
Gastric artery
  left, 231, 257, 283, 284, 297, 298, 299, 300, 327, 390
    arteriogram of, 285
    attachment of, 266
    esophageal branch of, 231, 234, 283
    in gastropancreatic fold, 264
  right, 271, 280, 283, 284, 298, 300
    arteriogram of, 285
  short, 283, 284, 300
Gastric canal, longitudinal folds of, 268
Gastric folds (rugae), 230, 268
  transverse section of, 325
Gastric impression, 277
Gastric lymph drainage zones and pathways, 293
Gastric lymph nodes, 233, 293, 294
Gastric plexus, 390
  left, 297, 298, 299
  right, 298
Gastric vein
  blood from, 292
  left, 232, 289, 290, 291, 292, 327
    esophageal branches of, 232
  right, 232, 289, 290, 292
  short, 232, 289, 292
Gastric vessels, short, 266, 282, 327
Gastrocnemius muscle, 469, 490, 494, 495, 504, 505, 507, 510, 529
  lateral head of, 469, 482, 483, 499, 504, 506, 509, 510
    origin of, 479, 503
  lateral subtendinous bursa of, 499
  medial head of, 469, 483, 490, 499, 504, 505, 506
    origin of, 479, 503
  sural (muscular) branches of, 506
Gastrocolic ligament
  anterior and posterior layers of, 264
  gastro-omental arterial anastomosis enclosed in, 264
Gastroduodenal artery, 271, 280, 283, 284, 286, 287, 300, 301, 306
  arteriogram of, 285
  plexus on, 301
Gastroduodenal plexus, 301, 306
Gastroepiploic arterial anastomosis, 264
Gastroepiploic artery
  left, 283, 284, 300
  plexus on, 298, 299
  right, 283, 286, 287, 300
    attachment to transverse mesocolon, 266
    covered by peritoneum, 264
Gastroepiploic lymph nodes
  left, 293
  right, 293
Gastroepiploic vein
  left, 232, 289
  right, 232, 289, 291, 292
Gastrolienal ligament, 264, 265, 282
Gastro-omental arterial anastomosis, 264
Gastro-omental artery
  left, 283, 284, 300
  plexus on, 298, 299
  right, 266, 283, 284, 286, 287, 300
    attachment to transverse mesocolon, 266
    covered by peritoneum, 264
Gastro-omental lymph nodes
  left, 293
  right, 293

Gastro-omental vein
  left, 232, 289, 292
  right, 232, 289, 291, 292
Gastro-omental vessels, 282
Gastropancreatic fold, left gastric artery in, 264
Gastrophrenic ligament, 264, 266
Gastrosplenic ligament, 264, 265, 282, 308, 327
  short gastric vessels in, 282
Gemellus muscle
  inferior, 483, 490, 491, 498
    insertion of, 478
    nerve to, 485, 487, 491
    origin of, 478, 479
    transverse section of, 399
  superior, 483, 490, 491
    insertion of, 478
    nerve to, 485, 487, 491
    origin of, 478, 479
Gemellus tendon, superior, MRI of, 531
Genicular artery
  descending, 489
    articular branch of, 488, 489, 500
    saphenous branch of, 488, 489, 500
  inferior lateral, 500, 505, 506, 509
  inferior medial, 488, 489, 500, 505, 506, 507
  medial, 505
  superior lateral, 490, 500, 504, 505, 506, 507, 509
  superior medial, 488, 489, 490, 500, 504, 506
Geniculate body
  lateral, 106, 109, 110, 113, 114, 115, 131, 137, 142, 143
    of left thalamus
      lateral, 141
      medial, 141
  medial, 106, 109, 110, 113, 114, 137, 142, 143
Geniculate ganglion, 43, 45, 94, 115, 122, 134
Geniculate nucleus
  left dorsal, projection on, 119
  right dorsal, projection on, 119
Geniculum, 43, 45, 94, 97, 124
Genioglossus muscle, 48, 59, 60, 63, 127
  superior mental spine for origin of, 53
Geniohyoid muscle, 34, 48, 53, 59, 63, 65, 127, 128
Genital cord, 369
Genitalia
  external, 161
    development of, 368
    female, 356, 368, 393
    homologues of, 368
    innervation of, 160, 389
    male, 360, 361, 368, 389
    nerves of, 393
    undifferentiated, 368
  internal, homologues of, 369
  lymph vessels and nodes of
    female, 386
    male, 388
  undifferentiated
    female, 369
    male, 369
Genital tubercle, 53
  anal pit of, 368
  anal tubercle of, 368
  epithelial tag of, 368
  glans area of, 368
  lateral part of, 368
  urogenital fold of, 368
Genitofemoral nerve, 255, 260, 308, 389, 484, 485, 486, 527
  femoral branch of, 251, 255, 260, 389, 471, 485, 486
  genital branch of, 251, 253, 254, 260, 367, 389, 471, 485, 486
  right, 330
Gerdy's tubercle, 482, 501, 502
  insertion of iliotibial tract to, 495
Gerota's fascia, 317
Gimbernat's (lacunar) ligament, 244, 245, 247, 473
Gingiva, lamina propria of, 57
Gingival epithelium, 57
Gingival groove, 57
Glabella, 1, 4, 6

Glans, of clitoris, 356
Glans area, of genital tubercle, 368
Glans penis. See Penis, glans of
Glenohumeral joint, 410
  anterior view of, 410
  arthrogram of, 468
  capsule of, 420
  corona section through, 410
Glenohumeral joint (Continued)
  greater tuberosity of, 468
  lateral view of, 410
Glenohumeral ligament
  inferior, 410
  middle, 410
  superior, 410
Glenoid cavity, 179, 410
  computed tomography of, 468
  magnetic resonance imaging of, 468
  radiograph of, 409
Glenoid labrum, 410
  inferior, magnetic resonance imaging of, 468
  superior, magnetic resonance imaging of, 468
Glisson's capsule, 278
Globus pallidus, 107, 109
Glomerular arteriole
  afferent, 314
  efferent, 314
Glomerular capsule, 313
Glomerulus, 118, 313
  cortical, 314
  corticomedullary, 314
  juxtamedullary, 314
Glossoepiglottic fold
  lateral, 58
  median, 58
Glossopharyngeal nerve, 13, 33, 46, 47, 62, 69, 71, 103, 113, 115, 116, 122, 124, 125, 129, 130, 132, 133, 134
  branch of, 161
  carotid sinus branch (of Hering) of, 33, 124, 129, 130
    nerve to, 125
  communication to auricular branch of vagus nerve, 124
  communication to facial nerve, 124
  distribution of, 117
  efferent and afferent fibers of, 124
  inferior ganglion of, 46, 124, 134
  in jugular fossa, 12
  lingual branches of, 62
  pharyngeal, tonsillar, and lingual branches of, 71, 124
  schema of, 124, 204
  superior ganglion of, 124
  tonsillar branch of, 62, 64, 71
  tympanic branch of, 124
    in tympanic canaliculus, 12
Gluteal aponeurosis, 248, 490
  over gluteus medius muscle, 309, 482, 483
Gluteal artery
  inferior, 316, 378, 382, 487, 490
  superior, 257, 316, 378, 382, 383, 490
Gluteal fold, 149, 469
Gluteal line
  anterior, 336, 474
  inferior, 336, 474
  posterior, 336, 474
Gluteal nerve
  inferior, 157, 485, 487, 490, 491
  superior, 157, 485, 487, 491
Gluteal surface, 336
Gluteal tuberosity, 477
Gluteal vein
  inferior, 258
  superior, 258, 291, 490
Gluteus maximus muscle, 149, 168, 248, 309, 341, 358, 361, 362, 375, 376, 390, 391, 393, 398, 469, 482, 484, 488, 489, 490, 491, 493
  insertion of, 478, 479
  MRI of, 531
  origin of, 479
  transverse section of, 399

Gluteus medius muscle, 149, 469, 480, 484, 488, 489, 490, 491, 531
  gluteal aponeurosis over, 248, 309, 482, 483
  MRI of, 531
  origin of, 479
  transverse section of, 399
Gluteus minimus muscle, 483, 491, 498
  origin of, 479
Gonads, 369
  male, 366
Graafian follicle, 355
Gracile fasciculus, 113, 114
Gracile tubercle, 114
Gracilis muscle, 480, 481, 483, 488, 489, 490, 493, 494, 504, 527
  insertion of, 503
  origin of, 478
Gracilis tendon, 469, 480, 481, 494, 495
Granular foveola, 9, 99, 101
Granule cells, 118
Gray matter
  imaging of, 148
  intermediolateral nucleus of, 132
    preganglionic sympathetic cell bodies in, 131
    presynaptic sympathetic cell bodies in, 43
  lateral horn of, 133, 163, 321
  spinal, 162
Great auricular nerve, 2
Greater occipital nerve, 2
Greater vestibular (Bartholin's) gland
  opening of, 356, 384
Great toe
  distal phalanx of, 525
  medial side of, vein of, 471
  proximal phalanx of, 525
Groin
  left, 242
  right, 242
Gubernaculum, 366, 369
Gut
  enteric plexus of, 304
  prenatal, 223

H

Habenula, 109
Habenular commissure, 105
Habenular trigone, 110, 114
Hair cells
  inner, 96
  outer, 96
Hamate, 449
  anterior (palmar) view of, 440, 441, 444
  coronal section: dorsal view of, 443
  hook of, 430, 436, 442, 446, 454
    anterior (palmar) view of, 440, 444, 446
    radiograph of, 445
  posterior (dorsal) view of, 440, 443
  radiograph of, 445
Hand. See also Finger(s)
  in anatomical position, 441
  anterior (palmar) view of, 447, 453, 460
  arteries of, palmar view of, 454
  bones of, 444
  bursae of, 450
  cutaneous innervation of, 460
  deep dorsal dissection of, 457
  deep palmar dissection of, 448
  dorsal fascia of, 450
  dorsal venous network of, 456
  dorsum of, 441
    lymph vessels passing to, 405
  in extension, 441
  in flexion, 441
  lateral (radial) view of, 455
  lymphatic drainage pathways of, 456
  muscles of, 453
  nerves of, 454
  posterior (dorsal) view of, 453, 456, 457, 460
  radiograph of, 445

Hand (Continued)
  right
    anterior (palmar) view of, 444
    posterior (dorsal) view of, 444
  spaces of, 450
  superficial dorsal dissection of, 456
  superficial palmar dissection of, 447
  superficial radial dissection of, 455
  tendon sheaths of, 450
  veins of, 454
Hartmann's pouch (infundulum), 280
Hasner's valve, 82
Haustra, 273, 276
Head. See also Brain; Skull; specific parts of head
  autonomic nerves in, 130
  bones and ligaments of, 15
  cutaneous nerves of, 1
  lymph vessels and nodes of, 72
  surface anatomy of, 1
Heart, 125, 161
  anterior exposure of, 206
  apex of, 206, 208, 239
    radiograph of, 207
  base of
    posterior view of, 208
    posteroinferior view of, 208
  conducting system of, 219
  diaphragmatic surface of, 208
  in diastole, 216
  drawn out of pericardial sac, 209
  fibrous skeleton of, 216, 217
  inferior border (acute margin) of, 206
  in situ, 205
  left border of, 190, 206
  left bundle of, 219
  left side of, 219
  nerves of, 220
    schema of, 160
  in pericardium, 227
  right border of, 190
  right side of, 219
  in systole, 216
  valves of, 216, 217
Heiss, loops of, 349
Helicotrema, 92, 95
Helix, 1, 93
  crux of, 93
Helvetius, collar of, 230
Hematoma
  epidural, 99, 101
  subdural, 101
Hemiazygos vein, 186, 188, 210, 232
  accessory, 186, 201, 225, 232, 238
    junction with azygos vein, 232
Hemispheric vein, cerebellar inferior, 142
Henle's loop, 313
Hepatic artery
  branch of, 279
  common, 257, 264, 271, 280, 281, 286, 287, 297, 300, 306, 327
    arteriogram of, 285
    in peritoneal fold, 264
  fine branch of, 306
  intermediate, 284
  left, 280, 283, 284
  portal vein branch of, 278
  proper, 265, 266, 270, 271, 277, 278, 280, 281, 283, 284, 286, 300, 326
    arteriogram of, 285
    bifurcation, 327
    in right margin of lesser omentum, 323
  right, 280, 283, 284
Hepatic duct
  common, 277, 278, 280, 284, 327
  left, 280
  right, 280
Hepatic flexure, right. See Colic (hepatic) flexure, right
Hepatic lymph nodes, 294

Hepatic plexus, 125, 298, 299, 301
  anterior, 306
  branches to cardia, 299
  common, 297
  posterior, 306
  pyloric branch of, 125
  vagal branch of, 234, 298
Hepatic portal vein, 232, 265, 271, 277, 278, 279, 280, 281, 283, 284, 289, 290, 291, 292, 294, 323, 327
  prenatal, 223
  in right margin of lesser omentum, 323
  tributaries of, 292
Hepatic vein, 226, 232, 258, 266, 277, 278
  prenatal, 223
Hepatoduodenal ligament, 264, 265, 267, 270, 278
  transverse section of, 326
Hepatogastric ligament, 265, 267
Hepatopancreatic ampulla (of Vater), 280
  sphincter of, 280, 306
Hepatorenal recess, 327
Hering, carotid branch of, 33, 124, 129, 130
Hering-Breuer reflex, 204
Hesselbach's inguinal triangle, 247
Heubner, recurrent artery of, 137, 138, 139, 140
Hilar (bronchopulmonary) lymph nodes, 224
Hilum, of kidney, 311
Hip
  arthrogram of, 531
  bony attachments of, 479
    anterior view of, 478
    posterior view of, 479
  extension and flexion of, 470
  lateral view of, 474
  medial view of, 474
  MRI of, 531
  muscles of
    lateral view of, 482
    posterior view of, 483
  nerves of, 491
  radiograph of, 531
Hip bone
  auricular surface of, 474
  lateral view of, 474
  medial view of, 474
Hip joint, 475
  anterior view of, 475
  anteroposterior radiograph of, 476
  lateral view of, 475
  ligaments of, 480
  nerve to, 491
Hippocampal fimbria, 118
Hippocampal sulcus, 111
Hippocampus, 107, 109, 110
  alveus of, 111
  fimbria of, 105, 107, 109, 110, 111
  superior dissection of, 111
His, bundle of, 219
Horizontal cells, retinal, 119
Houston, valves of, 373
Humeral artery
  ascending branch of, 415
  circumflex
    anterior, 414, 417, 419, 420, 421, 422
    posterior, 415, 417, 420, 421, 422
  descending branch of, 415
  posterior circumflex, 414
Humeral ligament
  lesser, 410
  transverse, 410
Humeral vein, circumflex, 403
Humerus, 423, 424, 426
  anatomical neck of, 407
    radiograph of, 409
  anterior view of, 407
  capitulum of, 407
  condyles of
    lateral, 407
    medial, 407
  coronal fossa of, 407

Humerus (Continued)
deltoid tuberosity of, 407
epicondyles of
lateral, 419, 420, 433
medial, 407, 419, 420, 421, 433, 434
greater tubercle of, 407, 410, 414, 419
radiograph of, 409
head of, 407
articular cartilage of, arthrogram of, 468
articular cartilage of, MRI of, 468
computed tomography of, 468
intertubercular sulcus of, 407
lateral supracondylar ridge of, 407
left, shaft of, 236
lesser tubercle of, 407, 410, 419
radiograph of, 409
medial supracondylar ridge of, 407
muscle origins and attachments on, 408
olecranon fossa of, 424
radiograph of, 425
olecranon of, 400, 429, 432, 465
radiograph of, 425
posterior view of, 408
radial fossa of, 407, 424
radiograph of, 409
right, surgical neck of, 236
shaft of, 237, 238
surgical neck of, 407
radiograph of, 409
trochlea of, 407
radiograph of, 425
Hyaloid canal, 87
Hydatid of Morgagni, 355
Hymenal caruncle, 352, 356
Hyoepiglottic ligament, 77
Hyoepiglottic muscle, 63
Hyoglossus muscle, 26, 28, 33, 53, 59, 64, 127
Hyoid bone, 15, 26, 27, 28, 30, 33, 59, 60, 61, 63, 65, 67, 74, 76, 77, 80
body of, 15, 53
greater horn of, 15, 53, 68, 75
prominence caused by, 66
lesser horn of, 15, 53
Hypochondrium (hypochondriac) region
left, 242
right, 242
Hypogastric nerve, 303, 320, 389, 390, 394, 395, 396, 397
left, 297, 302, 392
right, 297, 302, 392
Hypogastric plexus, 160, 319, 389, 390, 392, 396
inferior, 160, 161, 303, 319, 389, 390, 392, 394, 395, 396
nerves to, 297, 487
nerve to sigmoid and descending colon, 302, 390
right, 302
superior, 297, 302, 303, 319, 320, 343, 389, 390, 392, 394, 395, 396, 397
Hypogastric (neurovascular) sheath, 345
Hypoglossal canal, 10, 12, 13
hypoglossal nerve in, 12
Hypoglossal fossa, 11, 50
Hypoglossal nerve, 13, 32, 33, 45, 46, 47, 59, 69, 71, 73, 103, 113, 128
distribution of, 117
in hypoglossal canal, 12, 127
meningeal branch of, 127
schema of, 127
vena comitans of, 70
Hypoglossal nucleus, 115, 116, 127
Hypoglossal sinus, 8
Hypoglossal trigone, 114
Hypoglossus muscle, 60, 65, 68
dorsal lingual vein coursing medial to, 70
Hypophyseal artery
inferior, 138, 146
superior, 138, 146
Hypophyseal fossa, 7

Hypophyseal portal system
primary plexus of, 146
secondary plexus of, 146
Hypophyseal portal vein
long, 138, 146
short, 146
Hypophyseal vein, efferent, 138, 146
Hypophysis, 103, 106, 145. *See also* Pituitary gland
arteries and veins of, 146
in sella turcica, 36
Hypothalamic area, lateral, 134
Hypothalamic artery, 138
Hypothalamic sulcus, 105, 114, 145
Hypothalamic vessels, 146
Hypothalamohypophyseal tract, 145
Hypothalamus, 107
arteries and veins of, 146
nuclei of, 145
arcuate (infundibular), 145
dorsomedial, 145
mammillary body, 145
paraventricular, 145
posterior, 145
supraoptic, 145
ventromedial, 145
parasympathtetic part of, 303
sympathetic part of, 303
Hypothenar eminence, 400
Hypothenar muscles, 447, 448, 450, 464
nerve to, 454
Hysterosalpingogram, of uterus, 354

I

Ileal artery, 287, 288
Ileal orifice, 276
muscle fibers of, 274
papillary, 274
Ileal vein, 290, 291
Ileal vessels, 290
Ileocecal fold, 273
Ileocecal junction, fibers around, 274
Ileocecal lips, 274
Ileocecal recess
inferior, 273
superior, 273
Ileocecal region, 273, 274
Ileocolic artery, 273, 287, 301, 302, 315
colic branch of, 273, 288
ileal branch of, 273, 288
Ileocolic lymph nodes, 296
Ileocolic plexus, 301, 302
Ileocolic vein, 290, 291, 292
Ileum, 261, 276, 324, 329
circular muscle of, 274
fibers to, 274
longitudinal muscle of, 274
mucosa of, 272
musculature of, 272
terminal part of, 263, 273, 274, 343, 347
Iliac artery
circumflex
ascending branch of, 249, 257
deep, 249, 257, 489, 500
superficial, 245, 257, 500
common, 257, 266, 315, 316, 378, 380, 381, 392
left, 297, 382
right, 308, 324, 382
ureteric branch from, 316
external, 257, 266, 297, 315, 378, 380, 381, 382, 392, 489, 500
right, 308
internal, 257, 288, 297, 315, 316, 352, 378, 380, 381, 382
anterior division of, 380, 382
posterior division of, 382
right, 308
Iliac crest, 149, 155, 168, 169, 170, 171, 240, 241, 248, 308, 309, 317, 332, 335, 469, 482, 483, 484, 490, 491

Iliac crest (Continued)
anterior superior, 531
radiograph of, 531
iliac tubercle of, 335
inner lip of, 241, 332, 335, 336, 474
intermediate zone of, 241, 332, 335, 336, 474
outer lip of, 241, 332, 335, 336, 474
radiograph of, 531
tuberculum of, 241, 332, 474
Iliac fossa, 335, 336, 343, 474
Iliac lymph nodes
common, 259, 296, 318, 386, 388
external, 259, 296, 318, 388, 473
lymphatic pathways to, 388
medial (inferior), 386
internal, 259, 296, 318, 388
lymphatic pathways to, 388
lateral (superior) external, 386
Iliac plexus, 392
external, 297
internal, 297
Iliac spine
anterior inferior, 241, 256, 332, 336, 340, 474, 475, 480, 481
anterior superior, 240, 241, 243, 244, 253, 254, 256, 331, 332, 335, 336, 357, 360, 469, 474, 475, 480, 481, 482, 484, 488
posterior inferior, 155, 474
posterior superior, 149, 155, 335, 336, 474
Iliac tubercle, 335, 336
Iliac tuberosity, 241, 332, 474
Iliacus muscle, 256, 308, 345, 372, 398, 480, 484, 486, 487, 526, 531
fascia of, 372
insertion of, 484
MRI of, 531
muscular branch of, 486
origin of, 478
Iliac vein
circumflex
deep, 250, 258
superficial, 240, 250, 258, 331, 471
tributaries to, 250
common, 258, 379
external, 258, 379, 489
internal, 258, 291, 352
Iliac vessels
circumflex
deep, 247, 255, 345, 383
superficial, 383, 488
common, 263, 381, 383, 392
external, 247, 253, 255, 273, 291, 342, 343, 344, 345, 346, 347, 354, 372, 381, 383
covered by peritoneum, 254
internal, 381, 383, 435
Iliococcygeus muscle, 337, 338, 339, 340
Iliocostalis cervicis muscle, 169
Iliocostalis lumborum muscle, 169
Iliocostalis muscle, 169, 327
Iliocostalis thoracis muscle, 169
Iliofemoral ligament, 475, 492
of hip joint, 484
Ilioinguinal nerve, 254
anterior scroal branch of, 251
Iliohypogastric nerve, 157, 171, 260, 308, 330, 389, 394, 484, 485, 486, 527
anterior branch of, 485
anterior cutaneous branch of, 251, 260, 389
lateral branch of, 485
lateral cutaneous branch of, 248, 472
Ilioinguinal nerve, 157, 260, 308, 309, 330, 389, 394, 484, 486, 487
anterior labial branches of, 260
scrotal branch of, 471
Iliolumbar artery, 257, 316, 382, 383
Iliolumbar ligament, 155, 309, 335
Iliolumbar vein, 258
Iliopectineal bursa, 475, 484

Iliopectineal line, 335, 372
 iliac part of, 340
 pubic part of, 340
Iliopsoas muscle, 247, 253, 398, 480, 481, 488
 direction of action of, 484
 insertion of, 479
 origin of, 478
 transverse section of, 399
Iliopubic eminence, 241, 332, 334, 335, 336, 340, 474, 475
Iliopubic tract, 253, 345, 347
 covered by peritoneum, 343
Iliotibial tract, 480, 490, 494, 495, 504, 507, 509
 blended into lateral patellar retinaculum and capsule, 496
 bursa deep to, 494
 bursa in, 495
 insertion of, 478, 495, 501, 503
iliotibial tract, 469, 482, 483
Ilium, 330, 474
 arcuate line of, 338
 body of, 336, 474
 radiograph of, 333, 476
 of right lung, 206
 wing (ala) of, 241, 332, 336, 340, 474
  gluteal surface of, 474
Incisive canal, 8, 36, 38, 41, 42, 63
 anastomosis in, 39
 greater palatine artery in, 40
Incisive fossa, 12, 16, 52, 56
Incisive papilla, 52
Incisor teeth, 227
Incus, 92, 96, 123
 lenticular long limb of, 94
 lenticular process of, 93
 long limb of, 93, 94
 medial view of, 93
 short limb of, 93, 94
 superior ligament of, 94
Index finger, 400
Inferior anastomotic vein of Labbé, 101
Inferior ganglion, 133
Inferior longitudinal muscle, of the tongue, 59
Inferior lymph nodes, vertical group of, 387
Inferior nasal concha, 8
Infraglottic region, 80
Infrahyoid artery, 74
Infrahyoid fascia, 27, 34
Infrahyoid muscles, 28
 fascia of, 27, 34
Infraorbital artery, 3, 35, 39, 69, 81, 85
Infraorbital canal, 44
Infraorbital foramen, 4, 35
 of newborn, 14
Infraorbital groove, 4
Infraorbital margin, 1
Infraorbital nerve (V₂), 2, 35, 43, 44, 46, 71, 81, 83, 120, 121
 entering infraorbital canal, 44
 nasal branches of, 41, 121
 superior alveolar branches of, 121
Infraorbital vein, 3, 70
Infrapatellar synovial fold, 495, 496
Infraspinatus muscle, 149, 174, 185, 236, 237, 238, 411, 413, 414, 415, 416, 420, 465
 computed tomography of, 468
Infraspinatus tendon, 420
Infratemporal crest, 6
Infratemporal fossa, 6
Infratrochlear artery, 35
Infratrochlear nerve, 35, 81, 86, 121
 from nasociliary nerve, 44
Infundibular process, 145
 capillary plexus of, 146
Infundibular recess, 107
Infundibular stem, 145
Infundibulum (Hartmann's pouch), 280
Infundibulum (pituitary stalk), 113, 138, 145
Inguinal canal, 254, 255
Inguinal falx, 244, 245, 247, 253, 254

Inguinal fold, 369
Inguinal ligament (Poupart's), 240, 243, 244, 245, 253, 255, 256, 331, 338, 357, 360, 387, 469, 471, 473, 480, 486, 488, 489
 reflected, 244, 245, 253
Inguinal lymph nodes
 deep, 259, 386, 387, 388, 473
  highest (of Cloquet), 259, 386, 387, 388
 superficial, 259, 296, 386, 388
  inferior nodes (vertical group), 259, 387, 473
  superolateral nodes (horizontal group), 259, 387, 473
  superomedial nodes (horizontal group), 259, 387, 473
Inguinal region, 253
Inguinal ring
 deep, 245, 247, 253, 343, 344, 345, 347, 366
 lateral, 253
 medial, 253
 superficial, 243, 253, 254, 357, 366, 367
Inguinal triangle (Hesselbach's), 247, 253
 fascia within, 253
Inion, 6, 8, 16
Inlet venule, 279
Insula (island of Reil), 104, 111, 139
 central sulcus of, 104
 circular sulcus of, 104
 limen of, 104
 long gyrus of, 104
 short gyri of, 104
Interalveolar septa, 17
Interarytenoid notch, 66
Interatrial septum, 214, 239
Intercalated lymph nodes, 72, 73
Intercapitular veins, 404, 456
Intercarpal ligament, interosseous, 443
Intercartilaginous ligament, 196
Intercavernous septum, 362
Intercavernous sinus
 anterior, 102, 103
 posterior, 102, 103
Interchondral joint, 180
Interchondral space, third, 239
Interclavicular ligament, 180, 406
Intercondylar area, anterior, 501, 502
Intercondylar eminence, 496, 501, 502
 radiograph of, 498
Intercondylar fossa, 477
Intercondylar tubercle
 lateral, 501, 502
 medial, 501, 502
Intercostal artery, 185
 anterior, 184, 185, 249
 collateral branches of, 184
 lower, anastomosis with, 249
 posterior, 164, 182, 183, 185, 224, 225
  dorsal branch of, 165, 185
  lateral cutaneous branch of, 165, 177
  right, 185
  spinal branch of, 185
  third right, 201, 231
  supreme, 135, 136
Intercostal lymph nodes, 233
Intercostal membrane
 external, 174, 183, 185, 252, 414
  anterior to internal intercostal muscles, 182, 183
 internal, 25, 174, 185
  deep to external intercostal muscle, 224
Intercostal muscle, 176, 192, 236, 237, 327
 cross section of, 236, 237, 238
 external, 170, 174, 182, 183, 185, 244, 249, 252, 414
 innermost, 184, 185, 249, 252
 internal, 174, 185, 224, 225, 249, 252
Intercostal nerve, 157, 174, 176, 183, 184, 185, 327, 485
 abdominal portions of, 182
 anterior branch of, 185
 anterior cutaneous branches of, 174, 182, 184, 185, 251, 414
 dorsal ramus of, 174
 dorsal root of, 185

Intercostal nerve (Continued)
 eighth, 203
 first, 418
 lateral cutaneous branches of, 171, 174, 182, 183, 185
 lower, 187
 posterior, 224, 225
 posterior cutaneous branch of, 174
 sixh, 203
 third, 234
 ventral ramus of, 163, 174, 252
 ventral root of, 185
Intercostal tributaries, to axillary nerve, 250
Intercostal vein
 anterior, 184, 186, 350
 collateral branches of, 184
 left superior, 232
 posterior, 186, 224, 225
 right posterior, 232
 right superior, 186, 224, 232
 superior
  left, 225
Intercostal vessels, 176, 327
Intercostobrachial nerve, 183, 251, 403, 414, 417, 461
Intercrural fibers, 243, 254
Intercuneiform ligament, dorsal, 515
Interfoveolar ligament, 247
Intergluteal (natal) cleft, 149
Interlobar artery, 312, 314
 lymph vessels along, 318
Interlobar lymph vessels, 202
Interlobar vein, 314
Intermaxillary suture, 10, 35
Intermediate bursa, 451
Intermediate nerve, 62, 103, 113, 122, 123, 130, 132, 134
 distribution of, 117
Intermediolateral nucleus
 of gray matter, 132, 133
 sympathetic presynaptic cell bodies in, 132, 133
Intermesenteric plexus, 260, 297, 301, 302, 303, 319, 330, 390, 392, 394, 395, 396
 renal and upper ureteric branches from, 319
Intermetacarpal joints, 443
Intermuscular septum, 419
 anterior, 480, 489
 anteromedial, 480, 489
 lateral, 420, 423, 433, 465
 medial, 419, 420, 421, 423, 433, 435, 436
 posterior, 510
 transverse, 510
Internal capsule, 107
 anterior limb of, 109
 genu of, 109
 posterior limb of, 109
Interosseous artery
 anterior, 422, 435, 436
  termination of, 433
 common, 422, 435, 436, 437
 interior, 436
 posterior, 422, 433, 436
 recurrent, 422, 433
Interosseous intercarpal ligament, 443
Interosseous membrane, 429, 431, 442, 499, 500, 502, 506, 510
 anterior view of, 502
 posterior (dorsal) view of, 443
Interosseous muscles, 452
 attachments of, 452
 deep, 524
 deep tibial nerve to, 529
 dorsal, 450, 458, 464, 519, 524
  bipennate, 453
  first, 433, 448, 453, 455
 of foot, 524, 525
  dorsal (bipennate), 525
  plantar (unipennate), 523, 525
 of leg, 529
 nerve to, 453
 palmar, 450, 464
  unipennate, 453

Interosseous muscles *(Continued)*
plantar, 524
superficial tibial nerve to, 529
Interosseous nerve
anterior, 436, 463
posterior, 433, 466
Interosseous palmar fascia, 450
Interosseous tendon slip, to lateral band, 452
Interpectoral lymph nodes, 178
Interpeduncular cistern, 108
Interphalangeal joint, 516
capsule and ligaments of, 446
distal
in extension: medial view of, 446
site of, 400
in extension: medial view of, 446
in flexion: medial view of, 446
proximal
in extension: medial view of, 446
site of, 400
Interphalangeal ligament, 446
Intersigmoid recess, 263, 315
Intersphincteric groove, 372, 373, 374
Interspinalis cervicis muscle, 170
Interspinalis lumborum muscles, 170
Interspinous ligament, 155, 156
Interspinous plane, 242
Intertendinous connections, 458
Interthalamic adhesion, 107, 109, 110, 114, 144, 145
Intertragic notch, 93
Intertransversarius muscle, 170
Intertransverse ligament, 181
Intertrochanteric crest, 475, 477, 491
radiograph of, 476
Intertrochanteric line, 475
Intertubercular plane, 242
Intertubercular tendon sheath, 410, 414, 419
Interureteric crest, 350
Interventricular artery, anterior, 211
Interventricular foramen (of Monro), 105, 107, 108, 110, 114, 144
left, 107
Interventricular septum, 218
membranous part of, 214
muscular part of, 210, 214, 215, 218, 219
Interventricular sulcus
anterior, 206, 239
posterior, 208, 209
Intervertebral disc, 156
cervical, 21, 22
lumbar, 152, 155, 329, 330, 429
lumbosacral, 336
thoracic, 188
cross-section of, 237, 238
transverse section of, 328
Intervertebral foramen, 174
for C3 spinal nerve, 21
lower margin of, 151
lumbar, 152, 155, 156
radiograph of, 153
sacral, 154
Intervertebral vein, 166, 167, 210
Intestinal artery, 287, 288
Intestinal gland, 305
Intestinal trunk, 259
Intestinal vein, 290, 291
Intestine, 161. *See also* Large intestine; Small intestine
innervation of, 160
intrinsic autonomic plexus of, 305
mesenteric relations of, 262, 263
Intraarticular sternocostal ligament, 180
Intraculminate vein, 142
Intralaminar nuclei, 110
Intramuscular plexus
circular, 305
longitudinal, 305
Intraparietal sulcus, 104

Intrapulmonary airway, schema of, 198
Intrapulmonary blood circulation, schema of, 199
Intrapulmonary lymph nodes, 202
Intrarenal artery, 312
Intratrochlear nerve, 2
Intrinsic autonomic plexus, of intestines, 305
Iridocorneal angle, 87, 88, 90
trabecular meshwork and spaces of, 88
Iris, 81, 87, 89, 90
arteries and veins of, 91
folds of, 88
major arterial circle of, 88, 90, 91
minor arterial circle of, 88, 90, 91
Irritant receptors, 204
Ischial spine, 241, 332, 334, 336, 338, 339, 340, 378, 391, 474, 475, 491
radiograph of, 531
Ischial tuberosity, 155, 334, 335, 336, 341, 357, 358, 360, 362, 363, 372, 375, 474, 475, 483, 490, 491
radiograph of, 333, 476, 531
Ischioanal fossa, 358, 372
anterior recess of, 247, 376
fat body of, 357, 360, 372, 398
posterior recess of, 376
preanal communication between right and left, 376
pus in, 376
roof of, 362
root of, 385
transverse fibrous septum of, 372, 374, 375
Ischiocavernous muscle, 342, 350, 352, 357, 358, 359, 361, 362, 363, 371, 375, 384, 385, 391
fascia of, 363
Ischiococcygeus muscle, 256, 341, 378, 382, 390, 392, 487
nerve to, 487
Ischiocondylar muscle, 527
Ischiofemoral ligament, 475
Ischiopubic ramus, 335, 336, 341, 346, 357, 358, 360, 362, 363, 364, 375, 475
Ischium, 474
body of, 474
radiograph of, 333, 476
ramus of, 474
spine of, 155
transverse section of, 399
Island of Reil. *See* Insula

J

Jejunal artery, 287, 288
anastomotic loop of, 272
Jejunal vein, 290, 291
anastomotic loop of, 290
Jejunal vessels, 290
Jejunum, 261, 262, 263, 270, 271, 272, 281, 328, 329, 330
mucosa of, 272
musculature of, 272
transverse section of, 326
Joint capsule, 492, 507, 516
attachment of, 499
Jugular foramen, 8, 13, 103, 124, 125, 126
Jugular fossa, 12, 94
jugular foramen in, 10
Jugular lymphatic trunk, 202
Jugular lymph nodes
anterior, 72
external, 72
Jugular nerve, 129
Jugular notch, 1, 27, 175, 179, 190
Jugular trunk, 72
left, 295
right, 295
Jugular vein
anterior, 3, 30, 31, 70, 74, 192, 200, 232
communication to, 70
termination of, 70
external, 3, 30, 31, 70, 74, 192, 200, 232
internal, 3, 27, 28, 29, 30, 32, 33, 34, 46, 47, 59, 60, 61, 70, 73, 74, 75, 76, 92, 97, 127, 183, 184, 192, 202, 205, 226, 232

Jugular vein, internal *(Continued)*
computed tomography of, 147
inferior bulb of, 75
in jugular fossa, 12
left, 206
right, 167, 200
right, superior bulb of, 167
Jugulodigastric lymph node, 72, 73
Juguloomohyoid lymph nodes, 72, 73
Jugum, 11
Juxtamedullary glomerulus, 314
Juxtamedullary renal corpuscle, 313

K

Kerckring, valves of, 271, 272
Kidney, 161, 270, 380
anterior relations of, 308
anterior surface of, 311
arteries and veins of, 314
base pyramid of, 311
blood vessels of, 311
cortex of, 311, 313, 314, 328
cross section of, 173
fibrous capsule of, 317
gross structure of, 311
hilum of, 311
inferior pole of, 311
in situ
anterior view of, 308
posterior view of, 309
innervation of, 160, 319, 320
schema of, 320
lateral border of, 311
left, 191, 281, 282, 308, 315, 317, 322, 327, 329
anterior surface of, 312
anterior view of, 312
axial CT image of, 324
cross section of, 265
frontal section of, 312
posterior surface of, 312
renal cortex of, 328
superior pole of, 326
lobulated, of infant, 311
lymph vessels and nodes of, 318
major calyces of, 311
medial border of, 311
medulla (pyramids) of, 311
minor calyces of, 311
parenchyma of, blood vessels in, 314
posterior relations of, 309
prenatal, 223
renal capsule of, 311
renal columns of, 311
renal sinus of, 311
retroperitoneal, 264, 267, 278, 281
right, 191, 266, 267, 277, 281, 308, 309, 315, 317, 322, 329
axial CT image of, 324
cross section of, 265
sagittal section through, 317
sectioned in several planes, 311
superior pole of, 328
superior pole of, 264, 311, 328
surface anatomy of, 311
Knee
anterior aspect of, 496
anterior view of, 495, 497
arteries of, schema of, 500
bursa of, 496
collateral ligaments of, 497
cruciate ligaments of, 497
extension and flexion of, 470
interior of, 496
joint capsule of, 494, 496
lateral view of, 494
medial view of, 494
posterior view of, 497, 499
radiograph of, 498

Knee (Continued)
  right
    in extension, 495, 497
    in flexion, 497
    posterior view of, 499
  sagittal view of, 499
  slightly in flexion, 495
  superior view of, 496
Kohn, alveolar pores of, 198

L

Labbé, inferior anastomotic vein of, 101
Labial artery
  inferior, 35
  posterior, 359, 384
  superior, 35, 69
Labial nerve
  anterior, 393
  posterior, 393, 394
Labial vein
  inferior, 70
  superior, 70
Labia majora
  anterior commissure of, 356
  groove or space between, 356
  posterior commissure of, 356
Labia minora, 342, 359
  frenulum of, 356
Labioscrotal swelling, 368
Labium majus, 342, 348, 352, 356, 368
Labium minus, 342, 348, 352, 356, 368
Labyrinth
  bony, 95
    right, 95
    right, superior projection of, 97
    schema of, 96
  membranous, 95
    posterolateral view of, 95
    right, lateral projection of, 97
    schema of, 96
  orientation of, within skull, 97
Labyrinthine artery, 13, 135, 137, 138, 139, 141
  left, 135
Lacrimal apparatus, 82
Lacrimal artery, 85, 136
  recurrent meningeal branch of, 100
Lacrimal bone, 4, 37, 50
  of newborn, 14
  orbital plate of, 6
Lacrimal canaliculi, 82
Lacrimal caruncle, 82
Lacrimal gland, 44, 86, 117, 132, 160
  excretory ducts of, 82
  orbital part of, 82
  palpebral part of, 82
  schema of, 161
Lacrimal lake, 82
Lacrimal nerve, 44, 83, 85, 86, 120, 121, 130
  communicating branch of, 44
  cutaneous branch of, 44
  meningeal branch of, 86
  palpebral branch of, 2
Lacrimal papilla
  inferior, 82
  superior, 81, 82
Lacrimal punctum
  inferior, 82
  superior, 82
Lacrimal sac, 81
  fossa for, 4, 6
Lacrimal unctum, 81
Lactiferous duct, 176
Lactiferous sinus, 176
Lacuna
  lateral (venous) of Trolard, 99, 100
  magna, 365
Lacunar (Gimbernat's) ligament, 244, 245, 247, 253, 255, 256
Lambda, 9

Lambdoid suture, 7, 8, 9, 14
Lamina
  cervical, 20
  internal medullary, 110
  lumbar, 152, 153, 155, 156
  posterior limiting, 88
  spiral
    hamulus of, 95
    osseous, 95
  of thyroid cartilage, 67, 77
Lamina affixa, 110
Lamina cribrosa, 87
Lamina propria, gingival, 57
Lamina terminalis, 105, 106, 114, 145
Large intestine
  arteries of, 288
  autonomic innervation of, 302, 303
    schema of, 303
  lymph vessels and lymph nodes of, 296
  mucosa and musculature of, 276
  veins of, 291
Laryngeal artery, superior, 33, 75, 76, 135, 229
Laryngeal inlet, 62, 66, 229
Laryngeal nerve (X)
  inferior, 80
    anterior branch of, 80
    posterior branch of, 80
  recurrent, 32, 34, 71, 80, 125, 129, 234
    left, 74, 76, 187, 200, 203, 204, 205, 206, 220, 225, 226, 234, 236, 237
    right, 74, 75, 76, 80, 125, 206, 220, 229, 234
  superior, 69, 74, 75, 80, 125, 129, 130, 134, 204, 234
    external branch of, 71, 75, 76, 80, 125
    internal branch of, 65, 66, 67, 71, 75, 76, 78, 80, 215, 229
Laryngeal prominence, 77
Laryngeal vein
  recurrent, 226
    left, 75
  superior, 70, 229
Laryngeal vessels, 78
Laryngopharynx, 63
  opened posterior view of, 66
Larynx, 134, 161, 204
  anterior view of, 77
  anterosuperior view of, 77
  cartilage of, 77
  innervation of, 160
  intrinsic muscles of, 78
    action of, 79
  medial view of, 77
  nerves of, 80
  normal: inspiration, 78
  posterior view of, 77, 78
  right lateral view of, 77, 78
  sensory branches to, 80
  superior view of, 78
Lateral aperture, 108
Lateral band, 452
Lateral direct vein, 143
Lateral dorsal cutaneous nerve, 471, 472, 530
Lateral ligament, 18, 515
Lateral recess, 114
Lateral sulcus, 104, 106
Latissimus dorsi muscle, 168, 171, 173, 174, 175, 182, 236, 239, 243, 244, 248, 252, 309, 327, 330, 407, 411, 412, 414, 416, 417, 419, 421, 423
  costal origin of, digitations of, 248
  MRI of, 468
  nerve to, 414
  transverse section of, 325
Latissimus dorsi tendon, 237, 238, 421
Left bundle, of heart, 219
Left lateral aperture, 107
Left lateral recess, 107
Leg
  anterior view of, 503
  cross section of, 510
  cutaneous innervation of, 530
  fascial compartments of, 510

Leg (Continued)
  interosseous nerve of, 529
  muscles of
    attachments of, 503
    deep dissection of, 506
    deep dissection of: anterior view of, 508
    intermediate dissection of: posterior view of, 505
    lateral view of, 509
    posterior view of, 506
    superficial dissection of: anterior view of, 507
    superficial dissection of: posterior view of, 504
  posterior view of, 503
  right, bones of, 501
Lens, 81, 83, 88, 90
  axis of, 89
  capsule of, 87, 88, 89
  cortex of, 89
  equator of, 89
  nucleus of, 88, 89
  supporting structures of, 89
  suspensory ligament of, 87
Lenticular process, 93
Lenticulostriate artery, 137, 138, 139, 141
  anterolateral, 139
  lateral, 137
Lentiform nucleus, 109, 139
  globus pallidus of, 107, 109
  putamen of, 107, 109
Leptomeninges, 163
Lesser occipital nerve, 2
Levator anguli oris muscle, 54, 122
Levator ani muscle, 247, 256, 276, 292, 303, 323, 339, 342, 349, 350, 357, 358, 362, 363, 371, 372, 373, 374, 376, 378, 382, 384, 390, 398, 487
  fibers to anal canal, longitudinal muscle from, 340, 341
  fibromuscular extension of, 341
  iliococcygeus part of, 338, 340, 341, 375
  levator plate of, 338
  medial border of, 341
  medial edge of, thickened, 323
  median raphe of, 339
  nerves to, 485, 487
  pubococcygeus part of, 338, 340, 341, 375
  puborectalis part of, 340, 341, 371, 375
  tendinous arch of, 256, 337, 338, 339, 341, 345, 348, 350, 352, 358, 372
  transverse section of, 399
Levator costarum muscle, 170
Levator labii superioris alaeque nasi muscle, 54
Levator labii superioris muscle, 25, 54, 122
Levator palpebrae superioris muscle, 81, 83, 84, 86, 120
  insertion of, 81
Levator plate, 338
Levator scapulae muscle, 26, 31, 34, 168, 171, 411, 414, 415, 465
  communication with cervical plexus, 32
  nerves to, 128
Levator veli palatini muscle, 47, 52, 64, 65, 67, 68, 94, 125
  fold caused by, 66
  interdigitating fibers of, 52
Lienorenal ligament, 264, 266, 282
Ligamenta flava, 22
Ligament of ovary, 343
Ligament of Treitz, 262
Ligaments. *See also specific ligaments*
  of ankle, 515
  of elbow, 426
  of foot, 516
  lumbosacral, 155
  of pelvis, 335, 336, 354
  of wrist, 442, 443
Ligamentum arteriosum, 200, 206, 215, 225
  aortic arch lymph node of, 202
  prenatal, 223
Ligamentum flavum, 155, 156, 330

Ligamentum nuchae, 22, 149
Ligamentum teres, 223, 247, 531
  with acetabular arterial branch, 531
  fissure for, 277
  MRI of, 531
Ligamentum teres uteri, 342
Ligamentum venosum, 223
  fissure for, 277
Limen, 104
Limen nasi, 36
Linea alba, 175, 182, 240, 243, 244, 245, 246, 252, 253, 324, 327, 330, 331, 343
Linea aspera
  lateral lip of, 477
  medial lip of, 477
Linea semilunaris, 240, 242, 331
Linea terminalis, 154, 345, 347
Lingual artery, 3, 33, 39, 59, 69, 75, 132, 135, 136
  deep, 51, 59
  dorsal, 59
    tonsillar branch of, 64
Lingual gyrus, 105
Lingual nerve, 18, 39, 45, 51, 53, 55, 59, 60, 61, 71, 121, 122, 130, 132, 133, 134
Lingual vein, 3, 59
  common trunk for, 59, 61, 70
  deep, 51
  dorsal, 59
    coursing medial to hyoglossus muscle, 70
Lingula, 17, 53, 142, 193
  of superior vermis, 112
Lip
  commissure of, 1
  frenulum of, 51
  philtrum of, 1
  superior, tubercle of, 1
  upper, frenulum of, 51
Lister's tubercle, 427
  posterior (dorsal) view of, 440
Liver, 125, 161, 190, 191, 232, 264, 270, 280, 317, 323, 327, 328, 329
  anterior view of, 277
  arteries of, 283, 284
  axial CT image of, 325
  bare area of, 277, 317
    area for, 308
    coronary ligament enclosing, 323
  bed of, 277
  caudate lobe of, 264, 277, 278
  central veins of, 279
  coronary ligament of, 266
  distributing vein of, 279
  ducts of, 277
    distribution of, 278
  inferior border of, 267
  in situ, 278
  inlet venula of, 279
  innervation of, 160
    schema of, 306
  intralobular arteriole of, 279
  left lobe of, 261, 267, 324
  left triangular ligament of, 266
  lymph vessels of, 279
  periportal space of, 279
  perivascular fibrous capsule of, 278
  portal arteriole of, 279
  posterior view of, 277
  prenatal, 223
  quadrate lobe of, 267, 277, 278
  right lobe of, 261, 267, 277, 278, 324
  round ligament of, 223, 247, 267, 277, 292, 330
    paraumbilical veins in, 250
  sinusoids of, 278, 279
  structure of, schema of, 279
  surface anatomy of, 277
  transverse section of, 325, 326
  vascular system of, 278
  veins of, 278, 279
  visceral peritoneum of, 327
  visceral surface of, 277

Lobule, 1
Locus caeruleus, 114
Longissimus capitis muscle, 169, 172
Longissimus cervicis muscle, 169
Longissimus muscle, 169, 327
Longissimus thoracis muscle, 169
Longitudinal bundle, 280
Longitudinal crease
  radial, 400
  right, 400
Longitudinal fissure
  imaging of, 148
Longitudinal intramuscular plexus, 305
Longitudinal ligament
  anterior, 22, 63, 65, 155, 156, 173, 327, 330, 335, 343
  posterior, 23, 155, 156
Longitudinal muscle, 305
  anterior, 63
  conjoined, 340, 341, 372
  of duodenum, 271, 280
  of esophagus, 228, 229, 230
    attachment of, 229
  inferior, 60
  of pharynx, 229
  rectal, 373
  superior, 60
  of tongue
    inferior, 127
    superior, 127
Longitudinal tendon, anterior, 181
Longus capitis muscle, 26, 29, 47, 60
  communication with cervical plexus, 32
  nerves to, 128
Longus colli muscle, 29, 34, 226, 418
  communication with cervical plexus, 32
  nerves to, 418
Loop of Heiss, 349
Lower limb. See also Ankle; Foot; Leg
  anterior view of, 469
  dermatomes of, 470
  lymph vessels and nodes of, 473
  posterior view of, 469
  segmental innervation of movements of, 470
  superficial nerves and veins of, 471
    posterior view of, 472
Lumbar artery, 164
  anastomosis with, 249
  right, first to fourth, 257
Lumbar curvature, 150
Lumbar disc protrusion, 158
Lumbar ganglion
  first, 160
  third, of sympathetic trunk, 297
Lumbar lymphatic trunk, 318
Lumbar lymph nodes, 259
  lateral, 386
Lumbar plexus, 157, 484, 485, 526, 527
  muscular branches from, 260
  schema of, 486
Lumbar region
  sagittal section through, 317
  vertebral ligaments of, 156
Lumbar spinal nerves, 163, 173
  dorsal and ventral roots of, 163
  dorsal rami of, 163, 171
    lateral cutaneous branches of, 248
  dorsal root of, 163
  L1, 157
    dorsal rami of, 248
    ventral rami of, 390, 486
  L2
    dorsal rami of, 171, 248
    ventral rami of, 155, 397, 484
  L3
    dorsal rami of, 171, 248
    ventral rami of, 395, 484
  L4, 155
    relation to lumbar vertebrae, 158
    ventral rami of, 484

Lumbar spinal nerves (Continued)
  L5, 157, 392
    relation to lumbar vertebrae, 158
    ventral rami of, 484
  L1-L5, schema of, 160
  origin of, 163
  relation to lumbar vertebrae, 158
  ventral ramus of, 163
  ventral root of, 163
Lumbar triangle (of Petit), 149, 168, 248
Lumbar trunk
  left, 259
  right, 259
Lumbar vein
  ascending, 258, 310
  right, first to fourth, 258
  second left, 310
Lumbar vertebrae
  anterior view of, 150
  assembled, 152
  cross section through, 163
  intervertebral disc of, 153
  L1, 157
    body of, 155
    superior articular process of, 153
    transverse process of, 189
  L2
    body of, 173
    inferior vertebral notch of, 153
    superior view of, 152
    transverse section through, 317
  L3
    articular process of, 153
    body of, 153, 343
    pedicle of, 153
    posterior view of, 152
    spinous process of, 330
    transverse process of, 153
    vertebral notch of, 153
  L4
    articular process of, 153
    body of, 336
    lamina of, 153
    posterior view of, 152
    spinous process of, 153
  L5, 157
    anterior view of, 150
    body of, 155, 336
    posterior view of, 150
    radiograph of, 333
  left lateral view of, 150, 152
  posterior view of, 150
  radiographs of, 153
  spinous process of, 173
  transverse process of, 241, 332
Lumbar vertebral body, 156
Lumbocostal triangle, 189
Lumbocostal trigone, 256
Lumbosacral plexus, 260, 485
Lumbosacral region, vertebral ligaments of, 155
Lumbosacral trunk, 260, 319, 390, 484, 485, 486, 487, 526, 527
Lumbosacral vertebrae, ligaments of, 155
Lumbrical muscles, 449, 451, 452, 453, 521, 522, 523
  in fascial sheaths, 450, 451
  first, 451, 463, 529
  fourth, 451, 464
    in fascial sheath, 448
  insertion of, 452
  nerves to, 453, 454
  schema of, 451
  second, 451, 463
    in fascial sheath, 448
  tendons of, 523
  third, 451, 464
    in fascial sheath, 448
Lumbrical tendons
  distal, 451
  proximal, 451
Lumen, 305

Lumobocostal ligament, 309
Lunate, 398, 442
  anterior (palmar) view of, 440, 441, 444
  articulation with radius, 47
  coronal section: dorsal view of, 443
  covered by ligament, 443
  posterior (dorsal) view of, 440, 443, 444
  radiograph of, 445
  sagittal section through, 441
Lunate sulcus (inconstant), 104
Lung, 161, 176, 317
  apex of, 190, 191, 193
  in situ, anterior view of, 192
  innervation of, 160
  left, 193, 205, 209
    anterior border of, 193
    apex of, 191, 193
    cardiac impression of, 193
    cardiac notch of, 190, 192, 193
    cross-section of, 236, 237, 238
    diaphragmatic fissure of, 193
    hilum of, 193, 206
    inferior border of, 190, 191, 193
    inferior lobe of, 192, 193, 194, 195, 325
    interior view of, 194
    lateral view of, 195
    lingula of, 192, 193
    lymphatic drainage of, 202
    medial view of, 195
    oblique fissure of, 190, 191, 193, 236
    posterior view of, 194
    root of, 187
    superior lobe of, 192, 193, 194, 195, 210, 235
    superior lobe of, lingula of, 192
  lymph vessels and nodes of, 202
  medial view of, 193
  right, 193, 205
    anterior border of, 193
    anterior view of, 194
    apex of, 193
    cardiac impression of, 193
    cross-section of, 236, 237, 238
    diaphragmatic surface of, 193
    hilum of, 193
    horizontal fissure of, 190, 191, 192, 193
    ilium of, 206
    inferior border of, 190, 191, 193
    inferior lobe of, 192, 193, 194, 195, 325
    lateral view of, 195
    lymphatic drainage of, 202
    medial view of, 195
    middle lobe of, 192, 193, 194, 195
    oblique fissure of, 193
    posterior view of, 194
    root of, 187
    superior lobe of, 192, 193, 194, 195, 235
  spinal nerves to, 163
  surface anatomy of
    posterior view of, 191
    superior view of, 190
Lunule, 459
Luschka, cleft of, 21
Luschka, foramen of, 108
Luschka, prerectal muscle fibers of, 341
Lymphatic drainage, of lungs, 202
Lymphatic duct, right, 202, 295
Lymphatic plexus, subscapular, 318
Lymphatic trunk
  intestinal, 295
  lumbar
    left, 295
    right, 295
Lymph follicle, of tongue, 58
Lymph nodes
  of abdomen, 330
  of abdominal wall, 259
  of esophagus, 233
  of genitalia
    female, 386
    male, 388

Lymph nodes *(Continued)*
  of head, 72
  of kidney, 318
  of large intestine, 296
  of lower limb, 473
  of lung, 202
  of mammary gland, 178
  of neck, 72
  of pancreas, 294
  of pelvis
    female, 386
    male, 388
  of perineum, 387
  of pharynx and tongue, 73
  pretracheal, 74
  of small intestine, 295
  of stomach, 293
  submandibular, 60
  of upper limb, 405
  of urinary bladder, 318
Lymphoid nodule
  aggregate, 272
  solitary, 272
Lymph vessels
  of abdominal wall, 259
  of esophagus, 233
  of genitalia, 388
  of head, 72
  of kidney, 318
  of large intestine, 296
  of liver, 279
  of lower limb, 473
  of lung, 202
  of mammary gland, 178
  of neck, 72
  of pancreas, 294
  of pelvis
    female, 386
    male, 388
  of perineum, 387
  of pharynx and tongue, 73
  of small intestine, 295
  of stomach, 293
  of upper limb, 405
  of urinary bladder, 318

M

Mackenrodt's ligament, 344, 345, 352, 353, 355
Macula, 90, 119
  fovea centralis in, 87
Macula densa, 313
Macular arteriole
  inferior, 90
  superior, 90
Macular venule
  inferior, 90
  superior, 90
Magendie, foramen of, 116
Magenstrasse, 268
Magnetic resonance imaging (MRI)
  of hip, 531
  sagittal pelvic, 377
  of shoulder, 468
Mallear fold
  anterior, 93, 94
  posterior, 94
Malleolar artery
  anterior lateral, 518, 519
  anterior medial, 518, 519
  lateral, 518
Malleolus
  lateral, 469, 501, 504, 505, 506, 509, 517
    articular facet of, 501, 502
    malleolar fossa of, 501
    radiograph of, 524
  medial, 469, 501, 502, 504, 505, 506, 507, 518
    anterior view of, 524
    lateral view of, 524
    radiograph of, 524

Malleus, 92, 96
  anterior ligament of, 93
  anterior process of, 94
  handle of, 93, 94
  head of, 93, 94, 123
  lateral part of, 93
  lateral process of, 93
  medial view of, 93
  superior ligament of, 93, 94
Malpighian corpuscle, 313
Mammary gland
  anterolateral dissection of, 176
  arteries of, 177
  lobules of, 176
  lymph nodes and vessels of, 178
  sagittal section of, 176
  subcutaneous tissue layer of, 176
  suspensory ligaments of, 176
Mammillary body, 105, 106, 107, 111, 113, 145
Mammillary process, 152
Mammillothalamic fasciculus, 105
Mammillothalamic tract (of Vicq d'Azyr), 145
Mandible, 6, 34, 63
  of aged person (edentulous), 17
  alveolar part (crest) of, 17
  angle of, 1, 5, 15, 17, 66
  base of, 17
  body of, 4, 6, 15, 17, 26, 48
  buccinator crest of, 68
  condylar process of, 15, 17
  condyle of, 7
  coronoid process of, 6, 7, 15, 17, 47
    temporalis muscle insertion for, 54
  digastric fossa of, 17
  head of, 17
  head of condylar process of, 6
  interalveolar septa of, 17
  lingula of, 17
  mandibular foramen of, 17
  mandibular notch of, 6, 17
  median section of, 63
  mental foramen of, 4, 6, 17
  mental protuberance of, 4, 17
  mental tubercle of, 4, 17
  mylohyoid groove of, 17
  mylohyoid line of, 17
  mylohyoid process of, 17
  neck of, 17, 47
  oblique line of, 6, 17, 68
  pterygoid fovea of, 17
  pterygomandibular raphe of, 17
  ramus of, 4, 5, 6, 15, 17, 26, 60
    horizontal section of, 24
  sublingual fossa of, 17
  submandibular fossa of, 17
  superior and inferior mental spines of, 17
Mandibular canal, 60
Mandibular foramen, 53
  inferior alveolar nerve entering, 45
Mandibular fossa, 6, 10, 14, 18, 98
Mandibular nerve, 2, 18, 45, 71, 86, 103, 120, 124, 130, 132, 133, 134
  anterior division of, 45
  lateral view of, 45
  medial view of, 45
  meningeal branch of, 45
  posterior division of, 45
Mandibular nerve (V₃), 12, 44, 121
  meningeal branch of, 12
Mandibular notch, 6, 15, 17
Mandibular periosteum, 57
Manubriosternal joint, 180
Manubriosternal junction, 238
Manubriosternal synchondrosis, 406
Manubrium, 179, 180, 406
  cross-section of, 236, 237
Marginal artery, 288, 302, 378
  left obtuse, 211

Marginal collecting vessels, 73
Marginal plexus, 302
Marginal sulcus, 105
Marshall, oblique vein of, 208, 209, 211, 215
Masseteric artery, 39, 54, 55, 69
Masseteric nerve, 39, 45, 54, 55, 71, 121
Masseter muscle, 26, 27, 47, 60, 61
  deep part of, 54
  horizontal section of, 24
  insertion of, 54
  superficial part of, 54
Mastication, muscles of, 54, 55, 117
Mastoid angle, 11
Mastoid antrum, 94
Mastoid canaliculus, 10, 12
Mastoid cells, 7, 46, 47, 94
Mastoid emissary vein, 3
  in mastoid fossa, 12
Mastoid foramen, 10, 12, 13, 16
Mastoid lymph nodes, 72
Mastoid notch, 10
Mastoid process, 10, 15, 16, 26, 27, 29, 53, 59, 98, 170
  horizontal section of, 24
  as posterior boundary of infratemporal fossa, 6
Maxilla, 4, 6, 50
  alveolar process of, 4, 6, 8, 16, 37, 48
  anterior nasal spine of, 4, 6, 8, 35, 37, 38
  frontal process of, 4, 6, 35, 37, 81
  incisive canal of, 8, 37, 38
  incisive fossa of, 10
  infraorbital foramen of, 4, 6, 14
  infratemporal fossa of, 16
  infratemporal surface of, 6
  intermaxillary suture of, 10
  nasal crest of, 38
  nasal surface of, 8
  of newborn, 14
  orbital surface of, 4
  palatine process of, 7, 8, 10, 36, 37, 38, 52, 56, 98
  tuberosity of, 6, 16
  zygomatic process of, 4, 10
Maxillary artery, 18, 33, 39, 40, 45, 46, 54, 55, 69, 71, 100, 130, 133, 135, 136
Maxillary bone, 47
Maxillary nerve (V₂), 2, 13, 44, 45, 46, 71, 86, 103, 120, 130, 132, 133, 134
  entering foramen rotundum, 43
  meningeal branch of, 86, 121
  pharyngeal branch of, 42
  posterior superior lateral nasal branch of, 41, 42
  schema of, 121
  with sphenopalatine foramen dissected away, 42
Maxillary ostium, 46
Maxillary periosteum, 57
Maxillary plexus, 130
Maxillary sinus, 5, 7, 43, 46, 49, 84
  growth throughout life, 50
  mucous membrane of, 44
  with opening into semilunar hiatus, 50
  opening of, 36, 37, 48, 49
  recesses of
    alveolar, 48
    infraorbital, 48
    zygomatic, 48
  transverse section of, 47
Maxillary sinus, growth of, 50
Maxillary vein, 70, 85
McBurney's point, 275
Median aperture (foramen of Magendie), 108, 114, 116
Median eminence, 114
Median nerve, 417, 418, 419, 421, 423, 434, 435, 436, 442, 448, 449, 453, 454, 461, 462, 463
  anterior view of, 460
  in arm, 467
  articular branch of, 463
  branches to lumbrical muscles, 453, 454
  branches to thenar muscles, 453
  communicating branch with ulnar nerve, 461, 463, 464

Median nerve *(Continued)*
  to cutaneous innervation, 463
  dorsal branches of, 463
  inconstant contribution of, 463
  muscular branch of, 421
  palmar branch of, 402, 404, 434, 435, 447, 460, 463
  palmar digital branches of, 402, 460, 461, 463
    common, 461, 463
  palmar view of, 463
  posterior view of, 460, 463
  recurrent branch of, 447, 448, 454, 461
Median sulcus, dorsal, 114
Mediastinal lymph nodes
  anterior, 178
  cross-section of, 236
Mediastinum
  anterior, 188
    fatty tissue of, 193
  cross sections of, 210
  left lateral view of, 225
  lymphatic routes to, 202
  right lateral view of, 224
  superior
    great vessels of, 200
Medulla
  of femur, 531
  renal, 313
Medulla oblongata, 13, 43, 47, 105, 114, 133, 134, 303, 320
  cross section of, 123
  in foramen magnum, 12
  lower part of, 134
  nuclear layer of, 112
Medullary artery
  anterior segmental, 164, 165
    major, 164
  posterior segmental, 164
Medullary capillary plexus, 314
Medullary lymph vessels, 318
Medullary vein
  anteromedian, 142
  segmental, 166
    anterior, 166
    posterior, 166
Medullary velum
  inferior, 105, 114
  superior, 105, 112, 113, 114
Meibomian (tarsal) gland, 81
  opening of, 81
Meissner's plexus, 305
Membranous labyrinth. *See* Labyrinth, membranous
Membranous septum
  atrioventricular part of, 210, 214, 215, 216, 217, 218, 219
  interventricular part of, 210, 215, 216, 217, 218, 219
Meningeal artery, 100
  accessory, 12, 13, 100
  anterior, 85
  middle, 13, 18, 39, 45, 55, 69, 71, 99, 100, 101, 103, 130, 135, 136
    branches of, 101
    frontal and parietal branches of, 100
    left, 135
  posterior, 3, 12, 13
Meningeal plexus, 130
Meningeal vein, middle, 13, 99, 101
Meningeal vessels
  anterior, groove for, 11
  middle, 12
    grooves for branches of, 8, 9, 11
    grooves for parietal branches of, 11
  posterior, groove for, 11
Meninges, 13, 101
  arteries to, 135
  coronal dissection of, 99
  spinal, 304
Meningohypophyseal trunk, 100
Meniscofemoral ligament, posterior, 496, 497

Meniscus
  coronal section: dorsal view of, 443
  lateral, 495, 496, 499
    attachment of horns of, 496
  medial, 495, 496
Mental foramen, 4, 6, 17
Mentalis muscle, 25, 54, 122
Mental nerve, 2, 45, 71, 121
Mental protuberance, 1, 4, 17
Mental tubercle, 4, 17
Mental vein, 70
Mesencephalic artery, superior, 317
Mesencephalic vein
  lateral, 142
  posterior, 142, 144
  superior, 317
Mesenteric artery
  inferior, 257, 262, 270, 288, 297, 302, 308, 310, 315, 316, 378, 380, 381
    ureteric branches of, 316
  superior, 125, 173, 271, 273, 281, 284, 286, 287, 288, 290, 294, 298, 300, 301, 307, 308, 310, 315, 316, 323, 329, 390
    prenatal, 223
    in root of mesentery, 262, 290
Mesenteric ganglion
  inferior, 160, 297, 302, 319, 389, 394, 395, 396, 397
  superior, 160, 161, 260, 297, 299, 300, 301, 302, 303, 304, 307, 389, 390, 394, 395, 396
Mesenteric lymph nodes
  inferior, 259, 296
  superior, 259, 293, 294, 295, 296
Mesentericoparietal recess (fossa), 262
Mesenteric plexus, 390
  inferior, 297, 302
  superior, 297, 299, 301, 307, 390
Mesenteric vein
  inferior, 232, 262, 281, 289, 291, 292, 294
    blood from, 292
  superior, 173, 271, 281, 287, 289, 290, 291, 292, 294, 328, 329
    blood from, 292
    in root of mesentery, 290
Mesenteric vessels, superior, 266, 270, 330
Mesentery, 173, 272
  of intestines, 262, 263
  peritoneal layers of, 305
  root of, 266, 281, 315, 343, 347
  of small intestine, 323, 330
Mesoappendix, 273, 301
Mesocolic taeniae, 273, 274
Mesocolon
  sigmoid, 263, 276, 288, 308, 315, 371
    attachment of, 277
  transverse, 261, 262, 264, 265, 270, 276, 288, 290, 308, 323
    attachment of, 266, 281
    elevated over pancreas, 263
Mesometrium, of broad ligament, 355
Mesonephric duct, 366, 369
  cranial, 369
Mesonephric tubule, 369
  caudal, 370
  cranial, 369
  vestigial, 370
Mesosalpinx
  of broad ligament, 344
  laminae of, 354
Mesothelial septum, 162
Mesovarium, 352
  laminae of, 354
Metacarpal artery
  dorsal, 457
  palmar, 453, 454
Metacarpal bone, 446, 452
  anterior (palmar) view of, 441, 444
  coronal section: dorsal view of, 443
  dorsal surface of, 446

Metacarpal bone (*Continued*)
fifth, 432, 433, 436
base of, radiograph of, 445
shaft of, radiograph of, 445
first, 433, 436, 449
palmar surface of, 446
palmar view of, 442
posterior (dorsal) view of, 443, 444
second, 433
third, sagittal section through, 441
Metacarpal ligament
deep transverse, 453
dorsal, posterior (dorsal) view of, 443
palmar, 442, 446
transverse
deep, 446
superficial, 404, 447
Metacarpal vein, dorsal, 456
Metacarpophalangeal ligaments, anterior (palmar) view of, 446
Metacarpophalangeal (MIP) joint, 446, 516
capsule and ligaments of, 446
in extension: medial view of, 446
in flexion: medial view of, 446
Metatarsal artery
dorsal, 518, 519, 524
anterior perforating arteries to, 523
posterior perforating branches of, 524
plantar, 521, 523, 524
anterior perforating branches of, 524
Metatarsal bones, 519, 524
fifth, 506, 509, 525
radiograph of, 514
tuberosity of, 511, 518, 523, 524, 525
first, 455, 506, 517, 525
radiograph of, 445
Metatarsal ligament
deep transverse, 524
dorsal, 515
first, 515
plantar, 524
superficial transverse, 520
Metatarsal vein, dorsal, 471
Midbrain
imaging of, 148
Midcarpal joint
coronal section: dorsal view of, 443
in extension, 441
in flexion, 441
sagittal section through, 441
Midclavicular line
left, 242
right, 242
Midline groove, 58
Midpalmar space, 448, 450, 451
septal separation from thenar space, 448
septum between, 450
Minute artery, of fingers, 459
Mitral cells, 118
Mitral valve, 207, 215, 217, 219
anterior cusp of, 210, 215, 216, 217, 218
commissural cusp of, 216, 217
fibrous ring of, 216
leaflet of, 239
posterior cusp of, 210, 215, 216, 217, 218
Moderator band (septomarginal trabecula), 214, 219
Modiolus, of cochlea, 96
Molar tooth, growth of, 50
Monro, interventricular foramen of, 105, 107, 108, 110, 114, 143, 144
left, 107
Mons pubis, 356
Morgagni
anal columns of, 373
hydatid of, 355
Morrison's pouch, 327

Mucosa
of duodenum, 271
of esophagus, 230
junction with gastric mucosa, 230
of intestine, 305
of large intestine, 276
olfactory, 42, 118
of small intestine, 272
of stomach, 268
junction with esophageal mucosa, 230
of urinary bladder, 315
Mucous glands
of nose, 161
of palate, 161
of paranasal sinus, 161
of tongue, 58
Mucous membrane, of maxillary sinus, 44
Müllerian duct, 369
Müller's (tarsal) muscle
superior, 81
Multifidus muscle, 170
Muscles. *See also specific muscles*
of airway, 198
anorectal, 374
of arm
anterior view of, 419
posterior view of, 420
of back
deep, axial CT image of, 324
deep layers of, 170
intermediate layers of, 169
superficial layers of, 168
of duodenum, 271
of esophagus, 228
of face, 122
of facial expression, 60
of foot
second layer of, 522
superficial dissection of, 518
of forearm
attachments of: anterior view of, 438
attachments of: posterior view of, 439
of hand, 453
of hip
lateral view of, 482
posterior view of, 483
of large intestine, 276
of larynx, 78
action of, 79
of leg
attachments of, 503
deep dissection of, 506
anterior view of, 508
lateral view of, 509
posterior view of, 506
superficial dissection of
anterior view of, 507
posterior view of, 504
of mastication, 54, 55
of neck
anterior view of, 26
infrahyoid and suprahyoid, 28
lateral view of, 26
scalene and prevertebral, 29
of orbit, 48
of pharynx
lateral view of, 68
partially opened posterior view of, 67
sagittal section of, 65
of rotator cuff, 413
of shoulder, 411
of small intestine, 272
of sole of foot, 521, 522
of stomach, 269
of thigh
anterior view of, 480, 481
lateral view of, 482
posterior view of, 483
of tongue, 60
Muscular artery, 90, 91

Muscularis mucosae, 305, 373
of anal canal, 374
of rectum, 374
Muscular vein, 90
Musculocutaneous nerve, 417, 418, 419, 421, 423, 436, 460, 461, 462, 463, 467
antebrachial cutaneous branch of, 437
anterior view of, 460
articular branch of, 462
posterior cutaneous, 404
posterior view of, 460
terminal part of, 402, 403, 434
Musculocutaneous vein, 417
Musculophrenic artery, 183, 184, 192, 205, 249
Musculophrenic vein, 183, 184, 250
Myelencephalon, 303. *See also* Medulla oblongata
Myenteric (Auerbach's) plexus, 305
Mylohyoid artery, 39
nerve to, 53
Mylohyoid groove, 17
Mylohyoid line, 17
Mylohyoid muscle, 26, 27, 28, 30, 33, 45, 48, 53, 59, 60, 61, 63, 65, 68, 117
median raphe between, 53
mylohyoid nerve to, 39
nerve to, 45, 53, 55, 60, 71, 121
Mylohyoid nerve, 18, 39
to mylohyoid muscle, 39
Myometrium, 355

N

Nail, body of, 459
Nail bed, 459
Nail matrix, 459
Nail root, 459
Nares, 1
Nasal aperture. *See* Choana
Nasal artery
dorsal, 3, 35, 39, 74, 81, 85, 136
external, 35
lateral, 35
Nasal bone, 1, 4, 6, 8, 35, 37, 38, 50
of newborn, 14
Nasal cavity, 82, 83
arteries of, 40
autonomic innervation of, 43
bones of, at birth, 50
coronal section of, 48
floor of, 36
growth of, 50
horizontal section of, 48
lateral wall of, 36, 37, 40, 41, 42
medial wall of, 38
nerves of, 42
speculum view of, 36
Nasal cleft, 149
Nasal concha
highest, 37
lower border of, 50
inferior, 4, 36, 37, 47, 49, 66, 82
growth of, 50
inferior (turbinate), 36
middle, 4, 36, 37, 48, 49, 50, 82
growth of, 50
superior, 36, 37
lower border of, 50
Nasalis muscle, 122
alar part of, 25, 35
transverse part of, 25, 35
Nasal meatus
airway to, 36
inferior, 36, 82
opening into, 50
middle, 36, 48
atrium of, 36
opening into, 49, 50
superior, 50
opening into, 36, 50

Nasal nerve
external, 35
lateral
inferior, 130
posterior, 130
superior, 130
posterior, 132
Nasal retinal arteriole, 90
Nasal retinal venule, 90
Nasal septum, 16, 38, 40, 42, 63, 66
bony, 8
coronal section of, 48
growth of, 50
schematic hinge of, 40
Nasal slit, 13
Nasal spine
anterior, 4, 8, 38
posterior, 38
Nasal vein
dorsal, 3
external, 70
Nasal vestibule, 36, 38, 47
Nasal wall, lateral, 8
Nasion, 4
Nasociliary nerve (V$_1$), 44, 83, 86, 120, 121, 130, 131
Nasofrontal vein, 3, 70, 85
Nasolabial sulcus, 1
Nasolacrimal canal, opening of, 37
Nasolacrimal duct, 82
in nasooptic furrow, 50
opening of, 36, 50, 82
Nasolacrimal foramen, 50
Nasooptic furrow, nasolacrimal duct in, 50
Nasopalatine nerve (V$_2$), 12, 41, 43
communication with greater palatine nerve, 41
groove for, 38
passing to septum, 42
Nasopalatine vessels, groove for, 38
Nasopharynx, 66, 92, 103
median section of, 63
opened posterior view of, 66
Navicular bone, 511, 515, 524, 525
lateral view of, 514
radiograph of, 514
tuberosity of, 511, 516, 524
Navicular fossa, 346
Neck
autonomic nerves of, 129
bones and ligaments of, 15
fascial layers of, 34
lymph vessels and nodes of, 72
muscles of
anterior view of, 27
infrahyoid and suprahyoid, 28
lateral view of, 26
scalene and prevertebral, 29
nerves and vessels of, 31, 32
posterior triangle of, 168, 172
right anterior dissection of, 32
superficial veins and cutaneous nerves of, 1, 30
surface anatomy of, 1
Nephron
Henle's loop of, 313, 314
schema of, 313
Nerve IX, 60
Nerves. See also specific nerves
of abdomen, 297
of abdominal wall, 251, 260
of back, 171
of buttocks, 491
of cranial base, 46
of cranial fossa, 142
of esophagus, 234
of external genitalia
female, 393
male, 389
of extrinsic eye muscles, 84
of female reproductive organs, 395
of fingers, 459

Nerves (Continued)
of hand, 454
of heart, 220
of hip, 491
of larynx, 80
of lower limb, 471, 472
of male reproductive organs, 396
of nasal cavity, 42
of neck, 31, 32
of oral cavity, 62
of oral region, 71
of orbit, 86
of pelvic viscera
female, 392
male, 390
of perineum
female, 393
male, 391
of pharyngeal region, 71
of pharynx, 62
of shoulder, 465
of upper limb, 461
of ureters, 397
of urinary bladder, 397
at wrist, 449
Nerve X, 60
Nerve XII, 60
Neurohypophysis, 138, 145, 146
Neuropathways, in parturition, 394
Neurovascular compartment, 423
Newborn, skull of, 14
Nipple, 175, 176, 331
Nose, 35. See also Nasal cavity
ala of, 1
anterolateral view of, 35
inferior view of, 35
mucous glands of, 161
transverse section of, 47
Nostril, 1
Nuchal line
inferior, 10, 16
superior, 10, 16, 168, 169, 170
Nucleus ambiguus, 115, 116, 124, 125, 126
Nucleus pulposus, 21, 152
Nutrient artery, 492
Nutrient foramen, 501

O

Obex, 114
Oblique aponeurosis
external, 330
internal, 330
Oblique capitis superior muscle, 172
Oblique fissure, 192
of left lung, 237
Oblique line, 17, 77, 501
Oblique muscle
external, 168, 169, 171, 173, 175, 176, 182, 185, 240, 244, 245, 246, 247, 248, 249, 251, 252, 253, 254, 256, 309, 327, 328, 330, 331, 343, 411, 412, 482
aponeurotic part of, 243, 244, 245, 246, 253, 255, 357, 361
costal origin of, digitations of, 248
fascia over, 360
muscular part of, 243
inferior, 84, 120, 182
internal, 168, 169, 173, 183, 244, 245, 246, 247, 248, 249, 253, 254, 256, 309, 330, 343
aponeurosis of, 246
fascial sheath of, 83
in lumbar triangle (of Petit), 168
tendon of origin of, 173
superior, 83, 84, 86, 117, 120
Oblique pericardial sinus, 209, 239
Oblique popliteal ligament, 499
Oblique popliteal membrane, 496
Oblique vein, of left atrium (of Marshall), 208, 209, 211, 215

Obliquus capitis inferior muscle, 169, 170, 172
Obliquus capitis superior muscle, 169, 170
Obturator artery, 257, 315, 316, 344, 345, 378, 380, 382, 383, 390, 398, 475, 500
accessory, 378, 382
acetabular branch of, 475, 492, 531
anterior branch of, 475
posterior branch of, 475
Obturator canal, 336, 338, 340, 344, 345, 348, 382, 489
Obturator crest, 336, 474
Obturator externus muscle, 479, 481, 489, 527
origin of, 478
transverse section of, 399
Obturator foramen, 241, 332, 335, 474
radiograph of, 333, 476
Obturator groove, 474
Obturator internus muscle, 247, 256, 337, 338, 339, 341, 350, 363, 372, 378, 382, 483, 487, 490, 491
fascia of, 338, 348, 372, 382, 391
MRI of, 531
nerve to, 485, 487, 491
origin of, 478, 479
transverse section of, 399
Obturator internus tendon, 341
MRI of, 531
Obturator lymph nodes, 386
Obturator membrane, 336, 352, 475
Obturator nerve, 247, 260, 315, 380, 390, 398, 484, 485, 486, 487, 526, 527
accessory, 260, 485, 486
anterior branch of, 489, 493
articular branch of, 527
cutaneous branches of, 471, 489, 527
muscles innervated by, 527
posterior branch of, 489, 527
Obturator vein, 258, 291, 379, 398
Obturator vessels, 247, 253
accessory, 253, 255
right, 383
Occipital artery, 3, 33, 69, 70, 100, 135, 136, 172
descending branch of, 33, 172
mastoid branch of, 100, 135
medial, 140
meningeal branch of, 3
occasional branch of, 13
occipital groove for, 10
sternocleidomastoid branch of, 33, 69
Occipital bone, 6, 8, 9, 14, 22
basilar part of, 8, 10, 11, 22, 29, 36, 37, 38, 52, 65, 67
clivus of, 11
condylar canal and fossa of, 10
condyle of, 11
external occipital crest of, 10
external occipital exuberance of, 10
external occipital protuberance of, 8, 10
foramen magnum of, 8, 10
groove for inferior petrosal sinus, 11
groove for posterior meningeal vessels of, 11
groove for superior sagittal sinus of, 11
groove for transverse sinus of, 11
hypoglossal canal of, 8, 10
inferior nuchal line of, 10
inferior petrosal sinus groove of, 8
internal occipital crest of, 11
internal occipital protuberance of, 11
jugular foramen of, 8
jugular process of, 29
occipital condyle of, 8, 10
pharyngeal tubercle of, 10, 63
superior nuchal line of, 10
superior view of, 14
transverse sinus groove of, 8
Occipital condyle, 8, 10, 16, 29, 98, 127
lateral mass for, 19
superior articular surface for, 19
Occipital crest
external, 10, 16
internal, 11

Occipital emissary vein, 99
Occipital groove, 10
Occipital horn, 108
Occipitalis muscle, 117, 172
Occipital lobe, 104
  left, projection on, 119
  right, projection on, 119
Occipital lymph nodes, 72
Occipital nerve
  greater, 171, 172
  lesser, 2, 31, 32, 128, 131, 171
  third, 2, 172
Occipital pole, 104
Occipital protuberance
  external (inion), 8, 10, 16, 149
  internal, 11
Occipital sinus, 102, 142
  groove for, 11
Occipital sulcus, transverse, 104
Occipital vein, 3, 70
  internal, 144
Occipitofrontalis muscle
  frontal belly of, 122
  occipital belly of, 122, 172
Occipitomastoid suture, 16
Occipitotemporal gyrus
  lateral, 105, 106
  medial, 105, 106
Occipitotemporal sulcus
  lateral, 106
  medial, 105
Oculomotor nerve (III), 13, 46, 84, 86, 103, 113, 115, 116, 120, 130, 142
  branch of, 161
  distribution of, 117
  inferior branch of, 83, 86, 120
  schema of, 120
  superior branch of, 83, 86, 120
Oculomotor nucleus, 115, 116, 120
  accessory, 115, 116, 120
Olecranon, 400, 429, 432, 465
  radiograph of, 425
Olecranon bursa, 426
Olecranon fossa, 424
  radiograph of, 425
Olfactory bulb, 42, 48, 106
  afferent fibers from, 118
  contralateral, fibers of, 118
  efferent fibers to, 118
Olfactory cells, 118
  schema of, 118
Olfactory mucosa, 42, 118
Olfactory nerve fibers, 118
Olfactory nerve (I), 13, 41, 118
  distribution of, 117
  schema of, 118
Olfactory nucleus, anterior, 118
Olfactory stria
  lateral, 118
  medial, 118
Olfactory sulcus, 106
Olfactory tract, 42, 105, 106, 113, 119
Olfactory tract nucleus, lateral, 119
Olfactory trigone, 119
Olfactory tubercle, 119
Olivary complex, inferior, 116
Olive, 113
Omental appendices, 263, 276, 330
Omental bursa, 323
  cross section of, 265
  lesser sac, 327
  lesser sac of, 265, 266
  posterior wall of, parietal peritoneum on, 327
  with stomach reflected, 264
  superior recess of, 266, 277
    probe in, 264
  superior recess of (lesser sac) of, 323
Omental foramen (of Winslow), 264, 265, 267, 278, 323, 327

Omental ligament, 278
  lesser, 278
    right free margin of, 271
Omental taenia, 273, 276
Omental vein, 232
Omentum
  greater, 261, 265, 267, 276, 278, 323, 329, 330
    elevated, 263
    overlying transverse colon and small intestine, 261
  lesser, 265, 267, 323, 327
    anterior layer of, 280, 298
    attachment of, 266
    hepatic branch of anterior vagal trunk in, 125
    posterior layer of, 298
    right free margin of, 270, 281
    right margin of, 264
Omohyoid bone, phantom, 33
Omohyoid muscle, 28, 30, 34, 53, 192, 407, 411, 416, 417
  inferior belly of, 1, 26, 27, 28, 31, 127, 128, 415
    communication with cervical plexus, 32
    nerve to, 71
  invested by cervical fascia, 182
  invested by fascia of infrahyoid muscle, 416
  superior belly of, 26, 27, 28, 127, 128
    communication with cervical plexus, 32
    nerve to, 71
Operculum
  frontal, 104
  orbital, 104
  parietal, 104
Ophthalmic artery, 3, 13, 39, 46, 85, 131, 135, 136, 138, 141
  continuation of, 85
  in optic canal, 83
  supraorbital branch from, 69
  supratrochlear branch from, 69
Ophthalmic nerve (V_1), 2, 44, 45, 46, 86, 102, 120, 130, 131, 132, 133, 134
  frontal branch of, 13
  lacrimal branch of, 13
  meningeal branch of, 86
  nasociliary branch of, 13
  schema of, 121
  tentorial branch of, 44, 86, 121
Ophthalmic vein
  inferior, 85
  superior, 13, 83, 85, 91, 103
Opponens digiti minimi muscle, 449, 453, 464
Opponens pollicis muscle, 449, 453, 454, 463
Optic canal, 8, 13, 83
Optic chiasm, 48, 103, 105, 106, 113, 119, 138, 139, 143, 144, 145
Optic disc, 90
Optic nerve (II), 13, 46, 48, 83, 86, 87, 90, 103, 106, 131, 141, 142
  distribution of, 117
  internal sheath of, vessels of, 91
  meningeal sheath of, 83, 84, 87, 91
  in optic canal, 13, 83
  schema of, 119
  in visual pathway, 119
Optic radiation, 119
Optic tract, 106, 107, 111, 113, 137, 142
Oral cavity, 38, 48, 63. See also Lip; Oral region; Teeth; specific parts of oral cavity
  afferent innervation of, 62
  floor of, 53
  inspection of, 51
  roof of, 52
Oral region
  arteries of, 69
  nerves of, 71
  veins of, 70
Ora serrata, 87, 89, 90
Orbicularis oculi muscle, 122
  orbital part of, 25
  palpebral part of, 25, 81
Orbicularis oris muscle, 25, 35, 54, 60, 122
Orbiculus ciliaris, 89

Orbit, 90
  arteries and veins of, 85
  fasciae of, 83
  fat in, 48, 83
  left, growth of, 50
  medial wall of, 48
  muscle attachments and nerves and vessels entering, 83
  muscles of, 48
  nerves of, 83, 86
  right, frontal and slightly lateral view of, 4
  superior view of, 86
  surface view of, 4
Orbital fat body, 83
Orbital fissure
  inferior, 4, 6, 16, 83
  superior, 4, 13, 83
Orbital gyri, 106
Orbital operculum, 104
Orbital plate, 14
Orbital septum, 81
Orbital sulci, 106
Orbitofrontal artery
  lateral, 137, 139, 140
  medial, 137, 139
Orbitofrontobasal artery, medial, 137, 139, 140
Oropharynx, 227
  medial view of, 64
  median section of, 63
  opened posterior view of, 66
Osseous cochlea, 96
Osseous spiral lamina, 95, 96
Ossicles, articulated, 93
Osteomeatal unit, 49
Otic capsule, 95, 96
Otic ganglion, 18, 45, 55, 121, 122, 124, 130, 132, 134, 161
  schema of, 133
Oval (vestibular) window, 14, 95
  base of stapes in, 92, 96
Ovarian artery, 316, 380, 392, 395
Ovarian plexus, 392, 395
Ovarian vein, 380
Ovarian vessels, 315, 343, 384
  tubal branches of, 384
Ovary, 315, 342, 343, 352, 369, 380, 392
  ligament of, 342, 343, 344, 352, 353, 355
  posterior view of, 355
  right, 354
  suspensory ligament of, 342, 343, 344, 354, 355, 369, 380
    ovarian vessels n, 345

P

Pain, referred, common area of, 306, 307
Palate
  growth of, 50
  hard, 48, 63, 64
  mucous glands of, 161
  soft, 38, 51, 63, 64, 66
  muscles of, 65
Palatine aponeurosis, 52, 65
Palatine artery
  ascending, 39, 64, 69
    tonsillar branches of, 39, 64
  greater (descending), 39, 40, 46, 52, 69
    left and right, 39
  lesser, 40, 46, 52, 64
    left and right, 39
    tonsillar branch of, 64
Palatine bone, 8, 50
  greater palatine foramen of, 10, 38
  horizontal plate of, 8, 10, 16, 36, 37, 38, 52, 56, 98
  lesser palatine foramen of, 38
  lesser palatine process of, 10
  nasal crest of, 38
  orbital process of, 4, 37
  perpendicular plate of, 8, 37, 38
  posterior nasal spine of, 10, 37, 38

Palatine bone (Continued)
pyramidal process of, 10, 14, 16
sphenoidal process of, 37
Palatine fold, transverse, 52
Palatine foramen
greater, 12, 37, 38, 40
lesser, 12, 37, 38, 40, 52
Palatine glands, 52, 63, 64
Palatine nerve
descending, 132
greater, 12, 41, 43, 44, 46, 52, 71, 121, 130, 132
communication with nasopalatine nerve, 41, 62
posterior inferior lateral nasal branch of, 41, 42
lesser, 12, 41, 43, 44, 46, 52, 62, 71, 121, 130, 132
Palatine process, 7, 8, 56, 98
Palatine raphe, 52
Palatine vein, 70
external, 70
Palatine vessels, 12
Palatoglossal arch, 51, 58, 60
Palatoglossus muscle, 52, 58, 59, 60, 64, 125
Palatomaxillary suture, 10
Palatopharyngeal arch, 51, 58, 64, 66
Palatopharyngeal muscle, 58, 125
Palatopharyngeal sphincter (Passavant's ridge), 65
Palatopharyngeus muscle, 52, 59, 64, 67, 229
Palpebral conjunctiva, 83
inferior, 81
superior, 81
Palm, 441
Palmar aponeurosis, 430, 434, 442, 447, 448, 450
septa from, 448
Palmar arterial arch
carpal, 453
deep, 453, 454
superficial, 448, 449, 454, 461
distal limit of, 454
Palmar carpal arterial arch, 453
Palmar carpal ligament, 448, 449
continuous with extensor retinaculum, 404, 434, 435, 447
Palmar carpometacarpal ligament, 442
Palmar crease, proximal, 400
Palmar digital artery, 447, 448, 454
common, 448, 450, 453, 454
to neighboring digit, 459
Palmar digital nerve, 404, 447, 448, 463, 464
branches to phalanges, 454
common, 450, 463, 464
dorsal branches of, 456
to fourth and fifth fingers, 448
from superficial branch of ulnar nerve, 447
of thumb, 448
Palmar digital vein, 404
Palmar interosseous muscle, 450
Palmaris brevis muscle, 447, 464
Palmaris longus muscle, 430, 434, 463
origin of, 438
Palmaris longus tendon, 400, 434, 435, 437, 442, 447, 448, 449
Palmar ligament, 452
plates of, 446
Palmar metacarpal artery, 453, 454
Palmar metacarpal ligament, 442, 446
Palmar radioulnar ligament, 442
radiocapitate part of, 442
radioscapholunate part of, 442
Palmar ulnocarpal ligament
ulnolunate part of, 442
ulnotriquetral part of, 442
Palmar venous arch, superficial, 448
Palmate folds, 355
Palpebral arterial arch
inferior, 85
superior, 85
Palpebral artery
lateral, 85
medial, 85

Palpebral artery (Continued)
superior lateral, 85
superior medial, 85
Palpebral ligament
lateral, 81
medial, 81, 83
Pampiniform venous plexus, 250, 367, 381, 383
Pancreas, 125, 266, 322, 323
acini of, 198
anterior view of, 294
arteries of, 284
autonomic innervation of, 307
body of, 264
cross section of, 173, 265
head of, 280, 281, 328
arteries of, 286
posterior view of, 286
reflected to left, 286
retroperitoneal, 264
in situ, 281
innervation of, 160
lymph vessels and nodes of, 294
posterior view of, 294
tail of, 282, 308
artery to, 284
intraperitoneal, 264
transverse section of, 326
uncinate process of, 281, 329
veins of, 289
Pancreatic artery
dorsal, 283, 284, 286, 287
greater, 284, 286
inferior, 284, 286, 287
Pancreatic duct
accessory (of Santorini), 271, 281
extrahepatic, 280
of Wirsung, 271, 281
Pancreatic lymph nodes, superior, 294
left, 293
right, 293
Pancreatic lymph vessels, 294
Pancreatic notch, 281
Pancreaticoduodenal artery
anastomotic branch of, 286
anterior inferior, 284, 286, 287, 288, 291, 300
plexus on, 298, 299
anterior superior, 283, 284, 286, 287, 291, 300
plexus on, 298, 299
retroperitoneal, 264
inferior, 284, 286, 288, 301
common portion of, 287, 288
posterior inferior, 284, 286, 287, 288, 291, 300
plexus on, 301
posterior superior, 283, 284, 286, 287, 300
plexus on, 301
Pancreaticoduodenal lymph nodes, 294
Pancreaticoduodenal plexus, 301
Pancreaticoduodenal vein
anterior inferior, 289, 292
anterior superior, 289, 292
posterior inferior, 289, 292
posterior superior, 289, 292
Pancreatic pain, common areas of, 307
Pancreatic vein
dorsal or superior, 291
great, 289
Papilla
duodenal
major (of Vater), 271, 280
minor, 271, 280
fibers to, 274
filiform, 58
foliate, 58, 134
fungiform, 58, 134
keratinized tip of, 58
parotid, 51
renal, cribriform area of, 313
vallate, 58, 134
Papillary duct, openings of, 313

Papillary muscle, 210, 239
anterior, 214, 215, 217, 219
left, 218
right, 218
posterior, 214, 215, 217, 219
left, 218
right, 218
septal, 214, 217, 218
Paraaortic plexus, 260
Paracentral artery, 139, 140
medial frontal branches of, 139
Paracentral sulcus, 105
Paracolic gutter
left, 263, 330, 343, 347
right, 263, 273, 330, 343
Paracolic lymph nodes, 296
Paradidymus, 369
Paraduodenal fossa, 262
Parahippocampal gyrus, 106, 107, 118, 150
Paramedian artery, 138
Paramesonephric duct, 369
Paranasal sinus
age-related changes in, 50
bones of, at birth, 50
coronal section of, 48
horizontal section of, 48
lateral dissection of, 49
mucous glands of, 161
sagittal section of, 49
Pararectal fossa, 343, 344, 347
Pararenal fat, 317
Parasternal lymph nodes, 178
Parasympathetic fibers, 120
of autonomic reflex pathways, 304
of stomach and duodenum, 300
of submandibular gland, 132
of tracheobronchial tree, 204
Parasympathetic nervous system, schema of, 161
Parathyroid gland
inferior, 76
posterior view of, 76
right lateral view of, 76
superior, 76
Paratracheal lymph nodes, 223, 233
left, 202
right, 202
Paraumbilical portocaval anastomosis, 292
Paraumbilical vein, 247, 292
in median umbilical fold, 247
tributaries of, 250
Paraurethral glands
openings of, 356
primordium of, 369
Paravertebral anastomosis, 165
Paravesical fossa, 344
Paravesical pouch, floor of, 352
Parenchyma, renal, 311
blood vessels entering, 311, 314
Parietal artery, 3
anterior, 139, 140
branch to angular gyrus, 139, 140
posterior, 139, 140
temporal branches of, 139
Parietal bone, 4, 9, 10
groove for middle meningeal vessels of, 11
lateral view of, 14
mastoid angle of, 11
of newborn, 14
squamous suture of, 14
superior view of, 14
tuber (eminence) of, 14
Parietal emissary vein, 3
Parietal foramen, 9
Parietal limb, 214
Parietal lobe, 104
Parietal lobule
inferior, 104
superior, 104

Parietal lymph nodes, posterior, 233
  intercostal, 233
  posterior mediastinal, 233
Parietal operculum, 104
Parietooccipital sulcus, 105
Parolfactory area, 118
Paroophoron, 369
Parotid duct (of Stensen), 24, 54, 55, 61, 69
  opening of, 51
Parotid gland, 24, 26, 27, 30, 47, 60, 61, 66, 92, 124,
    133, 161
  accessory, 61
  bed of, 60
  inferior, 75
  innervation of, 160
  superior, 75
Parotid lymph nodes
  deep, 72
  superficial, 72
Parotid papilla, 51
Parotid space, right lateral dissection of, 33
Pars distalis, 145
Pars flaccida, 93
Pars interarticularis, 152
Pars intermedia, 145
Pars tensa, 93
Pars tuberalis, 145
Parturition, neuropathways in, 394
Passavant's ridge, 65
Patella, 469, 480, 481, 482, 489, 494, 495, 499, 507,
    509
  posterior aspect of, articular surface on, 495
  radiograph of, 498
Patellar anastomosis, 488, 489, 500
Patellar ligament, 469, 480, 481, 482, 489, 495, 496,
    499, 507, 509
Patellar nerve plexus, 471
Patellar retinaculum
  blended into joint capsule, 496
  lateral, 480, 481, 482, 495, 509
  medial, 480, 481, 489, 494, 495
Pecten, 373
Pecten pubis, 241, 332, 335, 336, 340, 474
Pectinate line, 373
Pectinate muscle, 214
Pectineal (Cooper's) ligament, 88, 244, 245, 247,
    253, 255, 256
Pectineal line, 241, 332, 335, 336, 474
Pectineus muscle, 458, 480, 481, 488, 493, 526
  insertion of, 479
  origin of, 478
  transverse section of, 399
Pectoral fascia, 416
Pectoralis major muscle, 26, 30, 175, 176, 182, 185,
    192, 210, 239, 240, 243, 244, 400, 407, 412, 416,
    417, 419, 423
  abdominal part of, 411
  clavicular head of, 411
  cross-section of, 236, 237, 238
  fascia of, 416
  origin of, 406
  sternocostal head of, 411
Pectoralis major tendon, 423
Pectoralis minor muscle, 183, 192, 236, 238, 407,
    412, 417, 421
  fascia of, 416
  invested by clavipectoral fascia, 182, 416
Pectoralis minor tendon, 412, 414, 417, 419
Pectoral nerve
  lateral, 182, 416, 417, 418
  medial, 182, 416, 417, 418
Pedicle
  cervical, 20
  lumbar, 152, 153, 155, 156
  thoracic, 151
Peduncle
  cerebellar, 105
    decussation of, 112
    inferior, 123, 142
    middle, 113, 142

Peduncle, cerebellar (Continued)
    superior, 112, 113, 142
  cerebral, 105, 114
Pelvic brim, sacral part of, 154
Pelvic diaphragm, 342
  fascia of, 344, 348, 357, 358, 362, 372, 374, 376, 385,
    435
  female, 337, 338, 339
  male, 340, 341
Pelvic inlet
  female, 334
  male, 334
  radiograph of, 333
Pelvic organs, female, arteries and veins of, 380
Pelvic outlet, female, 334
Pelvic plexus. See Hypogastric plexus
Pelvic viscera
  female, 344
    nerves of, 392
  male, nerves of, 390
Pelvis
  anterior view of, 335
  arcus tendineus fasciae of, 353
  bones of, 332, 335, 336
  bony framework of, 332
  false, 336, 343
  female, 399
    anterior view of, 380
    arteries of, 382
    contents of, 343
    diaphragm of, 338
    lateral view of, 382
    linea terminalis of, 345
    lymph vessels and nodes of, 386
    measurements of, 334
    medial view of, 338
    radiographs of, 333
    right paramedian section of, 382
    sagittal MR images of, 377
    sagittal section of, 382
    superior view of, 338, 343
    veins of, 382
    viscera of, 342
  hemisected, medial and slightly anterior view of,
    487
  lateral view of, 336
  ligaments of, 335, 336, 354
  linea terminalis of, 347
  lunate (articular) surface of, 336
  male, 331
    arteries and veins of, 383
    bladder-prostate junction of, 398
    contents of, 347
    diaphragm of, 340
    left paramedian section: lateral view, 383
    lymph nodes and vessels of, 388
    measurements of, 334
    radiographs of, 333
    sagittal MR images of, 377
    superior view of, 347
    viscera of, 346
  median (sagittal) section of, 336
  posterior view of, 335
  renal, 311
  sex differences of, measurements of, 334
  transverse section of, 361
  true, 336
  viscera of, 342, 344, 346
Penis, 362
  body (shaft) of, 331, 368
  bulb of, 362, 363, 365
    artery of, 363, 385
  cavernous nerves of, 390, 396
  corpora cavernosa of, 362, 363, 377
  crus of, 350, 354, 362, 363
    ischiocavernosus muscle over, 361
  deep artery of, 361, 363, 385
  deep dorsal vein of, 341, 346, 363, 381, 385
    hiatus for, 340
  dorsal arteries of, 361, 363, 381, 383, 385

Penis (Continued)
  dorsal nerve of, 361, 363, 389, 390, 391, 396, 485,
    491
  fascia of
    deep (Buck's), 243, 360, 362, 381, 383, 385
    superficial (dartos), 243, 360, 361, 362
  frenulum of, 362
  fundiform ligament of, 243, 253, 346
  glans of, 331, 346, 362
    corona of, 362
    development of, 368
    MR sagittal images of, 377
    neck of, 362
  lateral superficial vein of, 361
  raphe of, 368
  skin of, 360, 361, 362, 367
  superficial dorsal vein of, 243, 250, 383
  suspensory ligament of, 244, 346
Perforated substance
  anterior, 106, 113
  lateral, 118
  posterior, 106, 113
Perforating artery
  anterior, to dorsal metatarsal arteries, 523
  first, 490
  fourth, 490
  posteromedial, 138
  second, 490
  third, 490
Perforating cutaneous nerve, 391, 393, 472, 485,
    487, 491
Perforating vein, 403, 404
  anterior, 186
  of kidney, 314
Perianal space, 372, 373, 376
Perianal tissue, 368
Pericallosal artery, 139, 140
  posterior, 141
Pericardiacophrenic artery, 184, 188, 200, 205, 206,
    210, 224, 225, 249
  left, 187
  right, 187
Pericardiacophrenic vein, 184, 188, 200, 205, 206,
    210, 224, 225
Pericardiacophrenic vessels, 209
Pericardial cavity, 210
Pericardial reflection, 208, 214, 215
Pericardial sac, 209
  with heart removed, 209
Pericardial sinus
  oblique, 209, 210, 239
  transverse, 206, 209, 214, 215
Pericardium, 34, 188, 200, 205, 206, 209, 226
  bare area of, 190
  diaphragmatic part of, 209
  fibrous, 225
    line of fusion to diaphragm, 205, 209
    over right atrium, 224
  heart in, 227
  at site of reflection from great vessels, 206
  sternocostal part of, 209
Perichoroidal space, 87, 88
Pericranium, 101
Periglandular plexus, 305
Periglomerular cells, 118
Perineal artery, 359, 383, 384, 385
  transverse, 385
Perineal body, 341, 346, 348, 349, 358, 362, 363, 364,
    375, 385
  perineal raphe over, 356
Perineal compartment, superficial, 376
Perineal fascia, 359
Perineal flexure, 398
Perineal ligament, transverse, 338, 340, 345, 348,
    357, 363, 385
Perineal lymph node, 296
Perineal membrane, 247, 256, 323, 341, 348, 350, 357,
    358, 359, 362, 363, 364, 371, 375, 376, 384, 385,
    391
  anterior thickening of, 340, 345, 348, 363, 385

Perineal muscle
  deep, fascia of, 338, 363
  deep transverse, 337, 342, 358, 359, 363, 364, 376, 384
    bulbourethral gland embedded in, 247
    deep, 363, 376
  superficial transverse, 337, 357, 358, 359, 361, 362, 363, 371, 375, 376, 384, 385
Perineal nerve, 359, 390, 391, 393, 485, 491
  deep branch of, 359, 391, 393
  posterior scrotal/labial branches of, 485
  superficial branch of, 359, 391, 393
Perineal raphe, 356, 368
Perineal space
  deep, 359
  female, 359
  male, 363
  perineal abscess in, 376
  superficial, 352, 357, 358, 359, 362, 384, 385, 391
Perineal vein, 385
Perineoplastic spaces, actual and potential, 376
Perineum
  arteries and veins of
    female, 384
    male, 385
  female, 342, 356, 358
    deep, 358
    interdigitating fibers of, 338
    lymph vessels and nodes of, 387
    nerves of, 393
    superficial dissection of, 357
  male, 331, 346, 360, 361
    deeper dissection of, 361
    frontal section, anterior view of, 363
    nerves of, 391
    surface topography of, 360
Periodontium, 57
Periorbita, 83
Periosteum
  alveolar, 57
  mandibular, 57
  maxillary, 57
Periportal space, 279
Perirenal fat, 317
Perisinusoidal space, 279
Peritoneal fold
  ductus deferens in, 347
  testicular vesicles in, 347
Peritoneal reflection, 371, 373
Peritoneum, 173, 254, 301, 308, 317
  abdominal, 247
  of abdominal wall, 266
  esophageal, 230
  forming floor of pararectal fossa, 372
  inferior extent of, 395, 396
  of large intestine, 276
  parietal, 255, 263, 265, 266, 323, 327, 330, 343, 346, 348
    of omental bursa, 327
    phrenic nerve to, 306
    of posterior abdominal wall, 323
    of urinary bladder, 350
  pelvic, 344, 380
    of pelvic viscera, 392
  perineal, female, 357
  of rectus sheath, 246
  visceral, 272, 305, 376
    of liver, 327
    of spleen, 282
    of stomach, 265
Perivascular fibrous (Glisson's) capsule, 278
Perivascular plexus, 304
Peroneal artery, 500, 504, 505, 506
Peroneal nerve, 506
  common, 506
  deep, 518
    lateral branch of, 519
Peroneal retinaculum, inferior, 506, 509, 515, 517
Peroneus brevis muscle, 509, 510, 517, 518, 528, 530

Peroneus brevis tendon, 469, 504, 506, 509, 515, 518, 523, 524
Peroneus longus muscle, 469, 495, 505, 509, 510, 517, 528, 530
Peroneus longus tendon, 469, 504, 505, 506, 509, 515, 518, 524
  groove for, 512
Peroneus muscle, 469
Peroneus tertius tendon, 509, 518, 524
Perpendicular plate, 8
Pes anserinus, 480, 481, 494, 495, 503
Pes hippocampus, 110, 111
Petit, lumbar triangle of, 149, 168, 248
Petropharyngeus muscle, 67
Petrosal nerve
  deep, 42, 43, 122, 124, 130, 132
  greater, 12, 13, 42, 43, 46, 62, 86, 94, 122, 123, 124, 132, 134
    groove for, 11, 97
    hiatus for, 13
  lesser, 12, 45, 86, 93, 121, 122, 124, 133
    groove for, 11
    hiatus for, 13
Petrosal sinus
  inferior, 13, 102, 103
    groove for, 8, 11
  superior, 46, 64, 97, 103
    groove for, 8, 11
Petrosal vein, 103
  draining to superior petrosal sinus, 142
Petrosquamous fissure, 14
Petrotympanic fissure, 10, 12
Peyer's patches, 272
Phalanx
  distal, 459, 511, 516
    anterior (palmar) view of, 444
    base of, 444
    in extension: medial view of, 446
    head of, 444
    posterior (dorsal) view of, 444
    of ring finger, radiograph of, 445
    shafts of, 444
    tuberosity of, 444
    ulnar nerve innervation of, 464
  middle, 511, 516
    anterior (palmar) view of, 444
    arteries to, 459
    base of, 444, 452
    in extension: medial view of, 446
    extensor tendon to, 452
    head of, 444
    nerves to, 459
    posterior (dorsal) view of, 444
    shafts of, 444
    ulnar nerve innervation of, 464
  proximal, 511, 516
    anterior (palmar) view of, 444
    base of, 444
    in extension: medial view of, 446
    head of, radiograph of, 445
    head of, 444
    posterior (dorsal) view of, 444
    shafts of, 444
Pharyngeal aponeurosis, 65, 229
Pharyngeal artery, 39
  ascending, 33, 46, 69, 135, 136
    meningeal branch of, 13, 100
    pharyngeal branch of, 64
    spinal segmental medullary branches of, 136
  left ascending, posterior meningeal branch of, 135
Pharyngeal constrictor muscle, 63, 80
  inferior, 26, 65, 67, 68, 75, 76, 80, 125, 227, 228
    cricopharyngeus part of, 229
  middle, 26, 59, 64, 65, 67, 68, 75, 125, 229
  superior, 39, 52, 55, 59, 60, 64, 67, 68, 69, 75, 125, 229
    glossopharyngeal part of, 59, 65
Pharyngeal muscle, longitudinal, 67
Pharyngeal nerve, 132
Pharyngeal plexus, 71, 124, 125, 129, 130
Pharyngeal raphe, 36, 63, 64, 65, 67, 75, 228

Pharyngeal recess, 36, 47, 64, 66
Pharyngeal region
  arteries of, 69
  nerves of, 71
  veins of, 70
Pharyngeal tonsil, 36
Pharyngeal tubercle, 10, 22, 38, 64, 65
Pharyngoepiglottic fold, 67, 229
  fibers to, 65
Pharyngoesophageal constriction, 227
Pharyngoesophageal junction, 229
Pharyngotympanic tube. See Auditory (pharyngo-tympanic, eustachian) tube
Pharynx, 34
  afferent innervation of, 62
  longitudinal muscles of, 229
  lymphatic drainage of, 73
  lymph nodes and vessels of, 73
  median section of, 63
  muscles of
    lateral view of, 68
    partially opened posterior view of, 67
    sagittal section of, 65
  opened posterior view of, 66
  posterior view of, 75
  posterior wall of, 51
  tonsil of, 36, 38, 63, 64, 66, 67
    imaging of, 148
Philtrum, 1, 51
Phrenic artery
  inferior, 226, 231, 257, 297, 390
    left, 264, 283, 284, 299, 310
      right, 283, 284, 298, 299, 310, 321
    left inferior, 89, 264, 266, 298
      recurrent branch of, 189, 283
      sympathetic fibers along, 234
    pericardial branch of, 187
    right inferior, 189, 299
Phrenic ganglion, 299, 306
Phrenic lymph nodes
  inferior (subdiaphragmatic), 178
  juxtaesophageal, 233
  superior, 233
Phrenic nerve, 29, 30, 31, 32, 34, 69, 71, 74, 128, 129, 183, 184, 187, 192, 200, 205, 206, 210, 220, 224, 226, 236, 249, 417
  afferent fibers of, 187
  anterior, 225
  efferent fibers of, 187
  inferior cervical cardiac branch of, 220
  left, 187, 189, 209, 225
    anterior branch of, 189
  nerve to, 418
  phrenicoabdominal branch of, 187
  right, 187, 188, 209, 237, 297, 306, 321
    anterior branch of, 189
Phrenicocolic ligament, 264, 266
Phrenic plexus, 390
  inferior, 297
  left inferior, 298, 299
  right inferior, 298, 299, 321
    branch to cardia, 298
Phrenic vein
  inferior, 258
    anastomosis with suprarenal vein, 248
  left inferior, 232, 310
Phrenoesophageal ligament, 230
Physeal closure, MRI of, 468
Pial arterial plexus, 165
  peripheral branches from, 165
Pial plexus, 164
Pial venous plexus, 166
Pia mater, 99, 101, 107
  overlying spinal cord, 162
  thoracic, 163
Pigment cells, retinal, 119
Pigment epithelium, of retina, 88
Pillar (rod) cells, 96
Pineal body, 105, 109, 110, 113, 114

Pineal gland
imaging of, 148
Pineal recess, 107
Piriform fossa, 66, 78, 227
Piriformis muscle, 256, 337, 338, 339, 382, 390, 391, 392, 435, 483, 487, 490, 491
insertion of, 478
nerve to, 485, 487
Piriform lobe, 118
Pisiform bone, 430, 434, 435, 436, 442, 447, 448, 449, 453, 454
anterior (palmar) view of, 441, 444, 446
radiograph of, 445
Pisohamate ligament, 442
Pisometacarpal ligament, 442
Pituitary gland, 105
adenohypophysis (anterior lobe) of, 138, 145, 146
cleft of, 145
imaging of, 148
neurohypophysis (posterior lobe) of, 138, 145, 146
in sella turcica, 36
Pituitary stalk, 113, 138, 145
Plantar aponeurosis, 517, 521, 522, 523
digital slips of, 520
Plantar arterial arch, deep, 523, 524
Plantar artery
deep, 518
to deep plantar arch, 524
from dorsalis pedis artery, 524
lateral, 506, 522, 523, 524
cutaneous branches of, 520
plantar metatarsal branch of, 521
medial, 506, 522, 523
cutaneous branches of, 520
deep branches of, 522, 523
superficial branch of, 520, 521, 522
superficial branch of, plantar digital branch of, 523
posterior perforating branches of, 524
Plantar calcaneonavicular ligament, 515, 516, 524
Plantar cuboideonavicular ligament, 516
Plantar digital artery, 521, 524
common, 521, 522, 524
dorsal branches of, 518
Plantar digital nerve, 520, 529
common, 522
dorsal branches of, 518
Plantar flexion, 470
Plantar interosseous muscle, 523
Plantaris muscle, 482, 483, 490, 494, 499, 504, 505, 506, 529
origin of, 479
Plantaris tendon, 483, 504, 505
Plantar ligament, 516, 524
long, 515, 524
plate of, 516
short, 515, 524
Plantar metatarsal artery, 521, 523
Plantar nerve
deep branch of, 529
lateral, 506, 522, 523, 529
cutaneous branches of, 520
deep branch of, 522, 523, 529
plantar cutaneous branches of, 472
plantar digital branches of, 521, 522
superficial branch of, 522, 523, 529
medial, 506, 517, 522, 523, 529
cutaneous branches of, 520
deep branches of, 523
plantar cutaneous branches of, 472
plantar digital branches of, 521, 522, 523
superficial branch of, 529
Platysma muscle, 25, 27, 30, 34, 122
Pleura
abdominal, 309, 327
costal, 225, 226
cupola (dome) of, 74
of lung, 193
mediastinal, 188, 206

Pleura *(Continued)*
parietal
cervical, 190, 191, 224, 225
costal, 187, 188, 191, 192, 200, 205, 224, 225
costal, left border of, 191
costal, right border of, 191
diaphragmatic, 225
diaphragmatic part of, 187, 188, 192, 200, 205, 226
mediastinal part of, 187, 188, 192, 200, 205, 206, 209, 224, 225, 226
spinal nerves of, 163
visceral, 199
Pleural cavity, 210
costodiaphragmatic recess of, 188, 191, 224, 225, 327
costomediastinal recess of, 188, 190
Pleural reflection, 190, 191, 192
Plica semilunaris, 81, 82
Poirier, space of, 442
Polar frontal artery, 139, 140
Polar temporal artery, 140
Pons, 105, 113, 114, 133
imaging of, 148
Pontine artery, 137, 138, 139
Pontine taste area, 134
Pontine vein
lateral, 142
transverse, 142
Pontomesencephalic vein, anterior, 142
Popliteal artery, 490, 500, 504, 506
deep, 505
Popliteal fossa, 469
Popliteal ligament, oblique, 499
Popliteal lymph nodes, 473
Popliteal membrane, oblique, 496
Popliteal vein, 473, 490
superficial, 504, 505
Popliteal vessels, 483
Popliteus muscle, 483, 499, 505, 506, 529
insertion of, 479, 503
nerve to, 529
origin of, 479
Popliteus tendon, 496
origin of, 495
Pores, of Kohn, 198
Porta hepatis, 277
Portal space, limiting plate of, 279
Portal triad, 265, 270, 278, 281, 326
Portal vein, 328
branch of, 279
hepatic, 265, 270, 277, 278, 279, 281, 283, 284
transverse section of, 326
Portocaval anastomosis, 292
Postanal space
deep, 376
superficial, 376
Postcaval lymph node, 318
Postcentral gyrus, 104
Posterior chamber, 81, 87, 89, 90
Posterior limiting lamina (Descemet's membrane), 88
Postganglionic fibers, 43, 131, 396
of autonomic reflex pathways, 304
parasympathetic, 43, 131
of stomach and duodenum, 300
of sympathetic nervous system, 160
Poupart's ligament, 240, 243, 244, 245, 253, 255, 256, 331, 338, 357, 360, 387, 469, 471, 473, 480, 486, 488, 489
reflected, 244, 245, 253
Preaortic lymph nodes, 296, 386, 388
Precaval lymph nodes, 318
Prececal lymph nodes, 296
Precentral artery, 139
Precentral cerebellar vein, 142
Precentral gyrus, 104
Prechiasmatic groove, 11
Precordial areas, of auscultation, 207
Preculminate vein, 142
Precuneus, 105

Prefrontal artery, 137
Preganglionic fibers, 43, 131, 396
of autonomic reflex pathways, 304
of stomach and duodenum, 300
of the sympathetic nervous system, 160
Premammillary artery, 138
Preoccipital notch, 104
Prepontine cistern, 108
Prepuce, 346, 368
of clitoris, 356
Preputial (Tyson's) gland, opening of, 362
Prepyloric vein, 289, 291
Prerectal muscle fibers (of Luschka), 341
Prerectal space, 376
Presacral space, 345
Presynaptic sympathetic cell body, 43
Pretracheal fascia, 34
Prevertebral anastomosis, 165
Prevesical lymph nodes, lateral, 318
Prevesical plexus, 388
Prevesical space, 348
fat in, 341
Princeps pollicis artery, 454
Procerus muscle, 25, 35, 122
Processus vaginalis, 366
Profunda brachii artery, 417, 420, 421, 422, 423
in triangular interval, 414
Profunda femoris artery, 488, 489, 490, 493, 500
openings for, 481
Profundus flexor tendon, 448
Promontorial (middle sacral) lymph nodes, 318, 386
common, 388
Promontory, 92
superior, 392
with tympanic plexus, 93
Pronator quadratus muscle, 428, 436, 453, 463
insertion of, 438
origin of, 438
Pronator teres muscle, 419, 421, 428, 434, 435, 436, 437, 461, 463
humeral head of, 461, 463
insertion of, 438, 439
medial head of, 435
origin of, 438
slip of insertion of, 433
ulnar head of, 435, 461
Prostate gland, 161, 323, 363, 364, 371, 398
apex of, 364
ascending anterior aspect of, 341
base of, 364
with benign hyperplasia, 383
capsule of, 350, 364
covered by fascia, 346
cross section through, 364
fibromuscular stroma of, 364
frontal section of, 364
inferolateral lobe of, 364
inferoposterior lobe of, 364
innervation of, 160
isthmus of, 364
lymphatic drainage from, 388
median lobe of, 364
MR sagittal images of, 377
posterior view of, 364
primordium of, 69
sagittal section of, 364
skeletal muscular band of, 364
utricle of, 364, 369
Prostate muscle, 247
Prostatic duct, opening of, 364, 365
Prostatic plexus, 319, 383, 390, 396
Prostatic sinus, 365
prostatic duct openings into, 364
Proximal interphalangeal (PIP) joint
in extension: medial view of, 446
site of, 400
Psoas major muscle, 173, 189, 256, 257, 258, 260, 270, 308, 309, 317, 329, 330, 343, 345, 347, 380, 480, 484, 486, 487, 526, 531

Psoas major muscle (Continued)
  area for, 309
  MRI of, 531
  origin of, 484
Psoas minor muscle, 256, 330, 343, 347, 484
  origin of, 484
Psoas muscle, 324, 484
  insertion of, 484
  muscular branch of, 486
  origin of, 478
Pterion, 6
Pterygoid artery, 39
  lateral, 39
  medial, 39
Pterygoid canal
  artery of, 39, 46
  nerve (vidian) of, 42, 43, 44, 46, 121, 122, 124, 130,
    132, 134
Pterygoid fossa, 16
  inferior view of, 10
  posterior view of, 16
Pterygoid fovea, 17
Pterygoid hamulus, 45, 50, 52, 55, 64, 65, 68, 98
Pterygoid muscle
  lateral, 39, 45, 47, 54, 55
    nerve to, 71
  medial, 24, 39, 45, 47, 52, 55, 60, 67, 71
    nerve to, 71
Pterygoid nerve
  lateral, 45, 121
  medial, 45, 55, 121
Pterygoid plate
  lateral, 6, 8, 10, 15, 16, 47, 55, 68
  medial, 8, 10, 16, 46, 50, 64, 65, 98
    hamulus of, 6, 15
Pterygoid plexus, 70, 85
  deep facial vein from, 3
Pterygoid process
  hamulus of, 10, 16, 52
  scaphoid fossa of, 10
Pterygomandibular raphe, 17, 39, 55, 60, 64, 68
Pterygomaxillary fissure, 6
Pterygopalatine fossa, 6, 16, 43, 49
  nasal branches in, 43
Pterygopalatine ganglion, 41, 42, 43, 44, 46, 62, 71,
    120, 121, 122, 124, 130, 132, 134, 161
  ganglionic branches of, 44
  schema of, 132
Pterymandibular raphe, 15
Pubic arch, 241, 332
Pubic bone, 323, 337, 338, 349, 363
  transverse section of, 399
Pubic crest, 340, 398
Pubic ligament, inferior, 241, 332, 338, 340, 341,
    345, 348, 357, 363
Pubic ramus
  inferior, 241, 332, 342, 350, 474, 475, 484, 531
    radiograph of, 531
    posterior, radiograph of, 531
  superior, 241, 332, 335, 336, 340, 342, 362, 363,
    474, 475, 484, 487
    radiograph of, 476
Pubic symphysis, 240, 241, 253, 256, 332, 338, 340,
    341, 342, 345, 348, 357, 359, 360, 363
  covered by fibers of external oblique aponeurosis, 254
  female, 334, 339
    MR sagittal images of, 377
  male, 334, 346
    MR sagittal images of, 377
  radiograph of, 333, 531
  superior portion of, 398
  transverse section of, 399
Pubic tubercle, 240, 241, 244, 245, 254, 256, 332,
    335, 336, 340, 341, 357, 362, 474, 480
Pubic vein, 258
Pubis, 331, 474
  body of, 398
  female
    radiograph of, 333
    symphyseal surface of, 392

Pubis (Continued)
  hypogastric region, 242
  male, radiograph of, 333
  superior ramus of, 481
Pubococcygeus muscle, 337, 338, 339, 340
Pubofemoral ligament, 475
Puboprostatic ligament, 348
Puborectalis muscle, 323, 339, 340
Pubovesical ligament
  lateral, 345, 348
  medial, 345, 348
Pudendal (Alcock's) canal, 372, 378, 385, 391
  internal pudendal artery in, 372, 382, 384, 385
  left internal pudendal vein in, 291
  perineal nerve in, 372
  pudendal nerve in, 385, 393
  pudendal vessels in, 372
Pudendal artery
  external
    deep, 249, 257, 500
    superficial, 245, 249
  internal, 257, 316, 359, 363, 378, 382, 383, 384, 385,
    398, 487
    passing superior to perineal membrane, 385
    in pudendal (Alcock's) canal, 372, 382, 384, 385
    on superior aspect of perineal membrane, 383
  perineal branch of, 363
  superficial external, 257
  transverse section of, 399
Pudendal canal, 378, 391
  internal pudendal artery in, 382
  internal pudendal vein in, 291
  internal pudendal vessels in, 385
  pudendal nerve in, 385, 393
Pudendal cleft, 356
Pudendal nerve, 157, 260, 303, 359, 390, 391, 394,
    395, 396, 398, 485, 490, 491
  in pudendal (Alcock's) canal, 385, 393
  transverse section of, 399
Pudendal vein
  external, 250, 258
  internal, 258, 379, 398
  superficial external, 471
Pudendal vessels
  deep external, 381, 488
  internal, in pudendal (Alcock's) canal, 385
  lymphatic pathways along, 388
  superficial external, 243, 381, 488
Pudendum, 356
Pulmonary artery, 199
  axial CT image of, 235
  left, 193, 200, 206, 208, 225, 238
    prenatal, 223
  left superior, 193
  radiograph of, 207
  right, 193, 200, 206, 208, 214, 215
    cross-section of, 238
    prenatal, 223
Pulmonary ligament, 193, 202, 224, 225
Pulmonary (intrapulmonary) lymph node, 202
Pulmonary plexus, 125, 161, 204, 234
  anterior, 203
  posterior, 203
Pulmonary trunk, 200, 206, 209, 214, 218, 219,
    238
  prenatal, 223
Pulmonary valve, 219
  anterior semilunar cusp of, 214, 216
  left semilunar cusp of, 214, 216
  right semilunar cusp of, 214, 216
Pulmonary vein, 199
  left, 200, 209, 218, 225
    prenatal, 223
  left inferior, 193, 208, 210
  left superior, 206, 208, 215
  right, 200, 209, 215, 224
    prenatal, 223
  right inferior, 193, 208, 210, 239
  right superior, 193, 206, 208, 214, 218
Pulmonic valve, 207

Pulp, of fingers, 459
Pulvinar, 110
  left, 142
  of thalamus, 109, 113
Pupil, 81
  muscles of, 117
Purkinje fibers, 219
Putamen, 107, 109
Pyloric antrum, 267
Pyloric canal, 267
  transverse section of, 326
Pyloric lymph node, 294
Pyloric orifice, 271
Pyloric sphincter, 268
  thickened, 269
Pylorus, 267, 268, 270
  transverse section of, 326
Pyramid, cerebellar, 112, 113
  of cerebellar vermis, 114
  decussation of, 113, 114
Pyramidal eminence, 93, 94
Pyramidalis muscle, 244, 254

Q

Quadrangular lobule, 112
Quadrangular space, 414
  axillary nerve in, 414
  posterior circumflex humeral artery in, 414, 415
Quadrate ligament, 426
Quadrate tubercle, 477
Quadratus femoris muscle, 490, 491
  insertion of, 479
  nerve to, 485, 487, 491
  origin of, 479
Quadratus femoris tendon, 469
Quadratus lumborum muscle, 170, 173, 189, 256,
    257, 258, 260, 308, 309, 317, 330, 343, 347, 484,
    486
  area for, 309
  fascia of, 173
Quadratus plantae muscle, 522, 523, 529
Quadratus plantae nerve, 529
Quadriceps femoris muscle, 483, 526
  insertion of, 478
Quadriceps femoris tendon, 480, 489, 494, 495, 499,
    509
  rectus femoris part of, 480
Quadrigeminal cistern, 108
  imaging of, 148
Quadrigeminal plate, 105

R

Radial artery, 421, 422, 433, 434, 437, 448, 449, 453,
    454, 455, 461
  in anatomical snuffbox, 455, 457, 458
  dorsal carpal branch of, 455
  palmar carpal branches of, 436, 453, 454
  superficial palmar branches of, . 435, 436, 442, 448,
    453, 454
Radial bursa, 448, 451
Radial collateral artery, 420, 422, 423
Radial collateral ligament, 426, 442
  posterior (dorsal) view of, 443
Radial fossa, 424
Radialis indicis artery, 454
Radial nerve, 402, 412, 414, 417, 418, 420, 423, 436,
    461, 462, 463, 467
  anterior view of, 460
  in arm, 465, 467
  communicating branches of, 456
  cutaneous innervation from, 466
  deep branch of, 435, 461, 466
  dorsal digital branches of, 402, 455, 460
  in forearm, 404, 466
  inconstant contribution, 465, 466
  inferior cutaneous, 403
  lateral branch of, 455
  medial branch of, 455

Radial nerve (Continued)
  posterior antebrachial branch of, 460
  posterior cutaneous, 403, 404
  posterior view of, 460
  superficial branch of, 402, 404, 435, 437, 455, 456,
    457, 460, 461, 466
Radial notch, of ulna, 424
Radial recurrent artery, 421, 422, 435
Radial styloid process
  anterior (palmar) view of, 440
  posterior (dorsal) view of, 440
Radial tubercle, distal, 400
Radial tuberosity, 419, 424, 427
  radiograph of, 425
Radiate artery
  cortical, 312, 314
    cortical lymph vessels along, 318
  perforating, 312
Radiate ligament, 181
Radiate vein, cortical, 314
Radicular artery
  anterior, 165
  posterior, 165
Radicular vein, segmental, 166
  anterior, 166
  posterior, 166
Radiocarpal joint. See Wrist
Radiocarpal ligament, 443
Radiograph
  of ankle, 514
  of chest, 207
  of elbow, 425
  of hand, 445
  of hip, 531
  of hip joint, 476
  of knee, 498
  of lumbar vertebrae, 153
  pelvic
    female, 333
    male, 333
  of shoulder, 409
  of wrist, 445
Radioulnar joint, 443
Radioulnar ligament
  dorsal, posterior (dorsal) view of, 443
  palmar, 442
    radiocapitate part of, 442
    radioscapholunate part of, 442
Radius, 424, 428, 429, 430, 431, 433, 436, 437,
    453
  annular ligament of, 426
  anterior border of, 427
  anterior (palmar) view of, 441
  anterior surface of, 427
  articular surface of, radiograph of, 445
  articulation with lunate bone, 427
  articulation with scaphoid bone, 427
  carpal articular surface of, 427
  coronal section of, 427
    dorsal view of, 443
  distal end of, radiograph of, 445
  dorsal tubercle (Lister's) of, 440
  in flexion, 441
  groove for extensor digitorum muscle, 427
  groove for extensor indicis muscle, 427
  groove for extensor pollicis longus muscle, 427
  head of, 419, 424, 427
    radiograph of, 425
  interosseous border of, 427
  interosseous membrane of, 427
  muscle attachment and insertion sites on, 439
  neck of, 424, 427
    radiograph of, 425
  radiograph of, 425
  right
    in pronation: anterior view, 427
    in supination: anterior view, 427
  rotator muscles of, 428
  sagittal section through, 441
  sites of muscle origins and insertions on, 438

Radius (Continued)
  styloid process of, 427
    radiograph of, 445
  tuberosity of, 419, 424, 427
    radiograph of, 425
  ulnar notch of, 427
Rami communicantes, 394
  gray, 129, 131, 132, 133, 160, 162, 163, 174, 185,
    203, 224, 225, 234, 252, 260, 297, 300, 303,
    319, 320, 390, 392, 395, 396, 397, 486,
    487
  white, 129, 131, 132, 133, 160, 162, 163, 174, 185,
    203, 224, 225, 234, 252, 260, 297, 300, 303,
    304, 320, 390, 392, 395, 396, 397, 486
Rathke's pouch, vestigial remnant of, 50
Rectal artery
  inferior, 378, 382, 384, 385
  middle, 257, 288, 302, 315, 345, 378, 380, 382, 383
  superior, 257, 288, 297, 302, 303, 315, 345, 380,
    390
    bifurcation, 378
    branch of, 288
Rectal lymph nodes
  middle, 296
  superior, 296
Rectal nerve, 359, 390, 391, 393, 394
  inferior, 303, 390, 391, 393, 394, 485
  superior, 303
Rectal plexus, 258, 302, 303, 319, 390, 392
  external, 291, 373, 379
  internal, 373, 379
  middle, 302
  perimuscular, 291, 379
  superior, 297, 302
Rectal portocaval anastomosis, 292
Rectal vein
  inferior, 292
  left middle, 291
  left superior, 291, 292
  middle, 258, 292, 379
  right inferior, to internal pudendal vein, 291
  right middle, 291
  right superior, 292
  superior, 379
  tributaries of left and right superior veins, 291
Rectal vessels, superior, 266
Rectocervical space, 344
Rectococcygeus muscle, 256
Rectosigmoid artery, 378
Rectosigmoid junction, 276, 371, 373, 374
Rectourethralis superior muscle, 341
Rectouterine fold, 344
Rectouterine ligament, 344
Rectouterine pouch (of Douglas), 342, 355, 371
Rectovaginal space, 344, 345
Rectovesical pouch, 323, 346, 371
Rectovesical space
  prerectal, 376
  retroprostatic, 376
  retrovesical, 376
Rectropubic space, 323
  areolar tissue in, 346
  vesical venous plexus in, 346
Rectum, 161, 256, 263, 276, 308, 323, 338, 342, 343,
    345, 348, 364, 373, 380
  ampulla of, 348
  anterior view of, 379
  arteries of, 378
  circular muscle layer of, 373, 374
  in situ
    female, 371
    male, 371
  longitudinal muscle layer of, 373, 374
  lymphatic pathway along, 388
  MR sagittal images of, 377
  muscularis mucosae of, 373, 374
  nerves of, 160
  posterior view of, 378
  retracted, 392
  termination of, 398

Rectum (Continued)
  transverse folds of
    inferior, 373
    middle, 373
    superior, 373
  transverse section of, 399
  veins of, 379
    female, 379
    male, 379
Rectus abdominis muscle, 175, 182, 183, 185, 240,
    244, 245, 246, 247, 251, 252, 253, 254, 323, 327,
    330, 331, 343, 345, 346, 347, 357
  axial CT image of, 324
  MR sagittal images of, 377
  transverse section of, 325
Rectus capitis anterior muscle, 73
  communication with cervical plexus, 32
  nerves to, 128
Rectus capitis lateralis muscle, 29
  communication with cervical plexus, 32
  nerves to, 128
Rectus capitis major muscle, posterior, 170, 172
Rectus capitis minor muscle, posterior, 169, 170, 172
Rectus femoris muscle, 469, 480, 482, 488, 489, 493, 526
  insertion of, 478
  MRI of, 531
  origin of, 478, 479, 480
  transverse section of, 399
Rectus femoris tendon, 469, 480, 493, 495, 507
Rectus muscle
  inferior, 83, 84
  lateral, 83, 84, 86, 117, 120
    fascial sheath of, 83
    tendon of, 87
  medial, 83, 84, 86, 120
    cheek ligament of, 82
    fascial sheath of, 83
    tendon of, 87
  superior, 83, 84, 86, 120
    fascial sheath of, 83
    tendon of, 91
Rectus plane, right lateral, 242
Rectus sheath, 183, 243, 244, 253, 330, 357
  anterior layer of, 182, 244, 245, 246, 251, 346, 357
  cross section of, 246
  posterior layer of, 245, 246, 249
Recurrent artery
  of Heubner, 137, 138, 139, 140
  interosseous, 422
  radial, 421, 422, 436
  tibial
    anterior, 500
    posterior, 500
  ulnar
    anterior, 422, 436
    posterior, 422
Recurrent laryngeal nerve, 32, 34
Recurrent process, 118
Red nucleus, 106, 115, 116
  imaging of, 148
Reissner's membrane, 96
Renal artery, 311, 312, 316, 380
  anterior branch of, 312
  in situ, 130
  left, 257, 302, 308, 310, 317, 329, 390
    ureteric branch of, 310, 312
  pelvic branch of, 312
  posterior branch of, 312
  right, 257, 297, 300, 308, 310
    ureteric branch of, 313
  ureteric branch of, 312, 316
Renal capsule, 311, 313, 314
Renal column (of Bertin), 311, 314
Renal corpuscle, 313
  cortical, 313
  juxtamedullary, 313
Renal cortex, 313, 314, 328
Renal ganglion, 319, 396
  left, 321
  right, 321

Renal impression, 277, 282
Renal medulla, 313, 314, 328
  efferent glomerular arteriole descending into, 314
Renal pelvis, 311, 329
Renal plexus, 302, 319, 390
  left, 321
  right, 297, 321
Renal segments
  arteries of, 312
  vascular, 312
Renal sinus, 311
  fat in, 311
    interlobar artery and vein in, 314
Renal vein, 311, 316, 380
  in situ, 310
  left, 232, 258, 308, 310, 317, 322, 329
  right, 232, 308, 310, 329
Renal vessels, 323, 381
Reproductive organs. See also specific reproductive
    organs
  female, innervation of, 395
  male, innervation of, 396
Rete testis, 370
Reticular nucleus, of thalamus, 110
Retina, 90
  ciliary part of, 87, 88, 89
  iridial part of, 88
  nonpigmented and pigmented regions of, 91
  optic part of, 87, 89
  projection on, 119
  structure of, 119
Retinacular artery, 492
  anterior, 482
  inferior, 492
  superior, 492
Retinacular foramen, 477
Retinaculum, inferior extensor, 528
Retinal arteriole
  inferior nasal, 90
  inferior temporal, 90
  superior nasal, 90
Retinal artery, 90
  central, 85, 87, 90, 91
Retinal vein, 90
  central, 87, 90, 91
Retinal venule
  inferior nasal, 90
  inferior temporal, 90
  superior nasal, 90
Retinal vessels, right, 90
Retrobulbar fat, 83
Retrocecal recess, 263, 273
Retromandibular vein, 3, 30, 31, 47, 59, 60, 61, 85
  anterior branch of, 31, 61, 70
  common trunk for, 59, 70
  posterior branch of, 31, 61, 70
Retroperitoneal artery, 266
  common, 266
  external, 266
Retroperitoneal portocaval anastomosis,
    292
Retropharyngeal space, 34, 60, 63, 65
Retroprostatic space, 376
Retropubic space, 245, 345, 348, 376
  fat in, 245, 341
Retropubic venous plexus, 383
Retropyloric lymph nodes, 293
Retrotonsillar fissure, 112
Retrotonsillar vein
  inferior, 142
  superior, 142
Retrouterine pouch (of Douglas), 342, 344
Retrovesical space, 376
Retzius, cave of, 323
Retzius, retropubic space of, 245, 345, 348, 376
  fat in, 245, 341
Rhinal sulcus, 105, 106
Rhomboid fossa, 113
Rhomboid major muscle, 168, 171, 174, 185, 236,
    238, 248, 411, 465

Rhomboid minor muscle, 168, 171, 411, 465
Rhomboid muscle, 237
Ribs, 180
  angle of, 179, 180
  axial CT image of, 235, 324
  body of, 179
  costal cartilage of, 236
  cross section of, 236, 237, 238, 265
  eighth, 179
  eleventh, 179
    projection of, 309
  false, 179
  fifth, 179
  first, 15, 21, 74, 157, 179, 186, 190, 191, 205, 224,
      225, 226, 406, 417, 418
    computed tomography of, 468
    groove for, 193
    left, superior view of, 80
    synchondrosis of, 406
  floating, 179
  fourth, 179
  head of, 179, 180
    articular facet of, 181
    articulation of, 180
    interarticular ligament of, 181
    radiate ligament of, 181
  middle, posterior view of, 180
  muscle origin and insertion sites on, 180
  neck of, 179, 180
  ninth, 179, 282
  second, 176, 179, 406
    computed tomography of, 468
  seventh, 151
    head of, 239
    neck of, 239
  sixth, 176, 179
  tenth, 179
  third, 179
  true, 179
  tubercle of, 179, 180
  twelfth, 157, 168, 179, 189, 241, 317
    projection of, 309
Ring finger, 400
  distal phalanx of, radiograph of, 445
Risorius muscle, 25, 122
Rod cells, 96
Rods, retinal, 119
Rolandic artery, 139, 140
Rolando, central sulcus of, 104
Root canal, 57
Rosenthal, basal vein of, 142
Rotator cuff
  anterior view of, 413
  muscles of, 413
  posterior view of, 413
  superior view of, 413
Rotatores cervicis muscle
  brevis, 170
  longus, 170
Rotatores thoracis muscle
  brevis, 170
  longus, 170
Round (cochlear) window, 14, 92, 95
  closed by secondary tympanic membrane, 96
  fossa of, 93, 94
Round ligament
  of liver, 223, 267, 277, 330
    paraumbilical veins n, 250
  of uterus, 315, 343, 352, 354, 369, 380, 384

S

Saccule, 92, 95, 96, 123
Sacral artery
  lateral, 164, 257, 316, 378, 382, 383
  median, 164, 257, 288, 316, 345, 378, 382
Sacral canal, 154, 340
Sacral cornu, 154
Sacral crest
  intermediate, 154

Sacral crest (Continued)
  lateral, 154
  median, 154, 337
Sacral curvature, 150
Sacral foramen, 153
  anterior, 154
  fourth posterior, 337
  margins of, radiograph of, 531
  posterior, 154, 335
  radiograph of, 333
Sacral ganglion, 160, 297
Sacral hiatus, 154
Sacral lymph nodes
  lateral, 259, 386, 388
  middle, 259, 388
Sacral nerve, 485, 487
Sacral plexus, 157, 390, 395, 396, 485, 487
  right, 302
Sacral promontory, 334, 336, 338, 342, 344
Sacral spinal cord, schema of, 303, 397
Sacral spinal nerves
  dorsal and ventral roots of, 163
  S1, 157, 390
    dorsal ramus of, 171
    relation to lumbar vertebrae, 158
    ventral ramus of, 394
  S2
    dorsal ramus of, 171
    relation to lumbar vertebrae, 158
  S3
    dorsal ramus of, 171
    relation to lumbar vertebrae, 158
  S4, relation to lumbar vertebrae, 158
  S5, 157
  S6, relation to lumbar vertebrae, 158
  S1-L5, schema of, 160
Sacral tuberosity, 154
Sacral vein
  lateral, 258
  median, 291, 374
Sacral vertebrae, radiographs of, 153
Sacral vessels, median, 344, 380, 383
Sacrococcygeal ligament
  anterior, 335, 338, 345
  lateral, 155, 335
  posterior, 155, 335
    deep, 335
    superficial, 335
Sacrogenital fold, 266, 347, 372
Sacroiliac joint, 334, 340
  radiograph of, 333, 531
Sacroiliac ligament
  anterior, 335
  posterior, 155, 335, 336
Sacrospinous ligament, 335, 336, 337, 339, 341, 390,
    483, 491
Sacrotuberous ligament, 155, 335, 336, 337, 339,
    341, 358, 376, 382, 390, 391, 393, 483, 490, 491
Sacrum, 149, 155, 157, 158, 332, 340
  ala of, 154
    radiograph of, 333
  anterior inferior view of, 154
  apex of, 154
  articular facet of, 152, 154
  articular process of, 154
  articular surface of, 155
  base of, 154
  dorsal surface of, 154
  lumbosacral articular surface of, 154
  median sacral crest of, 154
  median sagittal section of, 154
  MR sagittal images of, 377
  pelvic surface of, 154
  posterior superior view of, 154
  promontory of, 154
  radiograph of, 333
  S1-5
    anterior view of, 150
    left lateral view of, 150
    posterior view of, 150

Sacrum (Continued)
superior articular surface of, 154
transverse ridge of, 154
transverse section of, 154
Sagittal sinus
inferior, 99, 102, 103, 142, 143, 144
superior, 99, 100, 101, 102, 103, 105, 108, 142
computed tomography of, 147
groove for, 9, 11
imaging of, 148
Sagittal suture, 9, 14
Salivary glands, 61. *See also* Sublingual gland;
Submandibular gland
coronal section of, 60
lingual minor, 51
molar minor, 52
Salivatory nucleus
inferior, 115, 116, 133
superior, 43, 115, 116, 122, 132
Salpingopharyngeal fold, 64, 66
Salpingopharyngeus muscle, 64, 65, 67, 125
Santorini, accessory pancreatic duct of, 271, 281
Saphenous nerve, 471, 488, 489, 493, 510, 526, 529
branches of, 472, 526
infrapatellar branch of, 471, 488, 489, 526
Saphenous opening, 244, 250, 357, 471
cribriform fascia within, 473
falciform margin of, 255
Saphenous vein
accessory, 471, 472
great, 243, 244, 250, 258, 469, 471, 472, 473, 493, 510
transverse section of, 399
small, 469, 471, 472, 473, 490, 504, 510
Sartorius muscle, 398, 469, 480, 482, 483, 488, 489,
493, 494, 504, 526
insertion of, 478, 503
MRI of, 531
origin of, 478, 479, 480
transverse section of, 399
Sartorius tendon, 480, 481, 494, 495
Scala tympani, 92, 95, 96
Scala vestibuli, 92, 95, 96
Scalene muscle, 28
anterior, 29, 32, 69, 74, 183, 187, 192, 200, 224, 225,
226, 414, 415
origin of, 180
slips of origin of, 29
communication with cervical plexus, 32
middle, 29, 180, 183, 414
origin of, 180
posterior, 29, 180, 183, 226, 414
origin of, 180
slips of origin of, 29
Scalene muscles, 27, 418
anterior, 26, 29, 31, 34, 70, 71, 184, 205, 417
middle, 26, 29, 31, 34, 69, 70, 71
nerves to, 128
nerves to, 418
posterior, 26, 29, 34
Scalene node, 72
Scalp
skin and subcutaneous tissue of, 3, 25
superficial arteries and veins of, 3
Scaphoid bone, 455
anterior (palmar) view of, 440, 441, 444
articulation with radius, 47
coronal section: dorsal view of, 443
middle third of, fracture of, 455
posterior (dorsal) view of, 440, 443, 444
radiograph of, 445
tubercle of, 442
anterior (palmar) view of, 440, 444
Scaphoid fossa, 93, 98
inferior view of, 10
Scapula, 174, 185, 236, 414
acromion of, 179
anastomoses around, 415
anterior view of, 407, 415
blade of, computed tomography of, 468
body of, 416

Scapula (Continued)
coracoid process of, 179
radiograph of, 207
cross section of, 236, 237, 238
glenoid cavity of, 179
radiograph of, 409
inferior angle of, 149, 239
medial border of, 149
muscle origins and attachments on, 408
neck of, 179
posterior view of, 408, 415
spine of, 149, 160, 171, 179, 191, 411, 413, 414, 415, 416
radiograph of, 409
subscapular fossa of, 179
superior border of, 413
suprascapular notch of, 179
vertebral body of, computed tomography of, 468
Scapular artery
circumflex, 414, 415, 417, 419, 422
dorsal, 31, 32, 167, 415, 417
Scapular ligament
superior transverse, 412, 414
transverse, 410, 413, 414, 415
Scapular nerve, dorsal, 417, 418, 465
Scapulohumeral dissection, 414
anterior view of, 414
lateral view of, 414
posterior view of, 414
Scapulothoracic dissection, 414
anterior view of, 414
lateral view of, 414
posterior view of, 414
Scarpa, vestibular ganglion of, 95
Scarpa's layer, 243, 323, 346, 357, 360, 361
attachment to fascia lata, 243
line of attachment of, 360
Schlemm, canal of, 87, 88, 90, 91
veins draining, 91
Schwalbe's line, 88
Sciatic foramen
greater, 155, 335, 336, 337
lesser, 155, 335, 336
Sciatic nerve, 157, 483, 485, 487, 490, 491, 493, 528
as adductor magnus muscle innervation, 527
articular branch of, 490
common fibular division of, 485, 487
left, 398
muscular branches of, 490
right, 398
tibial division of, 485, 487
transverse section of, 399
Sciatic notch
greater, 241, 332, 474
lesser, 241, 332, 474
Sclera, 81, 83, 87, 88, 89, 90, 91
lamina cribrosa of, 87
Scleral spur, 87, 88
Scleral venous sinus, 87, 88, 90, 91
veins draining, 91
Scrotal artery, posterior, 383, 385
Scrotal ligament, 369
Scrotal nerve
anterior, 389
posterior, 390, 391, 491
Scrotal septum, 370
Scrotal vein, anterior, 250
Scrotum, 331, 367, 368
contents of, 367
fascia of, 243, 244, 360, 367, 385
septum of, 346, 367, 375, 385
skin of, 367, 370
Sebaceous gland, 81
Segmental artery
anterior inferior, 312
inferior, 312
posterior, 312
superior
anterior, 312
apical, 312
capsular and perirenal branches of, 312

Sella turcica, 7, 8, 38, 63
dorsum fossa of, 11
hypoglossal fossa of, 11
posterior clinoid process of, 11
tuberculum sellae of, 11
Semicircular canal
anterior, 46, 95, 96, 97
plane of, 97
lateral, 95, 96, 97
prominence of, 92, 94
posterior, 95, 96, 97
plane of, 97
Semicircular duct, 92
anterior, 96
lateral, 95, 96
ampulla of, 123
posterior, 95, 96
ampulla of, 123
Semilunar cusp, 214, 215
commissure of, 494
left, 217, 218
posterior, 217, 218
right, 217, 218
Semilunar fissure, 112
Semilunar fold, 64, 276
Semilunar ganglion. *See* Trigeminal ganglion
Semilunar hiatus, 36, 37, 49, 50
Semilunar valve. *See also* Semilunar cusp
nodule of, 217
Semimembranous bursa, 499
Semimembranous membrane, 496, 505
Semimembranous muscle, 482, 483, 493, 504
insertion of, 479, 503
origin of, 479
Semimembranous tendon, 499, 506
groove for insertion of, 501
Seminal colliculus, 350, 364
Seminal vesicle, 247, 346, 347, 364, 369, 371
Seminiferous tubule, 370
Semispinalis capitis muscle, 168, 169, 170, 172
Semispinalis cervicis muscle, 169, 170, 172
Semispinalis thoracis muscle, 170
Semitendinosus muscle, 469, 481, 483, 490, 491, 493,
504
insertion of, 503
origin of, 479
Semitendinosus tendon, 480, 494, 495
Sensory cortex, 134
Sentinel lymph nodes of Virchow or Troisier, 72
Septal cartilage, 35
Septal papillary muscle, 217
Septomarginal trabecula, 214, 219
Septum, 199
Septum pellucidum, 105, 107, 109, 110, 111, 139,
141, 143, 145
anterior vein of, 143, 144
posterior veins of, 144
Serosa, 272
of spleen, 282
visceral, 305
Serous glands, of von Ebner, 58
Serratus anterior muscle, 168, 174, 175, 176, 185,
236, 238, 239, 240, 243, 244, 248, 251, 252, 331,
400, 407, 411, 412, 414, 417
digitations of, 182, 183
transverse section of, 325
Serratus muscle
first digitation of, 180
origin of, 180
Serratus posterior inferior muscle, 168, 169, 173,
248, 309
Serratus posterior superior muscle, 168, 173
Sesamoid bones, 516, 522, 523, 525
anterior (palmar) view of, 441, 444
Shenton's line, 531
Shoulder
anterior view of, 403, 410, 411
arthrogram of, 468
computed tomography of, 468
cutaneous nerves of, 403

Shoulder (Continued)
glenohumeral joint of, 410
joint capsule of, 414
magnetic resonance imaging of, 468
muscles of, 411
posterior, nerves of, 465
posterior view of, 403
deeper layer, 411
superficial layer, 411
radiograph of, 409
superficial veins of, 403
Sigmoid arteries, 378
Sigmoid artery, 257, 288, 302, 315
Sigmoid lymph node, 296
Sigmoid plexus, 302
Sigmoid sinus, 13, 46, 97, 102, 103
computed tomography of, 147
groove for, 8, 11
Sigmoid vein, 291, 292, 379
Sigmoid vessels, attachment of, 277
Signal lymph node of Virchow or Troisier, 72
Sinuatrial nodal artery, 219
Sinuatrial node, 211, 219
Sinuses
confluence of, 97, 103, 142, 143
frontal, 5, 7, 8, 36, 37, 38, 48, 49, 63
growth throughout life, 50
maxillary, growth of, 50
paranasal
age-related changes in, 50
bones of, at birth, 50
coronal section of, 48
horizontal section of, 48
lateral dissection of, 49
mucous glands of, 161
sagittal section of, 49
petrosal, 8, 11, 13, 46, 64, 97, 102, 103
prostatic, 365
prostatic duct openings into, 364
renal, 311
fat in, 311
sphenoidal, 7, 8, 36, 38, 48, 49, 63, 64, 83, 103
within bony shell, 50
opening of, 8, 36, 37
straight, 97, 102, 103, 108, 142, 143, 144
computed tomography of, 147
in tentorium cerebelli, 105
transverse, 97, 102, 103, 143
computed tomography of, 147
groove for, 8, 11
left, 142
Sinusoids, 278
Skene's glands
openings of, 356
primordium of, 356
Skin
of head, 101
of neck, 34
over rectus sheath, 246
of penis, 360, 362, 367
perianal, 374
sweat glands and hair in, 373
of scrotum, 367, 370
spinal nerve to, 304
Skull
anterior view of, 4
anteroposterior radiograph of, 5
base of, 157, 158
horizontal section through, 103
lateral radiograph of, 7
lateral view of, 6
midsagittal section of, 8
of newborn, 14
regional scan of, 147
superior nuchal line of, 169, 170
Small intestine, 125, 261, 323, 330
area for, 308
arteries of, 287
autonomic innervation of, 301, 303
schema of, 303

Small intestine (Continued)
lymph vessels and nodes of, 295
mesentery of, 323, 330
mucosa and musculature of, 272
veins of, 290
Smooth muscle, of airway, 198
Snuffbox, anatomical. See Anatomical snuffbox
Soleal line, 501
Sole (foot)
cutaneous innervation of, 529
muscles of, 521
second layer of, 522
third layer of, 523
superficial dissection of, 520
Soleus muscle, 483, 494, 504, 506, 507, 509, 510, 517, 529
inserting into calcaneal (Achilles) tendon, 503, 505
insertion of, 503
nerve to, 504, 505
tendinous arch of, 505, 506
Solitary tract nucleus, 115, 116, 122, 124, 125, 134, 320
Sound reception, pathway of, 92
Space of Poirier, 442
Spence, axillary tail of, 177
Spermatic cord, 247, 254, 381, 398
fascia on, 243, 253, 254, 255, 385
testicular vessels in, 381
Sphenoethmoidal recess, 36, 37
Sphenoidal concha, 50
Sphenoidal emissary foramen of Vesalius (inconstant), 13
Sphenoidal fontanelle, 14
Sphenoidal sinus, 7, 8, 36, 38, 46, 48, 49, 63, 64, 83, 103
within bony shell, 50
opening of, 8, 36, 37, 49
probe in, 36
Sphenoid bone, 6, 15, 47
anterior clinoid process of, 8
body of, 8, 38, 50
jugum, 11
prechiasmatic groove, 11
sella turcica, 11
carotid groove of, 11
clivus of, 11
crest of, 38
foramen ovale of, 10
foramen spinosum of, 10
greater wing of, 4, 5, 6, 8, 10, 14
groove for middle meningeal vessels, 11
greater wing of, orbital surface of, 4
infratemporal crest of, 6
lateral plate of pterygoid process, 6
lesser wing of, 4, 5, 8
anterior clinoid process of, 11
orbital surface of, 4
midsagittal section of, 8
optic canal of, 8
pterygoid process of, 10
hamulus of, 6, 8, 10, 14, 37
lateral plate of, 8, 10, 14, 37, 38
medial plate of, 8, 10, 14, 37, 38
pterygoid fossa of, 10
scaphoid process of, 10
sella turcica of, 8, 11
dorsum sellae, 11
hypoglossal fossa, 11
posterior clinoid process, 11
tuberculum sellae, 11
sphenoidal sinus of, 8, 37
spine of, 10, 16, 98
Sphenomandibular ligament, 18, 39, 55
phantom, 18
Sphenooccipital synchondrosis, 63
Sphenopalatine artery, 39, 69
posterior lateral nasal branch of, 39, 40
posterior septal branches of, 39, 40
Sphenopalatine foramen, 6, 8, 16, 37, 39, 40, 41
Sphenopalatine vessels, 12
Sphenoparietal sinus, 102, 103
Spherical recess, 95

Sphincter muscles, 349. See also Anal sphincter muscles
of bile duct, 280
external, 349, 373
subcutaneous part of, 373
of hepatopancreatic ampulla (of Vater), 280
internal
loop of Heiss of, 349
posterior loop of, 349
trigonal ring of, 349
pyloric, 268
Sphincter pupillae muscle, 88, 117, 120, 131
Sphincter urethrae muscle, 247, 341, 346, 349, 358, 364, 376
continuation of, 364
Sphincter urethrovaginalis muscle, 348, 357, 358
Spinal accessory lymph node, 72
Spinal artery
anastomotic loop to, 164
anterior, 136, 137, 139, 164, 165
left posterior, 141
posterior, 137, 139, 164, 165
left, 165
right, 165
Spinal cord, 43
arteries of
intrinsic distribution of, 165
schema of, 164
central canal of, 107, 108, 114
cross-section of, 236, 237
CT axial image of, 235
descending tracts to, 204
imaging of, 148
membranes and nerve roots of, 162
in situ, 157
thoracic
anteroposterior view of, 165
schema of, 132, 204
thoracic part of, 131, 306, 307
thoracolumbar, schema of, 303
veins of, 166
Spinal dura mater, 173
Spinal ganglion, dorsal root, 163, 174, 252, 300, 303, 304, 306, 307, 320
Spinalis muscle, 169, 327
Spinalis thoracis muscle, 169
Spinal membranes, 162
Spinal nerve roots
posterior view of, 162
relation to vertebrae, 158
Spinal nerves. See also Cervical spinal nerves; Lumbar spinal nerves; Sacral spinal nerves; Thoracic spinal nerves
associated radicular arteries of, 164
associated segmental medullary arteries of, 164
dorsal ramus of, 162, 174
lateral branch of, 163
medial branch of, 163
dorsal root of, 162, 174
filament of, 162
origin of, cross section of, 163
recurrent meningeal branch of, 163
schema of, 222
ventral ramus of, 162
ventral root of, 162, 300
filaments of, 162
ventral roots of, 113
Spinal nerve trunk, 252
Spinal vein
anterior, 142, 166
posterior, 142, 166
Spinoumbilical line, McBurney's point on, 275
Spinous process
axial CT image of, 235
cervical, 20
lumbar, 152, 155, 156
of L3 vertebra, 152
of L4 vertebra, 153
thoracic, 151

Spiral ganglion, 96, 123
Spiral lamina
  hamulus of, 95
  osseous, 95, 96
Spiral ligament, 96
Spiral organ of Corti, 92, 96
Splanchnic nerves
  lumbar, 160, 303, 389, 392, 394, 395
    fifth, 390
    first, 320, 390, 397
    first left, 321, 390
    first right, 321
    fourth, 297
    second, 297, 319, 390, 397
    third, 297, 390
    upper, 396
  pelvic (parasympathetic), 161, 302, 303, 319, 390,
    392, 394, 395, 396, 485
    to inferior hypogastric plexus, 487
  sacral (sympathetic), 160, 303, 319, 390, 392,
    397
    to inferior hypogastric plexus, 487
  thoracic
    greater, 160, 189, 203, 225, 234, 252, 256, 260, 299,
      301, 303, 304, 319, 389, 390, 394, 395, 396
    least, 89, 160, 203, 256, 260, 299, 300, 301, 302,
      303, 304, 389, 390, 394, 395
    left, 298
    left greater, 188, 210, 234, 297, 298, 300, 302, 306
    left lesser, 297, 302
    lesser, 89, 160, 203, 252, 256, 260, 299, 301, 304,
      319, 389, 390, 394, 395, 404
    preganglionic fibers of, 321
    right greater, 188, 234, 297, 298, 300, 306, 307,
      321
    right least, 297, 321
    right lesser, 297, 300, 321
Spleen, 191, 264, 267, 278, 281, 322, 327, 328
  anterior extremity of, 282
  area for, 308
  arteries of, 283, 284
  axial CT image of, 324
  cross section of, 265, 282
  diaphragmatic surface of, 282
  hilum of, 282
  inferior border of, 282
  in situ, 282
  posterior extremity of, 282
  superior border of, 282
  transverse section of, 325, 326
  veins of, 289
  visceral surface of, 282
Splenic artery, 270, 281, 282, 283, 284, 286, 287, 297,
    298, 299, 300, 306, 307
  arteriogram of, 285
  left, 257
  retroperitoneal, 266
  splenic branches of, 283
  transverse section of, 326
Splenic lymph nodes, 293
Splenic plexus, 297, 298, 299
Splenic pulp, 282
Splenic vein, 232, 282, 287, 289, 290, 291, 292, 294,
    328
  blood from, 292
  cross section of, 265
  transverse section of, 326
Splenic vessels, 266, 323
Splenium, of corpus callosum, 141
Splenius capitis muscle, 26, 168, 169, 172
Splenius cervicis muscle, 168, 169, 172
Splenorenal ligament, 264, 266, 282, 308
  with splenic vessels, 327
Spring ligament, 515, 524
Stapedius muscle, 117
  nerve to, 122
  tendon of, 93, 94
Stapes, 93
  base of, 92
    in fossa of oval window, 94

Stapes *(Continued)*
  footplate of, 93
  limbs of, 92, 94
  medial view of, 93
  in oval window, 92, 96
Stellate ganglion, 203, 220, 234
Stellate veins, 311, 314
Stensen, parotid duct of, 51, 54, 55, 61
Stensen's duct, 24, 54, 55, 61, 69
  opening of, 51
Sternal facet, of clavicle, 406
Sternal head, 175
Sternalis muscle (inconstant), 182
  sternal part of, 184, 189
Sternoclavicular joint, 190, 406
  articular cavities of, 406
  cross section of, 236
Sternoclavicular ligament, anterior, 406
Sternocleidomastoid lymph node, 72
Sternocleidomastoid muscle, 26, 30, 31, 33, 34, 60,
    61, 73, 126, 128, 168, 172, 175, 182, 192, 240,
    411, 412, 417
  clavicular head of, 1, 26, 27, 240
  innervation of, 117
  medial margin of, 74
  origin of, 406
  sternal head of, 1, 26, 27, 240
Sternocostal articulations, 180
Sternocostal joint, 406
Sternocostal ligament
  intraarticular, 180
  radiate, 180, 406
Sternocostal triangle, 184, 189
Sternohyoid muscle, 26, 27, 28, 30, 34, 53, 65, 127,
    184, 192, 406
  communication with cervical plexus, 32
  insertion of, 406
  invested by cervical fascia, 182
  nerve to, 71
Sternothyroid muscle, 28, 30, 34, 80, 127, 128, 184,
    192
  communication with cervical plexus, 32
  invested by cervical fascia, 182
  nerve to, 71
Sternum, 174, 185, 188, 210, 411
  angle of, 179
  body of, 175, 179, 182, 184, 186, 239, 240, 241
  CT axial image of, 235
  jugular notch of, 179
  lateral view of, 25
  manubrium of, 26, 27, 34, 63, 179, 184
  xiphoid process of, 175, 179, 182
Stomach, 161, 190, 226, 231, 261, 265, 277, 278, 280,
    281, 323, 327
  angular notch of, 267
  area for, 308
  arteries of, 283
  axial CT image of, 324
  body of, 267
    vagal branch to, 234
  cardiac orifice of, 268
  cardiac part of, 227, 230, 267
    vagal branch to, 234
  cardiac zone of, 268
  circular muscle layer of, 230
  fundus of, 227, 230, 267, 268
    transverse section of, 325
  gastric zone of, 268
  in situ, 267
  innervation of, 160, 298, 299
    schema of, 300
  lesser curvature of, 267
    vagal branch to, 234
  lymph vessels and nodes of, 233, 293
  mucosa of, 268
    junction with esophageal mucosa, 268
  musculature of, 230, 269
    innermost oblique layer of, 230
    outer longitudinal layer of, 230
  posterior surface of, 264

Stomach *(Continued)*
  pyloric part of, 267
    hepatic plexus vagal branch to, 298
  pyloric zone of, 268
  transverse section of, 326
  veins of, 289
  zigzag line of, 268
Straight artery, 272, 287, 288
  branch to intestine and accompanying nerves, 305
Straight gyrus, 106
Straight sinus, 97, 102, 103, 108, 142, 143, 144
  computed tomography of, 147
  in tentorium cerebelli, 105
Straight vein, 290
Strap muscles, 117
Stretch receptors, 204
Stria, olfactory
  lateral, 118
  medial, 118
Stria medullaris, 105, 110, 114
Striate artery, distal medial, 137, 138, 139, 140
Stria terminalis, 107, 110, 111
Striatum, 109
Stroma, fibromuscular, 364
Styloglossus muscle, 39, 47, 59, 60, 65, 127
Stylohyoid ligament, 15, 59, 64, 68
Stylohyoid muscle, 26, 27, 28, 33, 39, 53, 60, 61, 67,
    68, 117, 122
Styloid mastoid foramen, 124
Styloid mastoid muscle
  nerve to, 24
Styloid process, 6, 10, 14, 15, 16, 18, 29, 33, 47, 53,
    59, 66, 67, 68
  radial
    anterior (palmar) view of, 440
    posterior (dorsal) view of, 440
    radiograph of, 445
  ulnar
    anterior (palmar) view of, 440
    posterior (dorsal) view of, 440
    radiograph of, 445
Stylomandibular ligament, 18
Stylomastoid foramen, 10, 12, 98, 122
  facial nerve emerging from, 24, 94
Stylopharyngeus muscle, 59, 60, 64, 65, 67, 68, 124,
    125, 229
  with branch from glossopharyngeal nerve, 124
Subacromial space, arthrogram of, 468
Subaponeurotic space, dorsal, 450, 456
Subarachnoid space, 87, 99, 101, 108, 163
  imaging of, 148
Subcallosal area, 105, 118
Subcallosal gyrus, 105
Subcapsular lymphatic plexus, 318
Subcapsular zone, 314
Subclavian artery, 29, 31, 32, 69, 70, 71, 74, 76, 129,
    135, 136, 164, 177, 182, 184, 192, 205, 206, 226,
    231, 249, 414, 415, 417
  groove for, 180, 193, 406
  left, 75, 167, 187, 200, 208, 225, 236
  right, 75, 125, 167, 200, 224
Subclavian groove, 180, 193, 406
Subclavian lymphatic trunk, 202
Subclavian lymph nodes, 72
Subclavian trunk, 72
  left, 295
  right, 259, 295
Subclavian vein, 29, 31, 32, 70, 74, 183, 184, 192,
    202, 205, 206, 226, 232, 250, 414, 417
  groove for, 180
  left, 75, 167, 200, 225
  right, 75, 187, 200, 224
Subclavicular nerves, 31
Subclavius muscle, 180, 183, 224, 225, 406, 412, 417
  fascia of, 416
  insertion of, 406
  invested by fascia, 182, 416
  nerve to, 418
Subcostal artery, 257
  anastomosis with, 249

Subcostal muscle, 252
Subcostal nerve, 157, 260, 308, 309, 389, 394, 484, 485, 486
  anterior branch of, 485
  lateral branch of, 485
  lateral cutaneous branch of, 248, 251, 471
  lateral subcutaneous branch of, 260
  right, 308
Subcostal plane, 242
Subcostal vein, 258
Subcutaneous infrapatellar bursa, 499
Subcutaneous prepatellar bursa, 499
Subcutaneous space, 450
Subcutaneous tissue
  of abdomen, 243
  Camper's layer, 243, 323, 346, 357, 360
  fatty membranous, 357
  of mammary gland, 176
  of neck, 34
  of rectus sheath, 246
  Scarpa's layer, 243, 323, 346, 357, 360, 361
    attachment to fascia lata, 243
    line of attachment of, 360
  of skull, 3
Subcutaneus calcaneal bursa, 517
Subdeltoid bursa, 410, 419
Subdural hematoma, 99, 101
Subendocardial branches, of heart, 219
Subependymal vein, 144
Subhiatal fat ring, 230
Sublingual artery, 59, 61
Sublingual caruncle, with opening of submandibular duct, 51, 61
Sublingual duct, openings of, 51
Sublingual fold, 51, 61
Sublingual fossa, 17
Sublingual gland, 45, 48, 51, 53, 60, 61, 122, 132, 161
  bed of, 60
  innervation of, 160
Sublingual muscle, 117
Sublingual nerve, 45
Sublingual vein, 59, 61
Sublobular vein, 278, 279
Submandibular duct (of Wharton), 51, 53, 59, 60, 61
  opening of, 51
Submandibular fossa, 17
Submandibular ganglion, 45, 59, 61, 71, 121, 122, 130, 161
  schema of, 132
Submandibular gland, 1, 26, 27, 30, 45, 53, 61, 66, 69, 70, 122, 132, 161
  bed of, 60
  innervation of, 160
Submandibular lymph nodes, 60, 73
Submandibular muscle, 117
Submental artery, 39, 69
Submental lymph nodes, 72
Submental node, 73
Submental vein, 30, 70
Submucosa, 305
  with duodenal (Brunner's) glands, 271
  esophageal, 230
  of small intestine, 272
Submucosal glands, 305
Submucosal plexus, 305
Submucous plexus, 232
Submucous space, 372, 376
  internal rectal venous plexus in, 373
Suboccipital nerve, 22, 172
Suboccipital triangle, 172
Subparotid lymph nodes, 72
Subpleural lymphatic plexus, 202
Subpopliteal recess, 486, 495
Subpubic angle, radiograph of, 333
Subpyloric lymph nodes, 293
Subscapular artery, 414, 415, 417, 422
  lower, 414
Subscapular fossa, 179
Subscapularis muscle, 174, 185, 236, 237, 238, 407, 412, 413, 414, 416, 419, 421

Subscapularis muscle (Continued)
  computed tomography of, 468
  subtendinous bursa of, opening of, 410
Subscapularis tendon, 410, 413, 414
Subscapular nerve
  lower, 412, 414, 417, 418, 465
  middle, 418
  upper, 412, 417, 418
Subscapular recess, arthrogram of, 468
Subserous connective tissue, 305
Subserous plexus, 305
Substantia nigra, 106, 116
Subtendinous bursa, 499
  opening of, 410
  of tendocalcaneus, 509
Subtrapezial plexus, 171
Subungual space, 459
Sulcal artery
  central (rolandic), 140
  postcentral, 139, 140
  precentral (prerolandic), 139, 140
  prefrontal, 140
Sulcal vein
  anterior, 166
  posterior, 166
Sulcus
  calcarine, 104
  central (of Rolando), 104
  collateral, 105
  of corpus callosum, 105
  dorsal median, mesothelial septum of, 162
  frontal
    inferior, 104
    superior, 104
  hypothalamic, 105, 145
  intertubercular, 407
  intraparietal, 104
  lateral (of Sylvius), 104, 139
    anterior ramus of, 104
    ascending ramus of, 104
    posterior ramus of, 104
  lunate (inconstant), 104
  marginal, 105
  median, 58
    dorsal, 114
  naoslabial, 1
  occipitotemporal, 105
  olfactory, 106
  paracentral, 105
  parietooccipital, 105
  rhinal, 105
  temporal superior, 104
  terminalis, 58, 208
  transverse occipital, 104
Sulcus limitans, 114
Superciliary arch, 1
Superficialis flexor tendon, 448
Superior anastomotic vein (of Trolard), 101
Superior bulb, in jugular fossa, 12
Superolateral lymph nodes, horizontal group of, 387
Supinator muscle, 428, 433, 435, 436, 437, 461, 466
  insertion of, 438, 439
  origin of, 439
Supraclavicular lymph nodes, 72
Supraclavicular nerve, 2, 30, 32
  from cervical plexus, 402, 403
  intermediate, 128, 403
  lateral, 128, 403
  medial, 128, 403
Supracondylar line, lateral, 477
Supracondylar ridge
  lateral, 407, 424
  medial, 407, 424
Supraduodenal artery, 283, 284, 286, 287
Supraglenoid tubercle, 407
Suprahyoid artery, 59, 69
Suprahyoid lymph nodes, 72
Suprahyoid muscle, 28
Supralevator space, 372
Supramarginal gyrus, 104

Supraopticohypophyseal tract, 145
Supraoptic recess, 105, 107
Supraorbital artery, 3, 35, 39, 69, 81, 85, 136
Supraorbital nerve, 2, 35, 44, 81, 121
  branches of, 86
  lateral branch of, 86
  medial branch of, 86
Supraorbital notch, 1, 4, 6, 14
Supraorbital vein, 3, 70, 85
Suprapatellar bursa, 495, 496, 499
Suprapatellar fat body, 499
Suprapineal recess, 107
Suprapleural membrane, 225
Suprapyloric lymph node, 293
Suprarenal artery
  inferior, 257, 312, 322
  left inferior, 310
  left middle, 310
  left superior, 189, 310
  middle, 257, 322
    branches of, 322
  right inferior, 310
  right middle, 310
  right superior, 310
  superior, 257, 322
Suprarenal gland, 270, 281, 282, 317, 322, 366
  arteries of, in situ, 322
  autonomic nerves of, dissection and schema of, 321
  capsule of, 322
  cortex of, 321, 322
  cross section through, 322
  left, 191, 264, 308, 326, 327, 328
  medulla of, 321, 322
  postganglionic fibers of, 321
  preganglionic fibers of, 321
  right, 191, 266, 308, 321, 326, 328
    abdominal exposure of, 322
  veins of, in situ, 322
Suprarenal impression, 277
Suprarenal plexus, right, 297
Suprarenal vein
  anastomosis with inferior phrenic vein, 258
  left, 232, 258, 310
  right, 310
  right inferior, 258
Suprascapular artery, 31, 32, 74, 75, 76, 136, 414, 415, 417
  infraspinous branch of, 415
Suprascapular foramen, 410, 413, 414, 415
Suprascapular nerve, 414, 417, 418, 465
  MRI imaging of, 468
Suprascapular notch, 179, 414
Supraspinatus muscle, 168, 171, 407, 410, 411, 412, 413, 416, 420, 465
  magnetic resonace imaging of, 468
Supraspinatus tendon, 410, 413, 414, 420
  fused to capsule, 410
Supraspinous ligament, 22, 155, 156, 173, 174, 336
Suprasternal space (of Burns), 27, 34, 63
Supratonsillar fossa, 64
Supratrochlear artery, 3, 35, 39, 69, 81, 85, 136
Supratrochlear nerve, 2, 35, 44, 81, 86
Supratrochlear vein, 3, 70, 85
Supraventricular crest, 214
Supraventricular cusp, 218
Supravesical fossa, 247
Sural cutaneous nerve
  lateral, 504, 510, 528, 530
    branches of, 471, 528
    sural communicating branch of, 510
  medial, 472, 490, 504
Sural nerve, 472, 529
  continuation of, 518
  lateral calcaneal branches of, 472, 506, 529
  lateral dorsal cutaneous nerve branch of, 471, 472, 530
  medial calcaneal branch of, 529
  via lateral calcaneal and lateral dorsal cutaneous branches, 529
  via lateral dorsal cutaneous branch, 528

Suspensory ligament, 244
    of axilla, 416
    of breast, 176
    of clitoris, 357, 358, 359
    of ovary, 369, 380
    of penis, 346
Sustentaculum tali, 511, 514, 515, 516
Sutural (wormian) bone, 6, 9
Suture
    coronal, 4, 6
    frontal (metopic), 14
    occipitomastoid, 16
    palatomaxillary, 10
    sagittal, 9
Sweat glands, of skin, innervation ot, 160
Sylvius
    cerebral aqueduct of, 15, 108
    sulcus of, 104, 139
        anterior ramus of, 104
        ascending ramus of, 104
        lateral, 104, 106
        posterior ramus of, 104
Sympathetic fibers, 120
    of autonomic reflex pathways, 304
    of stomach and duodenum, 300
    of submandibular gland, 132
    of tracheobronchial tree, 204
Sympathetic ganglion, 174, 319, 389, 395
    cervical, 60
        middle, 32, 129, 220, 234
        superior, 124, 129, 130, 132, 133, 220, 234
    lumbar, 163, 390, 392
    sacral, 392
    thoracic, 174, 185, 394, 396
        first, 131
        fourth, 220
        third, 220, 234
Sympathetic nerve
    adrenergic, schema of, 204
    pharyngeal branch of, 71
Sympathetic nervous system, schema of, 160
Sympathetic preganglionic cell bodies, 133
Sympathetic trunk, 34, 43, 47, 69, 70, 133, 189, 203,
    224, 225, 252, 256, 260, 303, 306, 319, 343, 389,
    392, 395, 396, 485, 486
    cervical, 71, 124, 130, 234
    ganglion of, schema of, 304, 320
    left, 188, 210, 297, 307, 321, 330
    lumbar, 390, 487
        left, 302
        third, 297
    right, 188, 297, 307, 327
    sacral, 302
        first ganglion of, 297
        left, 392
        right, 392
    schema of, 204, 304
    thoracic, 132, 185, 188, 234, 394
        left ninth ganglion of, 300
        right, 188
        right 6th ganglion of, 300
Symphyseal surface, 474
Synovial bursa, 495, 496, 499
Synovial cavity, 23
Synovial fold, infrapatellar, 495
Synovial joint, 406
Synovial membrane, 410, 426, 495, 496, 499
    attachment of, 496
    line of attachment of border of, 477
    line of reflection of, 477
    protrusion of, 475
Synovial tendon sheath, 449
    of fingers, 459

T

Taenia
    fibers of, 274, 374
    of fourth ventricle, 114
    free, 263, 273, 274, 276, 371, 374

Taenia *(Continued)*
    mesocolic, 273, 274, 276
    omental, 273, 276
Talocalcaneal ligament
    interosseous, 515
    lateral, 515
    medial, 515
    posterior, 515
Talofibular ligament
    anterior, 502, 515
    posterior, 502, 515
Talonavicular ligament, dorsal, 515
Talus, 511
    anterior view of, 524
    head of, 512
        radiograph of, 514
    lateral process of, 512
    lateral view of, 514, 524
    neck of, 512
    posterior process of, 512, 514, 515
        groove for flexor hallucis longus tendon,
            511
        lateral tubercle, 511
        medial tubercle, 511
        radiograph of, 514
    trochlea of, 512
        radiograph of, 514
Tarsal artery
    lateral, 518, 524
    medial, 518, 524
Tarsal gland, 81
    opening of, 81
Tarsal joint, transverse, 511, 512
Tarsal (Müller's) muscle, superior, 81
Tarsometatarsal joint, 511
Tarsometatarsal ligament, dorsal, 515, 524
Tarsus, 83
    inferior, 81
    superior, 81, 84
Taste
    area of tongue responsible for, 124
    nerves for, 62, 117
Taste buds, 58
Taste pathways, schema of, 134
Tectal (quadrigeminal) plate, 105
Tectorial membrane, 23, 96
    deeper part of, 23
Tectospinal tract, 131
Tectum
    imaging of, 148
Teeth
    apical foramina of, 57
    canine, 56
    cement of, 57
    crown of, 57
    deciduous, usual age of eruption of, 56
    dentinal tubules of, 57
    dentine of, 57
    enamel of, 57
    incisors, 56, 57
    interglobular spaces between, 57
    interproximal spaces between, 57
    molars, 56
        first, 56, 57
        second, 56, 57
        third, 56, 57
    neck of, 57
    nerves to, 57
    odontoblast layer of, 57
    papilla of, 57
    permanent
        left lower, 57
        left upper, 57
        lower, 56
        upper, 56
    premolars, 56, 57
    primary, usual age of eruption of, 56
    root canals of, 57
    roots of, 49, 57
Tegmen tympani, 92, 93

Tela choroidea, 107, 110
Temporal artery
    deep, 69, 99
        anterior, 39
        posterior, 39
    middle, 3, 99
    polar, 140
    superficial, 33, 35, 39, 47, 61, 69, 70, 71, 99, 100,
        133, 135, 136
        branches of, 3
        frontal and parietal tributaries of, 99
        frontal branch of, 85
Temporal bone, 6, 8, 15
    articular tubercle of, 6, 10
    carotid canal (external opening) of, 10
    external acoustic meatus of, 6
    groove for posterior deep temporal artery, 6
    groove for sigmoid sinus of, 8
    groove for superior petrosal sinus, 8
    internal acoustic meatus of, 8
    jugular fossa of, 10
    lambdoid suture of, 6, 8
    mandibular fossa of, 6, 10, 14
    mastoid caniculus of, 10
    mastoid foramen of, 10
    mastoid notch of, 10
    mastoid process of, 6, 10
    occipital groove of, 10
    opening of vestibular aqueduct of, 8
    oval (vestibular) window of, 14
    petrosquamous fissure of, 14
    petrotympanic fissure of, 10
    petrous part of, 8, 10, 97, 98
        accessory muscle bundle from, 67
        arcuate eminence, 11
        groove for greater petrosal nerve, 11
        groove for lesser petrosal nerve, 11
        groove for sigmoid sinus, 11
        groove for superior petrosal sinus, 11
        trigeminal impression, 11
    round (cochlear) window of, 14
    squamous part of, 6, 8, 11, 14
    styloid process of, 6, 10, 14
    stylomastoid foramen of, 10
    supramastoid crest of, 6
    tympanic part of, 14
    zygomatic process of, 6, 10, 14
Temporal fossa, 6, 15
Temporal gyrus
    inferior, 104, 106
    middle, 104
    superior, 104
Temporalis muscle, 45, 54, 61, 99, 101
    insertion of, 54
Temporal line, inferior, 6
Temporal lobe, 104, 113, 139
    imaging of, 148
Temporal nerve, deep, 71, 121
    posterior, 39, 45
Temporal pole, 104
Temporal sulcus
    inferior, 104, 106
    superior, 104
Temporal vein
    middle, 3
    superficial, 60, 70
        branches of, 3
        frontal and parietal tributaries of, 99
        tributary of, 101
Temporofacial division, 24
Temporomandibular joint, 18, 55
    articular disc of, 54, 55
    joint capsule of, 18
    lateral and medial views of, 18
Temporomandibular ligament, 18
Tendinous arch, 68
Tendinous intersection, 175, 240, 244, 331
Tendinous slips, to extensor expansions, 453
Tendocalcaneus, subtendinous bursa of, 509

Tendons. *See also specific tendons*
  of ankle, 515
  of foot, plantar view of, 516
Tendon sheaths, 449
  of ankle, 517
Tenon's capsule, 87
Tensor fasciae latae muscle, 398, 469, 480, 482, 488,
    490, 491, 493, 531
  MRI of, 531
  origin of, 479, 480
  transverse section of, 399
Tensor tympani muscle, 45, 93, 94, 117
  tendon of, 93
Tensor tympani nerve, 45, 121
Tensor veli palatini muscle, 45, 64, 65, 68, 93, 117, 121
  nerve to, 71
  palatine aponeurosis from, 52
  tendon of, 52, 65
Tensor veli palatini nerve, 45
Tentorial artery, 103
Tentorium cerebelli, 86, 102, 103, 142, 143
Teres major muscle, 149, 168, 171, 174, 236, 237,
    238, 407, 411, 412, 414, 415, 416, 417, 419, 420,
    421, 423, 465
  lower margin of, 422
  MRI of, 468
  nerve to, 414
Teres major tendon, 420
Teres minor muscle, 168, 171, 236, 237, 411, 412,
    413, 414, 415, 416, 420, 465
Teres minor tendon, 410, 413, 420
Testicular artery, 249, 257, 367, 383, 389, 396
  left (ovarian), 308, 310
  right (ovarian), 297, 310
Testicular plexus, 389, 396
  right, 297
Testicular vein, 258
  left, 308, 310
  right, 310
Testicular vessels, 247, 253, 255, 266, 315, 330, 347,
    381
  covered by peritoneum, 254
  left (ovarian), 291
  lymphatic pathways along, 388
  in peritoneal fold, 347
  right (ovarian), 291
  in spermatic cord, 381
Testis, 323, 370, 396
  appendix of, 367, 369
  arteries and veins of, 381
  descent of, 366
  frontal section of, 370
  lobules of, 370
  mediastinum, rete testis in, 370
  MR sagittal images of, 377
  pathways from, 388
  schema of, 370
  spermatic fascia over, 385
  tunica albuginea of, 370
  tunica vaginalis of, 323, 367
Thalamic veins, posterior, 144
Thalamogeniculate artery, 141
Thalamoperforating artery, 138, 141
Thalamostriate vein
  inferior, 142, 144
  posterior, 144
  superior, 99, 110, 143, 144
Thalamotuberal artery, 138
Thalami, 111
Thalamus, 105, 107, 109, 110, 111, 145, 303
  left, 142
  nuclei of, 110
  posterolateral view of, 113
  pulvinar of, 106, 113, 114, 137, 143
  schema of, 110
  stria medullaris of, 105
  in third ventricle, 114
  ventral posteromedial nucleus of, 134
Thenar eminence, 400
Thenar muscle, 447, 448

Thenar muscle *(Continued)*
  abductor pollicis brevis, 463
  innervation of, 464
  nerves to, 448, 453
  opponens pollicis, 463
  superficial head of flexor pollicis brevis, 463
Thenar space, 450, 451
  septal separation of, 448
  septum between, 450
Thigh
  arteries of
    anterior view of, 488, 489
    posterior view of, 490
    schema of, 500
  bony attachments of
    anterior view of, 478
    posterior view of, 479
  cutaneous innervation of, 527, 528
  deep dissection of, 489, 490
  fascia lata of, 357
  intermuscular septa of, 493
  muscles of
    anterior view of, 480, 481
    lateral view of, 482
    posterior view of, 483
  nerves of, 526
    posterior, 528
  serial cross section of, 493
  veins of
    anterior view of, 488, 489
    posterior view of, 490
Thoracic aortic plexus, 203
Thoracic artery
  internal, 75, 136, 177, 183, 184, 185, 192, 200, 205,
    206, 210, 226, 231, 239, 249, 415
    anterior intercostal branches of, 183
    cross-section of, 237, 238
    left, 187, 225
    medial mammary branches of, 177
    perforating branches of, 177, 182, 184, 185
    perforating branch of, 414
    right, 187, 224
  lateral, 177, 182, 183, 414, 415, 417, 422
  left, 75, 188
  superior, 183, 414, 415, 417
Thoracic cardiac nerve, 187
Thoracic constriction, 227
Thoracic duct, 72, 183, 188, 192, 200, 202, 203, 205,
    210, 225, 226, 232, 233, 236, 237, 238, 239, 259,
    295, 297, 327
  lumbar lymph nodes to, 318
  transverse section of, 325
Thoracic ganglion
  first, 160
  sixth, right, 300
Thoracic muscle
  transverse, 210
  transversus, 174
Thoracic nerve
  dorsal ramus of
    lateral branch of, 185
    medial branch of, 185
  long, 182, 184, 251, 414, 417, 418
Thoracic spinal cord
  anteroposterior view of, 165
  schema of, 132, 204
Thoracic spinal nerves, 133, 160
  dorsal root of, 132, 133, 163
  origin of, 163
  relation to thoracic vertebrae, 158
  roots of, filaments of, 157
  T1, 131, 132, 133, 157
    relation to thoracic vertebrae, 158
  T2, 132, 133
    relation to thoracic vertebrae, 158
  T3, relation to thoracic vertebrae, 158
  T4, relation to thoracic vertebrae, 158
  T5, relation to thoracic vertebrae, 158
  T6, relation to thoracic vertebrae, 158

Thoracic spinal nerves *(Continued)*
  T7
    dorsal rami of, 171
      lateral cutaneous branch of, 248
      medial cutaneous branch of, 248
    relation to thoracic vertebrae, 158
    ventral rami of, 394
  T8
    dorsal rami of, 171
    relation to thoracic vertebrae, 158
  T9
    dorsal rami of, 171
    relation to thoracic vertebrae, 158
  T10
    dorsal rami of, 171
    relation to thoracic vertebrae, 158
    ventral rami of, 390
  T11
    dorsal rami of, 171
    relation to thoracic vertebrae, 158
    ventral rami of, 394
  T12, 157
    dorsal rami of, 171
    relation to thoracic vertebrae, 158
    ventral rami of, 248
  T1-T12, schema of, 160
  typical, 174
  ventral rami of, 185
  ventral root of, 132, 133, 163
Thoracic sympathetic cardiac nerves, 129
Thoracic sympathetic ganglion
  fourth, 220
  third, 220
Thoracic vein
  internal, 183, 184, 186, 206, 210, 239, 250
    cross-section of, 237, 238
    perforating branches of, 184
    perforating tributaries to, 250
  lateral, 250
  left, 75, 188
  right internal, 188
Thoracic vertebrae, 151
  cross action through, 163
  posterior view of, 150
  radiographs of, 153
  T1, 15, 22, 157
    spinous process of, 191
  T2, body of, 468
  T3
    body of, 236
    lower levels, transverse section of, 236
    transverse cross-section of, 236, 237
  T6
    lateral view of, 151
    superior view of, 151
  T7
    body of, 239
    posterior view of, 151
    spinous process of, 151
  T8, 210
    posterior view of, 151
  T9, posterior view of, 151
  T10, body of, 325
  T12, 157
    anterior view of, 150
    body of, 327
    lateral view of, 151, 153
    left lateral view of, 150
    posterior view of, 150
    radiograph of, 153
    spinous process of, 149, 168, 169, 171, 411
Thoracic vertebral body, fourth, 224
Thoracic wall
  anterior, 182, 183
    internal view of, 184
  internal, veins of, 186
Thoracis muscle, transverse, 183, 184, 185
Thoracoabdominal nerve, 252
  cutaneous branches of, 182

Thoracoacromial artery, 183, 415, 416, 417, 422
  acromial branch of, 415, 417
  clavicular branch of, 415, 417
  deltoid branch of, 411, 415, 417
  pectoral branch of, 182, 415, 417
Thoracoacromial vein, 403
Thoracodorsal artery, 414, 415, 417, 422
Thoracodorsal nerve, 412, 417, 418
Thoracoepigastric vein, 243, 250
Thoracolumbar spinal cord, schema of, 303
Thoracroacromial artery, 416
Thorax
  autonomic nerves of, 203
  bony framework of, 179
  cross section of
    at T4-5 level, 238
    at T7 level, 239
    transverse, 236, 237
  surface anatomy of, 175
Thumb, 400
  carpometacarpal joint of, 442
  digital arteries to, 454
  digital nerves to, 454
  metacarpal joint base, radiograph of, 445
  palmar digital nerves of, 448
Thymus, 205, 237
  area for, 193
  seen through mediastinal pleura, 224, 225
Thyroarytenoid muscle, 78, 80
  action of, 79
Thyrocervical trunk, 31, 32, 33, 69, 71, 74, 75, 76,
    135, 136, 226, 231, 415
  left, 167
  right, 167
Thyroepiglottic muscle, 78, 80
Thyrohyoid membrane, 28, 63, 65, 67, 68, 74, 76, 77,
    80, 229
Thyrohyoid muscle, 26, 27, 28, 30, 127
  nerve to, 71, 128
Thyroid artery
  inferior, 32, 33, 69, 74, 135, 136, 220, 232, 415
    esophageal branch of, 231
  superior, 30, 33, 69, 74, 75, 76, 135, 136
  superior laryngeal branch of, 33
Thyroid gland, 28, 30, 34, 63, 70, 80, 190, 192, 200
  anterior view of, 74
  articular surface of, 78, 80
  fibrous capsule of, 76
  isthmus of, 74
  left lobe of, 74, 76
  posterior view of, 75
  pyramidal lobe of, 74
  retracted, 32
  right lobe of, 74, 75, 76
Thyroid lymph nodes, superior, 72
Thyroid notch, superior, 77
Thyroid vein
  inferior, 30, 70, 74, 75, 76, 192, 205, 232
  middle, 30, 70, 74, 76
  superior, 30, 70, 74, 76, 80
Tiabialis posterior tendon, groove for insertion of, 501
Tibia, 499, 501, 515, 518
  anterior border of, 469, 502
  anterior view of, 501, 524
    with ligament attachments, 502
  Gerdy's tubercle of, 501
  inferior articular surface of, 501, 502
  interosseous border of, 501
  lateral condyle of, 482, 501
  lateral facet of, 496
  lateral surface of, 501, 502
  lateral view of, 514
  ligaments of, 502
  medial border of, 501, 502
  medial condyles of, 495, 497, 498, 501
  medial facet of, 496
  medial surface of, 501, 502
  nutrient foramen of, 501
  oblique line of, 495, 501
  posterior articular surface of, 501, 502

Tibia *(Continued)*
  posterior view of, 501
  radiograph of, 498, 514
  soleal line of, 501
  superior articular surface of, 496, 501
Tibial artery
  anterior, 500, 506, 510, 518
  posterior, 500, 504, 505, 506, 510, 522
    calcaneal branch of, 504, 505
    medial calcaneal branch of, 506, 520, 521
    medial malleolar branch of, 506
Tibial collateral ligament, 495, 499, 505, 506, 507
  oblique fibers of, 494
  parallel fibers of, 494
  superficial and deep fibers of, 496
Tibialis anterior muscle, 469, 482, 495, 503, 509,
    510, 528, 530
  insertion of, 503
  origin of, 503
Tibialis anterior tendon, 507, 515, 517, 518, 524
Tibialis anterior tendon sheath, 517
Tibialis posterior muscle, 506, 510, 529
  origin of, 503
Tibialis posterior tendon, 504, 505, 506, 515, 517,
    522, 523, 524
Tibialis posterior tendon sheath, 517
Tibial nerve, 483, 485, 487, 490, 493, 504, 505, 506,
    529
  lateral plantar, 529
  medial calcaneal branch of, 472, 520, 521, 529
  medial plantar, 529
  posterior, 522
Tibial recurrent artery
  anterior, 500
  posterior, 500, 506
Tibial tuberosity, 469, 480, 495, 496, 499, 501, 509
Tibial vein
  anterior, 510
  posterior, 504, 505, 510
Tibiofibular ligament
  anterior, 515
  posterior, 515
Toes. *See also* Phalanx
  dorsal view of, 525
  fifth
    distal phalanx of, 525
    middle phalanx of, 525
    proximal phalanx of, 525
  great
    distal phalanx of, 516, 525
    medial side of, vein of, 471
    proximal phalanx of, 516, 525
  plantar view of, 525
Tongue, 38, 58, 64
  anterior, as taste and somatic sensation area, 117
  apex of, 58
  body of, 48, 58, 63
  dorsum of, 58
  duct of gland of, 58
  frenulum of, 51, 61
  furrow of, 58
  horizontal section of, 60
  intrinsic muscle of, 58, 127
  lateral view of, 59
  lingual glands of, 58
  lymphatic drainage of, 73
  lymph follicles of, 58
  lymph nodes and vessels of, 73
  mucous glands of, 58
  muscles of, 60, 117
  posterior, as taste and somatic sensation area, 124
  root of, 58, 66, 67, 78, 229
  salivary glands and, 60, 61
  schematic stereogram of, 58
  taste and sensation area of, 58, 124
  taste buds of, 58
Tonsil
  cerebellar, 112
  of cerebellum, 114
  of cranial fossa, 142

Tonsil *(Continued)*
  lingual, 58, 63, 64, 78
  palatine, 51, 52, 58, 64, 66
  pharyngeal, 36, 38, 63, 64, 66, 67
    imaging of, 148
  root of, 63
Tonsillar artery, 39, 69
Torus levatorius, 66
Torus tubarius, 36, 38, 64, 66
Trabecula, 146
  artery of, 146
Trabeculae carneae, 214
Trachea, 15, 28, 34, 63, 65, 66, 68, 74, 75, 76, 77, 78,
    125, 161, 190, 192, 196, 200, 205, 224, 226, 227,
    228, 231
  area for, 193
  arteries of, 196
  cross section of, 196, 236, 237
  CT axial image of, 235
  elastic fibers of, 196
  epithelium of, 196
  innervation of, 160
  longitudinal folds of, 196
  pulled to left, 201
  radiograph of, 207
Trachealis muscle, 196
Tracheal wall
  anterior, 196
  posterior, 196
    mucosa of, 196
Tracheobronchial lymph nodes, 259
  inferior, 202, 233, 238
  superior, 233, 237
    left, 202
    right, 202
Tracheobronchial tree, innervation of, 204
Tragus, 1, 93
Transpyloric plane, 242
Transversalis fascia, 245
Transverse cervical nerve, 2
Transverse ligament, of atlas
  articular facet for, 19
  tubercle for, 19
Transverse metacarpal ligament, superficial, 404
Transverse process, 155, 173
  cervical, 20
    anterior tubercle of, 21
    posterior tubercle of, 21
  of coccyx, 154
  of lumbar vertebrae, 152, 156
  thoracic, 151
Transverse sinus, 97, 102, 103, 143
  computed tomography of, 147
  groove for, 8, 11
  left, 142
Transversospinalis muscle, 236
Trapezium, 449, 455
  anterior (palmar) view of, 440, 441, 444
  coronal section: dorsal view of, 443
  posterior (dorsal) view of, 440, 443, 444
  radiograph of, 445
  tubercle of, 442
    anterior (palmar) view of, 440, 444
Trapezius muscle, 1, 26, 27, 28, 30, 34, 126, 128, 149,
    168, 171, 172, 174, 182, 183, 185, 236, 237, 238,
    239, 240, 248, 400, 407, 411, 412, 416, 417
  cross section of, 236, 237, 238
  innervation of, 117
  reflected, 171
Trapezoid, 449
  anterior (palmar) view of, 440, 441, 444
  coronal section: dorsal view of, 443
  posterior (dorsal) view of, 440, 443, 444
  radiograph of, 445
Trapezoid ligament, 410, 413
  attachment of, 406
Trapezoid line, of clavicle, 406
Trapezoid muscle, insertion of, 406
Treitz, ligament of, 262
Treves, bloodless fold of, 273

Triangle
anal, 360
ausculatory, 248
of auscultation, 149, 411
cystohepatic (Calor's), 280, 284
deltopectoral, 240
inguinal (Hesselbach's), 247
lumbar (of Petit), 149, 168, 248
lumbocostal, 189
of neck, posterior, 168, 182
sternocostal, 184
urogenital, 360
Ward's, 531
radiograph of, 476
Triangular aponeurosis, 452
Triangular fold, 64
Triangular fossa, 93
Triangular interval, 414
Triangular ligament
left, 266, 277
right, 266, 277
Triangular space, 414
with circumflex scapular artery, 414
Triceps brachii muscle, 149, 175, 438
lateral head of, 149, 400, 411, 414, 415, 420, 423, 465
long head of, 149, 236, 237, 238, 400, 407, 411, 412, 414, 415, 420, 421, 423, 465
medial head of, 412, 421, 423, 465
nerve to, 420
origin of, 439
tendon of, 149, 420
Triceps brachii tendon, 400, 426, 432, 433, 465
Tricuspid area, 207
Tricuspid valve, 217
anterior cusp of, 210, 214, 216, 217, 218
orifice of, 239
posterior cusp of, 210, 214, 216, 217, 218
right fibrous ring of, 216, 219
septal cusp of, 210, 214, 216, 217, 218
Trigeminal ganglion, 44, 45, 86, 103, 115, 131, 132, 133, 134
Trigeminal impression, 11
Trigeminal nerve, 46, 97, 113, 115, 132, 133, 134, 142
dental and gingival branches of, 44
distribution of, 117
ganglion of, 116, 130
mandibular division of, 2
maxillary division of, 2, 62
meningeal branch of, 44
mesencephalic nucleus of, 115, 116, 121, 134
motor nucleus of, 115, 116, 121, 134
motor root of, 45, 130
ophthalmic division of, 2
principal sensory nucleus of, 115, 116, 121
schema of, 121
sensory root of, 45, 130
spinal nucleus of, 115, 116, 121, 124, 125
spinal tract of, 115, 116, 121, 124, 125
via pterygopalatine ganglion, 62
via superior alveolar nerves, 62
Trigeminal tubercle, 114
Trigone
collateral, 110
habenular, 110
Triquetrum bone
anterior (palmar) view of, 440, 441, 444
coronal section: dorsal view of, 443
posterior (dorsal) view of, 440, 443
radiograph of, 445
Trochanter
greater, 149, 241, 332, 469, 475, 480, 483, 484, 490, 491
arthrogram of, 531
radiograph of, 333, 476, 531
lesser, 241, 256, 332, 475
iliacus and psoas muscle insertion on, 484
radiograph of, 333, 476, 531
Trochanteric fossa, 477

Trochlea, 407, 424, 512
fibular (peroneal), 512
radiograph of, 425
Trochlea (pulley), 84
Trochlear nerve, 13, 46, 83, 84, 86, 103, 113, 114, 115, 116, 120, 142
distribution of, 117
schema of, 120
Trochlear notch, 424
radiograph of, 425
Trochlear nucleus, 115, 116, 120
Troisier, signal lymph nodes of Virchow, 72
Trolard, lateral lacuna of, 99, 100
Trolard, superior anastomotic vein of, 101
Tuber cinereum, 105, 106, 113
median eminence of, 145
Tubercle
anterior, 110
auricular (of Darwin), 93
carotid, of Chassaignac, 21
cervical
anterior, 20, 21
inconspicuous anterior, 20
posterior, 20, 21
conoid, of clavicle, 406
cornuate, 67, 78
cuneate, 113
cuneiform, 67, 78
distal radial, 400
pharygneal, 64, 67
pubic, 241
of rib, 179
Tuberculum sellae, 11
Tufted cells, 118
Tunica albuginea, 361, 365, 370
Tunica vaginalis, 323
cavity of, 366
parietal layer of, 367, 370
visceral layer of, 367, 370
Tympanic artery
anterior, 69, 136
inferior, 46
Tympanic canaliculus, 10, 12
Tympanic cavity, 43, 92, 94, 96, 123, 124
coronal oblique section of, 93
lateral wall of, 94
medial wall of, 94
right
lateral view of, 93
otoscopic view of, 93
Tympanic cells, 94
Tympanic membrane, 92, 93, 94, 96
secondary, 96
Tympanic nerve (of Jacobson), 46, 93, 94, 122, 124, 133
Tympanic plexus, 94, 122, 124, 131, 133
on promontory, 93
tubule branch of, 124
Tyson's gland, opening of, 362

U

Ulna, 428, 429, 430, 431, 433, 442, 453
anterior border of, 427
anterior (palmar) view of, 440, 441
anterior surface of, 427
carpal articular surface of, 427
coronal section: dorsal view of, 443
coronoid process of, 424, 427
radiograph of, 425
groove for abductor pollicis longus muscle, 427
groove for extensor carpi radialis longus muscle, 427
interosseous border of, 427
muscle origin and attachment sites on, 439
oblique cord of, 427
olecranon of, 400, 420, 424, 427, 433
posterior (dorsal) view of, 440, 443
radial notch of, 424, 427

Ulna *(Continued)*
radiograph of, 425
right
in pronation: anterior view, 427
in supination: anterior view, 427
sites of muscle origins and insertions on, 438
styloid process of, 427
radiograph of, 445
trochlear notch of, 424, 427
tuberosity of, 419
Ulnar artery, 421, 422, 434, 435, 436, 437, 442, 447, 448, 449, 453, 454, 461
deep branch of, 442, 453
deep palmar branch of, 435, 436, 442, 447, 448, 453, 454, 461
palmar carpal branch of, 436, 453, 454
with venae and ulnar nerve, 448
Ulnar bursa, 448, 449, 450, 451, 454
Ulnar collateral artery, 421
inferior, 421, 422
superior, 422, 423, 432
Ulnar collateral ligament, 426
posterior (dorsal) view of, 443
Ulnar nerve, 417, 418, 420, 421, 423, 432, 433, 434, 435, 436, 437, 442, 448, 449, 453, 454, 461, 462, 463
anterior view of, 460, 464
in arm, 467
articular branch of, 464
branches to interosseous muscles, 453
branches to lumbrical muscles, 453
communicating branches of, 454, 456, 461
to cutaneous innervation, 464
deep branch of, 435, 447, 454, 461, 464
deep palmar branch of, 448
dorsal branch of, 402, 404, 432, 436, 437, 456, 460, 461, 464
to dorsum of middle and distant phalanges, 464
dorsal carpal branch of, 457
dorsal digital branches of, 402, 457, 460
groove for, 424
inconstant contribution, 464
muscles innervated by, 464
palmar branch of, 404, 435, 447, 460, 464
palmar digital branches of, 54, 402, 460, 461
common, 461
palmar view of, 464
patent branch of, 402
posterior view of, 460, 464
superficial branch of, 363, 435, 447, 448, 454, 461
Ulnar notch, 427
Ulnar recurrent artery
anterior, 422, 435, 436
posterior, 422
Ulnar styloid process
anterior (palmar) view of, 440
posterior (dorsal) view of, 440
Ulnar tuberosity, 427
Ulnocarpal ligament
dorsal, posterior view of, 443
palmar
ulnolunate part of, 442
ulnotriquetral part of, 442
Umbilical artery(ies), 223, 257, 315, 378
left, obliterated, 247
median, 345, 348
obliterated, 247, 354
occluded part of, 223, 247, 254, 255, 257, 266, 315, 343, 345, 380, 382, 383
patent part of, 316, 380, 382
right, patent part of, 383
Umbilical fold
lateral, 247, 266, 343
inferior epigastric vessels in, 247
medial, 266, 343, 347, 380
right, 247
median, 246, 266

Umbilical ligament
  medial, 223, 245, 253, 254, 255, 257, 315, 316, 343,
    345, 347, 380, 382, 383
    left, 247
    right, 247
  median, 23, 246, 247, 253, 254, 255, 348, 380
Umbilical region, 242
Umbilical vein, 223
  obliterated, 223
  obliterated left, 267
Umbilicus, 240, 247
Umbo, 93, 96
Uncal vein, 143
Uncinate process, 36, 49
  cervical, 20
    articular surface of, 20
  of ethmoidal bone, 37, 50
  left, 20
    area for articulation of, 20
  of pancreas, 281
Uncovertebral joint, 20, 21
Uncus, 105, 106, 118
Upper limb. *See also* Arm; Hand
  anterior (palmar) view of, 402
  anterior view of, 400
  arteries of, 461
  cutaneous innervation of, 402
  dermatomes of, 401
  lymph vessels and nodes of, 405
  nerves of, 461
  posterior view of, 400, 402
  topographic anatomy of, 400
Urachus, 23, 254, 255, 343, 345, 346, 347, 348, 357,
  380, 383
  in median umbilical fold, 266
  obliterated, 246, 247
Ureter, 247, 255, 258, 263, 311, 316, 342, 343, 344,
  348, 355, 364, 371, 372, 380, 382, 384, 390, 392
  arteries of, 316
  autonomic nerves of, 319, 320
  diagonal course through bladder wall, 315
  in female, superior view of, 315
  left, 315, 330
  lower, nerves of, 397
  in male, 346
    in the abdomen and pelvis, 315
  retroperitoneal, 266, 315
  right, 297, 308, 315, 354
  upper, autonomic innervation of, 320
Ureteric fold, 343, 344
Ureteric orifice, 348, 364
  left, 360
  right, 350
Ureteric plexus, 390
  right, 297
Ureteropelvic junction, 329
Urethra, 256, 338, 341, 342, 348, 349, 358, 363, 365
  beginning of, 398
  fascial support for, 353
  female, 339, 350, 399
  floor of, 365
  hiatus for, 340
  lacuna magna of, 365
  membranous
    intermediate part of, 365
    lymphatic pathway from, 388
  musculofascial extensions to, 339
  prostatic, 350, 364, 365, 398
  roof of, 365
  spongy
    bulbous portion of, 350, 364, 365
    pendulous portion of, 365
    transverse section of, 399
Urethrae muscle, compressor, 358, 384
Urethral artery, 363, 385
Urethral crest, 364, 365
Urethral fold, partly fused, 368
Urethral meatus, 346
Urethral orifice, external, 331, 342, 356, 359, 362,
  368, 375

Urethral raphe, 368
Urethral sphincter, internal, 350, 364, 365
Urethrovaginal muscle, 349
Urinary bladder, 161, 247, 254, 255, 261, 302, 308,
  315, 323, 342, 343, 344, 345, 349, 363, 364, 371,
  380, 392
  apex of, 346, 348
  arteries of, 316
  autonomic nerves of, 319
  body of, 346, 348
  fascial support for, 353
  female, 350
    midsagittal section of, 348
  fundus of, 346, 348, 350
  innervation of, 160, 397
  lateral ligament of, 345
  lymph vessels and nodes of, 318
  male, 346, 350
  MR sagittal images of, 377
  mucosa of, 315
  neck of, 346, 348, 350
  orientation and supports of, 348
  trigone of, 346, 348, 350, 364
  ureteric orifice of, 348
  uvula of, 350, 364, 365
Urinary bladder-prostate junction, 398
Urogenital fold, 368
Urogenital groove, 368
Urogenital hiatus, 349
Urogenital sinus, 369
Urogenital triangle, 360
Uterine artery, 315, 316, 354, 380, 382
  ovarian branches of, 384
  tubal branches of, 384
  vaginal branches of, 384
Uterine fold, 355
Uterine ligament, lateral, 343
Uterine ostium, 355
Uterine tube, 342, 343, 344, 346, 352, 353, 380, 392, 395
  ampulla of, 354, 355
  fimbriae of, 354
  infundibulum of, 354, 355
  right
    infection of, 354
  uterine part of, 355
Uterine vein, 258
  superior, 379
Uterine vessels, 344, 352, 384
  ovarian branches of, 354
Uterosacral fold, 315, 343, 372
Uterosacral ligament, 342, 353, 355, 435
Uterovaginal plexus, 392, 394, 395
Uterovesical pouch, 354
Uterus, 352, 355, 369, 371, 380, 392
  age changes and muscle pattern of, 353
  arteries and veins of, 384
  body of, 342, 344, 355
  cervix of, 342, 344, 352, 355
  external os of, 355
  fascial ligaments of, 353
  fascia of, 353
  frontal section of, 355
  fundus of, 342, 343, 344, 348, 355
  hysterosalpingogram of, 354
  internal os of, 355
  isthmus of, 355
  MR sagittal images of, 377
  os of, 355
  posterior view of, 355
  retracted, 392
  round ligament of, 258, 315, 342, 343, 344, 352,
    353, 357, 380
  supporting structures of, 352
Utricle, 92, 95, 96, 123, 364, 365, 369
Uvula, 51, 64, 66, 67
  of cerebellar vermis, 114
  of cranial fossa, 142
  of inferior vermis, 112
  of urinary bladder, 364, 365
Uvular muscle, 52

V

Vagal cardiac nerves, 129
Vagal nerve fibers, 125
Vagal nucleus, dorsal, 115
Vagal trigone, 114
Vagal trunk, 256
  anterior, 125, 203, 226, 234, 297, 298, 299, 300, 301,
    302, 306, 307, 319, 390
    anterior gastric branch of, 298
    celiac branch of, 125, 298, 299, 301
    gastric branches of, 125
    hepatic branch of, 125, 298, 299, 302, 306
  celiac branch of, 300, 390
  posterior, 234, 297, 299, 300, 301, 302, 306, 307,
    319, 321, 390
    celiac branch of, 125, 234, 298, 299, 301
    posterior gastric branch of, 299
Vagina, 337, 338, 342, 348, 349, 352, 355, 358, 375,
  380, 399
  fascial support for, 353
  fornix of, 342
  lower 1/5 of, 369
  MR sagittal images of, 377
  supporting structures of, 352
  transverse section of, 399
  upper 4/5 of, 369
  vertical portion of, 353
  vestibule of, 356
Vaginal artery, 315, 352, 354, 380, 382
  inferior, 345, 348
  inferior vesical branch of, 315
Vaginal fornix, 355
Vaginal orifice, 342, 359, 368
Vaginal wall, 353, 359
Vagus nerve, 13, 31, 32, 33, 34, 46, 47, 69, 70, 71, 74,
  75, 76, 103, 113, 115, 116, 124, 125, 126, 129,
  130, 161, 226, 234, 303, 320
  auricular branch of, 2, 125
    communication with glossopharyngeal nerve,
      124
    in mastoid canaliculus, 12
  branches to cardiac and pulmonary plexuses,
    203
  celiac branch of, 300
  communicating branch of, 125
  communication with cervical plexus, 32
  distribution of, 117
  dorsal nucleus of, 115, 125
  inferior cervical cardiac branch of, 125
  inferior (nodose) ganglion of, 46, 125, 126, 127,
    234
  in jugular fossa, 12
  left, 75, 187, 200, 206, 220, 225, 236, 237
  meningeal branch of, 125
  pharyngeal branch of, 71, 124, 125, 129, 130
  posterior (dorsal) nucleus of, 116, 303, 320
  right, 75, 187, 200, 206, 220, 224, 236
  schema of, 75, 125, 204, 220, 303, 304
  superior cervical cardiac branch of, 71, 125, 129,
    130
  superior ganglion of, 125, 234
  thoracic cardiac branch of, 125, 203, 220
Vallate papillae, 58, 134
Vallecula, 58, 64
Valsalva, aortic sinus of, 217
Valves of Houston, 373
Valves of Kerckring, 271, 272
Vasa rectae spuria, 314
Vasa rectae vera, 314
Vascular smooth muscle, innervation to, 160
Vas deferens. *See* Ductus (vas) deferens
Vastus intermedius muscle, 481, 489, 493, 495, 526
  insertion of, 478
  origin of, 479
Vastus lateralis muscle, 469, 480, 481, 482, 488, 489,
  490, 493, 495, 507, 509, 526
  insertion of, 478
  origin of, 478
  transverse section of, 399

Vastus medialis muscle, 469, 480, 488, 489, 493, 494, 495, 507, 526
  insertion of, 478
  nerve to, 488, 493
  origin of, 479
Vater
  ampulla of, 280
  papilla of, 281
Veins. *See also specific veins*
  of abdominal wall, 250, 258
  of anal canal
    female, 379
    male, 379
  of brain, 143
  bronchial, 201
  cardiac, 211
  of duodenum, 289
  of esophagus, 232
  of eye, 90
  of eyelid, 85
  of face, 3
  of female pelvic organs, 380
  of forearm, 404
  of hypothalamus and hypophysis, 146
  of internal thoracic wall, 186
  of kidney, 314
  of large intestine, 291
  of lower limb, 471, 472
  of neck, 30
  of oral and pharyngeal regions, 70
  of orbit, 85
  of pancreas, 289
  of pelvis
    female, 382
    male, 383
  of perineum, 384
    female, 384
    male, 385
  of rectum
    female, 379
    male, 379
  of scalp, 3
  of small intestine, 290
  of spleen, 289
  of stomach, 289
  of suprarenal glands, 322
  of testis, 381
  of thigh, 488, 489, 490
  of uterus, 384
  of vertebral column, 167
Velum, medullary
  inferior, 114
  superior, 112, 114
Vena cava
  inferior, 200, 203, 208, 209, 215, 219, 226, 232, 258, 266, 270, 277, 281, 286, 289, 308, 310, 317, 328, 329, 330, 343, 347, 378, 379, 380, 381, 382, 383, 392
    axial CT image of, 235, 324
    covered by parietal pleura, 224
    cross section of, 173, 265
    groove for, 193, 277
    opening of, 217
    prenatal, 223
    radiograph of, 207
    receiving hepatic veins, 188
    retroperitoneal, 264
    transverse section of, 325, 326
  superior, 74, 75, 186, 187, 200, 205, 206, 208, 209, 210, 214, 218, 219, 224, 232, 239
    cross-section of, 237, 238
    CT axial image of, 235
    groove for, 193
    prenatal, 223
    radiograph of, 207
    valve of, 214
Venae comitantes, 59, 448
Venae ectae, 290
Venous network, dorsal, 404
Venous plexus, 348

Venous plexus *(Continued)*
  areolar, 250
  basilar, 103
  external, 372
  in foramen magnum, 12
  of internal carotid artery, 46
  pampiniform, 250, 381, 383
  prostatic, 383
  rectal, 258
    external, 291, 373, 374, 379
    internal, 373, 374, 379
    perimuscular, 291, 379
  submucous, 232
  uterine, 354, 379
  uterovaginal, 258
  vaginal, transverse section of, 399
  vertebral
    anterior external, 167
    internal, 163
  vesical, 258, 350, 383
Ventral ramus, in situ, 157
Ventricle (cerebral), 107
  fourth, 107, 112, 142, 144
    choroid plexus of, 105, 108, 113
    imaging of, 148
    lateral and medial apertures of, 144
    median sagittal section of, 114
    outline of, 141
    posterior view of, 114
    rhomboid fossa of, 113
    vein of lateral recess of, 142
  imaging of, 148
  lateral, 107, 109, 111, 137, 144
    choroid plexus of, 99, 107, 108, 109, 137, 141, 143
    lateral vein of, 144
    medial vein of, 144
    occipital horn of, 109, 110, 111, 144
    right, 107
    temporal (inferior) horn of, 107, 110, 111, 144
    veins on, 144
  left lateral, 107
    central part of, 107
    frontal (anterior) horn of, 107
    occipital (posterior) horn of, 107
    temporal (inferior) horn of, 107
  medial wall of, veins on, 144
  right lateral, occipital horn of, 141
  third, 105, 107, 109, 110, 144
    choroid plexus of, 105, 107, 108, 110, 141
    imaging of, 148
    posterior view of, 114
    tela choroidea of, 107, 110, 143
    thalamus in, 114
Ventricle (heart), 218
  left, 206, 208, 209, 210, 212, 218, 239
    axial CT image of, 235
    posterior vein of, 211
    posterolateral wall of, 215
    radiograph of, 207
  right, 206, 208, 209, 210, 214, 218, 239
    axial CT image of, 235
Ventricular folds, 78
Ventricular vein
  hippocampal, 144
  inferior, 144
Venulae rectae, 314
Venule
  inferior macular, 90
  inferior nasal retinal, 90
  inferior temporal retinal, 90
  superior macular, 90
  superior nasal retinal, 90
  superior temporal retinal, 90
Vermian artery
  choroidal branch of, 141
  inferior *(phantom),* 141
  superior branch of, 141
Vermian vein
  inferior, 142
  superior, 142, 144

Vermis, 112
  central lobule of, 114
  culmen of, 114
  declive of, 114
  folium of, 114
  inferior
    nodule of, 112
    pyramid of, 112
    tuber of, 112
    uvula of, 112
  lingula of, 114
  nodulus of, 114
  pyramid of, 114
  superior
    central lobule of, 112
    culmen of, 112
    declive of, 112
    folium of, 112
    lingula of, 112
  tuber, 114
  uvula of, 114
Vertebrae. *See also* Cervical vertebrae; Lumbar vertebrae; Sacral vertebrae; Thoracic vertebrae
  body of, 163
    axial CT image of, 235, 324
  relation of spinal nerve roots to, 158
  spinous process of, axial CT image of, 235
Vertebral artery, 13, 22, 31, 32, 71, 75, 76, 136, 137, 138, 139, 164, 220, 231, 415
  atlantic part of, 172
  cervical part of, 135
  computed tomography of, 147
  in foramen magnum, 12
  groove for, 19
  imaging of, 148
  left, 135, 141
  meningeal branches of, 13
    anterior, 135, 141
    anterior branch, 100
    posterior, 135
    posterior branch, 100, 141
  right, 135, 167
  venous plexus of, 167
Vertebral body
  articular facets of, 180
  cervical, 20, 21
  lumbar, 152, 156
    L1, 265
    posterior surface of, 156
    radiograph of, 153
  thoracic
    fourth, 224
    origin of psoas muscle from, 484
Vertebral canal
  lumbar, 152
  thoracic, 151
Vertebral column
  anterior view of, 150
  left lateral view of, 150
  posterior view of, 150
  veins of, 166, 167
Vertebral foramen, 151
  cervical, 20
  lumbar, 152
Vertebral ganglion, 129, 220
  of cervical sympathetic trunk, 234
Vertebral ligament
  of lumbar region, 156
  lumbosacral, 155
Vertebral notch
  inferior, 151, 152
  lumbar
    inferior, 153
    superior, 153
  superior, 151, 152
Vertebral prominens, 20
Vertebral segments
  anterior, 156
  posterior, 156

Vertebral vein, 232
  accessory, 167
  anterior, 167
  forming, 167
  left, 167
  right, 167
Vertebral venous plexus
  external, 166
    anterior, 167
  internal, 166
    anterior, 167
  internal (of Batson), 102, 166
Vertebrocostal trigone, 256
Vesical artery
  inferior, 257, 315, 316, 345, 348, 378, 381, 382, 383
    capsular branches of, 383
    prostatic branches of, 383
    ureteric branches of, 316
    urethral branches of, 383
  superior, 247, 257, 315, 316, 345, 378, 380, 382, 383
    ureteric branch from, 316
Vesical fold, transverse, 247, 343, 354
Vesical lymph nodes, lateral, 318
Vesical plexus, 302, 319, 390, 392, 394, 396
Vesical vein, superior, 258, 379
Vesical venous plexus, 383
  in retropubic space, 346
Vesicocervical fascial fibers, 345
Vesicocervical space, 345
Vesicosacral fold, 347
Vesicoureteric pouch, 342, 344
Vesicouterine pouch, 348, 354, 371
Vesicovaginal space, 345
Vesicular appendix, 355, 369
Vestibular aqueduct, opening of, 8, 13, 97
Vestibular area, 114
Vestibular (Bartholin's) gland, greater, 358, 359, 384
Vestibular fold, 80
Vestibular fossa, 356
Vestibular ganglion, 95, 123
Vestibular (Bartholin's) gland, 358, 359, 384
  opening of, 356
Vestibular (Reissner's) membrane, 96
Vestibular nerve, 92, 95, 97, 117, 123
  inferior part of, 95, 97, 123
  superior part of, 95, 97, 213
Vestibular nuclei, 116
  inferior, 123
  lateral, 123
  medial, 123
  superior, 123
Vestibular window, 95
  base of stapes in, 92
Vestibule, 80, 92, 95, 96, 352, 369
  bulb of, 350, 352, 358, 359
  cochlear recess of, 95
  elliptical recess of, 95
  spherical recess of, 95
Vestibulocochlear nerve, 13, 92, 95, 97, 103, 113, 115, 116, 130
  distribution of, 117
  schema of, 123
Vicq d'Azyr, mammillothalamic tract of, 145
Vidian nerve, 42, 43, 44, 121, 124, 132
Vincula longa, 452
Vinculum breve, 452
Virchow, signal lymph nodes of, 72

Viscera
  abdominal, 261, 323
  pelvic
    female, 342, 344
    male, 346
Visceral lymph nodes
  celiac, 259
  inferior mesenteric, 259
  superior mesenteric, 259
Visceral pleura, 199
Visual fields, overlapping, 119
Visual pathway, 119, 131
Vitreous body, 87
Vitreous chamber, 90
Vocal fold, 63, 78, 80
Vocalis muscle, 78, 80
  action of, 79
Vocal ligament, 77, 78
  abduction of, 79
  adduction of, 79
  lengthening of, 79
  shortening of, 79
Voiding cystourethrogram
  female, 351
  male, 351
Vomer, 4, 8, 10, 38, 47
von Ebner, serous glands of, 58
Vorticose vein, 85, 90
  anastomosis with episcleral veins, 91
  anterior tributaries of, 91
  bulb of, 91
  posterior tributaries of, 91
  suprachoroidal tributaries of, 91
Vulva, 356

W

Ward's triangle, 531
  radiograph of, 476, 531
Wharton, submandibular duct of, 51, 53, 59, 61
White matter
  imaging of, 148
  spinal, 162
White rami communicantes, 129, 131, 132, 133, 160, 162, 163, 174, 185, 203, 224, 225, 234, 252, 260, 297, 300, 304, 390, 392, 395, 396, 486
Willis, cerebral arterial circle of, 137, 138
  inferior view of, 138
  vessels dissected out, 138
  vessels in situ, 138
Winslow, omental (epiploic) foramen of, 265, 267, 278, 327
Wirsung, pancreatic duct of, 271, 281
Wolffian duct, 366, 369
Wormian bone, 9
Wrisberg, intermediate nerve of, 113, 134
Wrist
  anterior (palmar) view of, 447, 460
  arteries of, 449
  articular disc of, sagittal section through, 441
  bones of, 444
  compartments of, 458
  coronal section: dorsal view of, 443
  cutaneous innervation of, 460
  deep dorsal dissection of, 457
  deep palmar dissection of, 448
  extensor muscles of, 429

Wrist *(Continued)*
  extensor tendons at, 458
  in flexion, 441
  flexor muscles of, 430
  flexor tendons of, 449
  lateral (radial) view of, 455
  ligaments of, 442, 443
  movements of, 441
  palmar view of, 445
  posterior (dorsal) view of, 443, 456, 457, 458, 460
  radiograph of, 445
  sagittal section through, 441
  superficial dorsal dissection of, 456
  superficial palmar dissection of, 447
  superficial radial dissection of, 455
  transverse section of, 445
  veins of, 449

X

Xiphoid process, 175, 179, 180, 182, 184, 190, 192, 240, 241, 243
  transverse section of, 325

Y

Y ligament of Bigelow, 475, 484

Z

Zigzag line, 230, 268
Zinn, common tendinous ring of, 84, 86, 120
Zona orbicularis, 475, 531
  arthrogram of, 531
Zone of sparse muscle fibers, 68, 75, 228, 229
Zonular body
  equatorial, 89
  postequatorial, 89
  preequatorial, 89
Zonular fibers, 87, 88, 89, 90
Zygapophyseal joint
  C2-3, 21, 23
  C3-4, capsule of, 22
  C4-5, 22
  C5-6, 22
  lumbar, capsule of, 156
Zygomatic arch, 6, 15, 16, 54
Zygomatic bone, 1, 4, 6, 10, 81
  frontal process of, 4
  orbital surface of, 4
  temporal process of, 4, 6
  zygomaticofacial foramen of, 4, 6, 14
Zygomatic nerve, 44, 120, 121
Zygomaticofacial artery, 3, 85
Zygomaticofacial foramen, 4, 6, 14
Zygomaticofacial nerve, 2, 44, 71
Zygomaticofacial vein, 3
Zygomaticoorbital artery, 3
Zygomaticotemporal artery, 3
Zygomaticotemporal nerve, 2, 44, 71, 121
Zygomaticotemporal vein, 3
Zygomatic process, 10, 14
Zygomaticus major muscle, 25, 54, 122
Zygomaticus minor muscle, 25, 54, 122
Zygopophyseal (facet) joint, 239